Animal Physiotherapy

Assessment, Treatment and Rehabilitation of Animals

Second Edition

Edited by

Catherine M. McGowan

Professor of Equine Internal Medicine
Head of Equine Division and Director of Veterinary Postgraduate Education
Institute of Ageing and Chronic Disease
Faculty of Health and Life Sciences
University of Liverpool, UK

Lesley Goff

Lecturer, Equine Science
School of Agriculture & Food Sciences
University of Queensland, Australia
and
Director
Active Animal Physiotherapy
Toowoomba
Queensland, Australia

 WILEY Blackwell

Contents

CHAPTER 1

Introduction

Catherine M. McGowan

University of Liverpool, Liverpool, UK

The aim of this book is to provide physiotherapists and interested others with a broad base of information on animal physiotherapy; the assessment, treatment and rehabilitation of animals. Physiotherapy (called physical therapy in some countries) is an established, independent profession with an excellent reputation for evidence-based practice. In the medical field, physiotherapists form an essential part of musculoskeletal, neurological and cardiorespiratory care from paediatrics to geriatrics and sports medicine. Physiotherapy research has led human medical advancement in areas such as back and pelvic pain, whiplash and women's health. The positive perception of physiotherapy in the human sphere, together with an increased awareness of options and expertise available for animals, has resulted in a demand for physiotherapy for animals.

Animal physiotherapy is an emerging profession, representing physiotherapists qualified to treat humans, who are applying their skills on animals. Physiotherapists, when working with animal patients, work on referral from a veterinary surgeon rather than autonomous first contact practice as with human patients. This presents the ideal situation where veterinarians and physiotherapists continue to practise within, and be regulated by, their own profession but work together as a multidisciplinary team in the assessment, treatment and rehabilitation of animals. This situation is also essential in an emerging profession where the evidence base is necessarily largely drawn from the medical field, and as such, physiotherapists when working with animal patients must draw upon their knowledge and experience in people in order to appropriately translate that knowledge to animals.

This new area of expertise has been embraced by both physiotherapy professional bodies and registration boards, as well as educational institutions. Leading universities in the United Kingdom and Australia have led the way in providing postgraduate university-based training for physiotherapists to specialise in treating animals. Formalised, special interest groups (SIGs) of animal physiotherapy have been established by many physiotherapy professional groups around the world, represented by the official subgroup of the World Confederation for Physical Therapy (WCPT), the International Association of Physical Therapists in Animal Practice (IAPTAP; www.wcpt.org/iaptap).

In this text we have used the terminology animal physiotherapy to designate the professional assessment, treatment and rehabilitation of animals by physiotherapists (or physical therapists). In some countries, the terminology veterinary physiotherapy is also used, but we have continued with animal physiotherapy in accordance with the WCPT.

Physiotherapists provide a functional assessment to identify pain or loss of function caused by a physical injury, disorder or disability and they use techniques to reduce pain, improve movement and restore normal muscle control for better motor performance and function. Physiotherapists can provide equivalent levels of care and follow-up treatment for their animal patients, as they can for people. In small animal surgery, the demand for postoperative physiotherapy has paralleled the increase in surgical options for small animal patients. Elite equine athletes and their riders now access a team of professionals including the veterinarian–animal physiotherapist team. More and more people prefer to opt for treatments where they can see progressive results, professional teamwork and high levels of care and expertise.

The text begins with essential applied background information on animal behaviour, nutrition, biomechanics and exercise physiology. Following this are chapters focusing on the assessment of the musculoskeletal and neurological systems in animals from both a veterinary and physiotherapy perspective, including chapters on lameness and neurological conditions in the dog and horse and physiotherapy assessment. The next section reviews physiotherapy techniques, drawing from both the human and animal literature in their discussion. The final chapters apply this information to an evidence-based clinical reasoning model describing the physiotherapy approaches to treatment and rehabilitation of animals, giving case examples. The last chapter

Animal Physiotherapy: Assessment, Treatment and Rehabilitation of Animals, Second Edition. Edited by Catherine M. McGowan and Lesley Goff.
© 2016 John Wiley & Sons, Ltd. Published 2016 by John Wiley & Sons, Ltd.

outlines outcome measures in animal physiotherapy, reminding us all that assessment and reassessment of physical dysfunction, with accurate measurement of the response to treatment, are fundamental principles of physiotherapy.

This textbook is not a handbook of physiotherapy but rather a text aiming to cover the scientific and clinical principles behind animal physiotherapy. For animal physiotherapists, it will be a valuable reference text in their profession. For veterinarians and others who work with animals, it will be a valuable insight into the profession of physiotherapy and what it can achieve.

CHAPTER 2

Applied animal behaviour: assessment, pain and aggression*

Daniel Mills[1] and Fiona Williams[2]

[1] University of Lincoln, Lincoln, UK
[2] Dogs at Donyatt Canine Hydrotherapy, Ilminster, Somerset, UK

Summary

It is important for the animal physiotherapist to understand animal behaviour both in terms of the assessment of signs of pain and the safe and appropriate delivery of physiotherapeutic interventions. Here we discuss the importance of considering both genetic and environmental factors when assessing animal behaviour in general as well as factors influencing the identification and assessment of pain more specifically. The mechanisms underlying pain and pain management are also considered with reference to their relationship with behaviour. Finally, we discuss aggression in terms of potential triggers and its management whilst administering treatments.

2.1 Introduction

Understanding animal behaviour is important for animal physiotherapists to ensure safe handling of animals that may be in pain and therefore aggressive, and to facilitate a more complete and accurate assessment of the animal's pain. Often, we only know that an animal is in need of physiotherapeutic intervention because of its behaviour. The behaviour may be overt, such as a non-weight-bearing lameness, or more subtle, such as a decline in activity or in the vigour of the activity. In

---

*Adapted from the first edition chapter, which was written by Daniel Mills, Susan Millman and Emily Levine

either case, the challenge may be to distinguish pain from a pain-free loss of physical function or mobility.

In horses, pain may manifest as training problems or poor performance. If we wish to address the cause of this behaviour (rather than simply contain the problem), then we need to be aware of the full range of potential factors that interact with and influence behaviour. This involves at least some appreciation of many diverse branches of zoology as well as various branches of psychology, veterinary medicine, animal management and nutrition. This might seem a bit daunting, and is why it is often most effective to work as part of a multidisciplinary team, with everyone respecting each other's expertise.

Since there are two elements to the expression of pain, that is, a sensory-discriminative component (i.e. processing of the nature of the aversive stimulus and its bodily location) and an affective-motivational component of pain (i.e. the emotional and behavioural response to pain or its anticipation) (Craig 2006), it is important to recognise their differing behavioural expression. The former will largely relate to local changes such as lameness and local sensitivity to interference, whereas the latter will be expressed in more general behavioural changes such as increased aggressivity and avoidance.

Therefore, the animal physiotherapist should be aware that some animals might need behavioural therapy in order to treat the affective-motivational aspects of pain before the sensory-discriminative component of pain can be effectively addressed. Although animal physiotherapists are not expected

---

to be behaviour specialists and should not be tempted to practise beyond their own knowledge base and skill, a solid grounding and appreciation of the subject are essential to avoid putting themselves and others at risk of harm and to avoid threatening the well-being of their animals. Animal physiotherapists who have moved into the field from the human discipline may have a substantial awareness of the psychological effects of chronic pain, but it is important to understand the biological and cognitive differences that exist between humans and non-human animals and not assume that what applies to one species necessarily applies to another. Anthropomorphism (ascribing human characteristics to animals) may lead to superficial and/or inaccurate assessments with consequently inappropriate treatment. It is therefore important to always be thorough and assess all of the available information objectively in the light of the biology of the species being considered.

In this chapter, we begin with an initial guide to the principles that underpin the assessment of animal behaviour. Behaviour, like physiology, is a mechanism and expression of an animal's attempt to adapt to or cope with its environment. To survive and be successful within an evolutionary context, animals must be as efficient as possible, since those able to adapt most appropriately will outcompete those less efficient. Accordingly, the behaviour of a given individual should be viewed as an attempt by the animal to behave most appropriately in the current circumstances given previous experience.

There are three major considerations to the evaluation of an animal's behaviour: the nature of the individual concerned; its previous experience; and its current circumstance. Consideration of all three is fundamental to a complete understanding of why an animal is behaving in a particular way. After discussing these three considerations, we move on to discuss the concepts of pain, pain assessment, pain management and aggression within a context that is relevant to the animal physiotherapist.

2.1.1 Assessment of animal behaviour

As previously mentioned, there are three major principles that should be included in one's thought process when trying to evaluate an animal's behaviour.

1 The nature of the individual is influenced genetically at many levels.
2 Previous experience has both general and specific effects on behaviour.
3 The current circumstance of the individual refers to both its general motivational state and the internal and external factors which cause this state to dominate the animal's behaviour.

Genetic influence

Genetic effects lay the foundation for both species-typical behaviour but also individual differences within a given species. Species-typical behaviour refers to those activities that define a dog as a dog and a horse as a horse. One species is a predator-scavenger and the other a prey species. In order to reduce the risk of predation, natural selection is likely to have favoured a greater capacity to mask, where possible, the signs of pain, injury

and disease in horses compared with dogs. In other words, by the time a horse appears overtly sick or lame, its welfare is often already seriously compromised. Similarly, during treatment and rehabilitation, a horse might be expected to stop showing these signs before it has fully recovered, increasing the risk of relapse if the animal is returned to an inappropriate level of work too rapidly or too abruptly. The animal physiotherapist plays an essential role in ensuring that this does not happen and that the build-up to full fitness is appropriately managed.

It is also essential to be aware of the normal behaviours of the species in order to appreciate if something is genuinely disease related; for example, an inexperienced owner might mistakenly think that their cat is in pain because she is intermittently meowing with great intensity and rolling around on the floor, when in fact this is normal behaviour for a female cat in oestrus. It is not possible to go into detail here about species-typical behaviour patterns of companion animals, so the reader is referred to the many texts available on the different species and breeds, which should be essential reading according to the species being treated by the individual concerned.

There is also a large genetic contribution to the enormous variation that occurs within a species, for example between breeds and within a breed itself. So, although some generalisations about breeds may be easy to argue, such as selection favouring greater stoicism in breeds which are used to fight live game (e.g. terriers), it is important to appreciate that the variation within a breed may be greater than the variation that exists between breeds, i.e. it should not be assumed that because an individual is of a certain breed that it will necessarily be more or less stoical than an individual from another breed. Expressions of individual variation arise as a result of the interaction of different genetic and environmental factors throughout life; this serves to shape the temperament of the individual (Scott & Fuller 1965) and the way it perceives the world around it, including the personal significance of events (Weisenberg 1977). So whilst it is important to appreciate breed characteristics, they should not be rigid points of reference, especially when it comes to an individual's response to pain.

Suffering is a subjective experience and must always be respected when observed, and not dismissed as unworthy of consideration because the cause seems minor to the observer. This is perhaps one of the main challenges faced by those trying to devise generic guides to the recognition of pain in animals. Therefore, it is not surprising that in many cases the owner is the best assessor, since they recognise what is normal for that individual, and how it behaved before any change arose (Wiseman et al. 2001). Owners see a far wider range of behaviour in their animals than will be observed during a consultation by the physiotherapist; for example, an animal may display greater signs of pain in the evening or first thing in the morning and this can only be monitored at home.

It is therefore important that records of behaviour relevant to the individual are kept and that each subject acts as its own point of reference when trying to evaluate response to treatment.

This kind of record keeping is essential for the physiotherapist to be able to identify therapeutic progress and/or identify early signs of relapse, which may not have been noticed by the owner or the veterinarian. In addition, if progress reports show a steady improvement and then the physiotherapist identifies subtle changes during therapy, such as the dog resisting a bit more, or it being seemingly more tense or painful than normal for that individual, this should be relayed to the referring or supervising veterinarian.

Previous experience

The second major consideration is that previous experience has both general and specific effects on behaviour. It has already been mentioned that a large part of temperament arises as a result of interactions between the genetics of the animal and its early experience, and temperament might be considered a general factor reflecting the animal's behavioural predispositions in a wide variety of environments. For example, dogs that are poorly socialised are likely to be more fearful and aggressive towards the large range of items that may be unfamiliar to them (Appleby *et al.* 2002), but these unfamiliar items may seem very 'normal' to us, such as a man wearing a hat or with facial hair. Specific effects include individual learned responses that have been effective from the animal's perspective in the past. If a fearful dog growls at someone who approaches it and the person (understandably) leaves the dog alone as a result, then the dog will learn that growling helps achieve its goal and may use this strategy in other contexts. The sensible thing to do is to recognise the early signs of unease such as turning the head away, yawning and blinking, and avoid an unnecessary escalation to overt aggression (Shepherd 2009), assess why this has occurred and take appropriate remedial steps.

Within a clinical context, it is obviously important to be able to differentiate an animal that is generally (i.e. temperamentally) fearful and does not like being approached by strangers from one which is perhaps protecting a painful body region (specific response). Both may threaten aggressively when initially approached for assessment, but in only one of them is the behaviour related to a potential physiotherapeutic problem. Similarly, horses are often generally predisposed to behave fearfully towards any novelty they encounter, which might be a new individual or an unfamiliar form of handling and this does not necessarily mean they are in pain. However, if the animal is not handled sensitively on this first encounter, it will create stronger aversion in future similar circumstances, which may be reflected in a general irritability and specific aversive behaviour. Many horses become protective of a particular region of the body as a result of insensitive handling, when that region has been irritated by another process. For example, harsh handling to put a bridle on when a horse has a mouth or ear irritation may soon produce a head-shy animal. In these situations, the animal learns that the safest response is to always avoid handling even when there is no longer any pain, perhaps because the handling is likely to be rough and unpleasant. With time, this will also lead to more general changes in irritability.

The inappropriate use of a twitch or painful restraint like a lip chain, or physical punishment at any time, might also result in head shyness or protective avoidance in relation to any body part. From a physiotherapeutic perspective, ensuring handling is appropriate not only applies to assessment but also to the introduction of interventions; a dog can be shaped to stand on a wobble cushion rather than being manually handled onto it (Box 2.1) or introduced to apparatus such as an underwater treadmill using positive reinforcement or target training.

It is important to identify and acknowledge the possible role of any condition in the animal's history which might result in general irritability, including episodes of low-grade general pain, such as subclinical rhabdomyolysis in the horse, and any history of a change in temperament in adult life should be viewed with a concern for the possible role of underlying disease. As already mentioned, more than one factor may of course occur concurrently, and temperamentally fearful individuals who are being treated for painful lesions may require considerable training beforehand to allow effective handling. The animal physiotherapist should not be afraid to point this out to the owner, following an initial assessment, and refer to a qualified behaviourist if necessary, although the procedures involved in desensitising animals to being approached are relatively straightforward and easily learned (Box 2.2). This

---

Box 2.2   Desensitisation and counter-conditioning a dog that is fearful of an approaching stranger (including the physiotherapist)

1 Identify the 'safe distance'

The safe distance is the distance at which the stranger can stand in front of the animal (but not looking directly at the animal) without causing the animal to show any behavioural signs of anxiety, fear or aggression. Common behavioural signs shown by dogs that are anxious include yawning, lip licking, lifting a paw and panting. In addition, body postures such as ear and tail position can provide information about the animal's underlying emotional state.

2 Counter-condition the dog at the safe distance

As long as the animal is showing no signs of anxiety, fear or aggression, it is possible to change its perception of the stranger by associating the stranger's presence with something positive (e.g. a highly valued treat that the animal does not normally receive). If the animal is not food motivated, toys or attention/praise provided by the owner may be used. Once the animal is willing to take the treats, make sure the owner asks the dog to 'sit' or 'down' before getting any more treats in the presence of a stranger.

3 Desensitise and counter-condition to the stranger getting closer

Once the dog is willing to take treats in a 'sit' or 'down' position in the presence of the stranger, the next stage may be started. The stranger may take one small step closer to the animal and the animal's reaction should be carefully observed. It is expected that the animal may now show some signs of anxiety. The animal needs time to learn that the stranger getting closer is not associated with anything negative. It is important *not* to punish any anxious or aggressive behaviour at this stage. The animal may be distracted with a command and treat. The owner may show the treat (or toy) but it should not be given until the dog sits. Once the animal sits, the reward is given (counter-conditioning). *It is important that the stranger should not be making direct eye contact with the dog or raising arms up, as both of these can be seen as threatening gestures.*

4 Small steps forwards

Step 3 should be repeated with the stranger getting steadily closer to the dog, without the dog showing any sign of anxiety or fear. It is important that very small steps are made and the progress is made at the dog's pace. Too often, these exercises are done too fast and the dog is not given a sufficient amount of time to learn. For some dogs, it may be possible to do this relatively swiftly; however, for others several sessions attending to the behavioural issues may have to be scheduled before actually doing any physiotherapy work. Particular attention should be paid to getting to within 1–2 metres of the dog, as this is when the dog's personal space is being entered.

5 Make the stranger a source of good things

Before taking the final steps, the stranger should offer a highly valued reward, which can be rolled to the dog at a comfortable distance. The dog should start making the association that not only is the stranger nothing to be afraid of but also that the stranger has something positive to offer. This should make the animal willing to approach the stranger. (It is better to allow a nervous animal to do the approaching than being approached.) *When the stranger is giving the treat, he/she should kneel down and look away as the treat is rolled at first as this is a less threatening posture. The stranger can then progress to a more normal position as long as the dog is comfortable.*

6 Stranger approaches dog

Once the dog has learned to approach the stranger, the stranger can try to approach the dog. The stranger should show the dog that he/she has a treat to offer, give a relevant obedience command and pay attention to the dog's body language. If at any time the dog appears anxious, earlier stages of the programme need repeating first.

7 Stranger touching the dog

It is obviously important for a physiotherapist to not only get within the dog's personal space, but also to be able to touch it (another reactive point). It is important to realise that just because the dog may be OK with a stranger being in close physical proximity, this does not mean that it will be OK with being touched. In order to desensitise and counter-condition the dog to being touched, the same principles are involved as described above, with every body part that is to be examined or manipulated. Always give the command first and then the treat, as this helps to relax the animal.

8 'Overlearning'

Once this is successfully done, the final steps should be repeated so the dog 'overlearns' that this stranger is a source of pleasure, i.e. responds without hesitation in a positive way.

---

procedure can be applied to overtly aggressive animals and any that are tense in response to initial examination. A relaxed animal is both easier and safer to examine.

A brief behavioural history will help determine how the animal might be expected to behave and should review a range of external and internal factors that can influence behaviour (see Askew 2002 for details of more extensive behavioural history taking). External factors include the general management and any specific triggers of aggression or known fears of the animal. Internal factors include the signalment of the individual (age, breed, sex, etc.), which might be of relevance. Obtaining basic information regarding triggers prior to the initial consultation can be helpful in managing behaviour from the outset and avoiding early negative experiences of the treatment environment, e.g.

controlling exposure to other dogs when arriving at a centre for treatment if a dog is known to be aggressive towards or afraid of its own species.

In some cases, animals learn particular behaviours as a result of sustaining an injury. These learned behaviours range from aggression in order to prevent contact with the injured area to attention-gaining behaviours such as sham lameness. The latter can be quite problematic in some dogs, but can usually be recognised by its disappearance in the absence of the owner or when the animal is relaxed. Horses, on the other hand, are far less likely to produce such vestigial behaviour since the expression of lameness for psychological reasons is likely to have been heavily selected against in evolution as it is likely to result in a greater risk of predation. However, previous poor experience during, for example, shoeing may manifest as very poor behaviour on the picking up of hindlimbs, which may need to be differentiated from a hindlimb pain process. Or, a horse may learn behaviour to avoid being saddled or ridden, resulting in it appearing 'cold backed' or demonstrating adverse reaction to the tightening of the girth.

Current circumstance

The third consideration is the current circumstance of the animal – both its motivational state and the internal and external factors which cause this state to dominate the animal's behaviour. Motivational states may be thought of as general predispositions for behaviour towards a certain goal. For example, an animal that is hungry is motivated to seek and consume food. Low blood sugar and the presence of food are internal and external factors that would encourage the animal to start eating in such circumstances, but the presence of a predator might intervene and cause a switch in motivation towards self-preservation. It may be that a given goal (self-preservation) can be achieved in many different ways behaviourally (fight, flight or freeze response) or that a given behaviour (biting) may be associated with achieving different goals (eating or self-preservation). Therefore, there is not necessarily a perfect relationship between behaviour and motivational state.

When trying to understand behaviour, it is important to be able to justify the inferred motivational state on the basis of the available information and not assume that one is necessarily associated with the other. An animal's priorities and motivational predispositions may also vary due to seasonal factors, since both bitches and mares may become more irritable around the time they become sexually receptive. Additionally, it is important to bear in mind that animals undergoing treatment and rehabilitation are often restricted in terms of exercise which can also alter the animal's priorities, having potential physical, psychological and behavioural consequences such as obesity, frustration and overactivity (Corridan 2009). Interventions such as physiotherapy and hydrotherapy may provide an opportunity for physical and mental stimulation in such cases.

It is also important to recognise that behaviour does not happen independently of environment; animals are rarely aggressive without good reason. Although it might be obvious why a horse attempts to kick you when you touch its painful leg, defensive behaviours may be inadvertently triggered in a number of other contexts, which, if they are not recognised, may result in serious injury. For example, entering into the animal's personal space or moving into a blind spot are all commonly perceived as potentially dangerous situations and so trigger defensive behaviour. If the animal cannot retreat, it will often resort to an attempt to repel the perceived threat. Defensive behaviour, because it is associated with self-preservation in the face of a perceived threat, will quickly dominate behavioural output regardless of the potential alternatives or competing motivations. It is, therefore, essential to make sure that your presence is recognised and

acknowledged by the animal before intervening too closely. A horse is likely to kick out or a dog snap if it is spooked for any reason, regardless of the presence of any pain focus.

Anthropomorphism can be dangerous when dealing with animals. For humans, the natural way to greet each other in a friendly way is directly, while making eye contact, but this can appear very threatening to dogs and horses. Sudden movement of the arms vertically, such as to put your arms around a horse or to withdraw them from a sniffing dog, and looming over an animal can provoke a fear response, and so it is important to consider carefully your own initial approach behaviour towards the animal. It is generally advisable to encourage and allow the animal to approach you in the first instance rather than the reverse, and give them time to investigate so they can establish that you are not a direct threat. An animal that has made this appraisal of the situation is far more likely to be tolerant of you than one that is still uncertain when initial physical assessment is undertaken (see Chapter 11). Initial contact should also be structured similarly to give the animal confidence.

Just as insensitive handling can provoke aggression, so can indecisive handling. If the therapist is nervous for any reason, then there will be changes in behaviour, which the animal will detect. The animal is most likely to interpret the uncertainty in the behaviour of others in its environment as a sign of potential danger and not realise that nervousness may be caused by the physiotherapist's fear of the animal itself. The animal may then, at best, try to avoid contact with the physiotherapist and at worst seek to repel the physiotherapist by whatever means it deems appropriate! Unfortunately, if the cause is not recognised, the interaction becomes a self-fulfilling prophecy for the handler, which impacts on future attempts at interaction. Initial contact before commencing any palpation or treatment techniques should therefore help to reassure both parties. The physiotherapist may utilise soft tissue techniques such as stroking, kneading, skin rolling, and/or circular finger/hand motion in a region away from the region of pain or lesion. The physiotherapist must adjust their 'touch' to the behaviour accordingly, making sure hand pressure is not ticklish but definite, using a mild-to-moderate depth of pressure and where possible, preferably with both hands.

Understanding some of these basic tenets that influence how an animal will behave will help the physiotherapist to make a more accurate and thorough assessment of the animal's behaviour.

2.2 Pain

The International Association for the Study of Pain defines pain as 'an unpleasant sensory and emotional experience associated with actual or potential tissue damage, or described in terms of such damage' (Paul-Murphy *et al.* 2004). Pain is a potent negative affective state that focuses an animal's attention and biases its behaviour.

One of the problems with assessing pain in animals is that pain can only be measured indirectly; while humans can self-assess their levels of pain and verbally report pain scores, the subjective experiences of animals are particularly difficult to assess. An animal in pain will withdraw from the source of the insult if it can be identified, protect the area affected both through immobilisation and active defensive aggression and may communicate the pain to others through changes in facial expression, body postures and vocalisation. By contrast, health and happiness are identifiable by an open and relaxed posture, facial expressions of contentment and production of chemicals that are associated with pleasure, such as endorphins.

The ability to recognise and to respond to painful stimuli has evolved to protect individuals against tissue damage and provides information to safeguard against dangerous or threatening stimuli in the future (Nesse & Williams 1994). Pain may be associated with suffering at many different levels, depending on both the circumstance and the cognitive ability of the animal concerned. At its simplest, it may be a temporary negative state, which guides the animal's withdrawal from a noxious stimulus. Some animals may be able to anticipate pain and generate feelings of anxiety when faced with a predictably painful stimulus and will take avoidance action as appropriate. This will cause the activation of the hypothalamic-pituitary axis and behaviourally might include threatening behaviour or attempts at escape (fight or flight response). The intensity of the response is usually directly related to the intensity of the perceived threat. It is important to realise that the perceived threat arises from a combination of factors (e.g. previous experience, sensitivity to pain, emotional state) without a single cause, and as a result of the accumulation of several risk factors within the three levels of behaviour assessment discussed in the previous section. Therefore, simply approaching the animal may not seem threatening from the person's perspective, but very threatening from the animal's perspective.

It is also thought by some that certain species such as horses and dogs may be capable of pain phobia; this involves the generation of an ungraded and extreme reaction in response to even the most low-grade painful stimuli. While pain phobias may exist, they should be distinguished from extreme responses that have been conditioned and allodynia. Allodynia is an exaggerated pain response to normally innocuous stimuli. Although the mechanisms are unknown, it probably arises in the structures of the limbic system of the brain, such as the amygdala and periaqueductal grey, associated with the processing of emotions (Craig 1999).

Animals showing an extreme response for whatever reason are potentially very dangerous and require specialist intervention in consultation with a veterinary behaviourist. An even higher cognitive level of response to pain is pain empathy, i.e. responding to the pain of others. Owners may report that their pets are capable of this and, although it remains to be demonstrated scientifically, there is growing evidence of empathy in relevant species (Custance & Mayer 2012).

Pain is also often classified according to its temporal pattern and this is associated with different psychological impacts and behavioural tendencies, which might be apparent in a range of species. In humans, individual painful episodes may be referred to as peracute pain episodes and are behaviourally characterised by vocalisation and withdrawal of the painful area. Acute pain refers to episodes that last up to about 3 weeks and are associated with fear and anxiety, reduced activity and care-soliciting behaviour. Subacute pain lasts for between 3 and 12 weeks and is characterised by oscillating bouts of activity and inactivity, signs of frustration (including irritability) and the development of coping strategies associated with longer term adaptation to the pain. Early signs of depression may also become apparent at this time. Beyond this, the pain may be considered chronic and depression, together with other passive coping strategies, is more likely. Subacute episodes may occur against a background of chronic pain in individuals with long-standing musculoskeletal lesions, and in the horse this may present as periodic bucking set against a 'loss of spirit' or poor performance. While the changes over time may partly reflect natural adaptive developmental changes to an unresolved lesion, it is important to recognise that learning will also occur as a consequence of the responses made over time and affect the response that is shown.

Pain is sometimes also characterised as adaptive and maladaptive, with adaptive pain referring to normal responses to tissue damage, such as inflammation, whilst maladaptive pain is associated with changes within the nervous system due to continued adaptive pain, such as neuropathic and central pain (Hellyer *et al.* 2007).

2.2.1 Mechanisms of pain

Pain sensation is a dynamic process with highly organised neural and chemical circuits (Watkins & Maier 2000). Sensory information is transmitted to the central nervous system from afferent neurons, a process termed 'nociception'. These incoming pain signals are processed within the dorsal horn of the spinal cord and result in reflexive actions, such as withdrawal from the source of injury. Reflexive actions facilitate a rapid response while, concurrently, pain signals are transmitted to the brain to produce an emotional response and memory. The motivational responses to pain, which provoke a goal-directed action of avoidance, result from activity within the hypothalamus, periaqueductal grey area and thalamus, whereas the anterior cingulate cortex evaluates the hedonic value of pleasure and of pain (Sewards & Sewards 2002). Within the midbrain, the pain system interacts closely with the fear system at several locations, such as within the amygdala and periaqueductal grey (Panksepp 1998), facilitating consolidation of memories that will be important for recognising potentially dangerous stimuli in the future and developing flexible responses of avoidance.

Pain signals are suppressed or amplified by coordinated neural connections between the brain and spinal cord (Watkins & Maier 2000). During sympathetic nervous system activation or the fight-flight-freeze response, when animals may be scared, pain sensations are suppressed – a phenomenon referred to as 'stress-induced analgesia'. Suppression of pain serves an adaptive function, allowing the animal to escape from or resolve the conflict. The 'gate control theory' suggests that sensory inputs of pain are modulated through ascending and descending pathways in the central nervous system (Melzak & Wall 1965). Descending neural pathways potentiate or attenuate pain signals, influencing the amount of neurotransmitter released by the incoming neurons or by changing the sensitivity of the ascending nerves in the spinal cord to these neurotransmitters. Analgesia is not just a response to pain but can also be classically conditioned to avoid painful sensation. When stimuli are perceived that are predictive of pain from past experience, descending signals may be sent to inhibit pain sensation (antinociception). Conversely, conditioned safety signals can increase pain sensation by resulting in the release of peptides such as cholecystekinin in the cerebrospinal fluid surrounding the spinal cord, which suppress pain-controlling mechanisms (antianalgesia), including opioid analgesic drugs, acupuncture and placebo effects. Thus, administering painful physiotherapeutic interventions to an animal in the presence of a safety signal (most often the owner) may actually exacerbate the pain of the procedure.

Hyperalgesia refers to exaggerated pain states with increased responsiveness to signals within the spinal cord (Watkins & Maier 2000). The pain threshold is lowered, and sensory nerve fibres release large quantities of neurotransmitter in the spinal cord in response to afferent signals. It may arise for many reasons, but chronic compression of pain fibres within the spinal cord due to a vertebral lesion is a common cause in animals. In these cases, the pain may be sensed as arising from the point of compression or the area innervated by the nerve. Similarly, 'wind-up' refers to a heightened sensation of both peripheral and central pain (Hellyer *et al.* 2007) and has been linked to activation-dependent plasticity in dorsal horn neurons due to high-frequency discharge of primary afferent nociceptors as a result of prolonged or intense noxious stimuli (Woolf & Salter 2000).

Neuropathic pain refers to a pain that arises as a result of nerve damage and can be extremely painful. Causalgia is a particular form of hyperalgesia associated with nerve damage (neuropathy), particularly stretching (Gregory 2004). It is sensed as a burning pain following trauma local to the nerve. It is an important differential in cases presenting with attempts at self-mutilation. A history of trauma to the region and exacerbation by warmth with remission in response to cooling of the affected area may help identify the problem, which often resolves within a year. Infection may also result in hyperalgesia, both with and without neuropathy. For example, it has been suggested that herpes virus infection of the trigeminal nerve in horses may be a cause of headshaking, a severe, involuntary tossing of the head by the ridden horse (see Mills *et al.* 2005 for a review of this and other repetitive behaviours in the horse). It is also known that two types of glial cells, astrocytes and microglial cells, that act as immune cells within the central nervous system,

specifically recognise and bind to bacteria and viruses, and when activated they release nitric oxide, prostaglandins and proinflammatory cytokines, such as interleukin-1 and tumour necrosis factor. These chemicals excite neurons and are key mediators within the spinal cord of exaggerated pain states (Milligan *et al.* 2003; Weiseler-Frank *et al.* 2005).

Phantom limb pain is a common sequel to limb amputation in humans and usually develops several days following surgery. It is reportedly more common in individuals who experienced pain in the limb before amputation (Codere *et al.* 1986). An animal experiencing phantom limb pain might be expected to present with self-mutilation of the wound site and this must be differentiated from direct wound site problems such as irritation from sutures; alternatively, the animal may show a more general pain response.

Pain sensation may be suppressed by competing motivational systems. For example, in poultry it has been found that expression of feeding and of prelaying behaviour produces a degree of analgesia (Gentle & Corr 1995). While there are no scientific reports known to the authors of this being tested experimentally in a physiotherapeutic context, this is often applied in practice by feeding or distracting an animal during examination. This is most effectively achieved if the food is offered before any painful procedure is administered, and also if the animal is given a familiar command to obey, so it builds an expectation of rewards which will buffer against the negative affective state. It would also be interesting to examine the effects of enriched environments on rehabilitation, especially in horses that often undergo box rest in very barren environments.

The processing of pain is also affected by background mood. For example, pain reports are lower in human subjects when stimuli are paired with positive or pleasant odours (Marchand & Arsenault 2002). Therapeutically, the creation of a relaxing environment for treatment is, therefore, to be advised for many reasons. Suppression of pain also occurs during and following intense aerobic activity, and is probably mediated by endogenous opioids. This may be one of the benefits of exercise-based therapies, e.g. hydrotherapy. However, not all interventions producing analgesia are necessarily positive and it is important to be aware that when an animal is faced with inescapable aversion, as might occur as a result of intense restraint during painful manipulation, learned helplessness may occur (Seligman & Maier 1967). This results in emotional biasing of behaviour towards passivity, active inhibition of skeletal muscles and opioid-mediated analgesia (Maier 1993). Thus, if an animal initially struggles and is then overzealously restrained, it may be harder to identify the source of pain.

2.2.2 Assessing pain in animals

Pain assessment involves the integration of measurements of behaviour and physiology together with knowledge of the bidirectional mechanisms that control pain. Morton and Griffiths (1985) proposed a framework for the recognition of pain, distress and discomfort based on a combined assessment of appearance, food and water intake, behaviour, cardiovascular functioning, digestive system activity and neurological/musculoskeletal signs. This provides a useful framework but the correlation between physiological measures such as heart rate, respiratory rate and pupil dilation versus subjective pain scores may be poor (Holton *et al.* 1998) and there is a need for greater validation of pain scales. These are beginning to appear in the literature in relation to specific problems; for example, Wiseman-Orr *et al.* (2004) have developed and validated a scale for the assessment of chronic pain from chronic degenerative joint disease in dogs – the Canine Brief Pain Inventory (CBPI). The Helsinki Chronic Pain Index (HCPI) has also been validated in dogs with osteoarthritis (Brown *et al.* 2007, 2008, 2013; Hielm-Björkman *et al.* 2003, 2009). There is growing interest in the facial expression as an affective component of pain and in many species this involves a tightening of the facial musculature around the muzzle alongside other changes which can be recognised with experience. Dalla Costa *et al.* (2014) have recently reported on this in the horse. It is now being increasingly well recognised that as pain is a subjective experience, animals vary enormously in their individual responses and so it is essential that assessment is focused around an assessor who is very familiar with the animal's normal behaviour, such as the owner or caretaker/groom.

Given the enormous range of individual factors that can affect pain perception and expression in a given context, it should be apparent that it is difficult to accurately assess the pain of an individual without a thorough history, including baseline assessments of behaviour and temperament (Sanford *et al.* 1986). In addition, given the differences that inevitably exist between assessors (Mathews 2000), it is also important that assessment is repeated by the same assessor on all possible occasions, in order to reduce this possible source of error. Laboratory methods to assess pain in domesticated animals might be thought of as being more objective and are increasingly sophisticated. However, these techniques are not necessarily practical for clinical situations, and further research is needed to determine how these measures may be integrated for a more complete assessment and how to interpret conflicting results. Nonetheless, some of the parameters measured using these techniques might be very informative and potentially adapted for use in a clinical setting with companion animal species (Table 2.1).

Clinical assessment generally relies on evaluating a range of behavioural signs of pain (Table 2.2), and these may be integrated into subjective scoring systems. Verbal rating scales involve qualitative description of behaviour observed, and simple quantitative scales involve subjectively rating pain as *no pain, mild, moderate* or *severe*. These assessment protocols have been criticised not only for the large variation between different observers, but also for their lack of sensitivity (Mathews 2000). Numeric scales rating pain between 0 and 10, and visual analogue scales marking pain on a ruler on which 0 = no pain present and 100 = worst pain imaginable are generally considered to provide better sensitivity and reliability

Table 2.1 A selection of non-invasive laboratory techniques and parameters used to assess pain responses in animals

Technique	Parameter measured	Species (reference)
Algometer	Pressure sensitivity	Equine (Varcoe-Cocks *et al.* 2006)
		Feline (Ko *et al.* 2007)
		Canine (Krimins *et al.* 2012)
Sonogram	Frequency and pitch of distress vocalisations	Swine (Weary *et al.* 1996)
		Cattle (Watts & Stookey 2000)
Thermal threshold assay	Foot lift response	Cattle (Machado-Filho *et al.* 1998; Veissier *et al.* 2000)
Inflatable forelimb tourniquet	Heart rate variability	Sheep (Stubsjøen *et al.* 2010)

Table 2.2 A selection of behavioural signs of acute pain

Source of pain	Behavioural response
General responses	Lethargy
	Reduction in grooming
	Depression
	Reduced feeding, drinking
	Protection of painful site
	Vocalisation (dog: whining, growling; equine: groaning)
	Aggression
	Hiding
	Inappropriate elimination
	Hanging tail
	Ear position (equine: pinned ears)
	Facial expression (canine: furrowed brow; equine: clenched jaw, wrinkled muzzle)
	Restlessness/weight shifting between all limbs
Limb	Avoidance or reduction in weight bearing
	Abnormal gait
	Head bobbing during locomotion
	Rubbing, licking wound site
	Weight shifting away from painful limb
Abdominal/ spinal/visceral pain	Tucked-up posture
	Glancing at or nosing abdomen
	Abnormal stance, stretching of hindlimbs
	Restlessness
	Sweating
	Trembling
Head pain	Head shaking and facial rubbing
	Head shyness
	Grimacing
	Signs often exacerbated by exercise
Intranasal pain	Snorting and sneezing
	Turning of the upper lip
Intraoral pain	Reduced appetite and/or dropping of food being chewed
	Teeth grinding

Source: Data from Morton & Griffiths 1985; Sanford *et al.* 1986; Molony & Kent 1997; Dobromylskyj *et al.* 2000; Mathews 2000; Mills *et al.* 2002; Hansen 2003; Price *et al.* 2003; Rietmann *et al.* 2004; Hellyer *et al.* 2007.

(Mathews 2000; Paul-Murphy *et al.* 2004). However, the validity of these systems may be questioned owing to a lack of transparency regarding pain parameters considered by observers, and these are weighted in the final score. As Mathews (2000) points out, observers may reliably weight vocalisations heavily because of ease of measurement and anthropomorphism, but these vocalisations may not correlate well with pain experiences since dogs occasionally vocalise while under anaesthesia when pain is presumably prevented. In a survey of equine practitioners, respondents cited personal experience to be the most important source of information about pain in horses, but respondents varied in how they rated pain associated with various procedures (Price *et al.* 2002).

Although the science of valid pain assessment in animals has some way to go, this does not negate the responsibility of those who work with animals in pain to institute and apply pain assessment criteria within their practice based on best available scientific evidence (Gaynor & Muir 2009). Given current knowledge, the physiotherapist should at the very least use some form of pain scale that both the owner and the physiotherapist can complete and keep a behavioural diary of therapy sessions to monitor pain responses. Should there be any doubt that a certain condition is painful, it is good practice to assume that what would be painful for a person is painful for that animal (IRAC 1985).

Further information on the recognition and assessment of animal pain is hosted by the University of Edinburgh at: www.vet.ed.ac.uk/animalpain/ and readers may wish to refer to this for further detail of some of the principles that have been discussed in this chapter.

2.2.3 Management of pain

It is sometimes suggested that if pain is an evolved response to minimise damage to injured tissues, analgesia may not be in the animal's interest. However, Flecknell (2000) points out that in situations where we take responsibility for an animal's injury and provide therapeutic treatment, the evolved pain responses are not necessary and more benefit is derived from providing pain relief. Pain slows recovery from surgery and may limit the efficacy of physiotherapeutic interventions due to very limited exercise tolerance. In addition, the associated reductions in feeding, drinking and self-maintenance behaviours cause increased risks of harm from dehydration and catabolism. Furthermore, analgesics reduce but do not eliminate pain sensations. Pain management is, therefore, in the animal's interest.

In addition to obvious pharmaceutical and physical interventions designed to reduce pain, social intervention may be important, especially grooming and other physical contact therapies. Social support has been shown to reduce physical pain in humans (Eisenberger & Lieberman 2004), and it seems reasonable to suggest that a similar mechanism may occur in social domestic species. If an animal is in pain as a result of a non-infectious agent, unless there is risk of bullying, there may be little need to isolate the individual, as the stress imposed by social isolation of an animal such as a horse can have detrimental effects. In addition, from what has already been discussed above, encouraging other behaviours through a stimulating environment matched to the animal's comfortable mobility may also be considered as part of a pain management and rehabilitation strategy. Diet may also play a role, not only in encouraging another motivational system but also more directly, and this is discussed in the next chapter.

2.3 Aggression

Aggression has been referred to several times in this chapter in relation to pain and an understanding of aggressive behaviour is important for those working with animals in distress. Aggression is not a unitary phenomenon. Clearly, the emotion underlying predatory behaviour (sometimes referred to as *predatory aggression*) is quite different from that underlying defence of a resource from a conspecific (*affective aggression*), or bouts of '*apparent aggression*' arising during acts of play. These three types of activity belong to functionally different behavioural systems and are directed towards very different goals. While they might all (in the case of carnivores in particular) share the potential to cause harm to another individual, it is potentially confusing to link them with each other through the use of the term 'aggression'. Injury that arises during play might be a result of *aggressive* play, but that does not make it a form of aggression; it is first and foremost a form of play.

Further subdivision of affective aggression is possible. It may be divided according to descriptive context, such as '*owner-directed aggression*', or according to motivation/mechanism, such as '*defensive aggression*', or according to underlying emotion. In the case of affective aggression, there are two important distinctions to be made here: aggression related to fear (i.e. threat of aversive behaviour) and aggression related to frustration (i.e. denial of something desired, including access to safety). Contextual labels do not reliably correlate with the underlying mechanism or emotion, nor the associated treatment of these. This is something that is frequently overlooked in the literature. A challenge with inferring the underlying emotion is the tendency to seek the signs that confirm your initial beliefs, but a more rigorous scientific process has been described (Mills *et al.* 2014) and although the contingencies associated with these are described below, the reader is referred to the former reference for details of further evidence to evaluate for a more confident assessment of the individual.

Archer (1976) highlighted that affective aggression tends to occur in a range of well-defined contexts, and these are listed below together with their associated emotion.

1 When a territorial boundary is crossed (fear with elements of frustration).
2 When the personal space is entered (fear with elements of frustration if escape is not possible).
3 The body is touched (frustration possibly with elements of pain and possibly fear).

4 The animal is faced by uncertainty/novelty or threats (fear/anxiety).

5 An expected reward is absent or withdrawn (frustration).

6 An expected reward is reduced (frustration).

7 Behaviour is prevented from being executed (frustration).

These circumstances may all arise within the context of a physiotherapist trying to treat an animal. A number of individual factors determine whether overt aggression rather than freezing, flight or some form of appeasement is offered. These include the following.

1 *The emotional state (mood) of the animal* – fearfulness in the absence of an easy route for escape greatly increases the probability that aggression will be used as frustration also arises. However, there are a wider range of factors that can increase irritability (an enhanced predisposition towards aggression), including low-grade chronic/subclinical pain. This is particularly worth investigating when the pattern is not entirely predictable, and probably underestimated in veterinary practice.

2 *The animal's appraisal of the situation* – this depends on the animal's perceived ability to win the contest, the value of any resource that is being disputed and the expected cost of defence. Learning can be very important in this, as an owner who always gives way to their dog will be perceived both as an inferior competitor and as an individual who does not put up much of a fight. It is perhaps for this reason that clinicians and therapists are often able to handle an animal in a way that would be impossible for the owner. This can obviously be to the physiotherapist's advantage, but must also be taken into consideration when making recommendations for treatment. Owners may not only lack the skill to undertake certain procedures in the home, but also the necessary authority.

Therapists should ensure that the risks to others of injury from an aggressive episode are minimised by:

- informing owners of their responsibility to prevent injury to others
- advising owners to avoid situations that are likely to exacerbate the problem. This may include identifiable trigger stimuli, such as approach towards a particularly painful area, uncertainty in handling the animal, frustrating or fearful situations
- ensuring the animal is not approached when it has no opportunity to retreat
- if it is safe to do so, encouraging the owner to muzzle-train an aggressive dog away from arousing or dangerous environments. A basket muzzle is preferable to a nylon one, as it allows the dog to pant and drink but not bite while it is on. The most common problem with muzzles is that they are only used when the dog is already showing aggression and will resent restraint. So training should begin away from distractions and be associated with rewards placed in the muzzle. Once trained, the dog should be muzzled before the problem arises, i.e. before arriving at the treatment centre.

While handouts, such as those by Landsberg *et al.* (2001), can be very useful in the management of such problems, they should not be used without understanding the fundamental nature of the problem faced. Therapists should also consider the potential need for specialist intervention in handling aggression, and ensure that the risks to others of injury from an aggressive episode are minimised.

Animals may become temperamentally more aggressive if they are in chronic pain. This may resolve once the pain is eliminated, but the animal may also learn to use displays of aggression in a wider range of contexts as a result of this episode. In this situation, specialist assistance should be sought to help resolve the problem.

There are many other circumstances and situations when an animal physiotherapist may need behaviour and/or training support, and the two can work very well together. For example, enormous benefit can be gained by proactively preparing animals for physiotherapy and management changes associated with elective procedures, such as hip surgery. To this end, Ryan *et al.* (2014) have recently produced an excellent, owner-friendly text outlining a range of exercises for animals to prepare them for a period of reduced or controlled exercise, such as might follow surgery.

2.4 Conclusion

For behaviours caused by underlying diseases or disorders for which physiotherapy is needed, the physiotherapist should have an understanding of how pain or the anticipation of pain can affect an animal's behaviour and how this behaviour may compromise therapeutic progress. The science of identifying and assessing pain is rapidly growing and so it is essential to keep up to date with the most recent findings and innovations which will optimise the welfare of animals. Yet with a basic and sound understanding of behaviour and its assessment, alongside a recognition of the factors that influence it, and how individuals differ in both their physical and emotional response to pain, the physiotherapist can be confident that appropriate steps are being taken to maximise the health and well-being of each individual animal.

References

Appleby, D.L., Bradshaw, J.W., Casey, R.A. 2002, Relationship between aggressive and avoidance behaviour by dogs and their experience in the first six months of life. *Vet. Rec.* 150: 434–438.

Archer, J. 1976, The organisation of aggression and fear in vertebrates. In: Bateson P.P.G., Klopfer P.H. (eds), *Perspectives in Ethology*, vol. 2. Plenum Press, New York, pp. 231–298.

Askew, H.R. 2002, *Treatment of Behaviour Problems in Dogs and Cats*, 2nd edn. Blackwell Science, Oxford.

Brown, D.C., Boston, R.C., Coyne, J.C. *et al.* 2007, Development and psychometric testing of an instrument designed to measure chronic pain in dogs with osteoarthritis. *Am. J. Vet. Res.* 68: 631–637.

Brown, D.C., Boston, R.C., Coyne, J.C. *et al.* 2008, Ability of the canine brief pain inventory to detect response to treatment in dogs with osteoarthritis. *J. Am. Vet. Med. Assoc.* 233: 1278–1283.

Brown, D.C., Boston, R.C., Farrar, J.T. 2013, Comparison of force plate gait analysis and owner assessment of pain using the canine brief pain inventory in dogs with osteoarthritis. *J. Vet. Intern. Med.* 27: 22–30.

Codere, T.J, Grimes, R.W., Melzack, R. 1986, Autonomy after nerve sections in the rat is influenced by tonic descending inhibition from *locus coeruleus. Neurosci. Lett.* 67: 82–86.

Corridan, C. 2009, Basic requirements for good behavioural health and welfare in dogs. In: Horwitz D.F., Mills, D.S. (eds), *BSAVA Manual of Canine and Feline Behavioural Medicine*, 2nd edn. BSAVA, Quedgeley, UK, pp. 24–34.

Craig, K. 1999, Emotions and psychobiology. In: Patrik, E., Wall, D. (eds), *Textbook of Pain*, 4th edn. Harcourt, Edinburgh, pp. 331–344.

Craig, K. 2006, Emotions and psychobiology. In: McMahon, S.B., Koltzenburg, M. (eds), *Wall and Melzack's Textbook of Pain*, 5th edn. Elsevier/Churchill Livingstone, Edinburgh, pp. 231–239.

Custance, D., Mayer, J. 2012, Empathic-like responding by domestic dogs (Canis familiaris) to distress in humans: an exploratory study. *Anim. Cogn.* 15(5):851–859.

Dalla Costa, E., Minero, M., Lebelt, D. *et al.* 2014, Development of the Horse Grimace Scale (HGS) as a pain assessment tool in horses undergoing routine castration. *PLoS ONE* 9: e92281.

Dobromylskyj, P., Flecknell, P.A., Lascelles, B.D. *et al.* 2000, Pain assessment. In: Flecknell, P., Waterman-Pearson, A. (eds), *Pain Management in Animals*. Harcourt, Edinburgh, pp. 53–79.

Eisenberger, N.I., Lieberman, M.D. 2004, Why rejection hurts: a common neural alarm system for physical and social pain. *Trends Cogn. Sci.* 8: 294–300.

Flecknell, P.A. 2000, Animal pain – an introduction. In: Flecknell, P., Waterman-Pearson, A. (eds), *Pain Management in Animals*. Harcourt, Edinburgh, pp. 1–8.

Gaynor, J.S., Muir, W.W. (eds) 2009, *Handbook of Veterinary Pain Management*, 2nd edn. Mosby Elsevier, St Louis, MO.

Gentle, M.J., Corr, S.A. 1995, Endogenous analgesia in the chicken. *Neurosci. Lett.* 201: 211–214.

Gregory, N.G. 2004, *Physiology and Behaviour of Animal Suffering*. Blackwell Publishing, Oxford.

Hansen, B.D. 2003 Assessment of pain in dogs: veterinary clinical studies. *ILAR* 44: 197–205.

Hellyer, P., Rodan, I., Brunt, J. *et al.* 2007, AAHA/AAFP pain management guidelines for dogs and cats. *J. Am. Anim. Hosp. Assoc.* 43: 235–248.

Hielm-Björkman, A.K., Kuussela, E., Liman, A. *et al.* 2003, Evaluation of methods for assessment of pain associated with chronic osteoarthritis in dogs. *J. Am. Vet. Med. Assoc.* 222: 1552–1558.

Hielm-Björkman, A.K., Rita, H., Tulamo, R.M. 2009, Psychometric testing of the Helsinki chronic pain index by completion of a questionnaire in Finnish by owners of dogs with chronic signs of pain by osteoarthritis, *Am. J. Vet. Res.* 70: 727–734.

Holton, L.L., Scott, E.M., Nolan, A.M. *et al.* 1998, Relationship between physiological factors and clinical pain in dogs scored using a numerical rating scale. *J. Small Anim. Pract.* 39: 469–474.

IRAC (Interagency Research Animal Committee) 1985, *U.S. Government Principles for Utilization and Care of Vertebrate Animals Used in Testing, Research, and Training*. Federal Register, May 20, 1985. Office of Science and Technology Policy, Washington, DC.

Ko, J.C., Abbo, L.A., Weil, A.B. *et al.* 2007, A comparison of anesthetic and cardiorespiratory effects of tiletamine-zolazepam-butorphanol and tiletamine-zolazepam-butorphanol-medetomidine in cats. *Vet Ther.* 8: 164–176.

Krimins, R.A., Ko, J.C., Weil, A.B. *et al.* 2012, Evaluation of anesthetic, analgesic, and cardiorespiratory effects in dogs after intramuscular administration of dexmedetomidine-butorphanol-tiletamine-zolazepam or dexmedetomidine-tramadol-ketamine drug combinations. *Am. J. Vet. Res.* 73: 1707–1714.

Landsberg, G., Horwitz, D., Mills, D. *et al.* 2001, *Lifelearn Client Handouts*. Available at: www.lifelearn.com

Machado-Filho, L.C., Hurnik, J.F., Ewing, K.K. 1998, A thermal threshold assay to measure the nociceptive response to morphine sulphate in cattle. *Can. J. Vet. Res.* 62: 218–223.

Maier, S.F. 1993 Learned helplessness: relationships with fear and anxiety. In: Stanford, S.C., Salmon, P., Gray, J.A. (eds), *Stress: From Synapse to Syndrome*. Academic Press, San Diego, CA, pp. 207–243.

Marchand, S., Arsenault, P. 2002, Odours modulate pain perception: a gender-specific effect. *Physiol. Behav.* 76: 251–256.

Mathews, K.A. 2000, Pain assessment and general approach to management. *Vet. Clin. North Am. Small Anim. Pract.* 30: 729–755.

Melzak, R., Wall, P. 1965 Pain mechanisms: a new theory. *Science* 150: 971–973.

Milligan, E.D., Maier, S.F., Watkins, L.R. 2003 Review: neuronal-glial interactions in central sensitisation. *Sem. Pain Med.* 1: 171–183.

Mills, D., Karagiannis, C., Zulch, H. 2014, Stress – its effects on health and behavior: a guide for practitioners. *Vet. Clin. North Am. Small Anim. Pract.* 44: 525–541.

Mills, D.S., Cook, S., Taylor, K. *et al.* 2002, Analysis of the variations in clinical signs shown by 254 cases of equine headshaking. *Vet. Rec.* 150: 236–240.

Mills, D.S., Taylor, K.D., Cooper, J.J. 2005, Weaving, headshaking, cribbing and other stereotypes. *Proc. Am. Assoc. Eq. Pract.* 51: 221–230.

Molony, V., Kent, J.E. 1997, Assessment of acute and chronic pain in farm animals using behavioural and physiological measurements. *J. Anim. Sci.* 75: 266–272.

Morton, D.M., Griffiths, P.H.M. 1985, Guidelines on the recognition of pain, distress and discomfort in experimental animals and a hypothesis for assessment. *Vet. Rec.* 116: 431–436.

Nesse, R.M., Williams, G.C. 1994, *Why We Get Sick: The New Science of Darwinian Medicine*. Random House, New York.

Panksepp, J. 1998 *Affective Neuroscience*. Oxford University Press, New York.

Paul-Murphy, J., Ludders, J.W., Robertson, S.A. *et al.* 2004, The need for a cross-species approach to the study of pain in animals. *J. Am. Vet. Med. Assoc.* 224: 692–697.

Price, J., Marques, J.M., Welsh, E.M. *et al.* 2002, Attitudes towards pain in horses – a pilot epidemiological survey. *Vet. Rec.* 151: 570–575.

Price, J., Catriona, S., Welsh, E.M. *et al.* 2003, Preliminary evaluation of a behaviour-based system for assessment of post-operative pain in horses following arthroscopic surgery. *Vet. Anesth. Analg.* 30: 124–137.

Rietmann, T.R., Stauffacher, M., Bernasconi, P. *et al.* 2004, The association between heart rate, heart rate variability, endocrine and behavioural pain measures in horses suffering from laminitis. *J. Vet. Med. Assoc.* 51: 218–225.

Ryan, S., Zulch, H., Baumber, P. 2014 *No Walks? No Worries! Maintaining Wellbeing in Dogs on Restricted Exercise*. Veloce, Dorchester, UK.

Sanford, J., Ewbank, R., Molony, V. *et al.* 1986, Guidelines for the recognition and assessment of pain in animals. *Vet. Rec.* 118: 334–338.

Scott, J.P., Fuller, J.L. 1965, *Genetics and the Social Behavior of the Dog*. University of Chicago Press, Chicago, IL.

Seligman, M.E., Maier, S.F. 1967 Failure to escape traumatic shock. *J. Exp. Psychol.* 74: 1–9.

Sewards, T.V., Sewards, M.A. 2002, The medial pain system: neural representations of the motivational aspect of pain. *Brain Res. Bull.* 59: 163–180.

Shepherd, K. 2009, Behavioural medicine as an integral part of veterinary practice. In: Horwitz, D.F., Mills, D.S. (eds), *BSAVA Manual of Canine and Feline Behavioural Medicine*, 2nd edn. BSAVA, Quedgeley, UK, pp. 10–23.

Stubsjøen, S.M., Bohlin, J., Skjerve, E. *et al.* 2010, Applying fractal analysis to heart rate time series of sheep experiencing pain. *Physiol. Behav.* 101: 74–80.

Varcoe-Cocks, K., Sagar, K., Jeffcott, L. *et al.* 2006, Pressure algometry to quantify muscle pain in racehorses with suspected sacroiliac dysfunction. *Equine Vet. J.* 38(1): 70–75.

Veissier, I.I., Rushen, J., Colwell, D. *et al.* 2000, A laser-based method for measuring thermal nociception of cattle. *Appl. Anim. Behav. Sci.* 66: 289–304.

Watkins, L.R., Maier, S.F. 2000, The pain of being sick: implications of immune-to-brain communication for understanding pain. *Annu. Rev. Psychol.* 51: 29–57.

Watts, J.M., Stookey, J.M. 2000, Vocal behaviour in cattle: the animal's commentary on its biological processes and welfare. *Appl. Anim. Behav. Sci.* 67: 15–33.

Weary, D.M., Lawson, G.L., Thompson, B.K. 1996, Sows show stronger responses to isolation calls of piglets associated with greater levels of piglet need. *Anim. Behav.* 52: 1247–1253.

Weiseler-Frank, J., Maier, S.F., Watkins, L.R. 2005, Immune-to-brain communication dynamically modulates pain: physiological and pathological consequences. *Brain Behav. Immun.* 19: 104–111.

Weisenberg, M. 1977, Pain and pain control. *Psychol. Bull.* 84: 1008–1044.

Wiseman, M.L., Nolan, A.M, Reid, J. *et al.* 2001, Preliminary study on owner-reported behaviour changes associated with chronic pain in dogs. *Vet. Rec.* 14: 423–424.

Wiseman-Orr, M.L., Nolan, A.M., Reid, J. *et al.* 2004, Development of a questionnaire to measure the effects of chronic pain on health-related quality of life in dogs. *Am. J. Vet. Res.* 65: 1077–1084.

Woolf, C.J., Salter, M.W. 2000, Neuronal plasticity: increasing the gain in pain. *Science* 228: 1765–1769.

Further reading

Horwitz, D.F., Mills, D.S. (eds) 2009, *BSAVA Manual of Canine and Feline Behavioural Medicine*, 2nd edn. BSAVA, Quedgeley, UK.

Horwitz, D.F., Ciribassi, J., Dale, S. (eds) 2014, *Decoding Your Dog: The Ultimate Experts Explain Common Dog Behaviors and Reveal How to Prevent or Change Unwanted Ones*. Houghton Mifflin Harcourt, Boston, MA.

McGreevy, P. 2012, *Equine Behavior: A Guide for Veterinarians and Equine Scientists*, 2nd edn. Saunders/Elsevier, Philadelphia, PA.

Mills, D., Nankervis, K. 1999, *Equine Behaviour: Principles & Practice*. Blackwell Science, Oxford.

Ryan, S., Zulch, H., Baumber, P. 2014 *No Walks? No Worries! Maintaining Wellbeing in Dogs on Restricted Exercise*. Veloce, Dorchester, UK.

CHAPTER 3

Applied animal nutrition*

Rosalind Carslake[1] and Teresa Hollands[2]

[1] University of Liverpool, Liverpool, UK
[2] University of Surrey, Guildford, UK

Summary

Nutrition plays an important role in the management of animals and animal physiotherapists need to be aware of some of the specific nutritional requirements of animals and how they may relate to performance, poor performance and disease. This chapter covers the nutritional requirements of dogs, cats and horses and health problems associated with nutritionally inappropriate diets, including obesity.

3.1 Applied small animal nutrition

3.1.1 Introduction and basic nutritional considerations

There is some debate over the exact timing of the first domestication of dogs but it is generally accepted that dogs and humans have been living in close proximity for over 10,000 years (Axelsson *et al.* 2013). For cats, domestication came a little later, with the earliest evidence dating to 9500 years ago (Driscoll *et al.* 2007). Despite this lengthy association, foods designed specifically for dogs and cats are a relatively recent development, with the nutritional requirements of these pets being given little consideration or understanding previously.

*Adapted from the first edition chapter, which was written by Linda Fleeman and Elizabeth Owens

Only 100 years ago, pets were fed primarily household leftovers and 'by-products' of human food production, such as offal. Since then, the role of dogs and cats within the community has changed from a peripheral role as scavengers of waste and hunters of vermin to a much more central role as companions and valued 'family members'. More than ever, the relationship between people and their pets is one of interdependence. Pet ownership is recognised as a non-human form of social support that helps to reduce stress and improve health (Takashima & Day 2014). This is associated with an increased responsibility of dog and cat owners for the healthcare and nutrition of their pets. In 2004, a survey on pet feeding practices showed that over 90% of pet owners in the US and Australia were feeding predominantly commercial pet food to their cats and dogs (Laflamme *et al.* 2008).

Owners' attitudes to feeding dogs and cats

Feeding is a major part of the human–animal bond. For many dog and cat owners, feeding is one of the most important methods of demonstrating a caring and loving relationship with the pet. The nutrition of their pet is very important to owners, and although the veterinarian is the most commonly cited source of information on pet nutrition, they also seek information from friends, family, breeders, pet shops, the internet and other media (Laflamme *et al.* 2008). Owners may see their pet as a reflection of their own identity. They often see their pets as reflections of

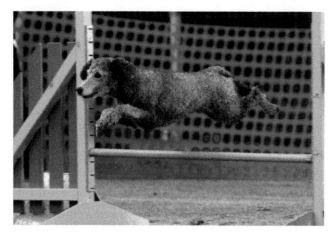

Figure 3.1 Dog in a flyball competition. *Source:* Photo courtesy of Päivi Heino.

3.1.2 Nutritional requirements of dogs and cats and evaluation of diets
Differences in nutritional needs between dogs and cats

There are some specific differences in the nutritional requirements of cats and dogs. Cats are strict carnivores, meaning that they must eat some animal-derived protein in order to remain healthy. In comparison, dogs are omnivores and can survive on a diet of either meat or plant material. Cats require a higher proportion of protein in their diet than dogs and require a dietary source of taurine, vitamin A and arachidonic acid, where dogs do not. If a dog food is fed to a cat, they may therefore become deficient in these nutrients, as well as thiamine, which cats require in higher levels (Armstrong *et al.* 2010). Dogs can taste sweet substances and so can distinguish ripe from unripe fruit, whereas cats lack the ability to identify sweet taste (Li *et al.* 2005).

General nutritional requirements and assessment of commercial feeds

Pet dogs and cats have become almost exclusively dependent on their owners for food. It is now much less acceptable for dogs to supplement their nutrition by scavenging and for cats to supplement by hunting. Owners have the responsibility of providing all the nutrients for their pet over its entire lifespan. Consequently, pet dogs and cats have become more vulnerable to diseases of nutritional origin and great care must be taken to provide them with complete and balanced nutrition during all stages of their lives. If pet dogs and cats are fed a complete and balanced diet throughout their lives, performance and longevity will be optimised. A *complete* food for dogs or cats is one that contains all the required nutrients in adequate quantities. A *balanced* diet requires that all the nutrients are present in the correct proportions (Armstrong *et al.* 2010; Debraekeleer *et al.* 2010).

The Association of American Feed Control Officials (AAFCO) is internationally recognised as the organisation that sets the most rigorous and comprehensive standard for pet food labelling claims (Roudebush *et al.* 2010). AAFCO dog and cat nutrient profiles define the minimum requirements of all nutrients for each species and life stage, as well as the maximum requirements of selected nutrients. AAFCO-approved products have a nutritional adequacy statement on the label, indicating that the food is complete and balanced for a particular life stage, such as growth, reproduction or adult maintenance, or that the food is intended for intermittent or supplemental feeding only. The labelling term 'nutritionally complete' indicates that all required nutrients are present in the food in adequate quantities, while 'complete and balanced' indicates that all required nutrients are present in the proper proportions as well as in adequate quantities. The pet food labelling term 'formulated to AAFCO standards' indicates that the food has been formulated to meet the AAFCO nutrient profile for that species and life stage. It is important to realise that if a label claims that a dog food is 'complete and balanced for adult maintenance', then that food will not necessarily be complete and balanced for dogs

their canine and feline wild ancestors. Owners may extrapolate from what they know of human nutrition, which is often irrelevant to dogs and cats. Everyone understands food, and pet owners generally like to discuss nutrition. It is likely to be a safe and comforting topic when owners are confronted with the news of a serious health problem in their pet. They may prefer to focus on nutrition rather than more time-consuming or costly therapies.

'Performance' of domestic dogs and cats

For the vast majority of domestic dogs and cats, 'performance' simply means that they must be healthy, long-lived pets. Some dogs and cats are required to perform as breeding or show animals, although often this function is secondary to their role as pets and companions. Working dogs are trained to perform tasks to assist their human counterparts and there is huge variety in how dogs are used in this way, including guard dogs, dogs working with livestock, assistance dogs that help people with disabilities and police and army dogs who may be trained in tracking and immobilising criminals or detecting drugs or explosives. Dogs also perform as competitive athletes in a wide variety of high intensity and endurance activities (Figure 3.1).

Comparison with wild species

Wild dogs and cats are not as long-lived as their domestic counterparts and the average life span is 5–7 years. Every individual endeavours to breed and all must 'work' to obtain food, whereas in contrast, most pet dogs and cats do not breed and have all of their food provided by their owners. Dogs are omnivores, which means that their diet naturally consists of foods of both animal and plant origin. Wild dogs will hunt and kill prey, in addition to seeking carrion, plant material, especially grass, and other foods (Stahler *et al.* 2005). They tend to feed in a pack, which means that the dominance hierarchy influences food intake. Cats are carnivores and their diet consists entirely of small prey. They tend to be solitary hunters and usually do not share food.

at other life stages, such as growing pups, breeding bitches or performance dogs.

If a diet contains all required nutrients, it does not automatically mean that those nutrients are available to the animal when the diet is consumed and digested. Pet food formulations that meet AAFCO standards can be additionally tested by AAFCO digestibility feeding trials. This is the preferred method for substantiating a nutritional adequacy claim. To meet these requirements, diets must be tested by long feeding trials where animals at the required life stages are fed only the test food and water while being monitored for nutrition-related disorders. When a dog or cat food meets this high standard, the following statement may be included on the product label: 'Animal feeding tests using AAFCO procedures substantiate that (Name of Product) provides complete and balanced nutrition for (life stage) of dogs/cats'. In certain circumstances, pet foods with very similar formulations may be considered comparable to those that have been tested by AAFCO digestibility feeding trials and this statement may appear on the label: '(Name of Product) provides complete and balanced nutrition for (life stage) and is comparable in nutritional adequacy to a product which has been substantiated using AAFCO feeding tests'.

In some countries, it is a requirement that pet food manufacturers include a brief nutrient profile on their product labels, which outlines percentages of crude protein, crude fat, crude fibre and moisture. This might take the form of a 'guaranteed analysis' of the *minimum* percentages for crude protein and crude fat and *maximum* for crude fibre and moisture. Importantly, this represents the 'worst case scenario' for levels of nutrients and does not reflect the exact or typical amounts of these nutrients. Alternatively, a 'typical analysis' might be supplied, indicating the *average* of the nutrient levels calculated from several samples. Actual nutrient levels might be within 10% (above or below) of the stated 'typical' level. Knowledge of the moisture content of pet foods is important for calculation of the dry matter content of individual nutrients. A common mistake is to confuse the percentage of crude protein, fat or fibre listed on the nutrient profile on the product label with percent dry matter (%DM) content for those nutrients.

Most pet food product labels also contain an 'ingredient list'. For products that meet AAFCO standards, all ingredients are listed in descending order by weight, and ingredient names conform to the AAFCO name (e.g. poultry by-product meal, corn gluten meal, powdered cellulose) or are identified by the common name (e.g. beef, lamb, chicken). These rules do not necessarily apply to ingredient lists of products that are not formulated to AAFCO standards.

As label information on the nutritive value of a pet food product may be quite limited, it is particularly useful if the full contact details for the manufacturer are supplied on the label. Ideally, a local telephone number should be included for each country in which the food is sold. This allows consumers to easily request additional information on the nutritive value of the product from the manufacturer.

Lists of nutritional requirements for dogs and cats refer to the lower limit of adequacy for each nutrient. Diets that contain nutrient concentrations that are close to the 'recommended' level should be considered marginally adequate.

Home-prepared diets

A survey of pet owners in the US and Australia conducted in 2004 showed that home-prepared diets represented at least half of the diet for approximately 10% of dogs and 3% of cats, although 30% of dogs consumed at least some non-commercial food (Laflamme *et al.* 2008). Home-prepared diets may be fed due to concerns about the commercial pet food industry, as a way of reinforcing the human–animal bond, or recommended by a veterinarian in order to manage a medical condition (Weeth 2013). Diets may be carefully formulated under the supervision of a veterinary nutritionist in order to provide a high-quality diet or may simply comprise 'left-overs' or table scraps. Home-prepared food may be cooked or raw when fed.

Advocates of home-cooked diets claim that these diets are safe and natural, and diets consisting of a high level of meat tend to be palatable and have increased digestibility and so are rewarding to feed. However, the major concern regarding home-prepared diets is nutritional adequacy. Published reviews evaluating home-prepared diets have found that less than half are complete and balanced. There are some consistent deficiencies that occur regardless of the ingredients used, unless the diet was developed by a nutritionist. Typically, these are deficient in calcium and other minerals and vitamins, and lack the essential fatty acids, linoleic and arachidonic acid (Larsen *et al.* 2012; Lauten *et al.* 2005; Streiff *et al.* 2002). They often contain excessive quantities of meat, which has a high protein and phosphorus content and low calcium. The added digestibility and palatability of home-prepared diets can also result in overfeeding and obesity. The result of feeding an unbalanced diet is that animals are at risk of nutrient deficiencies or excesses, which can present as poor skin and coat health, chronic diarrhea or anaemia, among others. This is a particular concern for growing puppies and kittens, or animals with increased requirements such as in pregnancy or lactation (Weeth 2013).

Feeding a raw food diet carries all the concerns of home-cooked diets, but also has the potentially disastrous risk of bacterial contamination to both the animal being fed the food and any person in the household involved in the preparation of it or who may come into contact with it. Raw meat ingredients can be a potential source of bacteria and parasites including *Salmonella*, *Campylobacter*, *Escherichia coli*, *Neospora*, *Toxoplasma* and *Cryptosporidium* spp. Most healthy adult cats and dogs appear to have adequate immunity to resist infection with these pathogens but young, elderly or immunocompromised individuals are at risk of disease following exposure, which may potentially result in death (Stiver *et al.* 2003). The risk of direct human exposure to these pathogens, and the animal being fed the diet becoming a potential source of environmental contamination, make feeding raw diets a public health concern, especially for pets that live with young children, the elderly or people with altered immune systems (e.g. cancer patients), and it is therefore strongly recommended that only adequately cooked food should be fed (Joffe & Schlesinger 2002; LeJeune & Hancock 2001).

Several problems are associated with feeding bones to dogs and cats. Although the actual incidence of these problems is unknown, oesophageal and intestinal obstruction, colonic impaction, gastrointestinal perforation, gastroenteritis and fractured teeth are all recognised complications of feeding bones to dogs and cats. Bones contain a very high amount of fat, particularly in the marrow cavity, and so contribute to an increased risk of obesity. It is a common perception that feeding raw bones to dogs and cats will provide some protection against the development of periodontal disease; however, comparison of dental disease in pet cats eating commercial foods and in free-roaming, feral cats found that a 'natural' diet based on live prey does not protect cats from developing periodontal disease (Clarke & Cameron 1998).

If home-prepared food is to make up the majority of a dog's or cat's diet for an extended period of time, owners require knowledge, motivation, additional financial resources and careful, consistent attention to recipe detail to ensure a consistent, balanced intake of nutrients.

Specific life stage and performance dietary requirements

Commercial dog and cat foods are available in different formulations to suit the varying nutritional requirements of individual animals. The majority of products are designed for long-term maintenance of adult dogs or cats. Specific formulations are also widely available for growth, performance and senior pets.

During pregnancy and lactation, energy requirements increase considerably, and pregnant dogs and cats should be fed a balanced commercial diet during this period. During the latter stages of pregnancy and throughout lactation, when energy and protein requirements are at their peak, a highly digestible and nutrient-dense diet should be fed, such as those formulated for growth or performance (Fontaine 2012).

Commercial diets designed for growth have higher levels of highly digestible protein when compared with maintenance adult diets. Certain micronutrients and macronutrients, when balanced with the other nutrients in the diet, can also promote the development of a healthier immune system, gastrointestinal system and improved hearing and vision, when fed during the growth life stages (Greco 2014).

Aged dogs and cats present a different set of dietary requirements from adults, in part due to normal physiological ageing changes and possibly also due to the presence of age-related disease such as arthritis, periodontal disease, cancer and cognitive dysfunction. Protein turnover is increased in older dogs, but energy requirements generally are reduced. There are many commercial senior diets available for dogs aged over 5–8 years of age, but the presence of concurrent disease should always be considered when assessing the suitability of these diets for the individual (Fahey *et al.* 2008; Larsen & Farcas 2014).

Dogs that are involved in high-intensity or endurance exercise require food with greater calorie density than sedentary dogs. Fat provides more than twice the calories provided by either protein or carbohydrate, so the most effective means of significantly increasing the calorie density of dog food is to increase the dietary fat content (Toll *et al.* 2010a). Commercial products formulated for working and performance dogs typically have higher dietary fat content than other adult maintenance diets. Products specifically designed for working and performance dogs provide benefit for dogs that habitually have a high activity level, and can promote obesity in more sedentary dogs. Sprint athletes such as agility dogs and racing greyhounds have only a modest increase in daily energy requirements and usually do not require these specific formulations. Increased calorie requirements can usually be met by increased consumption of an adult maintenance-type diet. Dogs involved in endurance, prolonged hunting and herding and other long-distance activities do require greater increases in their daily energy intake and therefore will benefit from a higher fat content to their diet (Wakshlag & Shmalberg 2014).

Important nutritional factors for large breed puppies

Growth rates vary greatly between small, medium, large and giant breed puppies and so nutritional requirements differ depending on the dog. As a result, there are many commercial diets available designed for different-sized dog breeds. Small breed dogs tend to reach physical and sexual maturity at a younger age, e.g. 6–8 months old, whereas some giant breed dogs, such as Great Danes, will not reach maturity until 24–36 months old, and the rate of growth in these dogs needs to be controlled. Whereas small breed puppy diets are high in energy and protein, large and giant breed diets should have a lower caloric content coupled with high enough protein levels for optimal growth and development.

The goal of feeding large and giant breed dogs is to achieve moderate calorie restriction and submaximal growth. Feeding controlled meals, rather than ad lib feeding, is the best way to achieve this. Calorie intake should be based on need and feeding instructions on commercial diets should be considered only as a guide. Rapidly growing, large and giant breed dogs have a very steep growth curve and their food requirements and growth rate can change dramatically in a short time. Owners should evaluate growth, using weight and body condition score (Figure 3.2), at least every 2 weeks and adjust food intake accordingly, decreasing calorie intake as the rate of growth decreases, maintaining a lean body condition.

Large and giant breed dogs are at increased risk of developmental orthopaedic disease, for which overnutrition, weight gain and nutrient imbalances, especially concerning calcium, phosphorus and vitamin D, are known to be risk factors (Dammrich 1991; Hazewinkel *et al.* 1991; Richardson *et al.* 2010; Schoenmakers *et al.* 2000). Developmental orthopaedic disease

Body Condition System

1. Ribs, lumbar vertebrae, pelvic bones and all bony prominences evident from a distance. No discernible body fat. Obvious loss of muscle mass.

2. Ribs, lumbar vertebrae pelvic bones easily visible. No palpable fat. Some evidence of other bony prominence. Minimal loss of muscle mass.

3. Ribs easily palpated and may be visible with no palpable fat. Tops of lumbar vertebrae visible; pelvic bones becoming prominent. Obvious waist and abdominal tuck.

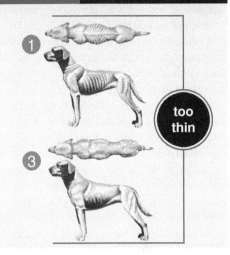

too thin

4. Ribs easily palpable, with minimal fat covering. Waist easily noted, viewed from above. Abdominal tuck evident.

5. Ribs palpable, without excess fat covering. Waist observed behind ribs when viewed from above. Abdomen tucked up when viewed from side.

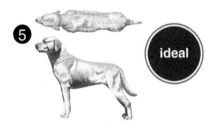

ideal

6. Ribs palpable with slight excess fat covering; waist is discernible viewed from above but is not prominent; abdominal tuck apparent.

7. Ribs palpable with difficulty; heavy fat cover. Noticeable fat deposits over lumbar area and base of tail. Waist absent. No abdominal tuck may be present.

8. Ribs not palpable under very heavy fat cover, or palpable only with significant pressure. Heavy fat deposits over lumbar area and base of tail. Waist absent. No abdominal tuck. Obvious abdominal distention may be present.

9. Massive fat deposits over thorax, spine and base of tail. Waist and abdominal tuck absent. Fat deposits on neck and limbs. Obvious abdominal distention.

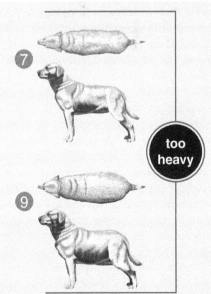

too heavy

Figure 3.2 Body condition scoring for dogs. *Source:* The Body Condition System is used with permission of Société des Produits Nestlé S.A.

encompasses a diverse group of musculoskeletal disorders that occur in growing animals, including hip dysplasia, osteochondrosis, osteochondritis dessicans, panosteitis and elbow dysplasia. The most critical period for development of these diseases occurs during the growth phase, before epiphyseal closure. Excessive dietary intake of calories causes rapid weight gain during growth and stress on developing bones. Overfeeding large breed puppies is associated with increased incidence of obesity and osteoarthritis whereas dietary restriction of calories during growth has been shown to minimise the development of hip dysplasia and osteoarthritis (Greco 2014; Kealy *et al.* 1992). An imbalance in dietary calcium and phosphorus during growth also has serious implications for bone development in large and giant breed dogs, and is perhaps the most important difference between small and large breed puppy nutrition. Excessive dietary calcium causes hypercalcitoninism and can result in abnormal skeletal development and osteochondrosis, while severely reduced calcium intake can result in reduced growth and weak bones (Schoenmakers *et al.* 2000). It is vital to ensure not only that the right amount of calcium is fed, but that the calcium/phosphorus ratio is optimal. Low dietary calcium is usually associated with feeding homemade foods containing meat. All meats are very low in calcium and have a Ca/P ratio in the range of 1/15 to 1/20. High dietary calcium is usually associated with feeding vitamin or mineral supplements to dogs that are fed complete and balanced foods. *If a nutritionally adequate food is being fed, supplementation is contraindicated.* Particular care must be taken to avoid supplements containing calcium, phosphorus, vitamin D and vitamin A.

Calculation of ideal daily energy requirements

Actual daily or maintenance energy requirements for an individual animal can only be estimated, not calculated exactly. Unfortunately, an individual's actual energy requirements may vary as much as 50% from the calculated value. However, this should still be calculated and used as a starting point when assessing how much food to give.

Maintenance energy requirements (MER) are often determined based on resting energy requirements (RER). The RER is the amount of calories required by an animal at rest in a thermoneutral environment, and does not support any exercise, growth or reproduction. This value is a function of metabolic bodyweight similar for all animals and is not markedly influenced by age, sex, neuter status, breed or activity level. However, because this calculation does not take into account age, sex, neuter status, breed or activity level, it does not give a reliable indication of the actual calorie requirement of an individual animal. Box 3.1 shows how the RER and MER can be calculated in cats and dogs to give a rough estimate of the requirements of an individual (Chandler & Takashima 2014). This is based on average energy needs and so may be too much or too little for an individual and real energy requirements may vary considerably from the calculated value. In reality, graphical

---

Box 3.1   Calculation of an estimated daily maintenance energy requirement

Maintenance energy requirements (MER) are based on resting energy requirements (RER) which can be calculated using bodyweight with the following equation:
The following are only a rough guide to the calculation of MER based on the average animal and may need to be adjusted up or down depending on the individual.

Canine MER (Kcal/day)

Intact adult	1.8 × RER
Neutered adult	1.6 × RER
Obese prone	1.4 × RER
Weight loss	1.0 × RER*
Light to moderate work	2 × RER
Moderate work	3 × RER
Heavy work	4–8 × RER
First 42 days of gestation	1.8 × RER
Last 21 days of gestation	3 × RER
Lactation	4–8 × RER
Growth	2–3 × RER

Feline MER (Kcal/day)

Intact adult	1.4 × RER
Neutered adult	1.2 × RER
Obese prone	1.4 × RER
Weight loss	1.0 × RER*
Pregnancy	1.6 × RER at breeding, increase to 2 × RER at queening
Lactation	2–6 × RER
Growth	2.5 × RER

*RER at ideal weight.
Source: Chandler and Takashima 2014. Reproduced with permission from Elsevier.

---

representation of the actual DER for a population of animals with the same body weight produces a wide, bell-shaped curve. Approximately 50% of the animals will have daily calorie requirements below the average DER and 50% will have requirements above it. If the population has a tendency to be more sedentary than average, then more than half the animals will have calorie requirements below the calculated DER. This can be quite confusing for pet owners.

When using the feeding recommendations on pet food packages as a guide, it must be considered that these guidelines are based on the average energy needs without any consideration of the age, sex or energy level of the individual, so may be too much or too little for an individual animal. They also assume that the pet food is the sole source of food being provided, and do not take into consideration any additional treats.

The key point when calculating the ideal amount of food for a cat or dog is to use these estimates only as a starting point, to evaluate the animal's body weight and body condition score regularly and adjust the food intake accordingly, to ensure an ideal lean body weight is maintained.

Evaluation of body condition

It is important to always record both body weight and body condition. Body weight does not correlate well with either body composition or body condition. Body composition refers to percentage of body fat and lean body mass. Body condition is a subjective evaluation of body composition.

Body condition scoring is a practical method for subjectively evaluating the animal's body fat that has been validated against a 'gold standard' method of measurement of body composition (Laflamme 1997a, 1997b). A variety of body condition score (BCS) systems are used to evaluate dogs and cats, and the system illustrated in Figures 3.2 and 3.3 uses a 9-point scale. Whatever system is used, it is important to consistently use a single system that is familiar. The evaluation of an animal's BCS entails visual examination from above and from the side, and palpation of the trunk, especially the ribs.

The goal for most pets is an ideal BCS of 4–5 of 9, whereby the ribs are easily palpated with minimal fat covering. For many pet owners, this may appear 'too thin', so client education is important. Dog and cat owners should be taught to evaluate their pet's body condition so that they can assess their pet's response to feeding and adjust food intake accordingly. The goal is to feed dogs and cats to achieve and maintain ideal body condition. Owners should be encouraged to monitor their pet's body condition continuously. If the animal starts to become fat, then the amount of food fed each day should be reduced. If the animal becomes thin, then more food should be fed.

A muscle condition scoring system is under development to specifically evaluate muscle mass, as opposed to body fat as assessed by BCS (Michel *et al.* 2011). Evaluation of muscle mass can be done by combining visual examination with palpation of bony prominences (temporal bones, scapulae, ribs, lumbar vertebrae and pelvic bones), and ranges from normal muscle condition to mild, moderate or severe muscle wasting. Muscle condition score (MCS) and BCS are not directly related, and an animal can be overweight yet have significant loss of muscle mass. Assessment of muscle mass is important as muscle loss is greater than fat loss in animals with many acute and chronic diseases, and loss of muscle mass can adversely affect strength, wound healing and immune function. Early identification of subtle muscle loss, as is possible by routinely evaluating MCS, can be valuable for successful and prompt intervention (Freeman *et al.* 2011).

3.1.3 Health problems associated with nutritionally inappropriate diets

Many diseases may be caused or influenced by nutrition. Some diseases may be the direct result of feeding an inappropriate diet, such as a poorly formulated diet resulting in deficiencies of excess of nutrients. This may be a particular problem in unbalanced home-prepared diets. Nutritional deficiencies or excesses can be responsible for a great range of disease presentations, depending upon the nutrients involved, for example, skeletal disorders in growing animals due to imbalances in calcium, phosphorus and/or vitamin D.

Nutritional secondary hyperparathyroidism is perhaps the most important of these diseases, and is a metabolic bone disorder occurring when an unbalanced diet with insufficient calcium or excessive phosphorus, or both, is fed. It typically occurs when cats or dogs are fed meat-only diets. It can cause clinical disease in growing dogs and cats, but can also occur occasionally in adults. The dietary imbalance causes progressive skeletal demineralisation and results in clinical signs of lameness and skeletal pain, and may result in bone fracture from relatively minor trauma (Johnson & Watson 2005).

Other diseases are nutrient sensitive, meaning that the pet's disease may benefit from a special diet for optimal disease management, e.g. chronic kidney disease, feline diabetes and many gastrointestinal conditions. However, by far the most commonly encountered nutritional problem in cats and dogs is obesity.

Obesity in cats and dogs

Obesity is now the most common form of malnutrition in dogs and cats, and one of the most common health problems seen. The lifestyles of pets are becoming more sedentary, resulting in a high incidence of excessive weight gain. It is estimated that 34–59% of dogs (Courcier *et al.* 2010b; Lund *et al.* 2006; McGreevy *et al.* 2005) and 27–63% of cats (Cave *et al.* 2012; Colliard *et al.* 2009; Courcier *et al.* 2010a) are overweight or obese. The most useful method of diagnosing obesity is to assess BCS (Figures 3.2 and 3.3). Pets with a BCS 7 out of 9 could be considered either very overweight or obese (Laflamme, 1997a, 1997b).

Although the risk factors for obesity include patient factors, such as age, breed and neuter status (Colliard *et al.* 2009; Lund *et al.* 2006), owner and lifestyle factors are likely to play more of a role, with owner feeding and exercise habits having a large bearing on the development of obesity (Courcier *et al.* 2010b; Linder & Mueller 2014). Owners are frequently likely to underestimate their pet's BCS (Courcier *et al.* 2011; White *et al.* 2011), and even when owners have correctly identified their pets as above ideal BCS, they still may not consider their pet to be overweight (Bland *et al.* 2009). Owner communication and education are therefore critical in managing obese patients.

Excess body weight has negative effects on health and evidence is mounting for strong associations between body fat content and numerous small animal diseases. Overweight dogs have an increased risk of osteoarthritis (Edney & Smith 1986; Kealy *et al.* 1997, 2002), pancreatitis (Hess *et al.* 1999), and urinary and mammary neoplasia (Alenza *et al.* 1998; Glickman *et al.* 1989). Fat cats are prone to diabetes mellitus (Rand *et al.* 2004), musculoskeletal problems and lameness (Scarlett & Donoghue 1998), non-allergic dermatitis (Scarlett & Donoghue 1998), lower urinary tract disease (Defauw *et al.* 2011; Segev *et al.* 2011) and hepatic lipidosis (Armstrong & Blanchard 2009).

Of particular note is the strong association between excess body fat and osteoarthritis in dogs. A 14-year lifespan study that

Body Condition System

PURINA®

1. Ribs visible on shorthaired cats; no palpable fat; severe abdominal tuck; lumbar vertebrae and wings of ilia easily palpated.

2. Ribs easily visible on shorthaired cats; lumbar vertebrae obvious with minimal muscle mass; pronounced abdominal tuck; no palpable fat.

3. Ribs easily palpable with minimal fat covering; lumbar vertebrae obvious; obvious waist behind ribs; minimal abdominal fat.

4. Ribs palpable with minimal fat covering; noticeable waist behind ribs; slight abdominal tuck; abdominal fat pad absent.

5. Well-proportioned; observe waist behind ribs; ribs palpable with slight fat covering; abdominal fat pad minimal.

6. Ribs palpable with slight excess fat covering; waist and abdominal fat pad distinguishable but not obvious; abdominal tuck absent.

7. Ribs not easily palpated with moderate fat covering; waist poorly discernible; obvious rounding of abdomen; moderate abdominal fat pad.

8. Ribs not palpable with excess fat covering; waist absent; obvious rounding of abdomen with prominent abdominal fat pad; fat deposits present over lumbar area.

9. Ribs not palpable under heavy fat cover; heavy fat deposits over lumbar area, face and limbs; distention of abdomen with no waist; extensive abdominal fat deposits.

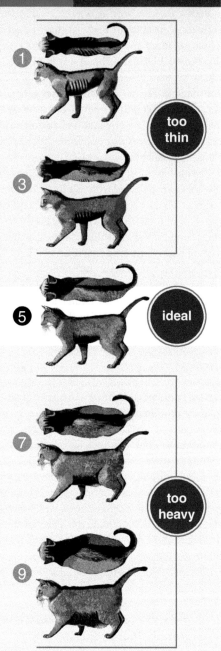

The BODY CONDITION SYSTEM was developed at the Nestlé Purina PetCare Center and has been validated as documented in the following publications:
Mawby D, Bartges JW, Mayers T et. al. **Comparison of body fat estimates by dual-energy x-ray absorptimetery and deuterium oxide dilusion in client owned dogs.** Compendium 2001; 23 (9A): 70
Laflamme DP. **Development and Validation of a Body Condition Score System of Dogs.** Canine Practice July/August 1997; 22: 10-15
Kealy, et. al. **Effects of Diet Restriction on Life Span and Age-Related Changes in Dogs.** JAVMA 2002; 220: 1315-1320

Call 1-800-222-VETS (8387), weekdays, 8:00 a.m. to 4:30 p.m. CT

Figure 3.3 Body condition scoring for cats. *Source:* The Body Condition System is used with permission of Société des Produits Nestlé S.A.

Table 3.1 Evidence of an association between obesity and osteoarthritis in dogs

	Control-fed dogs	Restricted-fed dogs
Dogs with radiographic evidence of hip dysplasia at 5 years of age	50%	13%
Dogs with >2 joints affected at 8 years of age	86%	24%
Age at which 50% of dogs required treatment of osteoarthritis	10.3 years	13.3 years
Median lifespan	11.2 years	13.0 years

evaluated the effect of calorie restriction on development and progression of hip osteoarthritis was performed in dogs predisposed to develop hip dysplasia (Kealy *et al.* 1997, 2000, 2002). The results provide strong evidence of an association between obesity and osteoarthritis in dogs. The dogs in the calorie restriction group had significantly less hip dysplasia, significantly less osteoarthritis of the hips and of other joints, lived for a significantly longer period before requiring medical treatment for the osteoarthritis, and lived significantly longer than the dogs in the control-fed group. The results are summarised in Table 3.1.

Dogs maintained in lean body condition have reduced prevalence and severity of osteoarthritis. The effect of weight loss in overweight dogs with existing radiographic evidence of osteoarthritis has also been found to be associated with significant reduction of lameness (Impellizeri *et al.* 2000). This indicates that improvement of the clinical signs of osteoarthritis can be achieved with weight loss alone. It has also been demonstrated that, when overweight, pets have a decreased quality of life that can be improved with successful weight loss (German *et al.* 2012).

Prevention of obesity is the most important goal of feeding dogs and cats. Owners require clear guidelines on how to feed their pets to achieve and maintain ideal, lean body condition. They need to understand how to calculate just how much food is enough food.

Management of obesity

The concept underlying obesity management is simple; weight loss occurs whenever daily energy expenditure exceeds daily consumption of calories. Yet it can be very challenging to implement successful weight loss programmes for pet dogs and cats. Owners frequently find it difficult to maintain compliance and motivation, even when they believe that their pet's health will be improved by reduction of excess body fat. The key is to use detailed evaluation of diet history and lifestyle to first identify the entire spectrum of specific owner and animal constraints that will affect implementation of a weight loss programme, and then to develop practical solutions that work within these constraints (Toll *et al.* 2010b). The aim is to make it as easy as

possible for owners to comply with their pet's obesity management regimen. It is important to consider the individual animal–human bond and to provide ongoing support and guidance so that owner motivation and compliance are optimised.

The primary goal is always to reduce the animal's daily consumption of calories and/or increase its daily energy expenditure. Monitoring of progress is crucial and regular reassessment of body weight and body condition score must be scheduled. Aim for a steady weight loss of approximately 1% (range 0.5–2.0%) of the animal's initial body weight per week. Once the ideal body weight has been reached, most cats and dogs require regular ongoing calorie control and monitoring of body condition to maintain the new ideal body weight (Linder & Mueller 2014; Toll *et al.* 2010b).

It is recommended that foods that are specifically formulated for obesity management of dogs and cats be fed to animals during weight loss. These products generally have reduced dietary fat content and increased fibre, air or moisture content. Importantly, they also have increased nutrient/calorie ratio, with more protein, essential fatty acids, vitamins and minerals per calorie compared with standard adult maintenance diets (Linder & Mueller 2014; Toll *et al.* 2010b). Attempting weight loss in a dog or cat by feeding a reduced portion of the usual diet could result in reduced intake of these essential nutrients and might result in deficiencies. A starting point for calorie restriction can be a 20% reduction in intake, if a full diet history is available. When current dietary intake is unknown, a starting point for the amount to feed for weight loss can be calculated as the resting energy requirement for an estimated target weight, and adjustments made from there as necessary (Linder & Mueller 2014).

Increased physical activity has been shown to allow dogs a higher energy intake while maintaining weight loss goals (Wakshlag *et al.* 2012) and exercise can be an important part of a weight loss programme. Recommendations for increasing the activity level of the dog or cat as part of an obesity management programme must be individually tailored to suit both the pet and the owner and the most appropriate advice will vary from case to case. In addition to increasing daily energy expenditure, benefits of incorporating activity into the daily routine include the introduction of a form of owner–pet interaction that does not involve feeding, and the perception by the owner that their pet's quality of life is improved. This is particularly important for owners who are concerned that calorie restriction will be an important welfare issue because they believe that they will be depriving their pet if they do not give the animal food when it appears to be hungry (Kienzle *et al.* 1998).

Owners of previously sedentary pets should be encouraged to increase their pet's activity gradually, starting with only 5–10 minutes of gentle activity a day, such as walking or swimming (Linder & Mueller 2014). Where there are exercise limitations, such as in dogs with orthopaedic disease, options to improve strength and mobility while limiting the risk of further injury may help. Studies indicate that physical therapy and aquatherapy may be a beneficial addition to weight management programmes in these patients (Chauvet *et al.* 2011; Mlacnik *et al.* 2006).

The introduction of physical activity in cats can be more challenging. The key for increasing activity in cats is to focus on environmental enrichment and encourage activity through play and by simulating natural hunting and stalking behaviour (Brooks *et al.* 2014). Hiding or placing food in multiple locations in the house or using food-dispensing toys can encourage exercise, as can using play with a rod or wand type toy or laser pointer that encourages the cat to mimic predatory behaviour (Ellis *et al.* 2013). Some cats can be easily encouraged to follow their owner around the house for 5–15 minutes per day. It is not necessary for the cat to be constantly moving throughout the exercise period. Physical activity in cats naturally occurs in sporadic stops and starts. Children often enjoy being given the task of exercising a cat.

3.1.4 Summary of important points

- Feeding is a major part of the human–animal bond. For many dog and cat owners, feeding is one of the most important methods of demonstrating a caring and loving relationship with the pet. In addition, pet owners generally like to discuss nutrition.
- *Dogs are omnivores; cats are strict carnivores.*
- A *complete* food for dogs or cats is one that contains all the required nutrients in adequate quantities.
- A *balanced* diet requires that all the nutrients are present in the correct proportions.
- The Association of American Feed Control Officials (AAFCO) is internationally recognised as the organisation that sets the most rigorous and comprehensive standard for pet food labelling claims.
- The major concern regarding home-prepared diets is nutritional adequacy. Published reviews evaluating home-prepared diets have found that less than half are complete and balanced.
- If home-prepared food is to make up the majority of a dog's or cat's diet for an extended period of time, owners require knowledge, motivation, additional financial resources and careful, consistent attention to recipe detail to ensure a consistent, balanced intake of nutrients.
- Feeding a raw food diet carries all the concerns of home-cooked diets, but also carries the risk of bacterial contamination to both the animal being fed the food and any person in the household involved in the preparation of it or who may come into contact with it.
- Commercial dog and cat foods are available in different formulations to suit the varying nutritional requirements of individual animals.
- The goal of feeding large and giant breed dogs is to achieve moderate calorie restriction and submaximal growth. Owners should evaluate growth, using weight and body condition score, at least every 2 weeks.
- Large and giant breed dogs are at increased risk of developmental orthopaedic disease, for which overnutrition, weight

gain and nutrient imbalances, especially concerning calcium, phosphorus and vitamin D, are known to be risk factors.

- Actual daily or maintenance energy requirements for an individual animal can only be estimated, not calculated exactly. An individual's actual energy requirements may vary as much as 50% from the calculated value. When calculating the ideal amount of food for a cat or dog, use these estimates only as a starting point, evaluate the animal's body weight and body condition score regularly and adjust the food intake accordingly, to ensure an ideal lean body weight is maintained.
- Body weight does not correlate well with either body composition or body condition.
- *Body composition* refers to percentage of body fat and lean body mass.
- *Body condition* is a subjective evaluation of body composition.
- *Body condition scoring* is a practical method for subjectively assessing the animal's body fat stores and muscle mass that has been validated against a 'gold standard' method of measurement of body composition.
- Owners should be encouraged to monitor their pet's body condition continuously. If the animal starts to become fat, then the amount of food fed each day should be reduced. If the animal becomes thin, then more food should be fed.
- Obesity is now the most common form of malnutrition in dogs and cats, and one of the most common health problems seen. It is estimated that 34–59% of dogs and 27–63% of cats are overweight or obese.
- There is a strong association between excess body fat and osteoarthritis in dogs. Dogs maintained in lean body condition have reduced prevalence and severity of osteoarthritis.
- When overweight, pets have a decreased quality of life that can be improved with successful weight loss.
- *Prevention of obesity is the most important goal of feeding dogs and cats.*
- The primary goal of weight management in cats and dogs is to reduce the animal's daily consumption of calories and/or increase its daily energy expenditure. Monitoring of progress is crucial and regular reassessment of body weight and body condition score must be scheduled.
- It is recommended that foods that are specifically formulated for obesity management of dogs and cats be fed to animals during weight loss.

3.2 Applied equine nutrition

3.2.1 Introduction

Opinions on nutrition are often based on personal experiences, partly because feeding horses is a daily activity. Whilst practical experience of feeding different animals is invaluable, the physiotherapist, like all scientists, also has to appreciate the limitations of 'n = 1'. They need to be able to help owners distinguish between information that has become 'folklore' and that which has grounding in research and science. Because of the ever-changing messages in the press on human nutrition, owners might either extrapolate misinformation and apply it to their horses or simply dismiss the importance of nutrition due to these conflicting views. However, nutritional support is a vital part of the physiotherapist's armoury because nutrition directly or indirectly affects all the body systems. Nutrition is an important adjunct for supporting health; correct nutrition will minimise the risk of diseases, support performance and aid recovery after exercise, after disease and from loss of function. Correct diet and meal management will ensure that nutrition is not the limiting factor in the performance animal whether during initial training, at the peak of its athleticism or during recovery.

Chapter 2 highlighted that it is necessary for a physiotherapist to recognise behavioural signs associated with pain. Equally important is an understanding of how inappropriate nutritional management might be contributing to both the pain and behaviour that the physiotherapist might be treating. Behavioural changes might be due in part to the feeding of large meals, resulting in hindgut acidosis, or might be an early warning sign of gastrointestinal disease. General lethargy could be a result of long-term micronutrient deficiency or under/oversupply of calories; resentment on tacking up and dullness could be a consequence of gastric ulceration. Loss of muscle/weight/condition along neck, back and quarters might be a result of poor-quality protein or a lack of fibre, which means that the horse spends more time exhibiting stereotypy than eating. In some instances, inappropriate meal management might be contributing to poor performance.

Whilst the animal physiotherapist should not be tempted to provide full nutritional support, they should have a solid grounding and appreciation of some of the more commonly encountered nutritional challenges. This awareness ensures that the physiotherapist can work in conjunction with a qualified equine nutritionist and/or veterinarian when necessary. It provides them with the knowledge of when nutrition might be contributing to the loss of function or performance or hindering recovery. This chapter will begin with a brief guide to assessment of equine nutrition followed by more in-depth discussion regarding appropriate nutritional support for the most common areas in which equine physiotherapy is deployed.

3.2.2 Taking of nutritional history

As with any examination, a systematic approach to recording nutritional information should be taken. In-depth details on systematic history taking are described in more depth in Chapter 11 and nutrition should be part of this history. Although you might prefer to involve a nutritionist for a detailed nutritional history, there are some steps that you can take to rule out the obvious and to check diet sufficiency and management.

Horse details

The signalment will share commonality with information that you or the referring vet might already have taken and therefore a database or app that allows you to add nutritional information

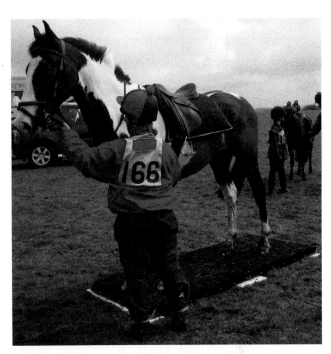

Figure 3.4 Weighing a horse on a weighbridge.

to current history saves duplication. Ensure that bodyweight and fat (condition) score and workload are included in the records.

Bodyweight

Knowing the bodyweight of the horse is important as it determines the energy (calorie/kilojoule) requirements of the horse. A weighbridge is the most accurate way of obtaining the bodyweight of the horse (Figure 3.4). However, a scientifically validated weigh tape (assuming the horse is an ideal fat score; see below) provides the owner with a weight that is not statistically significantly different from the weighbridge (Ellis & Hollands 1998, 2002).

Workload

Knowing the workload of the horse is important, as it is part of the calculation used to determine energy (calorie/kilojoule) requirements of the horse. The workload of a horse is often overestimated by owners and consequently the horse is often overfed. The National Research Council Committee on Nutrient Requirements of Horses (NRC 2007) has attempted to define more closely the workload of the horse (Table 3.2). However, if the horse continues to maintain or increase its fat score or bodyweight, it is highly likely that the workload has been overestimated and the horse is consuming too many calories.

Fat score

If a horse receives excess calories (energy) in its diet, then it will put on fat. Owners often find the term 'condition scoring' confusing as most define condition as 'fit, well rounded, shiny coat, well muscled, looking well, healthy'. They do not always appreciate that the score is simply a reflection of the

Table 3.2 Example weekly workloads of horses in light, medium, heavy and very heavy exercise

Exercise level	Mean heart rate of entire exercise bout beats/minute	Description	Types of activities
Light	80	$\frac{1}{2}$–1 h/day, 6 days a week;40% walk, 50% trot, 10% canter	Hacking Start of training Show horses Unaffiliated competitions School horses
Medium	90	1–2 h/day, 6 days/week; regular competitions.30% walk, 50% trot, 10% canter, 10% jumping, dressage, eventing	Affiliated competitions up to Novice Polo 8th week of training programmes
Hard	110	>2 h/day, 6 days/week;20% walk, 50% trot, 15% canter, 15% gallop/jumping, etc.	High goal poloMedium-level eventing, point-to-point
Very hard	110–150	Either minimum 1 h/week speed work plus schooling or >12 h/week slow long work	Endurance >50 miles, National Hunt, >2 days/week hunting

Source: Adapted from NRC 2007.

amount of fat palpated over specific areas of the horse's skeleton (Hollands *et al.* 2009). Research has identified that scoring each area of the horse's body (neck, middle and bottom) and not providing an average score increases owner's compliance and use of the fat scoring system. The modified Carroll and Huntington (1998) fat scoring index is described in Tables 3.3 and 3.4 together with an illustration of fat score 3,3,3 (ideal) (Figure 3.5).

No client knowingly makes their horse fat and the responsibility for the trend towards acceptance of the bulky outline of horses in many disciplines lies with professional and industry peers who have had interaction with the rider or the horse over the last 10 years: nutritionists, judges, veterinarians, physiotherapists or trainers. It is possible to access

a video which provides a step-by-step guide to fat scoring (www.youtube.com/watch?v=Zih1jT_pUgQ); this is a very useful tool for sharing with owner.

Diet details
Fibre
Whilst there is not a specific 'nutrient' requirement for fibre, most owners appreciate that the horse's gut is designed to process food for 16–18 out of each 24 hours; consequently fibre is important from both a physiological and a psychological perspective. Forage is the main source of fibre in a horse's diet and should provide a minimum of 50% of the dry matter (DM) intake even in competition horses (Figure 3.6). In human nutrition, cereals

Table 3.3 How to use the modified 0–5 fat scoring system

Action	Remarks
Divide the horse into three areas	**1** The neck (everything forward of the shoulder blade) **2** The middle (behind the shoulder blade to the hips) **3** The bottom (hips, pelvis and hindquarters)
Each area is given a separate score out of 5	Do not average as horses store fat in different places and lose fat from them at different rates. This is therefore a better method of monitoring changes in fat cover
Check what you are feeling against the standard descriptors in Table 3.4 and score accordingly	You can use half scores so, for example, if there is fat above the nuchal ligament (4) but the shoulder is easily felt (3) then the overall neck score is 3.5
Neck: crest and suprascapular fat deposits	• Start by finding the nuchal ligament and with your thumb and first finger, follow it along the neck • Run your hand along the horse's neck down towards the shoulder blade and feel around the shoulder • Check above the eyes (supraorbital fossa)
Middle: rib area and spinous back fat	• Run your hand diagonally across the horse's ribcage. Use a firm pressure but not so much that the horse moves away from your hand • Place your left hand at the bottom of the horse's withers at 90° to the backbone • Place your right hand next to it, with your fingers pointing across (not along) the backbone • Relax the fingers of your right hand
Bottom: sacrum and tailbone back fat; subcutaneous fat over the bony prominences of pelvis	• Place your hand flat on the top of the horse's bottom to feel the top of the pelvis • Run your hand from the hindquarters onto the tail, feeling for the tailbone • Find the 'hips' and curve your hand around to feel the outline of the bones

Source: Hollands *et al.* 2009.

Table 3.4 Modified fat scoring

	Neck				
Description	**1**	**2**	**3**	**4**	**5**
Nuchal ligament	Very fine, like a piece of string, easily felt but difficult to distinguish from skin. No fat cover Deep eye sockets	Feels like a piece of string, no fat on top Hollow above eyes	Feels like a plaited cord, sits on the top of the neck; no fat above. Horse pulls away slightly when palpated Firm rounded neck Hollow above eyes	Crest above the ligament. The ligament is thick and difficult to follow when a third of the way down the neck. The crest can be pulled over the ligament. Horse sensitive to palpation of ligament Infill above eyes, hollow disappearing	Very wide crest above the ligament. Unable to follow down the neck with fingers either side as too thick. When palpated behind the poll, the horse is normally very sensitive Complete infill above eyes, 'pocketed' with fat
Shoulder blade	When running hand down neck, abrupt stop at shoulder blade, almost sunken No fat cover Individual bones easily seen and felt Whole of the scapula easily visible, including scapula cartilage and shoulder joint Point of shoulder very prominent, angular and sharp	When running hand down neck, stops sharp at the shoulder blade No fat cover but individual bones cannot be seen Outline of scapula easily distinguishable. Scapula cartilage (under withers) rounded Point of shoulder easily cupped	When hand is run down neck, stops at scapula There is a distinct outline to the scapula although bones cannot be seen. There is less than 2 cm fat behind the shoulder blade Able to cup the point of shoulder	When the hand is run flat down the neck, it does not stop at the shoulder blade as the front of the blade is covered with fat Scapula is covered in fat and so bones cannot be felt It is possible to 'pinch' fat behind the shoulder blade; more than 2 cm Point of shoulder is very rounded as covered with fat	When running hand down the neck, the scapula is indistinguishable from the shoulder Shoulder blade cannot be felt and there is local accumulation of fat pads Roll of fat behind shoulder blade Sometimes fat behind shoulder cannot be 'pinched' due to excess amount Point of shoulder indistinguishable
	Middle (ribs and back)				
	1	**2**	**3**	**4**	**5**
Ribs	Individual ribs easily seen and ribcage is visible	Just visible and easily felt	Ribs easily felt, only visible when inhaling or turning on a circle	Ribs cannot be felt or only with firm pressure (horse will probably move away from pressure)	Cannot feel ribs and likely to be pockets of fat over ribcage
Backbone	Prominent backbone and vertebrae visible. Hand makes a sharp V shape when cupping backbone	Individual vertebrae can be felt but not seen. Cupped hand forms a rounded V over backbone	Vertebra felt easily but not seen When hand laid flat along backbone and relaxed, the hand forms a slight cup	Backbone starting to be buried, i.e. gutter starting to form. Hand stays flat on backbone when relaxed	Back is flat with gutter, backbone cannot be seen as is in gutter 'Tabletop back' – you can lay a pencil across the back or in the gutter and it stays there
	Bottom (pelvis and tailbone)				
	1	**2**	**3**	**4**	**5**
Pelvis	Pelvis well defined Hips prominent and defined, skin tight Deep cavity under tail.	Pelvis bones visible Hips defined but not prominent, can feel bones but skin is supple	Pelvis bones can be felt easily but not seen Hand can cup around the hip bones and feel them and skin is supple	Pelvis bones only found with firm pressure Cannot feel outline of hips, unable to cup hand around them	Pelvis buried Rump is bulging Cannot feel hip bones, likely to be cellulite type lumps near hips or a
Tail	Bum is sunken but skin supple. V shape to rear	Slight cavity under tail. Tailbone easily felt and visible. Rump flat either side of backbone, forming a slight V shape	Rump is an upside down 'C'. Tailbone easily felt	Tailbone cannot be felt. Gutter forming from rump to tailhead; apple shaped	dimpled appearance to the skin Lumps of fat either side of tailhead Very deep gutter from rump to tailbone

Source: Hollands *et al.* 2009.

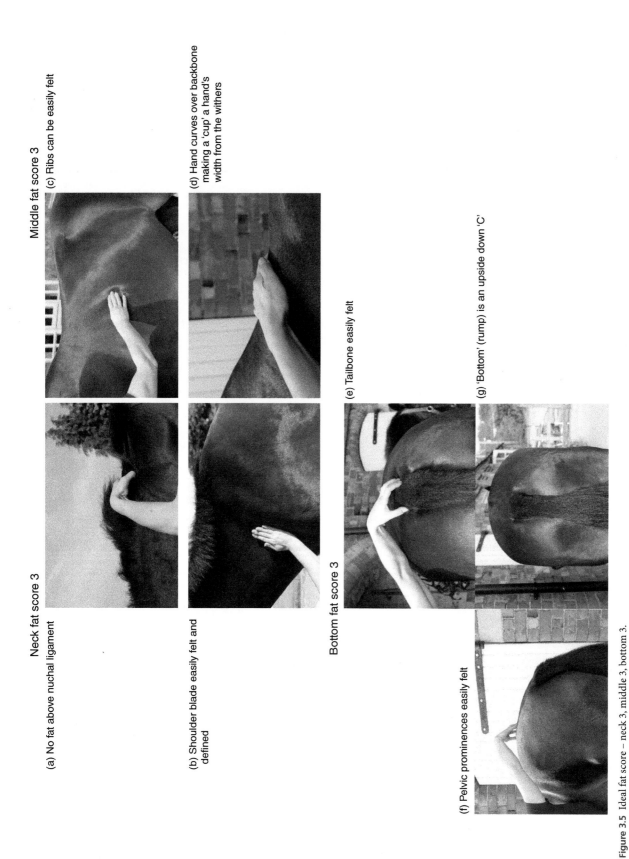

Middle fat score 3

(c) Ribs can be easily felt

(d) Hand curves over backbone making a 'cup' a hand's width from the withers

Neck fat score 3

(a) No fat above nuchal ligament

(b) Shoulder blade easily felt and defined

(e) Tailbone easily felt

(g) 'Bottom' (rump) is an upside down 'C'

Bottom fat score 3

(f) Pelvic prominences easily felt

Figure 3.5 Ideal fat score – neck 3, middle 3, bottom 3.
Neck fat score 3 (a) No fat above nuchal ligament (b) Shoulder blade easily felt and defined *Middle fat score 3* (c) Ribs can be easily felt (d) Hand curves over backbone making a 'cup' a hand's width from the withers *Bottom fat score 3* (e) Tailbone easily felt (f) Pelvic prominences easily felt (g) 'Bottom' (rump) is an upside down 'C'

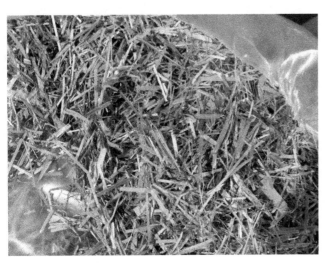

Figure 3.6 Fibre: forage should provide the foundation of the nutrient provision.

provide 45% of our fibre intake. This processed fibre in horse diets, whether in pellets or coarse mix, is of equal physiological benefit for the hindgut, but might have limitations in terms of saliva production and satisfying the horse's psychological need to chew.

Horses will receive sufficient energy (megajoules (MJ) per day) or 'calories' for maintenance on forage and can usually increase intake to compensate for low feed value (Edouard *et al.* 2008). Forage low in feed value can be improved by the addition of complementary feed. Low feed value forage should not be confused with forage of low hygienic quality (dusty/mouldy). Such forage is to be avoided as it can induce chronic respiratory disease such as recurrent airway obstruction or 'heaves'. The impact of poor hygiene quality can only be partially rectified by soaking (Moore-Colyer 1996).

Whilst forage should provide the foundation in any equine nutrition programme, its role in providing environmental enrichment is of equal importance and inadequate fibre is associated with the development of stereotypies (Bachmann *et al.* 2003; McGreevy *et al.* 1995; Videla & Andrews 2009; Waters *et al.* 2002). Stereotypies, in turn, are associated with clinical conditions that might require rehabilitation support from the physiotherapist, such as colic (Pinchbeck *et al.* 2008), gastric ulcers (Wickens & Heleski 2010) and abnormal dental wear (Maslak *et al.* 2013; Sarrafchi & Blokhuis 2013) resulting in weight loss.

Complementary feeds

Complementary feeds are so called as they are formulated to complement the forage/fibre portion of the diet to balance any deficiencies in the base forage. The type and nutrient content of the complementary feed will vary depending on the nutrients provided by the base forage, whether that be fresh grass or preserved forages (hay, haylage, straw). Feeds are formulated to be fed at several kg (800 g/100 kg BW) per day for horses undergoing hard work down to balancers which are designed to be fed at several hundred grams (100 g/100 kg BW) per day to provide vitamin, mineral and protein supplementation for horses receiving adequate 'calories' (energy or MJ/day) from their forage Most companies provide a selection of feeds within each range from a low intake balancer through to high intake feed (Table 3.5). The vitamin, mineral and protein intakes should be the same within the ranges, only the 'calorie' (energy or MJ/day) wrapper should vary. Make sure the client knows the recommended feeding rate to ensure adequate micronutrient intake.

The manufacturing, labelling and ingredients used for horse feed are governed by the EU Feeding Stuffs legislation. A common mistake is the reduction of intake (quantity fed) from a complementary feed in an attempt to reduce energy consumption, without altering the type of complementary feed, e.g. to a balancer. An unintended consequence is suboptimal intakes of micronutrients (vitamins and minerals) and quality protein which results in suboptimum nutrition.

Helpful hints

Encourage owners to weigh food at the very least when they change or increase products. Most owners simply 'guesstimate' forage intake and forage is often the main provision of 'calories' (energy or MJ/day).

Feeding by volume will lead to low DM intake if feeding haylages (Table 3.6) and up to 30% more energy if replacing a scoop of mix with a scoop of nuts.

Ensure that owners are feeding from the correct range, so a performance horse in work should not be fed a leisure/light

Table 3.5 Comparison of 'calorie' (as a colloquial term for energy or MJ) intake from different competition feeds all providing adequate vitamins and minerals (amounts shown for a 500 kg horse)

Product	Digestible energy MJ/kg feed	Feeding rate/ 100 kg BW	Feed intake	Scoops	Daily 'calorie' intake (MJ DE)
Competition balancer	11.5	100 g	500 g	0.5	5.75
Performance concentrate	12.5	300 g	1.5 kg	1.5	18.75
Slow-release performance mix	12	500 g	2.5 kg	2.5	30
Competition mix/cube	11.5	800 g	4 kg	4 scoops mix 2.7 scoops nuts	46

BW, bodyweight; DE, digestible energy; MJ, megajoule.

Table 3.6 The effect of feeding 4 kg haylage compared to hay on the dry matter (bulk/fibre) and nutrient intake of the horse

	Typical hay (dry matter 88%)	Typical haylage (dry matter 69%)	Dry haylage (dry matter 77.8%)	Wet haylage (dry matter 48%)
Energy MJ	33.9	29.5	32.9	19.2
Protein g	268.7	273.2	261.4	216.9
Dry matter (kg)/fibre	3.5	2.76	3.1	1.9

MJ, megajoule.

work feed as they will be deficient in micronutrients and quality protein.

3.2.3 An overview of nutritional support for specific conditions

Physiotherapists should be able to offer an overview of the principles of nutritional support for clinical problems and advice should be given in conjunction with an equine nutritionist and veterinarian. Equally important is a more in-depth understanding of the nutritional requirements and dietary management to support training programmes and the use of nutrition to help prevent reoccurrence of problems.

Musculoskeletal disease

Lameness and muscle disease as discussed in Chapters 7 and 10 are some of the most common problems for physiotherapy referral. Some of the specific areas where nutritional support and appropriate diet management can aid rehabilitation or indeed prevent further episodes are summarised below.

Equine intrinsic muscle disease

There are many causes of equine muscle damage, which cause episodes of tying up (exertional rhabdomyolysis/Monday morning disease): one or more episodes of acute stiffness, muscle cramping and pain. The literal definition of rhabdomyolysis is the 'dissolution of skeletal muscle' which may be due to an underlying metabolic disease, but may also occur sporadically associated with dietary deficiency of Vitamin E and selenium, acute overwork, immune-mediated disease or infection (bacterial or viral). More detail on instrinsic muscle disease is provided in Chapter 10.

Sporadic muscle disease should be investigated by a veterinarian, but dietary support for overwork injury such as delayed-onset muscle soreness (DOMS) might include checking electrolyte and antioxidant balance and making sure that the horse is on an appropriate ration for its workload. Advise products that are formulated for the good doer and appropriate electrolyte and micronutrient supplementation if necessary. This type of tying

up has no dietary link to carbohydrate intake; indeed, many of these horses are on low-energy products (i.e. low carbohydrate). There is some evidence in the literature that horses carrying 30% over their ideal bodyweight (and this includes the rider contribution) have higher lactate for up to 10 min after exercise, increased muscle soreness and tightness and higher creatine kinase (Powell *et al.* 2008). It is therefore important that clients appreciate that horses need to be fit enough for the work required and that carrying extra weight might predispose them to muscle damage.

Metabolic muscle disease

Recurrent episodes of tying up which have a metabolic cause (i.e. there is something wrong with the muscle metabolism) can be managed or minimised with an appropriate diet and exercise plan.

Recurrent exertional rhabdomyolysis (RER) and polysaccharide storage myopathy (PSSM) are different intrinsic muscle diseases (see also Chapter 10) and the general dietary recommendation is that they should be managed with a high-fat, low-starch diet, although the biology behind the dietary support is different.

A small study (Finno *et al.* 2010) suggests that high-starch diets fed to fit RER horses result in higher cortisol and insulin compared to an isocalorific high-fat diet. The authors hypothesise that this might indicate increased stress in these horses and that the potential predisposing effect of a high-starch diet on RER may be through its ability to exacerbate nervous behaviour as a result of alterations in central nervous system (CNS) neurotransmitters.

The feeding of a high-fat diet to horses with the glycogen storage disease PSSM has more of a biological explanation as it reduces the horse's reliance on glycogen and uses fat as the energy source. High-fat diets decrease insulin response to feeding in PSSM horses which lowers uptake of glucose into muscle cells. High-fat diets also increase the availability of fatty acids in the bloodstream for muscle to use as fuel (Ribeiro *et al.* 2004).

Some researchers recommend providing 20% of the horse's energy intake as oil (Valentine *et al.* 2001). However, in a horse with PSSM, prone to weight gain, this results in a significant compromise in DM intake and an excessive amount of 'calories' and good results have been achieved by feeding lower amounts of dietary fat (12.7% total energy intake; Ribeiro *et al.* 2004).

Nutritional support for equine gastric ulcer syndrome (EGUS)

From a dietary perspective, gastric ulcers occur when the acid production exceeds the protective factors, namely buffering. It is appropriate that clients understand that the aetiology of EGUS is multifactorial and numerous feeding management practices have been associated with EGUS. Ulcers have been recorded in a huge variety of horses undertaking very different levels of exercise and being fed very different diets. Importantly, however, the severity of ulcers is very different, and the veterinarian will make a clinical decision as to whether the ulcers are of clinical significance. If the only signs are poor performance, then often the physiotherapist is called upon for support and elimination of other factors. We know that restricting fibre is linked to incidence of EGUS (Murray & Eichorn 1996) and that feed deprivation of 12 hours causes gastric ulcers in some horses (Husted *et al.* 2008). If the horse is a frequent traveller that takes time to settle in unfamiliar surroundings and doesn't eat up then this might be a contributory factor, despite an otherwise 'balanced diet'.

Generally, the most successful approach to dietary management of EGUS is to ensure that clients understand the need to minimise acidification of the stomach by meal management that reflects the digestive physiology and function of the equine stomach. Saliva, the main buffering agent in the stomach, is only produced when the horse physically chews and 1 mL of saliva is produced per chew (Meyer *et al.* 1985). Horses that crib produce less saliva compared to horses that don't and therefore might be at greater risk of gastric ulcers (Moeller *et al.* 2008). Fifteen to 30 times more saliva is produced while eating compared to when cribbing (Houpt 2012). Horses take around 4500 chews/kg forage compared to 1200 chews/kg of concentrates and 5200 chews/kg short chop/chaff. Saliva has a buffering capacity of 50 mmol/L (Frape 2010) so a slice of hay (1 kg) producing 4.5 litres of saliva when eaten provides substantially more buffering than any supplement fed at 200 mL/day!

Lethargy/ poor performance related to gastric ulcers may be due to reduced forage intake or when meals are fed infrequently as buffering will be compromised. A kilo of fibre produces up to four times more saliva (and buffering) compared to the same weight of compound feed, but fibre type, quantity and frequency of feeding need to be considered and discussed with the client.

Fibre quantity

Even when only hay is fed, acid is still produced in the stomach (Sandin *et al.* 1998). Large 'meals' of hay have a similar effect as large meals of concentrates and increase the gastric acid production. Horses fed just hay (bulky intake) had a lower pH 2–5 hours after feeding, but a higher pH 12 hours after feeding compared to those fed hay and grain (smaller intake) (Nadeau *et al.* 2000). However, the horses fed the hay and grain mix had lower EGUS scores compared to just hay. The hay alone diet was bulkier and it has been shown that diets (whether large concentrate meals or nets of low-quality forage) higher in bulk increase plasma gastrin concentration, increase gastric acid secretion and lower stomach pH (Wickens *et al.* 2013).

Fibre frequency

If forage is withheld, the pH of the upper stomach, which is normally between 5–7, will drop to below 4 (Husted *et al.* 2008). Feeding forage every 6 hours or more decreases the risk of non-glandular ulcers, compared to gaps of more than 6 hours (Luthersson *et al.* 2009).

Fibre type
Straw

A study in Denmark showed that eating straw was associated with increased risk of EGUS (4.5 times greater risk) (Luthersson *et al.* 2009), but the study included horses that had no access to forage except their straw bed, which possibly confounds the association. It is likely that horses with access to only a straw bed would have lower fibre intake compared to horses with other sources of forage; however, the authors suggested that straw might irritate the stomach lining or doesn't buffer the stomach acid because straw is low in calcium and protein.

There is evidence that a fibrous mat, which aids buffering, sits at the bottom of the upper part of the stomach. Some people consider that the fibre acts as a physical barrier preventing the acid from the lower stomach splashing up into the upper stomach. Others consider that it is the minerals in the fibre that act as a buffer when they dissociate from the fibre.

Some degree of stomach acid is needed to free ingested calcium from the fibre mat or food matrix before it can be absorbed in the small intestine. The free calcium in the stomach then acts as a buffer before the food moves into the small intestine.

It is quite possible that fibre low in calcium (e.g. straw) might not have the buffering capacity of forage that contains more calcium. A simple solution if straw is being fed as a low-calorie forage for fat horses is to recommend the addition of a balancer, which is formulated to provide the necessary protein and vitamins and minerals, including calcium.

Haylage

Haylage can vary greatly in water content. If clients feed according to volume/perceived weight, then they may be compromising the horse's fibre intake (see Table 3.6). It is important that haylage is analysed and adjustment to weight made, to ensure adequate DM intake.

Alfalfa/lucerne

There is some evidence that feeding alfalfa with grain reduces the incidence of gastric ulcers in horses compared to hay alone, despite higher acid production. Whether this is due to meal size (see above), increased calcium or protein buffering or some other factor is unknown (Nadeau *et al.* 2000).

Top tips
- Dietary solutions to buffer the acid in the stomach include:
  - where possible, encourage ad lib fibre, but offered in small haynets frequently
  - recommend good-quality hay to encourage chewing and saliva production but reduce the amount of gastrin produced compared to large haynets of lower quality forage
  - adjust haylage quantities according to water content to ensure adequate fibre intake (see Table 3.6)

- add alfalfa chaff (protein and minerals) to small meals or feed before a meal
- ensure horse has access to grazing, at least 2–3 h/day
- add antioxidants, in feed or as a supplement.

- Feeding in relation to exercise has been shown to have a direct influence on the pH of the proximal stomach. A small meal 2 h before exercise may provide a protective effect and increase pH/reduce acidity in the upper stomach and protection against the splashback from the lower stomach during fast work (Lorenzo-Figueras & Merritt 2002).
- When travelling, owners must factor in rest periods for feeding and watering at least every 6 h (they should stop more frequently for themselves).
- If horses are on a predominantly forage diet, they must be given a balancer to provide adequate minerals, including calcium. Spring and summer grazing and preserved forages do not meet maintenance requirements of several minerals.
- Ensure water is available all the time.

Box-rested horses

Box resting a horse is necessary for numerous reasons, but is challenging from a physiotherapy perspective as muscle loss and fat gain associated with the sedentary environment are inevitable. In people, inactivity results in nitrogen (protein) loss from the whole body and average nitrogen lost through urine can reach 2 g/day (Teasell & Dittmer 1993) and inactivity can predispose to gut stasis in both humans and horses. Cutting back on DM intake of fibre should be discouraged for all the reasons discussed in the EGUS section, but it is essential to ensure micronutrient adequacy and control calorie intake. This is achievable by advising the feeding of low-calorie (but good hygienic quality) forages such as oat or barley straw or soaking hay for 8–16 h to remove the water-soluble carbohydrates (which supply a large percentage of the 'calories'). Soaking hay for 12 h as opposed to 30 min does not further improve the hygienic quality of the hay but does result in up to 1 kg of water-soluble carbohydrates being leached out of the hay (Longland et al. 2011).

Consideration needs to be given to how the forage is provided to the horse and the impact on the horse's health and welfare; the length of box rest might be the deciding factor as some short-term impact might be considered acceptable. Feeding forages in haynets has been linked to reduced lateral movement and decreased efficiency of chewing (Masey O'Neil et al. 2010) as well as an increased risk of respiratory disease. In the horse, mucociliary clearance is faster when the horse's head is lowered, due to the effects of gravity and the anatomical positioning of the airways (Racklyeft & Love 1990). Yet feeding hay in nets reduces rate of intake (Glunk et al. 2014) and keeps a horse occupied for a longer duration. Glunk et al. (2014) compared three different sized haynets (large, 15.2 cm openings; medium, 4.4 cm; and small, 3.2 cm) with the feeding of hay from the floor. The small holed haynet almost halved the horses' intake rate down to 0.9 kg/h compared to 1.5 kg/h when the hay was fed on the floor.

If the horse is to be boxed rested for a long period, it is vital to consider the role of nutrition in terms of feed enrichment and to encourage owners to replicate natural foraging behaviour. Meal management is as important for the health and welfare of the horse as the actual dietary intake. A study looked at the impact of feeding 1 kg of each of three long-chop (hay in nets) and three short-chop commercially available feeds (in buckets on the floor) and compared it to the same weight of a single forage (Thorne et al. 2005). Multiple choice forages increased foraging but decreased searching behaviour compared to the single forage source, suggesting that box-rested horses might spend more time eating if given a choice of multiple forages. The researchers suggested that 'sensory specific satiety, in which the horse becomes satiated by one food type but still motivated to consume others, may have left the horses satiated by hay on the Single Forage treatment but still motivated to consume other forages' when fed multiple forages. One way of satisfying foraging behaviour but not increasing intake is to provide hay in several small haynets (or floor mangers) at multiple points around the stable rather than in a single net.

Other successful meal management techniques to consider is the use of foraging balls which change the time budget of stabled horses so that it is more in line with their natural grazing behaviour (Winskill et al. 1996). However, other researchers (Goodwin et al. 2007) showed an increase in frustration when horses were given 5 min access to feed in a selection of foraging devices. These options should be discussed with owners and adapted to their individual horses.

Whilst it is important to control 'calories', most box-rested horses are convalescing and therefore need nutritional support, specifically quality protein, micronutrients and vitamins. High-forage diets are deficient in some nutrients, therefore a high-quality balancer should be considered. This can be fed alongside low-calorie chaff to slow intake. Additional feed enrichment can be provided by succulents such as carrots (cut lengthways into six slivers) and root vegetables hung from the ceiling. Sloppy unmolassed sugarbeet helps maintain water intake which is important as conserved forages only provide 150 g water/kg compared to grass which will provide between 800–900 g water/kg.

3.2.4 Nutritional support for training programmes
Active competition
Energy

Performance horses need complementary feed in the form of cereals for energy and glycogen replacement. However, large meals of starch increase the DM in the stomach compared to small meals (Meyer et al. 1975, cited in Frape 2010). An increase in DM buffers the stomach acid and facilitates lactobacilli fermentation of the starch; the resultant products are the same as are produced during fermentation of fibre, i.e. lactate and volatile fatty acids (VFAs). Therefore, advise owners to feed small meals of concentrates to reduce DM accumulation in the stomach. Feeding 1 g starch/kg BW/meal reduces the risk of EGUS, increases small intestine digestion of starch and minimises starch overload in the hindgut. Remember that meal size will vary according to starch content of the feed; most manufacturers' nutritionists will be able to provide this information.

It is clear that even in the performance horse, fibre/forage should be the foundation of the feed programme. However, as workload increases, forage no longer provides sufficient micronutrients, protein or substrate for aerobic energy. Fatigue induced by physical activity can be caused by depletion of muscle glycogen, loss of muscle ATP, dehydration and inappropriate meal management. It has been shown (Sewell et al. 1992) that horses can lose up to 50% of their muscle ATP after galloping and that the losses are greater than in humans.

There has been much discussion in the literature about the negative effects of feeding starch from the perspective of digestive physiology. However, with improved understanding of diet management, it can be desirable to improve both availability of muscle glycogen and blood glucose during exercise and to replenish both after exercise in horses undergoing hard or very hard work. Lacombe et al. (2004) fed horses low-, medium- and high-starch isocalorific diets after glycogen-depleting exercise. They found that the high-starch diet replenished muscle glycogen more effectively than the other two diets (Table 3.7). The authors concluded that:

> horses performing endurance events or horses undertaking several events on successive days could benefit from high soluble carbohydrate diets after exercise to hasten muscle glycogen synthesis. However, because horses fed large amounts of soluble carbohydrate may be predisposed to gastrointestinal disorders, optimal nutritional strategies should be developed and careful feeding management ensured.

Endurance horses, however, require a predominantly forage-based diet to help support fluid balance during exercise, as the forage within the large bowel acts as a reservoir of water.

With the appropriate meal management, it is possible to feed a high-starch diet by providing small starch meals, removing the risk of any starch overload in the hindgut. An increase in the number but reduction in size of feeds fed per day should be prescribed. Less than 1.0–1.5 g starch/kg BW/meal should

be recommended to maximise small intestine digestion of starch and ensure that the glycaemic response is within normal physiological parameters (Vervuert et al. 2007, 2009). A 450 kg filly will commonly be fed 5 kg of racehorse cubes per day to meet her growing and racing requirements; typically these would provide1.4 kg starch/day, so this is a high-starch diet. But, by dividing the ration into four feeds, she is only getting 0.78 g starch/kg BW/meal. As a further incentive for your clients to feed four meals a day, Bezděková et al. (2008) showed that 75% of horses fed twice a day had EGUS whereas for those fed three times per day, the incidence was reduced to 58%.

The type of energy fed to the horse should depend upon its exercise effort. Horses that are undergoing fast, anaerobic work will have little need for high-fat diets; however, in disciplines where stamina and aerobic work are important, then fat can be fed up to 10% of the DM intake. Manufacturers tend to offer both high-starch, fast-release competition feeds for racing and fast work and high-fat and fibre competition feeds for stamina and slower work.

Protein

It is not unusual for clients to struggle to achieve topline through muscle development, particularly if fat above the nuchal ligament is confused with muscle. Remind clients that top athletes in almost every sport are lean, meaning they have the optimal amount of muscle for performance in their sport and a low level of body fat. Achieving a lean body composition is an important way to improve sports performance and all-round health. The same should hold true for horses regardless of the discipline

Dressage horses will perform better if their bulk outline comes from muscle and not fat. Heavy topline (fat-filled crests above the nuchal ligament) and bulky necks/shoulders (shoulder blade outline filled in with fat and skeleton not visible) (see Figure 3.5 for ideal fat cover) will increase susceptibility to equine metabolic syndrome and restricted movement respectively.

There are two main requirements for muscle development: resistance training and nutrition that supports muscle protein synthesis. High forage intakes tend not to contain sufficient quality protein and the quality will be variable, dependent on harvesting and the grass lay; on the other hand, clients need to

Table 3.7 The effect of starch intake on glycogen replenishment after exercise

Diet	Compound fed kg/day	Starch % (g starch/kg feed)	Kg starch/feed (g starch/kg BW) 3 feeds/day	Muscle glycogen % of preexercise		Amount of glycogen replaced mmol/kg/h	Water intake L/day
				24 h after exercise	72 h after exercise		
High starch	6.5	50.9 (509)	1.1 (2.3)	64.4	133	1.5	43
Medium starch	7.8	26.4 (264)	0.68 (1.4)	54.2	106	1.1	67
Low starch (hay only)	9.7	4.3 (43)	0.13 (0.2)	52.9	102	0.9	88

BW, bodyweight.
Source: Data from Lacombe *et al.* 2004.

Table 3.8 Electrolyte loss in sweat g/day and replenishment through diet for a 500 kg horse (additional electrolyte supplementation is fed over several days after exercise)

Electrolyte lost in sweat (g/day)	Rest	10 litres	25 litres
Sodium	10	43	93
Chloride	10	71	163
Potassium	25	43	70
Magnesium	10	13	19

Intake of electrolytes provided by 9 kg hay & 3 kg competition mix (500 kg horse)				Additional electrolyte supplementation needed (g/day) relative to sweat loss (L/day)				
g/day	Concentrate	Hay	Total	Rest	5 litres	10 litres	25 litres	40 litres
Sodium	13.5	24	37.5	0	0	5	55	104
Chloride	21.0	41	62	0	0	11	101	192
Potassium	19.5	127	146.5	0	0	0	0	0
Magnesium	6	10	16	0	0	0	3	8

be discouraged from thinking that a 'topline/conditioning' feed is the only answer.

In human athletes, the timing of protein consumption has a significant effect on the rate of muscle protein synthesis. Research has shown that protein consumed immediately before, during and immediately after exercise causes more muscle protein synthesis than equal amounts of protein consumed at other times (Aragon & Schoenfeld 2013; Pennings et al. 2011). This is because carbohydrate stimulates the release of insulin, which in turn transports the amino acids from dietary protein to the muscle cells, initiating muscle protein synthesis. Research indicates that the provision of amino acids (protein) and glucose after exercise initiates the same biochemistry in the horse and is therefore likely to improve glycogen storage and muscle development (Urschel et al. 2010).

Water and electrolytes

Dehydration is strongly linked to poor performance and impairment of cognitive function. Even short periods of fluid restriction (1–2% body mass loss) have been reported to decrease performance in people (Maughan 2003). Clients don't always appreciate the importance of horses drinking before electrolyte supplementation. Advising electrolyte replenishment before the

horse has rehydrated is dangerous. Clients also need reminding that electrolytes are simply minerals that dissociate in solution, and competition and racing feeds have higher levels of minerals in recognition of the increased need that these horses have for electrolytes.

Work carried out at Burghley found that dehydration bodyweight losses after the dressage were similar in magnitude to those lost after the cross-country phase in some horses (Ellis & Hollands 2001). Electrolyte replenishment cannot be achieved immediately (Table 3.8) but clients need to monitor dehydration by using either a weigh tape or weighbridge, and loss during travelling needs to be taken into consideration.

Top tips for feeding for active competition

- Support clients in feeding the correct product appropriate for the horse's workload.
- Discourage the feeding of leisure feeds or reduced quantities of competition mix/cube to a performance horse; both will result in nutrient deficiencies although the horse may carry enough weight.
- Recommend that meals should contain less than 1 g starch/kg BW.
- Quality protein is essential for muscle development.

Table 3.9 The amount of 'calories' (as a colloquial term for energy or MJ) consumed by a 500 kg horse eating 1.5% BW as dry matter

Forage	Dry matter intake	Fresh weight	'Calorie' intake/day (MJ DE)	% of 'calorie' requirement
Winter pasture 17 h average grass	7.5	30	47	69
Late-cut meadow hay	7.5	8.9	52.5	77
High-fibre haylage	7.5	12.5	75	110
Straw	7.5	8.9	37.5	55
Summer grazing, 8 h, plenty of grass	7.5	38	76	111
Good-quality meadow hay	7.5	8.9	75	110
Spring grazing, average grass; out all night	7.5	50	90	132

DE, digestible energy; MJ, megajoule.

- Electrolytes will need replenishing over a period of days after hard work.
- Time of feeding can aid in muscle glycogen and amino acid replenishment.

Light work/rehabilitation

Overweight horses are at increased risk of musculoskeletal problems; an epidemiological study looking at the incidence of obesity in south east England found that chronic musculoskeletal conditions and body fat were related to a 2.5 times increased risk per unit increase of fat score (Salonen *et al.* 2009). With only 35% of horse owners recognising that their horses are overweight (Ireland *et al.* 2013), it is highly likely that the physiotherapist will need to support owners in accepting that weight loss is part of the rehabilitation plan.

Weight loss can only be achieved if energy intake is less than energy output. Many owners confuse reduction in energy with DM (bulk restriction). It is quite clear that fibre restriction is detrimental to the horse's health and welfare. For example, in order to minimise the risk of EGUS, the literature suggests that hay should never be fed at less than 1.5 kg/100 kg BW (Videla & Andrews 2009). However, when more than 1.5% BW is fed as forage, this is contrary to the current advice for feeding overweight horses, which recommends no more than 1.5% BW, at least in the short term (Dugdale *et al.* 2010). In practice, it is possible to provide a low-calorie forage-based diet which can be fed at more than 1.5% BW by taking the 'calories' into consideration (Table 3.9). Feed restriction can lead to ponies eating their shavings (Curtis *et al.* 2011); 250 kg ponies restricted to 1.5% BW ate up to 3 kg of wood shavings/day. It is also essential to ensure that micronutrient intake is adequate by advising a balancer. Being overweight is recognised as being a chronic inflammatory disease and as such, antioxidant support is as important for the rehabilitating/leisure horse as for the elite competition horse (Marlin *et al.* 2002; Williams & Burke 2010).

3.3 Conclusion

It is clear that nutrition is more than just a balanced diet. Feed or meal management, enrichment and appropriate feed materials contribute to the overall health and welfare of the horse as well as its performance. Every system in the horse's body is either directly or indirectly influenced by nutrition; whole textbooks are written on the subject and this chapter can only provide an overview. However, when providing advice or passing on nutritional information, always ask yourself, can you explain the biology behind the advice; does it make sense from a physiological and anatomical perspective and can you ensure client compliance? If not, no amount of research will make it work in the field. Obesity is one of the top three global economic and social burdens generated by human beings (McKinsey Global Institute 2014). Globally, governments are starting to recognise that nutrition should be one of the cornerstones of preventive medicine, particularly as the cost and effectiveness of new drugs become more constrained due to legislation and resistance. Similarly, equine nutrition should be the cornerstone between the nutritionist, veterinarian, the rider, the horse and the physiotherapist.

References

Alenza, D.P., Rutteman, G.R., Pena, L., Beynen, A.C., Cuesta, P. 1998, Relation between habitual diet and canine mammary tumors in a case–control study. *J. Vet. Intern. Med.* 12: 132–139.

Aragon, A.A., Schoenfeld, B.J. 2013, Nutrient timing revisited: is there a post-exercise anabolic window? *J. Int. Soc. Sports Nutr.* 10: 5–16.

Armstrong, P.J., Blanchard, G. 2009, Hepatic lipidosis in cats. *Vet. Clin. North Am. Small Anim. Pract.* 39: 599–616.

Armstrong, P.J., Gross, K.L., Becvarova, I., Debraekeleer, J. 2010, Introduction to feeding normal cats. In: Hand, M.S., Thatcher, C.D., Remillard, R.L., Roudebush, P., Novotny, B.J. (eds), *Small Animal Clinical Nutrition*, 5th edn. Mark Morris Institute, Topeka, KS, p. 364.

Axelsson, E., Ratnakumar, A., Arendt, M.-L. *et al.* 2013, The genomic signature of dog domestication reveals adaptation to a starch-rich diet. *Nature.* 495: 360–364.

Bachmann, I., Audigé, L., Stauffacher, M. 2003, Risk factors associated with behavioural disorders of crib-biting, weaving and box-walking in Swiss horses. *Equine Vet. J.* 35: 158–163.

Bezděková, B., Jahn, P., Vyskoči, M. 2008, Gastric ulceration, appetite and feeding practices in standardbred racehorses in the Czech Republic. *Acta Vet.* 77: 603–607.

Bland, I.M., Guthrie-Jones, A., Taylor, R.D., Hill, J. 2009, Dog obesity: Owner attitudes and behaviour. *Prev. Vet. Med.* 92: 333–340.

Brooks, D., Churchill, J., Fein, K. *et al.* 2014, 2014 AAHA weight management guidelines for dogs and cats. *J. Am. Anim. Hosp. Assoc.* 50: 1–11.

Carroll, C.L., Huntington, P.J. 1988, Body condition scoring and weight estimation of horses. *Equine Vet. J.* 20: 41–45.

Cave, N.J., Allan, F.J., Schokkenbroek, S.L., Metekohy, C.A.M., Pfeiffer, D.U. 2012, A cross-sectional study to compare changes in the prevalence and risk factors for feline obesity between 1993 and 2007 in New Zealand. *Prev. Vet. Med.* 107: 121–133.

Chandler, M.L., Takashima, G. 2014, Nutritional concepts for the veterinary practitioner. *Vet. Clin. North Am. Small Anim. Pract.* 44: 645–666.

Chauvet, A., Laclair, J., Elliott, D.A., German, A.J. 2011, Incorporation of exercise, using an underwater treadmill, and active client education into a weight management program for obese dogs. *Can. Vet. J.* 52: 491–496.

Clarke, D.E., Cameron, A. 1998, Relationship between diet, dental calculus and periodontal disease in domestic and feral cats in Australia. *Aust. Vet. J.* 76: 690–693.

Colliard, L., Paragon, B.-M., Lemuet, B., Benet, J.-J., Blanchard, G. 2009, Prevalence and risk factors of obesity in an urban population of healthy cats. *J. Feline Med. Surg.* 11: 135–140.

Courcier, E.A., O'Higgins, R., Mellor, D.J., Yam, P.S. 2010a, Prevalence and risk factors for feline obesity in a first opinion practice in Glasgow, Scotland. *J. Feline Med. Surg.* 12: 746–753.

Courcier, E.A., Thomson, R.M., Mellor, D.J., Yam, P.S. 2010b, An epidemiological study of environmental factors associated with canine obesity. *J. Small Anim. Pract.* 51: 362–367.

Courcier, E.A., Mellor, D.J., Thomson, R.M., Yam, P.S. 2011, A cross sectional study of the prevalence and risk factors for owner misperception of canine body shape in first opinion practice in Glasgow. *Prev. Vet. Med.* 102: 66–74.

Curtis, G., Barfoot, C., Dugdale, A., Harris, P.M., Argo, C.M. 2011, Voluntary ingestion of wood shavings by obese horses under dietary restriction. *Br. J. Nutr.* 106: S178–S182.

Dammrich, K. 1991, Relationship between nutrition and bone growth in large and giant dogs. *J. Nutr.* 121: S114–S121.

Debraekeleer, J., Gross, K.L., Zicker, S.C. 2010, Introduction to feeding normal dogs. In: Hand, M.S., Thatcher, C.D., Remillard, R.L., Roudebush, P., Novotny, B.J. (eds), *Small Animal Clinical Nutrition*, 5th edn. Mark Morris Institute, Topeka, KS, pp. 251–255.

Defauw, P.A.M., Van De Maele, I., Duchateau, L., Polis, I.E., Saunders, J.H., Daminet, S. 2011, Risk factors and clinical presentation of cats with feline idiopathic cystitis. *J. Feline Med. Surg.* 13: 967–975.

Driscoll, C.A., Menotti-Raymond, M., Roca, A.L. *et al.* 2007, The Near Eastern origin of cat domestication. *Science* 317: 519–523.

Dugdale, A.H.A., Curtis, G.C., Cripps, P. *et al.* 2010, Effect of dietary restriction on body condition, composition and welfare of overweight and obese pony mares. *Equine Vet. J.* 42: 600–610.

Edney, A.T.B., Smith, P.M. 1986, Study of obesity in dogs visiting veterinary practices in the United Kingdom. *Vet. Rec.* 118: 391–396.

Edouard, N., Fleurance, G., Martin-Rosset, W. *et al.* 2008, Voluntary intake and digestibility in horses: effect of forage quality with emphasis on individual variability. *Animal* 2: 1526–1533.

Ellis, J.M., Hollands, T. 1998, Accuracy of different methods of estimating the weight of horses. *Vet. Rec.* 143: 335–336.

Ellis, J.M., Hollands, T. 2001, A preliminary investigation into the use of weightapes for the detection of dehydration in the performance horse. Abstract: 40th British Equine Veterinary Association Congress, p. 221.

Ellis, J.M., Hollands, T. 2002, Use of height-specific weighs tapes to estimate the bodyweight of horses. *Vet. Rec.* 150(20): 632–634.

Ellis, S.L.H., Rodan, I., Carney, H.C. *et al.* 2013, AAFP and ISFM feline environmental needs guidelines. *J. Feline Med. Surg.* 15: 219–230.

Fahey, G.C.,Jr., Barry, K.A., Swanson, K.S. 2008, Age-related changes in nutrient utilization by companion animals. *Annu. Rev. Nutr.* 28: 425–445.

Finno, C.J., McKenzie, E., Valberg, S.J. *et al.* 2010, Effect of fitness on glucose, insulin and cortisol responses to diets varying in starch and fat content in Thoroughbred horses with recurrent exertional rhabdomyolysis. *Equine Vet. J.* 42(suppl. 38): 323–328.

Fontaine, E. 2012, Food intake and nutrition during pregnancy, lactation and weaning in the dam and offspring. *Reprod. Domest. Anim.* 47: 326–330.

Frape, D. 2010, *Equine Nutrition and Feeding*, 4th edn. Wiley-Blackwell, Oxford.

Freeman, L., Becvarova, I., Cave, N. *et al.* 2011, WSAVA nutritional assessment guidelines. *Compend. Contin. Educ. Vet.* 33: E1–E9.

German, A.J., Holden, S.L., Wiseman-Orr, M.L. *et al.* 2012, Quality of life is reduced in obese dogs but improves after successful weight loss. *Vet. J.* 192: 428–434.

Glickman, L.T., Schofer, F.S., Mckee, L.J., Reif, J.S., Goldschmidt, M.H. 1989, Epidemiologic study of insecticide exposures, obesity and risk of bladder cancer in household dogs. *J. Toxicol. Environ. Health* 28: 407–414.

Glunk, E., Hathaway, M., Weber W. *et al.* (2014). The effect of hay net design on rate of forage consumption when feeding adult horses. *J. Equine Vet. Sci.* 34: 986–991.

Goodwin, D., Davidson, H.B., Harris, P. 2007, A note on behaviour of stabled horses with foraging devices in mangers and buckets. *Appl. Anim. Behav. Sci.* 105: 238–243.

Greco, D.S. 2014, *Pediatric Nutrition. Vet. Clin. North Am. Small Anim. Pract.* 44: 265–273.

Hazewinkel, H.A., Vandenbrom, W.E., Vantklooster, A.T., Voorhout, G., Vanwees, A. 1991, Calcium metabolism in Great Dane dogs fed diets with various calcium and phosphorous levels. *J. Nutr.* 121: S99–S106.

Hess, R.S., Kass, P.H., Shofer, F.S., Van Winkle, T.J., Washabau, R.J. 1999, Evaluation of risk factors for fatal acute pancreatitis in dogs. *J. Am. Vet. Med. Assoc.* 214: 46–51.

Hollands, T., Ellis, J.M., Allen, D.E. *et al.* 2009, An assessment of 2 visual methods of fat scoring in the equine to determine the most suitable for client recognition of obesity in their horses. Proceedings of 48th BEVA Annual Congress, pp. 247–248.

Houpt, K. 2012, A preliminary answer to the question of whether cribbing causes salivary secretion. *J. Vet. Behav. Clin. Appl. Res.* 7: 322–324.

Husted, L., Sanchez, L.C., Baptiste, K.E. *et al.* 2008, Effect of feed/fast protocol on pH in the proximal equine stomach. *Equine Vet. J.* 41: 658–662.

Impellizeri, J.A., Tetrick, M.A., Muir, P. 2000, Effect of weight reduction on clinical signs of lameness in dogs with hip osteoarthritis. *J. Am. Vet. Med. Assoc.* 216: 1089–1091.

Ireland, J.L., Wylie, C.E., Collins, S.N. *et al.* 2013, Preventive health care and owner-reported disease prevalence of horses and ponies in Great Britain. *Res. Vet. Sci.* 95: 418–424.

Joffe, D.J., Schlesinger, D.P. 2002, Preliminary assessment of the risk of Salmonella infection in dogs fed raw chicken diets. *Can. Vet. J.* 43: 441–442.

Johnson, K.A., Watson, A.D. 2005, Skeletal diseases. In: Ettinger, S.J., Feldman, E.C. (eds), *Textbook of Veterinary Internal Medicine*, 6th edn. Elsevier Saunders, St Louis, MO, pp. 1965–1991.

Kealy, R.D., Lawler, D.F., Ballam, J.M. *et al.* 1997, Five-year longitudinal study on limited food consumption and development of osteoarthritis in coxofemoral joints of dogs. *J. Am. Vet. Med. Assoc.* 210: 222–225.

Kealy, R.D., Lawler, D.F., Ballam, J.M. *et al.* 2000, Evaluation of the effect of limited food consumption on radiographic evidence of osteoarthritis in dogs. *J. Am. Vet. Med. Assoc.* 217; 1678–1680.

Kealy, R.D., Lawler, D.F., Ballam, J.M. *et al.* 2002, Effects of diet restriction on life span and age-related changes in dogs. *J. Am. Vet. Med. Assoc.* 220: 1315–1320.

Kealy, R.D., Olsson, S.E., Monti, K.L. *et al.* 1992, Effects of limited food consumption on the incidence of hip dysplasia in growing dogs. *J. Am. Vet. Med. Assoc.* 201: 857–863.

Kienzle, E., Bergler, R., Mandernach, A. 1998, A comparison of the feeding behavior and the human–animal relationship in owners of normal and obese dogs. *J. Nutr.* 128: 2779S–2782S.

Lacombe, V.A., Hinchcliff, K.W., Kohn, C.W. *et al.* 2004, Effects of feeding meals with various soluble-carbohydrate content on muscle glycogen synthesis after exercise in horses. *Am. J. Vet. Res.* 65: 916–923.

Laflamme, D.P. 1997a, Development and validation of a body condition score system for cats: a clinical tool. *Feline Pract.* 25: 13–18.

Laflamme, D.P. 1997b, Development and validation of a body condition score system for dogs. *Canine Pract.* 22: 10–15.

Laflamme, D.P., Abood, S.K., Fascetti, A.J. *et al.* 2008, Timely topics in nutrition – pet feeding practices of dog and cat owners in the United States and Australia. *J. Am. Vet. Med. Assoc.* 232: 687–694.

Larsen, J.A., Farcas, A. 2014, Nutrition of aging dogs. *Vet. Clin. North Am. Small Anim. Pract.* 44: 741–759.

Larsen, J.A., Parks, E.M., Heinze, C.R., Fascetti, A.J. 2012, Evaluation of recipes for home-prepared diets for dogs and cats with chronic kidney disease. *J. Am. Vet. Med. Assoc.* 240: 532–538.

Lauten, S.D., Smith, T.M., Kirk, C.A., Bartges, J.W., Adams, A.M. 2005, Computer analysis of nutrient sufficiency of published home-cooked diets for dogs and cats. *J Vet. Intern. Med.* 19: 476–477.

Lejeune, J.T., Hancock, D.D. 2001, Public health concerns associated with feeding raw meat diets to dogs. *J. Am. Vet. Med. Assoc.* 219: 1222–1225.

Li, X., Li, W.H., Wang, H. *et al.* 2005, Pseudogenization of a sweet-receptor gene accounts for cats' indifference toward sugar. *Plos Genetics.* 1: 27–35.

Linder, D., Mueller, M. 2014, Pet obesity management: beyond nutrition. *Vet. Clin. North Am. Small Anim. Pract.* 44: 789–804.

Longland, A.C., Barfoot, C., Harris, P.A. 2011, Effects of soaking on the water-soluble carbohydrate and crude protein content of hay. *Vet. Rec.* 168: 618.

Lorenzo-Figueras, M., Merritt, A.M. 2002, Effects of exercise on gastric volume and pH in the proximal portion of the stomach of horses. *Am. J. Vet. Res.* 63: 1481–1487.

Lund, E.M., Armstrong, P.J., Kirk, C.A., Klausner, J.S. 2006, Prevalence and risk factors for obesity in adult dogs from private US veterinary practices. *Int. J. Appl. Res. Vet. Med.* 4: 177–186.

Luthersson, N., Hou Nielsen, K., Harris, P. *et al.* 2009, Risk factors associated with equine gastric ulceration syndrome (EGUS) in 201 horses in Denmark. *Equine Vet. J.* 41: 625–630.

Marlin, D.J., Fenn, K., Smith, N. *et al.* 2002, Changes in circulatory antioxidant status in horses during prolonged exercise. *J. Nutr.* 132: 1622S–1627S.

Masey O'Neill, H.V., Keen, J., Dumbell, L. 2010, A comparison of the occurrence of common dental abnormalities in stabled and free-grazing horses. *Animal* 4(10): 1697–1701.

Maslak, R., Sergiel, A., Hill, B. 2013, Some aspects of locomotory stereotypies in spectacled bears (Tremarctos ornatus) and changes in behavior after relocation and dental treatment. *J. Vet. Behav.* 8: 335–341.

Maughan, R. 2003, Impact of mild dehydration on wellness and on exercise performance. *Eur. J. Clin. Nutr.* 57(suppl 2): S19–S23.

McGreevy, P.D., Cripps, P.J. French, N.P. *et al.* 1995, Management factors associated with stereotypic and redirected behaviour in the Thoroughbred horse. *Equine Vet. J.* 27: 86–91.

McGreevy, P.D., Thomson, P.C., Pride, C., Fawcett, A., Grassi, I., Jones, B. 2005, Prevalence of obesity in dogs examined by Australian veterinary practices and the risk factors involved. *Vet. Rec.* 156: 695–702.

McKinsey Global Institute. 2014, Overcoming obesity: an initial economic analysis. Available at: www.mckinsey.com

Meyer, H., Coenen, M., Gurer, C. 1985, Investigations on saliva production and chewing effects in horses fed various feeds. *Proc. Equine Nutr. Physiol. Soc.* 9: 38–42.

Michel, K.E., Anderson, W., Cupp, C., Laflamme, D.P. 2011, Correlation of a feline muscle mass score with body composition determined by dual-energy X-ray absorptiometry. *Br. J. Nutr.* 106: S57–S59.

Mlacnik, E., Bockstahler, B.A., Mueller, M., Tetrick, M.A., Nap, R.C., Zentek, J. 2006, Effects of caloric restriction and a moderate or intense physiotherapy program for treatment of lameness in overweight dogs with osteoarthritis. *J. Am. Vet. Med. Assoc.* 229: 1756–1760.

Moeller, B.A., McCall, C.A., Silverman, S.J. *et al.* 2008, Estimation of saliva production in crib-biting and normal horses. *J. Equine Vet. Sci.* 28: 85–90.

Moore-Colyer, M.J.S. 1996, Effects of soaking hay fodder for horses on dust and mineral content. *Animal Sci.* 63: 337–342.

Murray, M.J., Eichorn, E.S. 1996, Effects of intermittent feed deprivation, intermittent feed deprivation with ranitidine administration, and stall confinement with ad libitum access to hay on gastric ulceration in horses. *Am. J. Vet. Res.* 57: 1599.

Nadeau, J.A., Andrews, F.M., Mathew, A.G. *et al.* 2000, Evaluation of diet as a cause of gastric ulcers in horses. *Am. J. Vet. Res.* 61: 784–790.

National Research Council (NRC) Committee on Nutrient Requirements of Horses. 2007, *Nutrient Requirements of Horses*, 6th edn. National Academies Press, Washington, DC.

Pennings, B., Koopman, R., Milou Beelen, M. *et al.* 2011, Exercising before protein intake allows for greater use of dietary protein-derived amino acids for de novo muscle protein synthesis in both young and elderly men. *Am. J. Clin. Nutr.* 93: 322–331.

Pinchbeck, G.L., French, N.P., Proudman, C.J. *et al.* 2008, Risk factors for epiploic foramen entrapment colic in a UK horse population: a prospective case-control study. *Equine Vet. J.* 40: 405–410.

Powell, D.M., Bennett-Wimbush, K., Peeples, A. *et al.* 2008, Evaluation of indicators of weight-carrying ability of light riding horses. *J. Equine Vet. Sci.* 28: 28–33.

Racklyeft, D.J., Love, D.N. 1990, Influence of head posture on the respiratory tract of healthy horses. *Aust. Vet. J.* 67: 402–405.

Rand, J.S., Fleeman, L.M., Farrow, H.A., Appleton, D.J., Lederer, R. 2004, Canine and feline diabetes mellitus: nature or nurture? *J. Nutr.* 134: 2072S–2080S.

Ribeiro, W.P., Valberg, S.J., Pagan, J.D. *et al.* 2004, The effect of varying dietary starch and fat content on serum creatine kinase activity and substrate availability in equine polysaccharide storage myopathy. *J. Vet. Intern. Med.* 18: 887–894.

Richardson, D.C., Zentek, J., Hazewinkel, H.A. 2010, Developmental orthopaedic disease of dogs. In: Hand, M.S., Thatcher, C.D., Remillard, R.L., Roudebush, P., Novotny, B.J. (eds), *Small Animal Clinical Nutrition*, 5th edn. Mark Morris Institute, Topeka, KS, p. 679.

Roudebush, P., Dzanis, D.A., Debraekeleer, J., Watson, H. 2010, Pet food labels. In: Hand, M.S., Thatcher, C.D., Remillard, R.L., Roudebush, P., Novotny, B.J. (eds), *Small Animal Clinical Nutrition*, 5th edn. Mark Morris Institute, Topeka, KS, p. 199.

Salonen, L.K., Hollands, T., Piercy, R.J. *et al.* 2009, Epidemiology of equine obesity in south east England: preliminary findings. Proceedings of 48th BEVA Congress, p. 247.

Sarrafchi, A., Blokhuis, H.J. 2013, Equine stereotypic behaviors: causation, occurrence, and prevention. *J. Vet. Behav.* 8: 386–394.

Sandin, A., Girma, K., Sjoholm, B., Lindholm, A., Nilsson, G. 1998, Effects of differently composed feeds and physical stress on plasma gastrin concentration in horses. *Acta Vet. Scand.* 39(2): 265–272.

Scarlett, J.M., Donoghue, S. 1998, Associations between body condition and disease in cats. *J. Am. Vet. Med. Assoc.* 212: 1725–1731.

Schoenmakers, I., Hazewinkel, H.A., Voorhout, G., Carlson, C.S., Richardson, D. 2000, Effect of diets with different calcium and phosphorus contents on the skeletal development and blood chemistry of growing great danes. *Vet. Rec.* 147: 652–660.

Segev, G., Livne, H., Ranen, E., Lavy, E. 2011, Urethral obstruction in cats: predisposing factors, clinical, clinicopathological characteristics and prognosis. *J. Feline Med. Surg.* 13: 101–108.

Sewell, D.A., Harris, R.C., Hanak, J. *et al.* 1992, Muscle adenine nucleotide degradation in the thoroughbred horse as a consequence of racing. *Comp. Biochem. Physiol.* 101B: 375–381.

Stahler, D.R., Smith, D.W., Guernsey, D.S. 2005, Foraging and feeding ecology of wolves: lessons from Yellowstone. Waltham International Nutritional Sciences Symposium, pp. 4–5.

Stiver, S.L., Frazier, K.S., Mauel, M.J., Styer, E.L. 2003, Septicemic salmonellosis in two cats fed a raw-meat diet. *J Am. Anim. Hosp. Assoc.* 39: 538–542.

Streiff, E.L., Zwischenberger, B., Butterwick, R.F., Wagner, E., Iben, C., Bauer, J.E. 2002, A comparison of the nutritional adequacy of home-prepared and commercial diets for dogs. *J. Nutr.* 132: 1698S–1700S.

Takashima, G.K., Day, M.J. 2014, Setting the one health agenda and the human–companion animal bond. *Int. J. Environ. Res. Public Health.* 11: 11110–11120.

Teasell, R., Dittmer, D.K. 1993, Complications of immobilization and bed rest. Part 2: Other complications. *Can. Fam. Physician* 39: 1445–1446.

Thorne, J.B., Goodwin, D., Kennedy, M.J. *et al.* 2005, Foraging enrichment for individually housed horses: practicality and effects on behaviour. *Appl. Anim. Behav. Sci.* 94: 149–164.

Toll, P.W., Gillette, R.L., Hand, M.S. 2010a, Feeding working and sporting dogs. In: Hand, M.S., Thatcher, C.D., Remillard, R.L., Roudebush, P., Novotny, B.J. (eds), *Small Animal Clinical Nutrition*, 5th edn. Mark Morris Institute, Topeka, KS, pp. 321–352.

Toll, P.W., Yamka, R.M., Schoenherr, W.D., Hand, M.S. 2010b, Obesity. In: Hand, M.S., Thatcher, C.D., Remillard, R.L., Roudebush, P., Novotny, B.J. (eds), *Small Animal Clinical Nutrition*, 5th edn. Mark Morris Institute, Topeka, KS, pp. 501–542.

Urschel, K., Geor, R.J., Waterfall, H.L., Shoveller, A.K., McCutcheon, L.J. 2010, Effects of leucine or whey protein addition to an oral glucose solution on serum insulin, plasma glucose and plasma amino acid responses in horses at rest and following exercise. *Equine Vet. J.* 42(suppl. 38): 347–354.

Valentine, B.A., van Saun, R.J., Thompson, K.N., Hintz, H.F. 2001, Role of dietary carbohydrate and fat in horses with equine polysaccharide storage myopathy. *J. Am. Vet. Med. Assoc.* 219: 1537–1544.

Vervuert, I., Voigt, K., Hollands, T. *et al.* 2007, The effect of feeding a single starch source (oats) or a high and a low starch compound to provide 2g starch/kgBW on the glycaemic and insulinaemic response of horses. Proceedings of 46th BEVA Congress, p. 294.

Vervuert, I., Voit, K., Hollands, T. *et al.* 2009, Effect of feeding increasing quantities of starch on glycaemic and insulinaemic responses in healthy horses. *Vet. J.* 182: 67–72.

Videla, R., Andrews, F.M. 2009, New perspectives in equine gastric ulcer syndrome. *Vet. Clin. North Am. Equine Pract.* 25: 283–301.

Wakshlag, J.J., Shmalberg, J. 2014, Nutrition for working and service dogs. *Vet. Clin. North Am. Small Anim. Pract.* 44: 719–740.

Wakshlag, J.J., Struble, A.M., Warren, B.S. *et al.* 2012, Evaluation of dietary energy intake and physical activity in dogs undergoing a controlled weight-loss program. *J. Am. Vet. Med. Assoc.* 240: 413–419.

Waters, A.J., Nicol, C.J., French, N.P. 2002, Factors influencing the development of stereotypic and redirected behaviours in young horses: findings of a four-year prospective epidemiological study. *Equine Vet. J.* 34: 572–579.

Weeth, L.P. 2013, Focus on nutrition: home-prepared diets for dogs and cats. *Compend. Contin. Educ. Vet.* 35: E3–E3.

White, G.A., Hobson-West, P., Cobb, K., Craigon, J., Hammond, R., Millar, K.M. 2011, Canine obesity: is there a difference between veterinarian and owner perception? *J. Small Anim. Pract.* 52: 622–626.

Wickens, C.L., McCall, C.A., Bursian, S. *et al.* 2013, Assessment of gastric ulceration and gastrin response in horses with history of cribbiting. *J. Equine Vet. Sci.* 33: 739–745.

Wickens, C.R., Heleski, H.O. 2010, Crib-biting behavior in horses: a review. *Appl. Anim. Behav. Sci.* 128: 1–9.

Williams, C.A., Burke, A.O. 2010, Nutrient intake during an elite level three-day event competition is correlated to inflammatory markers and antioxidant status. *Equine Vet. J.* 42(Suppl. 38): 116–122.

Winskill, H., Waran, N.K., Young, R.J. 1996, The effect of a foraging device (a modified 'Edinburgh Foodball') on the behaviour of the stabled horse. *Appl. Anim. Behav. Sci.* 48: 25–35.

CHAPTER 4

Applied canine biomechanics*

Caroline Adrian

VCA Animal Hospitals, Los Angeles, USA and VCA Veterinary Specialists of Northern Colorado, Loveland, USA

Summary

An understanding of the concepts of functional biomechanics is vital to the application of physiotherapy to animals. The aim of this chapter is to introduce key concepts of applied biomechanics in the dog and horse based on the limited research into animal functional biomechanics and kinematics.

4.1 Introduction

The aim of this chapter and the following chapter (Applied Equine Biomechanics) is to introduce key concepts of applied biomechanics in the dog and horse based on the limited research into animal functional biomechanics and kinematics. The chapters do not address pure biomechanics, nor are they intended to replicate the theoretical basis of biomechanics or summarise current biomechanics literature and texts. The authors aim to direct the reader towards some of the applied principles of functional biomechanics in relation to animal physiotherapy assessment and treatment, based on evidence where possible.

Movement is the foundation for life. Without movement, the mammalian species would not survive. When movement becomes altered, pathology may ensue. An understanding of concepts of neuromotor control, musculoskeletal physiotherapy and rehabilitation is vital to the application of physiotherapy to animals. To enable the animal to achieve a complete functional sports-specific outcome through rehabilitation, the animal physiotherapist must be able to apply treatment techniques and management strategies based on an understanding of the mechanisms behind the cause of musculoskeletal injury in the cursorial mammal. Thus, animal physiotherapists require an understanding of each species' anatomy and biomechanics, as well as the requirements of the animal's sport. A working knowledge of the mechanical demands and constraints under which animals operate during locomotion is essential to enable the clinician to assess the compensations, secondary neuromuscular and skeletal problems and pathology that ensue following failure of one or more elements. The reader is urged to review additional literature and texts referenced.

---

*Adapted from the first edition chapter, which was written by Lesley Goff and Narelle Stubbs

---

Biomechanics refers to the application of mechanical principles in the study of living organisms. Kinematics is the measurement and description of motion, including considerations of space and time, without looking at the forces, whereas kinetics is the measurement of force and the relationship of force and mass (Hall 1995; Wilson *et al.* 2003). Locomotion is a result of a force (e.g. via the limbs, particularly hindlimb in quadrupeds) being applied to a mass (trunk) that it accelerates. This chapter will cover canine joint biomechanics and species-specific biomechanics of locomotion, and give examples of applied sports-specific biomechanics in the dog. The following chapter will address the same in the horse, including the biomechanics of the equine distal limb related to pathology. For species-specific biomechanics of locomotion in animals, the greatest amount of research and knowledge has centred on the athletic horse, with research regarding the same in the canine notably lacking. Section 4.2 pertains to both this chapter and Chapter 5.

4.2 Joint biomechanics

This section focuses on biomechanics related to individual joint motion in the animal, as joint movements indicate how the musculoskeletal system is working. Knowledge of the normal pattern and amount of movement allows the physiotherapist to detect abnormalities of movement (Lee 1995).

According to Lee (1995), there are three parameters required for a full definition of movement at a joint:

- location of the axis of motion, including information about how this location changes during the movement
- amount of rotation – the angle through which the joint rotation occurs about the axis during movement
- amount of translation – the displacement that occurs along the axis during the movement.

The way we describe joint motion can only be an approximation, as many aspects of joint dynamics such as torques and forces acting at the joints are not readily available to us. *Axis of rotation* or *axis of motion* is a term for a central imaginary line that is orientated perpendicular to the plane in which the rotation occurs (Hall 1995). It is difficult to know the axis of joint rotation at any instant in a movement (the instantaneous axis, or instantaneous centre of rotation (ICR)). This is because very few joints have a fixed axis of motion, as biological joint movements are complex (Denoix 1999). Denoix (1999) states that the establishment of the ICR reveals several functional aspects of vertebral structures and associated ligaments during dorsoventral movements of the vertebral column. When a canine stifle is flexed, the instantaneous centre of rotation of the joint moves caudally and then cranially when the joint extends (Ireland *et al.* 1986). In the horse, Denoix (1999) has shown the ICR of thoracolumbar vertebrae to be variable in different dorsoventral positions of the thoracolumbar spine and cervical spine. For example, with cervical flexion, the ICR of each thoracolumbar vertebral body tends to move cranially and ventrally, and during

thoracolumbar flexion the ICR is centred in the vertebral body. In the lumbosacral joint during flexion, the ICR moves to a more ventral position than during extension.

In three-dimensional joint kinematics, coupled movements are known to occur (Denoix 1999; Lee 1995). To deal with the complexity of three-dimensional movement, it is useful to consider the joint motion as consisting of rotations in three orthogonal planes: sagittal, frontal and horizontal (or yaw, pitch and roll) and three components of translation – caudocranial, mediolateral and dorsoventral (Figure 4.1).

For physiological motion, where rotation is the desired motion, one of the rotations is designated as the main movement. All other movements, including rotations in other planes and translations in any direction, are called coupled movements (Lee 1995). For example, in dogs and humans, axial rotation of the cervical spine between C3 and C7 is coupled with ipsilateral lateral flexion (Breit & Kunzel 2002). Axial rotation is the main movement and lateral flexion is the coupled or accessory movement.

4.2.1 Joint stiffness

The range of motion of a joint is defined as its entire range of physiological movement, measured from the neutral position. It is divided into the neutral zone and the elastic zone (Panjabi 1992b). The neutral zone is the region of low stiffness, where joint motion is produced with minimal internal resistance, to allow physiological movements to occur freely within a certain range. The elastic zone is measured from the end of the neutral zone up to the physiological limit and is the zone of higher stiffness. When a joint is translated as in a passive accessory movement, the low stiffness zone is smaller than for a physiological movement, and resistance is likely through the entire movement, increasing linearly with degree of translation (Lee 1995). There is little information as to which anatomical structures are responsible for the tissue resistance perceived by the physiotherapist in either type of passive joint movement. The tissues involved in resistance may be muscles/fascia, ligaments, neuromeningeal structures and joint capsule.

4.2.2 Joint instability

It is worth noting here the difference between 'mechanical instability', 'clinical instability' and 'functional instability'. In physical terms, an unstable structure is one that is not in an optimal state of equilibrium (Pope & Panjabi 1985). Where there is mechanical joint instability, small initial movements will result in further movement until a position of stability is reached and potential energy is at a minimum (Lee 1995). In a physiological situation, muscles and other restraining soft tissues provide resistance and tend to restore the joint to its original position. In veterinary terminology, luxation is synonymous with dislocation, which is defined as displacement of a bone from a joint, compared with subluxation, which is defined as a partial dislocation (Blood & Studdert 1999). This may be the case in humans with a glenohumeral joint prone to subluxation or a dog with a patella

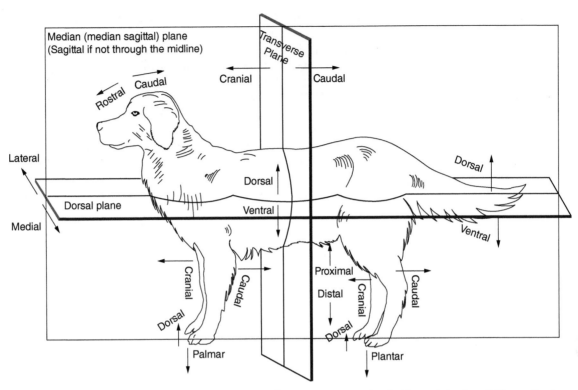

Figure 4.1 Directional terminology for the dog. *Source:* C. Riegger-Krugh, Canton, OH. Reproduced with permission from C. Riegger-Krugh.

that tends to subluxate, or where segmental spinal muscles do not perform the action of maintaining intervertebral motion (Panjabi *et al.* 1989).

4.2.3 Clinical instability

Clinical instability has been suggested by Lee (1995) to be alternatively named pathological hypermobility, where there may be damage to structures restraining a joint's movement. An example of a clinical instability is excessive motion at a vertebral level that may compromise the spinal cord, such as a Doberman with cervical vertebral malformation requiring surgical stabilisation (see Chapter 9). However, clinical instability of a spinal motion segment, as defined by Panjabi (1992b), is 'a significant decrease in the capacity of the stabilising system of the spine to maintain the intervertebral neutral zone within the physiological limit' such that there may not be altered neurological function, or no major deformity and no incapacitating pain. Therefore, size of the neutral zone of a given vertebral motion segment is a better indicator of clinical or functional instability than is the overall range of motion or current clinical symptoms alone, i.e. sensorimotor disturbances. Methods with which to measure the neutral zone *in vivo* are yet to be well established (Panjabi 1992b).

Thus the neutral zone, at least in the vertebral column, is a clinically important measure of spinal stability and overall *functional instability*. Human *in vitro* studies, animal *in vivo* studies and mathematical simulations have shown that the neutral zone is a parameter that correlates well with other parameters indicative of instability of the spinal system (Panjabi 1992b). In the vertebral column, the neutral zone has been shown to increase with injury or secondary weakness of the spinal muscles, due to a decrease in intersegmental dynamic muscle stability. For example, lumbosacral intervertebral motion has been extensively investigated in humans via a series of biomechanics and neuromotor control studies, in normal and low back pain subjects (Hides *et al.* 1992, 1994, 1996; Hodges 2003; Lee 2004; Moseley *et al.* 2002; Panjanbi 1992a,b; Panjabi *et al.* 1989). In human (Hides *et al.* 2001; Hodges & Richardson 1996; Hodges *et al.* 2001; Panjabi 1992a,b; Panjabi *et al.* 1989) and porcine (Hodges 2003; Kaigle *et al.* 1995, 1998) studies, the role of the deep stabilising muscles of the vertebral column has been investigated. These are the anteriorly situated *transversus abdominis* (hypaxial muscle in the quadruped) and the posteriorly located *multifidus* (epaxial muscle). The activity of the deep stabilising muscles of the vertebral column and pelvis muscle appears to be both preparatory and dynamic in the way they limit the neutral zone, and have been shown to affect both motion and stiffness of the intervertebral segments of the spine and pelvis. The multifidus muscle is directly associated with dysfunction and atrophy of this muscle has been shown to be closely linked with thoracolumbar and lumbosacral pathology in human back pain (Hides *et al.* 1994, 1996; Lee 2004; Moseley *et al.* 2002). Further, poor dynamic control of these muscles has been shown to be a predictor for lower back pain in humans (Cholewicki *et al.* 2005).

There is limited neuromotor control data for the equine and canine vertebral column, and the role of muscle in dynamic control of stability is virtually unknown (Peham *et al.* 2001). Equine electromyography studies have focused on the large trunk and epaxial muscles only, such as *longissimus dorsi* in relation to trotting on a treadmill (Licka *et al.* 2004; Peham *et al.* 2001; Robert *et al.* 2002).

The activity of the human multifidus muscle has been shown to increase intervertebral stiffness at L4–5 in multiple directions owing to the principal agonist muscles, the abdominal oblique muscles, simultaneously flexing the lumbar spine (Wilke *et al.* 1995). Kaigle *et al.*'s (1995, 1998) work shows that electrical stimulation of multifidus improves the quality of control of intervertebral motion around the neutral position during movement in the sagittal and frontal planes. It is hypothesised that the multifidus may provide a similar role in control of intervertebral stability in horses, as there is a similarity in muscle morphology and architecture in the thoracolumbar and lumbosacral and pelvic regions compared with the human (Stubbs *et al.* 2006).

In the canine vertebral column, the role of muscle in dynamic control of spinal stability is also virtually unknown (Peham *et al.* 2001). However, it has been suggested that aberrant neuromotor control mechanisms may be related to cranial cruciate ligament (CCL) disease (Adrian *et al.* 2013).

In humans, the patterns and timing of muscle activation influence the rate and magnitude of loading on knee structures. During the early stance phase of gait, proper attenuation of impact loads in the normal knee is due to coordinated timing of appropriate muscles (Bennell *et al.* 2008), especially the quadriceps muscle which is an important knee stabiliser in both humans (Johansson *et al.* 1991) and dogs (de Rooster *et al.* 1998; Johansson *et al.* 1991). In the presence of weak knee stabilising muscles, a reduction in the protective muscular activity that normally provides stability to the knee may increase joint loading and ultimately the risk of anterior cruciate ligament (ACL) rupture (Brandt 2004).

4.3 Biomechanics of the vertebral joints

The aim of the section that follows is to summarise the functional anatomy of the articulations of the vertebral column in the dog, so that the physiotherapist may identify alterations in patterns of joint movement from the normal. In understanding the normal directions and planes of joint motion, the physiotherapist can apply passive movement tests during assessment, with a reasonable amount of accuracy. Understanding the physiological loads experienced by any individual structure is also difficult because the associated moments and forces cannot be measured with any degree of accuracy.

The biomechanical function of the vertebral column is to allow movements between vertebral bodies, carry and transmit loads and protect the spinal cord and nerve roots (Panjabi

1992a). Panjabi (1992a) classifies the vertebral stabilising system into three parts:

- passive musculoskeletal subsystem
- active musculoskeletal subsystem
- he neural and feedback subsystem.

The passive musculoskeletal subsystem includes the vertebrae, facet articulations, intervertebral discs, spinal ligaments and joint capsules, plus the passive mechanical properties of muscle.

The mechanical properties of facet joints are determined by the inclination of angle of the facets, and also by any hypertrophy or degeneration due to dysfunction (Panjabi 1992a). Ligamentous components of the passive subsystem do not contribute significantly to stability near the neutral position of the joint. Ligaments develop reactive forces towards the end of physiological range of motion – their role in the neutral position becomes an active feedback function, thus they become part of the neural and feedback systems (Panjabi 1992a).

The passive range of motion varies along the length of the vertebral column within individuals and also between species, with higher flexibility in dogs compared with horses. This is partly because intervertebral discs influence the extent of the motion available at any given level of the vertebral column (Breit *et al.* 2002). The intervertebral discs in the dog contribute up to 20% of the length of the vertebral column (Dyce *et al.* 2002).

Following unilateral transection of the anterior longitudinal ligament, *nucleus pulposus* and *annulus fibrosus* of the T6–7 intervertebral discs in dogs, a significant increase in range of motion (ROM) in flexion–extension, lateral flexion and rotation occurred (Takeuchi *et al.* 1999). This suggests the disc and the anterior longitudinal ligament together may have a role in limiting movement in the thoracic spine.

The greatest combined passive and active vertebral range of motion occurs in cats, rather than the dog. In comparison, the equine spine is extremely limited and is often referred to as being a balance of stability and mobility (Jeffcott & Dalin 1980). In dogs, sagittal flexion and extension of the lumbar spine is used to increase stride length during gallop, but the horse is unable to apply this mechanism to any substantial level because of its larger musculoskeletal scaling (Dyce *et al.* 2002).

4.4 Canine vertebral column

Many of the studies regarding the biomechanics of the canine vertebral column are based on imaging techniques (Benninger *et al.* 2006; Breit & Kunzel 2002; Breit *et al.* 2002). There is some limited *in vivo* kinematic vertebral column research during gait (Schendel *et al.* 1995) and in cadaver specimens (Benninger *et al.* 2004; Hofstetter *et al.* 2009; Johnson *et al.* 2011). Limited cadaveric biomechanical studies are available that evaluate torsion and shear forces on the spine (Hediger *et al.* 2009; Reber *et al.* 2013). This section pertains to biomechanics of the vertebral column of the dog, based mainly on anatomical dissection and imaging techniques in specimens both normal and with varying conditions of the vertebral column. Before the application of these biomechanical principles to the examination and treatment of a dog, the physiotherapist is encouraged to refer to the chapters on manual therapy, orthopaedic and neurological examination, for information regarding contraindications and precautions for the canine vertebral column.

4.4.1 Cervical spine (O/C1–7)

Although the amount of movement between any two adjacent vertebrae is minimal, the cervical spine, as well as the spine as a whole, allows for considerable flexibility. The entire vertebral column protects, supports and acts as a flexible rod through which forces transmitted through the limbs are transmitted to the rest of the body. The cervical vertebrae allow for six degrees of freedom in all three planes of motion (Evans 1993).

Atlantooccipital joint

The first cervical vertebra (atlantooccipital) joint, or atlas, is atypical in both structure and function. It lacks a spinous process and its body size is greatly reduced. Large, readily palpable transverse processes protrude from each side. In dogs, the atlantooccipital joint is formed by the convex condyles of the occiput and the corresponding concave articulating surfaces of the atlas (C1). It allows for up-and-down nodding movements of the head, and thus is referred to as the 'yes' joint. In humans, it is suggested that there is lateral flexion (lateral tilt) and contralateral conjunct rotation, or an oblique tilt due to sliding of the occipital condyles (Kapandji 1974; Penning & Wilmink 1987). Information regarding such movement at the canine condyles has not yet been confirmed.

Atlantoaxial joint

The second cervical vertebra, or axis, includes an elongated dorsal spinal process. The atlantoaxial joint is a pivot joint, which primarily allows rotation of the head around the axis (C2) of the spine (Figure 4.2a). Movement of the atlas (C1) occurs around the dens, or odontoid process of the axis (Figure 4.2b). Human studies report that there may be some degree of flexion–extension available at C1–2 (Worth 1995), but this has not been documented in the dog. Mechanical instability of the atlantoaxial joint can result from loss of ligamentous support of the dorsal atlantoaxial ligament, due to excess stress from abnormality or absence of the dens. This may result in cranial cervical myelopathy, or dorsal displacement of the axis into the spinal canal.

Atlantoaxial stability is thought to be primarily achieved through the ligamentous complex, which includes the apical, transverse, alar and dorsal atlantoaxial ligaments and the joint capsule, due to the horizontal position of the neck causing greater shear loading (Reber *et al.* 2013). The role of individual atlantoaxial ligaments was evaluated to determine their stabilising function under sagittal shear loading (Reber *et al.* 2013). The alar ligaments, which connect the cranial portion of the dens with the ventral portion of the occipital condyles and foramen magnum, provided the most stabilisation during shear loads in

the canine atlantoaxial joint. Disruption of the alar ligaments is believed to be a main contributor to dorsal displacement of the dens and resultant cervical myelopathy.

C3–7

The spinous processes of the caudal cervical vertebral column (C3–7) increase in height and cranial inclination with increasing vertebral number (Dyce *et al.* 2002) (Figure 4.2c). The sixth cervical vertebra possesses a longer spine than vertebrae 3–5, while the seventh vertebra lacks transverse foramina (Evans 1993). The caudal cervical vertebrae have large, oval planar caudal articular processes, which face ventrolaterally and are angled at approximately 45° and less to the horizontal plane. The planar nature of the caudal articular processes varies slightly between breeds of dog and with age, and joint surfaces have been described as planar, slightly concave, severely concave, convex and sigmoid. Larger dogs tend to have steeper angles of inclination and more concave caudal articular processes in this region of the vertebral column (Breit & Kunzel 2002). The relative horizontal orientation of the caudal cervical facet joint suggests a weight-bearing function, as well as providing movement in sagittal rotation and lateral bending directions. It is suggested also that dogs with more concave facets have more ability for axial rotation to occur concurrently with lateral bending (Breit & Kunzel 2002). It is thought that a high degree of concavity is a risk factor for relative or absolute stenosis of the vertebral foramen and may be associated with instability, misalignment and degenerative changes in the facet joints and discs.

Limited information regarding kinematics of the canine cervical spine is available. The canine cervical spine has a greater degree of coupled motion compared to humans (Johnson *et al.* 2011). The coupled motion of axial rotation and lateral bending was confirmed in the cranial (C2–4) and caudal (C5–T2) cervical spine segments (Johnson *et al.* 2011), as well as at the C4–5 level (Hofstetter *et al.* 2009). A larger degree of cervical rotation was believed to be possible in larger dogs, compared to smaller breeds (Breit & Kunzel 2002). Flexion and extension range of motion is believed to increase when descending the spine (Breit & Kunzel 2004); however, another study showed C5–6 decreasing in range of motion compared to higher cervical levels, though these results were not statistically significant. C6 and C7 were found to have the most axial rotation and this correlates with the vertebral levels most commonly associated with neurological compromise (Breit & Kunzel 2002).

4.4.2 Thoracic spine (T1–13)

The bodies of thoracic vertebrae are short, but increase in length caudally from T10 (Dyce *et al.* 2002). In the upper to mid thoracic spine, the spinous processes overlap the body of the next most caudal vertebra. The orientation of facet joints changes from the lower cervical spine to the thoracic spine. In the cranial thoracic spine, the facet joints are orientated in a frontal plane, with the cranial articular processes facing dorsally and

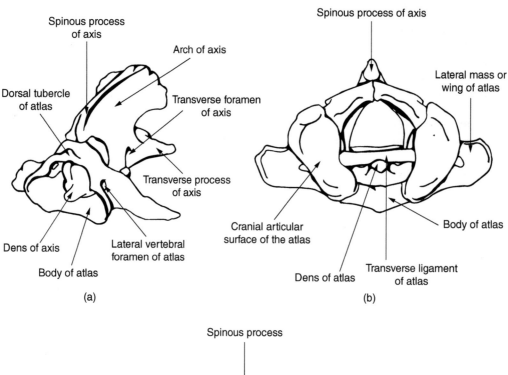

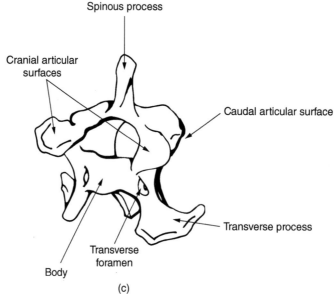

Figure 4.2 (a) Skeletal anatomy of the atlas and axis from a craniolateral view. (b) Skeletal anatomy of the atlas and axis from a cranial view. (c) Skeletal anatomy of the C5 vertebra from a craniolateral view. *Source:* C. Riegger-Krugh, Canton, OH. Reproduced with permission of C. Riegger-Krugh.

the caudal processes facing ventrally. This tends to allow lateral movement to occur (Dyce *et al.* 2002). At T11, the spinous process is vertical (the anticlinal vertebrae) and vertebrae caudal to T11 tend to have spinous processes directed cranially. At roughly the anticlinal vertebrae, the orientation of the articular facets changes to a more sagittal alignment where the caudal processes face more laterally and the cranial process face more medially, allowing sagittal flexion and extension to occur (Dyce *et al.* 2002; Evans 1993).

There are variations in the degree of sagittal alignment at facet joints in the caudal thoracic spine – some of the caudal articular facets are directed in a truly sagittal alignment, whereas in some specimens it was found that facets have a greater ventral or caudal component (Breit 2002). In small dogs, the alignment tends to be more sagittal and in larger dogs, more oblique towards a transverse plane. This occurs most frequently at L3–4 (Breit 2002).

Costovertebral and costotransverse joints
Costovertebral joints are formed by the head of each rib and the costal facets on the vertebrae. They are described as spheroid joints (Budras *et al.* 2002). The coupled movement of rotation

and lateral flexion in the thoracic spine showed an increase in motion after resection of the rib-head joint, suggesting the costovertebral joint also has a role in limiting movement in the thoracic spine.

Costotransverse joints are a planar joint between the tubercle of each rib and the transverse process of the vertebrae.

4.4.3 Lumbar spine (L1–7)

The lumbar vertebral bodies are the longest in the vertebral column, increasing in length caudally. They have long transverse processes that project cranioventrally alongside the preceding vertebral body (Dyce *et al.* 2002). The lumbar spine facet joints display mostly sagittal alignment, with interlocking of the caudal and cranial articular processes. The caudal articular processes face laterally and the cranial articular processes face medially. In the caudal lumbar spine, Benninger *et al.* (2006) found that there are four variations of shapes of facet joint observed on CT scan – straight (28%), angled (14%), arcuate (29%) and round (14%). Some 15% of facet joints were asymmetrical contralaterally. The difference in shape was found to vary with breed. Facet joint angle tended to be more in the transverse plane in caudal segments compared with the more cranial levels of the lumbar spine. Intervertebral disc height increased from L4–5 to L7–S1. The L7–S1 level had a significantly more wedge-shaped disc, thicker ventrally.

According to Benninger *et al.* (2006), there are four major influences on motion pattern in the lumbar spine: height of intervertebral disc, facet joint angle in the transverse plane, facet joint angle difference between levels in the transverse plane, and length of lever arm (distance between the centre of facet joint and dorsal rim of intervertebral disc). Flexion–extension increased with disc height. Flexion–extension also increased with greater facet joint angle in the transverse plane, despite the motion guiding and limiting function of the facet joint. Differences in facet joint angle in the transverse plane between levels affected all motion in all planes. The short lever arm was associated with increased flexion–extension. In summary, the amount of flexion–extension, as the major movement present, increased caudally in the lumbar spine.

An *in vivo* kinematic study of canine lumbar intervertebral joints revealed the following values during gait (Schendel *et al.* 1995): axial rotation 1.3°, lateral flexion 4.25°, flexion–extension 1.8°. During ambulation, axial rotation was coupled with contralateral lateral bending.

A more recent *in vitro* study revealed that flexion–extension was variable throughout the lumbar spine, increasing from 5–10° at L4–5 to 40° at L7–S1. Flexion–extension was coupled with slight axial rotation, which increased from cranial to caudal. The greatest amount of lateral bend was at L4–5, and very little axial rotation was observed at all lumbar segments. Motion patterns in axial rotation differed between humans and dogs (Benninger *et al.* 2004). In humans, the most axial rotation was found in the midlumbar region (Panjabi *et al.* 1994), whereas Benninger *et al.* (2004) determined the amount of axial rotation to be smallest in

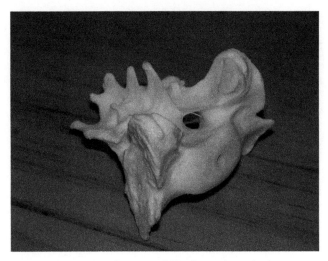

Figure 4.3 Orientation of canine caudal lumbosacral articular facets – cranio-oblique view.

the midlumbar region and highest at L4–5 and L7–S1 in dogs. Similar to humans at all levels, coupled axial rotation and lateral bending in dogs ranges between 1° and 2° (Benninger *et al.* 2004; Panjabi *et al.* 1994).

4.4.4 Lumbosacral and sacroiliac joint

Lumbosacral (LS) joint

The caudal facet joints face mediodorsally and cranial facets face lateroventrally – they are more angled to the transverse plane than the more cranial lumbar joints (Benninger *et al.* 2006) (Figure 4.3). Flexion–extension is significant at this articulation, up to three times as mobile as the human LS junction (Benninger *et al.* 2004). An exponential increase in flexion–extension motion was found from L5–6 to L7–S1. During lateral flexion and axial rotation, the coupling of these motions was greatest in the LS segment, followed by L4–5 (Benninger *et al.* 2006). Translation of the vertebrae at L7–S1 was found to move in either a dorsal or ventral direction, with the least amount detected at the LS junction, compared to L4–5 (Benninger *et al.* 2004). L7–S1 is a common site for the development of intervertebral disc disease; however, it is unknown whether disc degeneration precedes increased ventrodorsal translation or whether increased shear forces from increased translation lead to LS disc disease (Benninger *et al.* 2004). Asymmetry of the right and left facet joint angles was found in German Shepherd Dogs, though no association with disc degeneration was found (Seiler *et al.* 2002). *In vivo* forces acting on the LS spine are unknown in the dog and most likely differ between breed, age and gender (Hediger *et al.* 2009).

Sacroiliac joint (SIJ)

The canine SIJ has a synovial part and an interosseous part. The synovial part of the joint is planar, and crescent shaped on the

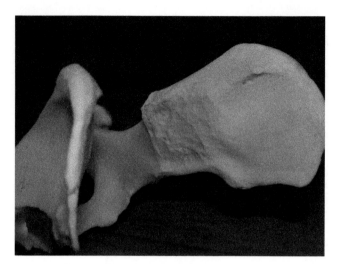

Figure 4.4 Iliac articular surface of canine sacroiliac joint.

sacral and iliac surfaces (Gregory *et al.* 1986). Alignment is basically sagittal, with variations in obliquity of alignment between breeds. Dorsal to the synovial part of the joint is a roughened area, the sacral tuberosity, at which an interosseous ligament unites the wings of ilium and sacrum (Evans 1993) (Figure 4.4).

The main movements available at the SIJ are flexion–extension, with a total of range of 7° thought to be available (Gregory *et al.* 1986). The sagittally aligned wings of ilium and sacrum permit very little lateral translation (Breit & Kunzel 2001); however, there may be some varying amounts of craniocaudal translation as accessory motion, depending on the conformation of the dog. Loading forces are transmitted through the coxofemoral joint, acetabulum and ilium to the sacrum and lumbar spine and thus the SIJ is significant in load transfer (Breit & Kunzel 2001).

The canine SIJ is affected by conformation, body weight and activity (Breit & Kunzel 2001). A group of researchers have described the orientation of joint surfaces and the variation in orientation that exists between large and small dogs. Using 1093 radiographs of German Shepherds (GSD), Rottweilers and Golden Retrievers, these researchers discovered a more oblique alignment of the sacroiliac joints in Rottweilers and a more sagittal alignment in GSDs and Golden Retrievers (Breit *et al.* 2002). In large dogs, inclination of wings of sacrum was more vertical (lower than 3.2° in 43% GSD), leading to an increased potential for craniocaudal translation at the SIJ. Large dogs, especially Rottweilers, had greater concavity of articular surface to improve interlock – this is thought to be related to high bodyweight. Relative to bodyweight, disproportionately low values of the size of SIJ contact area present, especially in large dogs, resulting in higher forces exerted on their SIJ. Forces in large breeds are approximately twice as high as in toy breeds (Breit & Kunzel 2001). A smaller proportion of sacral tuberosity area with respect to auricular surface was found in Bernese Mountain Dogs and Rottweilers compared with Dachshunds and Collies,

thus less interosseous ligament area. Due to less interosseous ligament area, the SIJ is less rigid in these breeds and during locomotion may place more strain on other SIJ ligaments (Breit & Kunzel 2001).

4.4.5 Common spinal injury – intervertebral disc degeneration (IVDD)

The function of an intervertebral disc is to form a cushion between adjacent bony vertebrae that allows limited motion in any plane, minimises shock, and joins vertebral column segments. Following the long axis of the vertebral column, the intervertebral disc resists compressive forces that are generated by the weight of the head and abdominal muscles (Jeffery *et al.* 2013). During disc compression, the nucleus pulposus is displaced in all directions and the annulus fibrosis is distended to absorb shock (Toombs & Bauer 1993). Degeneration of the discs due to age results in altered biomechanics of the vertebral column. In humans, the most likely cause of disc degeneration is degeneration of the blood supply that provides nutrition for the nucleus pulposus; however, in dogs, a genetic predisposition is the likely cause (Jeffery *et al.* 2013).

Two types of herniation have been described, each leading to a unique type of disc protrusion (Hansen 1952) (Figure 4.5). A Hansen Type I disc protrusion occurs predominantly in chondrodystrophic dogs between the ages of 2 and 7 years, with peak incidence between 4 and 5 years (Toombs & Bauer 1993). Chondroid degeneration is characterised by dehydration of the nucleus pulposus, leading to cellular degeneration and calcification of the whole structure. Degenerative changes cause

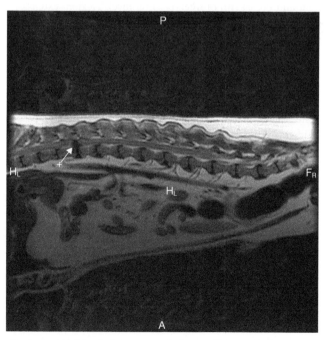

Figure 4.5 Example of a T12–13 disc extrusion on MRI in the sagittal plane. *Source:* A. Komitor, Loveland, CO. Reproduced with permission from A. Komitor.

alterations in intradiscal pressure which change mechanical stresses on the annulus fibrosis, leading to rupture of individual strands and eventual mechanical failure (Jeffery *et al.* 2013). Degeneration of the passive stabilising structures leads to instability in the spinal motion segments, resulting in significant deviations of range of motion from normal (Hediger *et al.* 2009). The degenerative process eventually leads to increased spine segment stiffness due to hypertrophic changes and facet joint osteoarthritis (Hediger *et al.* 2009). Type I IVDD tends to produce more acute clinical signs that can appear rapidly.

A Hansen Type II disc protrusion occurs primarily in non-chondrodystrophic dogs and develops at a slower rate, with clinical signs appearing between 5 and 12 years of age. Collagen content of the nucleus increases, exerting more mechanical pressure on the annulus, and fibres of the annulus split, allowing tissue fluid and plasma accumulation. Over time, thickening of the annulus develops, causing protrusion into the vertebral canal, commonly compressing the spinal cord or nerve roots (Jeffery *et al.* 2013). Fibroid degeneration typically produces a more insidious onset of clinical signs and dogs present with less severe neurological signs (Oliver *et al.* 1997).

Disc degeneration may occur throughout the vertebral column; however, in small breed dogs, acute (Type I) intervertebral cervical herniation typically occurs between C2 and C4, whereas T11 and L1 disc spaces are most commonly affected in the thoracolumbar spine (Brisson 2010; Jeffery *et al.* 2013). In large breed dogs, chronic, or Type II, herniation is most common in the caudal cervical spine from C6 to C7, and T13–L1 and L7–S1 (Brisson 2010; Jeffery *et al.* 2013). Susceptibility of the caudal cervical region to chronic disc herniation is believed to be caused by a higher range of motion in lateral bending, where the maximum increase in annulus stress occurs (Breit & Kunzel 2004). Higher disc length to cross-sectional area ratio, also found in large breed dogs, causes greater axial displacement whereas increased tensile stress in the annulus fibrosis and marked dorsolateral disc bulge were found in large breed dogs, due to their tendency to have longer discs (Breit & Kunzel 2004). The thoracolumbar junction lies between the rigid thoracic cage with rib attachments and a well-muscled, rigid lumbar region (Jeffery *et al.* 2013). The lumbosacral junction is the region of focus for forces transferred from the vertebral column to the pelvis. This may be a reason why this level of the lumbar spine is most susceptible to disc lesions (Jeffery *et al.* 2013).

The most common clinical signs associated with IVDD are pain, paresis and acute and chronic ataxia. Referred pain associated with the level of the lesion and lameness that mimics orthopaedic disease occurs in up to 50% of dogs (Seim & Prata 1982). The general consensus regarding treatment of IVDD remains controversial over the extent to which surgical intervention is necessary. Treatment decisions also depend on first-time occurrence or recurrence of clinical signs. It is beyond the scope of this chapter to review all of the imaging techniques and medical management for IVDD; however, the reader is encouraged to review the various diagnostics, surgical techniques and neuroprotective treatments for spinal cord injury related to IVDD.

4.4.6 Summary

There are many assumptions made regarding the contribution of facet joints, intervertebral discs and other structures to stability and/or movement of the vertebral column, based on morphology and observation. As some studies have shown, a given motion segment of the spine does not necessarily behave in the manner predicted by morphology. We can only be guided by the current knowledge of anatomy and morphology and the growing field of kinematics and motion analysis in the canine vertebral column.

4.5 Canine peripheral joints

Kinematic research in the peripheral joints has focused primarily on the pelvic limbs, related to cranial cruciate ligament rupture and repair. As with the vertebral column, physiotherapists can only be guided by the current knowledge of anatomy and morphology and the growing field of kinematics and motion analysis in the canine peripheral joints. Table 4.1 provides a summary of the peripheral joints, noting the type of articulation, the main direction of motion available at the joint, as well as conjunct motions available.

4.6 Biomechanics of locomotion: the dog

4.6.1 Kinematic data collection

Kinematic analysis of gait in the dog has been limited to date, but there is a growing interest in the area (Hottinger *et al.* 1996) motivated by responses of dogs to surgical procedures (Robinson *et al.* 2006), orthopaedic conditions (Evans *et al.* 2005) and breed differences (Besancon *et al.* 2005; Colborne *et al.* 2004).

Establishment of gait analysis in the normal subject has been attempted, using force-plate analysis and skin-mounted markers to describe flexion–extension movements in the joints of healthy Greyhounds, at the trot (DeCamp *et al.* 1993). Figure 4.6 shows a dog mounted with lightweight reflective markers. These authors point out that the shape of the joint angle/time curve is intrinsic to an animal's limb conformation. Thus, in dogs, analysis of gait will be specific for the breed of dog.

Despite choosing the Greyhound, because of uniformity of body conformation and temperament, DeCamp *et al.* (1993) discovered variances in joint angles during the swing phase, attributable to trial repetition, with the carpus showing most variance with a mean trial repetition variance. In stance phase, each joint was characterised by peaks of extension – the coxofemoral joint had a single peak towards the end of stance phase; the femorotibial joint had two peaks of extension with maximal extension preceding stance phase; the tarsal and elbow joints had two peaks of extension, as did the scapulohumeral joint. The carpal joint had one peak of extension early in the stance phase

Table 4.1 A summary of the canine extremity joints: joint type, articular surfaces, the primary motion of the joint and the accessory movements that occur at each complex

Joint	Joint type and articular surfaces	Main movement	Accessory movement
Glenohumeral	Spheroid, between the glenoid cavity of the scapula and the head of humerus, with the glenoid fossa on the scapula	Flexion and extension	Rotation
Elbow	Composite joint formed by the humeral condyle and the head of the radius (humeroradial joint) and the semilunar notch of the ulna (humeroulnar joint) – ginglymus joints. Proximal radioulnar joint communicates with the main elbow joint – trochoid joint	Flexion–extension. Rotation occurs at the radioulnar joint (and carpal joints) so that about 90° of supination of the forepaws can be achieved	Lateral translations minimal due to strong collateral ligaments and the anconeus of the ulna
Carpus	Composite articulation, which involves the proximal, middle, carpometacarpal and intercarpal joints. Proximal carpal joint is a ginglymus between the distal end of the radius and ulna and the proximal carpal row. The middle carpal joint is a compound condylar joint between the proximal and distal rows of carpals. The carpometacarpal joint is a compound plane joint between the distal carpals and the metacarpus. The intercarpal joints are compound planar joints between the carpal bones of each row	As a whole joint, flexion–extension. The majority of the movement occurs at the proximal and middle carpal joints	Lateral movement
Metacarpophalangeal joint	Compound articulation between proximal phalanges, proximal sesamoid bones, dorsal sesamoid bones and metacarpals	Flexion and extension	Ab/adduction and axial rotation
Proximal interphalangeal joint	Saddle joint between proximal and middle phalanges(forelimb and hindlimb)	Flexion and extension	Axial rotation and lateral movements
Distal interphalangeal joint	Saddle joint between middle and distal phalanges(forelimb and hindlimb)	Flexion and extension	Axial rotation and lateral movements
Coxofemoral joint (hip)	Spheroid joint, articulation between the femoral head and the acetabulum of the ilium, ischium and pubis. The acetabulum is deepened by a band of fibrocartilage on the rim of the acetabulum	Flexion and extension are the main movements	Abduction and adduction, multidirectional
Stifle	Complex joint comprising the tibiofemoral joint (condylar) and the patellofemoral joint (simple, sliding joint). At the tibiofemoral joint, the convex femoral condyles articulate with the planar tibial plateau. The incongruity of this joint is improved by the two menisci, into which each condyle fits. The patellofemoral joint is between the patella and the trochlea of the femur	The main movements at the stifle are flexion–extension at the tibiofemoral joint, with the patella gliding in the trochlea during the movement	Accessory craniocaudal movements are limited by the cruciate ligaments, the collateral ligaments and the concave nature of the menisci
Proximal tibiofibular	Simple plane joint between tibia and head of fibula	Minimal gliding movement	
Distal tibiofibular	Simple plane joint between distal tibia and fibula	Minimal gliding movement	
Tarsal joint (hock)	The hock complex includes the talocrural joint (cochlear joint), proximal and distal intertarsal joints, tarsometatarsal joint (compound plane joints) and intertarsal joints (perpendicular tight joints). The greatest amount of movement occurs at the talocrural joint	At the talocrural joint, flexion–extension, in a plane that deviates about 25° from the sagittal plane. This allows the hindpaws to pass the forepaws laterally in full gallop. Slight flexion–extension available at the proximal intertarsal joint. Little mobility at distal intertarsal, tarsometatarsal and intertarsal joints	Slight rotation at talocrural and proximal intertarsal joint
Metatarsophalangeal joint	See forelimb		
Proximal and distal interphalangeal joints	See forelimb		
Temporomandibular	A simple condylar joint which allows translatory movement, with an articular disc	Hinge – opening and closing	Lateromedial excursion. Increased opening is associated with upper cervical extension

Source: Adapted from Budras *et al.* (2002) and Evans (1993).

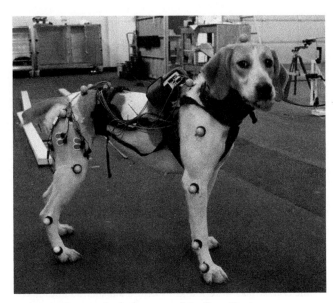

Figure 4.6 Photograph of a dog prepared for data collection, demonstrating kinematic reflective marker attachment sites and donning EMG equipment. Wireless EMG transmitter is depicted by the green box attached to the dorsum of the thoracic harness and electrode leads attached to the dorsum of the pelvic harness. Note also surface EMG electrode placement on left thigh musculature (*blue ovals*). *Source:* Photo courtesy of Dr Caroline Adrian.

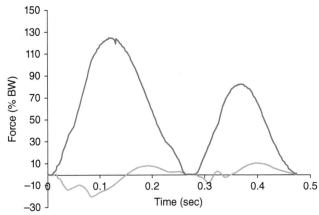

Figure 4.7 Example of a typical force-plate tracing. The most common data collected includes vertical forces (*red line*) and cranial-caudal forces (*green line*) for the thoracic and pelvic limbs, respectively.

and then rapid flexion initiated to the end of stance (DeCamp *et al.* 1993). Movement of skin markers due to skin movement, muscle contraction and other soft tissue movement may have contributed to the variance in measurement of joint angles during swing. It is as a result of such problems that McLaughlin (2001) reports that data for the swing phase in dogs are minimal.

4.6.2 Force-plate data collection

The dog is led across a force-plate by a handler, in a consistent manner, with no interference from the handler. Trials consist of ipsilateral forefoot and hindfoot strikes, and for each valid trial, three orthogonal ground reaction forces are recorded (McLaughlin 2001) (Figure 4.7). Velocity of the dog is measured and sometimes accelerometers are used as acceleration and deceleration affect force values. Ground reaction force data are presented in a force–time curve, or numerically (McLaughlin 2001). Vertical force is usually the largest of the orthogonal forces, with craniocaudal braking and mediolateral forces generally smaller. Force data are also normalised with respect to the dog's bodyweight (McLaughlin 2001), which means that dogs of different breeds can be compared.

4.6.3 Walking data

Walking in the quadruped involves a cyclic exchange of gravitational potential energy and kinetic energy of the centre of mass. In a study by Griffin *et al.* (2004), kinematic and ground reaction force data were collected from dogs walking over a

range of speeds. The authors found that the forequarters and hindquarters of dogs behaved like two independent bipeds, with the centre of mass moving up and down twice per stride. Up to 70% of the mechanical energy required to lift and accelerate the centre of mass was recovered via a mechanism likened to an inverted pendulum (Griffin *et al.* 2004). Using a model of two inverted pendulums, these authors concluded that there are two reasons why dogs did not walk with a flat trajectory of the centre of mass.

- Each forelimb lagged its ipsilateral hindlimb by only 15% of the stride time – this produced time periods when the forequarters and hindquarters moved up or down simultaneously.
- Forelimbs supported 63% of body mass during gait. (This is consistent with static four-legged weight bearing.)

The model proposed here predicts that the centre of mass of a dog will undergo two fluctuations per stride cycle.

In an attempt to establish some normative data in large breed dogs, Hottinger *et al.* (1996) have presented data on the stance and swing phase of gait at the walk, pertaining to the joint angles, total time of stance and swing phase of each limb. It is beyond the scope of this chapter to reproduce these data, but the reader is directed to this research as a useful resource.

4.6.4 Lameness data

Kinematic research in the peripheral joints has focused primarily on cranial cruciate ligament rupture and repair. A population of adult Labrador Retrievers – 17 subjects free of orthopaedic and neurological abnormalities, 100 with unilateral cranial cruciate ligament (CCL) rupture, and 131 studied 6 months after surgery for unilateral CCL injury, 15 with observable lameness – were walked over a force platform, with ground reaction force (GRF) recorded during the stance phase (Evans *et al.* 2005). The probability of visual observation detecting a gait abnormality was compared with that of force platform gait analysis. During the stance phase, it was determined that a combination of peak vertical force (PVF) and falling slope was optimal for discriminating sound and lame Labradors. After surgery, 75% of subjects with no observable lameness failed to achieve GRFs consistent with sound Labradors. The authors conclude that a force platform is an accurate method of assessing lameness in Labradors with CCL rupture and is more sensitive than visual observation. This has clinical relevance for animal physiotherapists as interventions for stifle lameness can be accurately and objectively evaluated using two vertical ground reaction forces obtained from a force platform.

Another group of researchers assessed the relationship between postoperative tibial plateau angle (TPA) and GRFs in Labrador Retrievers at least 4 months after tibial plateau levelling osteotomy (TPLO) surgery (Robinson *et al.* 2006). Thirty-two Labrador Retrievers with unilateral cranial cruciate ligament disease that had TPLO and concurrent meniscal surgery were studied. Both TPA and GRFs were measured before surgery and a time greater than or equal to 4 months after surgery. The GRFs, TPA, duration of injury preoperatively, postoperative TPA and degree of rotation were each compared with postoperative GRFs. No significant relationship was found between preoperative GRFs, preoperative TPA, duration of injury, postoperative TPA, degree of rotation or meniscal release/meniscectomy and postoperative function, suggesting limb function in Labrador Retrievers was not affected by postoperative TPA.

It is a general belief that dogs adapt well following amputation of a thoracic or pelvic limb; however, limited data exist on compensatory changes during gait post amputation. In thoracic limb amputees, kinetic data reported an increase of 17% additional bodyweight to the remaining thoracic limb and an additional 13% bodyweight to the remaining pelvic limb during stance phase, with no increase in peak vertical ground reaction forces (Kirpensteijn *et al.* 2000). However, these dogs significantly decreased their stance time, implying that the same force was distributed over a shorter time. This same result was found in pelvic limb amputees, resulting in increased limb cadence rather than an increase in overall velocity (Kirpensteijn *et al.* 2000).

In thoracic limb amputations, kinematic analysis addressing musculoskeletal compensatory strategies found a 14% increase in weight distribution on the remaining thoracic limb and a 17% combined increase on pelvic limbs (Jarvis *et al.* 2013). During stance phase, the carpus and ipsilateral hip and stifle joints had greater flexion. Range of motion increased in the cervicothoracic veterbral region in both the horizontal and sagittal planes; thoracolumbar vertebral region increased in the sagittal plane, but decreased in the horizontal plane; and increased flexion without a change in range of motion was found in the lumbosacral vertebral region (Jarvis *et al.* 2013).

Pelvic limb amputees showed an increased range of motion at the tarsal joint, cervicothoracic and thoracolumbar regions and increased lumbosacral extension at L7 in the sagittal plane (Hogy *et al.* 2013). Increased lateral bending toward the remaining pelvic limb was found in the horizontal plane, resulting in a laterally deviated gait pattern (Hogy *et al.* 2013).

Regardless of evaluating gait at a walk or trot, effects of hindlimb lameness on load redistribution and temporal changes showed similar compensatory mechanisms. The affected limb was consistently unloaded and the centre of mass was shifted to the contralateral side and rear in thoracic limb lameness and to the front in pelvic limb lameness (Fischer *et al.* 2013).

4.6.5 Breed-specific and sports-specific data

Comparisons of breeds have revealed some consistencies between breeds regarding PVF and vertical impulse in the pads of Greyhounds and Labrador Retrievers. Besancon *et al.* (2005) compared eight Greyhounds and eight Labrador Retrievers to discover that digital pads 3 and 4 are the major weight-bearing pads in dogs. The loads were found to be fairly evenly distributed between breeds, and digital pad 5 and the metacarpal or metatarsal pad were found to bear a substantial amount of load in both breeds.

Colborne *et al.* (2004) investigated the angular excursions, net joint moments and powers across the stifle, tarsal and metatarsophalangeal (MTP) joints in Labrador Retrievers and Greyhounds to investigate differences in joint mechanics between these two breeds of dogs. Not surprisingly, there were gross differences in kinematic patterns between Greyhounds and Labrador Retrievers. At the stifle and tarsal joints, moment and power patterns were similar in shape, but amplitudes were larger for the Greyhounds. The MTP joint was found to be a net absorber of energy, and this was greater in the Greyhounds. Greyhounds had a positive phase across the stifle, tarsal and MTP joints at the end of stance for an active push-off, whereas for the Labrador Retrievers, the only positive phase was across the tarsus, and this was small compared with values for the Greyhounds. This is clinically significant for animal physiotherapists, to take into consideration the conformation of the dog when considering biomechanics of locomotion, and the potential for certain pathologies to occur in different breeds. In addition, the occupation or sport of the dog needs to be considered.

Kemp *et al.* (2005) tested a hypothesis of functional trade-off in limb bones by measuring the mechanical properties of limb bones in two breeds of domestic dog that have undergone intense artificial selection for running (Greyhound) and fighting (Pit Bull) performance. They postulate that the physical demands of rapid and economical running would differ from the demands of fighting in ways that may prevent the simultaneous evolution of optimal performance in these two sports. The bones were loaded to fracture in three-point static bending. In Pit Bulls, the proximal limb bones differed from those of the Greyhounds in having relatively larger second moments of area of mid-diaphyseal cross-sections and in having more circular cross-sectional shape. The Pit Bulls exhibited lower stresses at yield, had lower elastic moduli, and failed at much higher levels of work. In the Greyhound, the stiffness of the tissue of the humerus, radius, femur and tibia was 1.5–2.4-fold greater

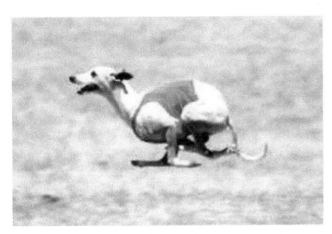

Figure 4.8 Picture of a whippet illustrating the extreme ranges of motion at a gallop. *Source:* Photo courtesy of Dr Robert Taylor.

than in the Pit Bulls. These differences between breeds were not observed in the long bones of the feet, metacarpals and metatarsals. These authors conclude that selection for high-speed running is associated with the evolution of relatively stiff limb bones, whereas selection for fighting performance leads to the evolution of limb bones with relatively high resistance to failure.

Epaxial musculature was also evaluated between the Greyhound and Pit Bull to determine muscular architecture of the vertebral column between the two breeds (Webster *et al.* 2014). Greyhound (sprinting breed) epaxial muscles, specifically the iliocostalis lumborum and longissimus dorsi, have a propensity to increase pelvic limb power production by 12% by facilitating lumbar extension during a gallop (Figure 4.8). Differences in cranial cervical muscles and deep thoracic muscles inserting on the ribs were also found between the breeds. Not surprisingly, Pit Bulls were found to have larger muscle mass in the cervical region, which may highlight selective breeding for different skull and neck conformations in a fighting dog. Muscles in the thoracic region of the spine, specifically the scaleni, serratus dorsalis and multifidus thoracis, were larger in the Greyhound. Originating and inserting on the ribs, these muscles function to facilitate ventilation by contributing to inspiration via expansion of the thoracic cavity by rotating the ribs cranially and laterally (Webster *et al.* 2014). It follows that adaptations of musculature to facilitate ventilation may be needed in an animal specialised for rapid sprinting. The Greyhound was also found to have a large volume of hip extensor muscle, an important requirement for power production in a sprinting canine athlete. Increased extensor moments found about the hip and tarsus also allow for increased power output and rapid acceleration (Williams *et al.* 2008).

Speed of running is constrained by the speed at which the limbs can be swung forwards and backwards, and by the force they can withstand while in contact with the ground. Regarding sprinting Greyhounds, Usherwood & Wilson (2005) have shown

that, on entering a tight bend, Greyhounds, unlike humans sprinting around banked bends, do not change their foot-contact timings. Greyhounds have to withstand a 65% increase in limb forces, whereas humans change the duration of foot contact to spread the time over which the load is applied, thereby keeping the force on their legs constant. These authors conclude that there is no force limit on Greyhound sprint speed – they suggest that Greyhounds power their locomotion by torque about the hips, so that the muscles that provide the power are mechanically divorced from the structures that support weight.

The majority of canine biomechanical research focuses on the walk and trotting gaits in dogs, though very little data exists on the initiation of movement from which all animal movement begins. One study reported on the kinematic quantification of maximal movement initiation of the Greyhound. A countermovement, or 'set position', was the first movement described where dogs negatively displace the centre of gravity in the y-direction by lowering the body to the ground from the standing position by flexing the shoulder, elbow, hip and stifle. A general sequence of maximal movement initiation is described allowing for successful quantification of movement initiation. This is the first step to better understanding the kinematics of maximal movement initiation in Greyhounds, possibly leading to additional research such as natural and synthetic surfaces and how rehabilitation and surgical techniques influence biomechanics of movement.

4.6.6 Electromyography

An additional technique for investigating neuromuscular dysfunction is electromyography (EMG), the study of an electrical signal associated with a muscle activity (Figure 4.9). In addition to kinematic and kinetic gait analysis, EMG provides insight into muscle activity and the biomechanical alterations associated with joint instability (Winter 2005) (see Figure 4.6).

In the human anterior cruciate ligament (ACL) injury, for example, changes in muscle activity, as well as limb kinetics and

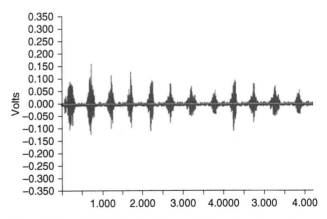

Figure 4.9 A typical EMG tracing of the canine biceps femoris muscle at a trot. *Source:* Courtesy of Dr Caroline Adrian.

kinematics, are common contributing factors in the development of osteoarthritis (OA) (Andriacchi *et al.* 2009; Hurd & Snyder-Mackler 2007; Rudolph *et al.* 2001). The on/off timing of muscle activity that spans the human knee contributes to stability and mobility of a joint. Muscle activity provides joint compressive forces that contribute to important additional joint stabilisation (Williams *et al.* 2001). Any change in muscle activity, such as muscle onset or intensity, may result in altered joint stiffness (change in force per unit change in displacement) (Johannson *et al.* 1991; Williams *et al.* 2001).

Neuromuscular control is defined as the 'ability to produce controlled movement through coordinated muscle activity' (Williams *et al.* 2001). Injury to the ACL produces asynchronous muscle firing prior to (Limbird *et al.* 1988), as well as post rupture characterised by weakness, impaired proprioception, incoordination ('microklutziness') and altered muscle firing patterns (Williams *et al.* 2004). These neuromuscular changes may be the result of disuse atrophy or decrease in voluntary muscle activation, which is speculated to be due to pain, fatigue or joint effusion (Snyder-Mackler *et al.* 1994).

In normal canine stifle biomechanics, a synergistic relationship exists between the CCL, quadriceps, gastrocnemius and biceps femoris muscles to provide stability (Goslow *et al.* 1981; Slocum & Slocum 1993). Cranial thigh muscles (stifle extensors) and the gastrocnemius muscle are active to prevent stifle flexion and pelvic limb collapse during weightbearing. Caudal thigh muscles (stifle flexors) stabilise the stifle by pulling the proximal tibia caudally and extending the hip to create forward propulsion (Slocum & Slocum 1993). However, the effect of cranial cruciate ligament rupture on this coordinated relationship is unknown.

4.7 Conclusion

Knowledge of the concepts of functional biomechanics of animals from the orientation and movements available at individual joints, to the way in which movement differs between conformation breeds and between sports, will assist the animal physiotherapist in achieving the best outcome for performance in an animal.

References

Adrian, C.P., Haussler, K.K., Kawcak, C. *et al.* 2013, The role of muscle activation in cruciate disease. *Vet. Surg.* 42(7):765–773.

Andriacchi, T.P., Koo, S., Scanlan, S.F. 2009, Gait mechanics influence healthy cartilage morphology and osteoarthritis of the knee. *J. Bone Joint Surg. Am.* 91:95–101.

Bennell, K.L., Hunt, M.A., Wrigley, T.V. *et al.* 2008, Role of muscle in the genesis and management of knee osteoarthritis. *Rheum. Dis. Clin. North Am.* 34:731–754.

Benninger, M., Seiler, G., Robinson, L. *et al.* 2004, Three-dimensional motion pattern of the caudal lumbar and lumbosacral portions of the vertebral column of dogs. *Am. J. Vet. Res.* 65(5):544–552.

Benninger, M., Seiler, G., Robinson, L. *et al.* 2006, Effects of anatomic conformation on the three-dimensional motion of the caudal lumbar and lumbosacral portions of the veterbral column of dogs. *Am. J. Vet. Res.* 67(1):43–50.

Besancon, M.F., Conzemius, M.G., Evans, R.B., Ritter, M.J. 2005, Distribution of vertical forces in the pads of Greyhounds and Labrador Retrievers during walking. *Am. J. Vet. Res.* 66(9):1563–1571.

Blood, D., Studdert, V. 1999, *Saunders Comprehensive Veterinary Dictionary*, 2nd edn. Saunders, London.

Brandt K.D. 2004, Neuromuscular aspects of osteoarthritis: a perspective. *Novartis Found. Symp.* 260:49–58.

Breit, S. 2002, Functional adaptations of facet geometry in the canine thoracolumbar and lumbar spine (T10–L6). *Ann. Anat.* 184(4):379–386.

Breit, S., Kunzel, W. 2001, On biomechanical properties of the sacroiliac joint in purebred dogs. *Ann. Anat.* 183:145–150.

Breit, S., Kunzel, W. 2002, Shape and orientation of articular facets of cervical vertebra (C3–C7) in dogs denoting axial rotational ability: an osteological study. *Eur. J. Morphol.* 40(1):43–51.

Breit, S., Kunzel, W. 2004, A morphometric investigation on breed-specific features affecting sagittal rotational and lateral bending mobility in the canine cervical spine (C3-C7). *Anat. Histol. Embryol.* 33(4):244–250.

Breit, S., Knaus, I., Kunzel, W. 2002, Use of routine ventrodorsal radiographic views of the pelvis to assess inclination of the wings of the sacrum in dogs. *Am. J. Vet. Res.* 63(9):1200–1255.

Brisson, B.A. 2010, Intervertebral disc disease in dogs. *Vet. Clin. North Am. Small Anim. Pract.* 40(5):829–858.

Budras, K., McCarthy, P., Fricke, W. *et al.* 2002, *Anatomy of the Dog – An Illustrated Text*, 4th edn. Iowa City, Iowa State University Press.

Cholewicki, J., Silfies, S.P., Shah, R.A. *et al.* 2005, Delayed trunk muscle reflex responses increase the risk of low back injuries. *Spine.* 30(23):2614–2620.

Colborne, G.R., Innes, J.F., Comerford, E.J. *et al.* 2004, Distribution of power across the hind limb joints in Labrador Retrievers and Greyhounds. *Am. J. Vet. Res.* 65(11):1497–1501.

DeCamp, C., Soutas-Little, R., Hauptman, R. *et al.* 1993, Kinematic analysis of the trot in healthy Greyhounds. *Am. J. Vet. Res.* 54(4):627–634.

Denoix, J.M. 1999, Spinal biomechanics and functional anatomy. *Vet.Clin. North Am. Equine Pract.* 15(1):27–60.

de Rooster, H., van Ryssen B, van Bree, H. 1998, Diagnosis of cranial cruciate ligament injury in dogs by tibial compression radiography. *Vet. Rec.* 142:366–368.

Dyce, K.M., Sack, W.O., Wensing, C.J.G. 2002, *Textbook of Veterinary Anatomy*, 3rd edn. Saunders, Philadelphia, PA.

Evans, H.E. (ed.) 1993, In: *Millers Anatomy of the Dog*, 3rd edn. W.B. Saunders, Philadelphia, pp. 292–318.

Evans, R., Horstman, C., Conzemius, M. 2005, Accuracy and optimization of force platform gait analysis in Labradors with cranial cruciate disease evaluated at a walking gait. *Vet. Surg.* 34(5):445–449.

Fischer, S., Anders, A., Notle, I., Schilling, N. 2013, Compensatory load redistribution in walking and trotting dogs with hind limb lameness. *Vet. J.* 197(3):746–752.

Goslow, G.E.J., Seeherman, H.J., Taylor, C.R. *et al.* 1981, Electrical activity and relative length changes of dog limb muscles as a function of speed and gait. *J. Exp. Biol.* 94:15–42.

Gregory, C., Cullen, J., Pool, R. *et al.* 1986, The canine sacroiliac joint – preliminary study of anatomy, histopathology and biomechanics. *Spine* 11(10):1044–1048.

Griffin, T.M., Main, R.P., Farley, C.T. 2004, Biomechanics of quadrupedal walking: how do four-legged animals achieve inverted pendulum-like movements? *J. Exp. Biol.* 207(20):3545–3558.

Hall, S. 1995, *Basic Biomechanics*, 2nd edn. Mosby-Year Book, St Louis.

Hansen, H.J. 1952, A pathologic-anatomical study on disc degeneration in dogs, with special reference to the so-called enchondrosis intervertebralis *Acta Orthopaed. Scand.* 11(suppl):1–117.

Hediger, K.U., Ferguson, S.J., Gedet, P. *et al.* 2009, Biomechanical analysis of torsion and shear forces in lumbar and lumbosacral spine segments of nonchondrodystrophic dogs. *Vet. Surg.* 38(7): 874–880.

Hides, J., Cooper, D., Stokes, M. 1992, Diagnostic ultrasound imaging for measurement of the lumbar multifidus muscle in normal young adults. *Physiother. Theory Pract.* 8:19–26.

Hides, J., Stokes, M., Saide, M. *et al.* 1994, Evidence of lumbar multifidus wasting ipsilateral to symptoms in patients with acute/subacute low back pain. *Spine* 19(2):165–172.

Hides, J., Richardson, C., Jull, G. 1996, Multifidus muscle recovery is not automatic after resolution of acute, first-episode low back pain. *Spine* 21(23):2763–2769.

Hides, J.A., Jull, G.A., Richardson, C.A. 2001, Long-term effects of specific stabilizing exercises for first-episode low back pain. *Spine* 26(11):243–248.

Hodges, P.W. 2003, Neuromechanical control of the spine. *Thesis, Kongl Karolinska Medico Chirurgiska Institiutet*, Stockholm, Sweden.

Hodges, P.W., Richardson, C.A. 1996, Inefficient muscular stabilization of the lumbar spine associated with low back pain. A motor control evaluation of transversus abdominus. *Spine* 21(22):2640–2650.

Hodges, P.W., Cresswell, A.G., Daggfeldt, K. *et al.* 2001, *In vivo* measurement of the effect of intra-abdominal pressure on the human spine. *J. Biomech.* 34:347–353.

Hofstetter, M., Gedet, P., Doherr, *et al.* 2009, Biomechanical analysis of the three-dimensional motion pattern of the canine cervical spine segment C4-C5. *Vet. Surg.* 38(1):49–58.

Hogy, S.M., Worley, D.R., Jarvis, S.L. *et al.* 2013, Kinematic and kinetic analysis of dogs during trotting after amputation of a pelvic limb. *Am. J. Vet. Res.* 74(9):1164–1171.

Hottinger, H., DeCamp, C., Olivier, N. *et al.* 1996, Noninvasive kinematic analysis of the walk in healthy large-breed dogs. *Am. J. Vet. Res.* 57(3):381–388.

Hurd, W.J., Snyder-Mackler, L. 2007, Knee instability after acute ACL rupture affects movement patterns during the mid-stance phase of gait. *J. Orthop. Res.* 25:1369–1377.

Ireland, W., Rogers, J., Myers, R. 1986, Location of the instantaneous centre of joint rotation in the normal canine stifle. *Am. J. Vet. Res.* 47(4):837–840.

Jarvis, S.L., Worley, D.R., Hogy, S.M. *et al.* 2013, Kinematic and kinetic analysis of dogs during trotting after amputation of a thoracic limb. *Am. J. Vet. Res.* 74(9):1155–1163.

Jeffcott, L.B., Dalin, G. 1980, Natural rigidity of the horse's backbone. *Equine Vet. J.* 12:101.

Jeffery, N.D., Levine, J.M., Olby, N.J., Stein, V.M. 2013, Intervertebral disk degeneration in dogs: consequences, diagnosis, treatment and future directions. *J. Vet. Intern. Med.* 27(6):1318–1333.

Johansson, H., Sjolander, P., Sojka, P. 1991, A sensory role for the cruciate ligaments. *Clin. Orthop. Relat. Res.* 268:161–178.

Johnson, J.A., da Costa, R.C., Bhattacharya, S. *et al.* 2011, Kinematic motion patterns of the cranial and caudal canine cervical spine. *Vet. Surg.* 40(6):720–727.

Kaigle, A.M., Sten, M.S., Holm, H. 1995, Experimental instability in the lumbar spine. *Spine* 20(4):421–430.

Kaigle, A., Ekstrom, L., Holm, S. *et al.* 1998, *In vivo* dynamic stiffness of the porcine lumbar spine exposed to cyclic loading: influence of load and degeneration. *J. Spinal Disord.* 11(1):65–70.

Kapandji, I. 1974, *The Physiology of the Joints. Vol. 3. The Trunk and Vertebral Column*, 2nd edn. Longman, New York, pp. 218–228.

Kemp T.J., Bachus, K.N., Nairn, J.A. *et al.* 2005, Functional trade-offs in the limb bones of dogs selected for running versus fighting. *J. Exp. Biol.* 208(18):3475–3482.

Kirpensteijn, J., van den Bos, R., van den Brom, W.E., Hazewinkel, H.A. 2000, Ground reaction force analysis of large breed dogs when walking after the amputation of a limb. *Vet. Rec.* 146(6):155–159.

Lee, D.G. (ed.) 2004, *The Pelvic Girdle: An Approach to the Examination and Treatment of the Lumbo-Pelvic-Hip Region*, 3rd edn. Churchill Livingstone, Edinburgh, pp. 138–139, 153–154.

Lee, M. 1995, Biomechanics of joint movements. In: Refshauge, K., Gass, L. (eds), *Musculoskeletal Physiotherapy – Clinical Science and Practice*. Butterworth Heinemann, Oxford, pp. 19–23.

Licka, T.F., Peham, C., Frey, A. 2004, Electromyographic activity of the longissimus dorsi muscles in horses during trotting on a treadmill. *Am. J. Vet. Res.* 65(2):155–158.

Limbird, T.J., Shiavi, R., Frazer, M. *et al.* 1988, EMG profiles of knee joint musculature during walking: changes induced by anterior cruciate ligament deficiency. *J. Orthop. Res.* 6:630–638.

McLaughlin, R. 2001, Kinetic and kinematic gait analysis in dogs. *Vet. Clin. North Am. Small Anim. Pract.* 31(1):193–201.

Moseley, G.L., Hodges, P.W., Gandevia, S.C. 2002, Deep and superficial fibres of the lumbar multifidus muscles are differentially active during voluntary arm movement. *Spine* 27(2):29–36.

Oliver, J.E., Lorenz, M.D., Kornegay, J.N. 1997, *Handbook of Veterinary Neurology*, 3rd edn. W.B. Saunders, Philadelphia.

Panjabi, M. 1992a, The stabilising system of the spine. Part 1. Function dysfunction, adaptation, and enhancement. *J. Spinal Disord.* 5(4):383–389.

Panjabi, M. 1992b, The stabilizing system of the spine. Part II. Neutral zone and instability hypothesis. *J. Spinal Disord.* 5(4):390–396.

Panjabi, M.M., Abumi, K., Duranceau, J. *et al.* 1989, Spinal stability and intersegmental muscle forces: a biomechanical model. *Spine* 14(2):194–200.

Panjabi, M.M., Oxland, T.R., Yamamoto, I. *et al.* 1994, Mechanical behavior of the human lumbar and lumbosacral spine as shown by three-dimensional load-displacement curves. *J. Bone Joint Surg. Am.* 76(3):413–424.

Peham, C., Frey, A., Licka, T. *et al.* 2001, Evaluation of the EMG activity of the long back muscle during induced back movements in stance. *Equine Vet. J.* 33(suppl):165–168.

Penning, L., Wilmink, J. 1987, Rotation of the cervical spine. A CT study in normal subjects. *Spine* 12:732–738.

Pope, M., Panjabi, M. 1985, Biomechanical definitions of spinal instability. *Spine* 10(3):255–256.

Reber, K., Burki, A., Reves, N.V. *et al.* 2013, Biomechanical evaluation of the stabilizing function of the atlantoaxial ligaments under shear loading: a canine cadaveric study. *Vet. Surg.* 42(8):918–923.

Robert, C., Valette, J.P., Denoix, J.M. 2002, The effects of velocity on muscle activity at the trot. In: Lindner, A. (ed.), *The Elite Dressage and Three Day Event Horse, Conference on Equine Sports Medicine and Science*, pp. 189–198.

Robinson, D.A., Mason, D.R., Evans, R. *et al.* 2006, The effect of tibial plateau angle on ground reaction forces 4–17 months after tibial plateau leveling osteotomy in Labrador Retrievers. *Vet. Surg.* 35(3):294–299.

Rudolph, K.S., Axe, M.J., Buchanan, *et al.* 2001, Dynamic stability in the anterior cruciate ligament deficient knee. *Knee Surg. Sports Traumatol. Arthrosc.* 9:62–71.

Schendel, M., Dekutoski, M., Ogilvie, J. *et al.* 1995, Kinematics of the canine lumbar intervertebral joints. *Spine* 20(23):2555–2564.

Seiler, G.S., Hani, H., Busato, A.R. *et al.* 2002, Facet joint geometry and intervertebral disk degeneration in the L5-S1 region of the vertebral column in German Shepherd dogs. *Am. J. Vet. Res.* 63(1):86–90.

Seim, H.B., Prata, R.G. 1982, Ventral decompression for the treatment of cervical disc disease in the dog: a review of 54 cases. *J. Am. Anim. Hosp. Assoc.* 18:233.

Slocum, B., Slocum, T.D. 1993, Tibial plateau leveling osteotomy for repair of cranial cruciate ligament rupture in the canine. *Vet. Clin. North Am. Small Anim. Pract.* 23:777–795.

Snyder-Mackler, L., DeLuca, P.F., Willams, P.R. *et al.* 1994, Reflex inhibition of the quadriceps femoris muscle after injury or reconstruction of the anterior cruciate ligament. *J. Bone Joint Surg. Am.* 76:555–560.

Stubbs, N.C., Hodges, P.W., Jeffcott, L.B. *et al.* 2006, Functional anatomy of the thoracolumbar and lumbosacral spine in the horse. *Equine Vet. J.* 36(suppl):393–399.

Takeuchi, T., Abumi, K., Shono, Y. *et al.* 1999, Biomechanical role of the intervertebral disc and costovertebral joint in stability of the thoracic spine. A canine model study. *Spine* 24(14):1414–1420.

Toombs, J.P., Bauer, M.S. 1993, Intervertebral disc disease. In: Slatter, D. (ed.), *Textbook of Small Animal Surgery*. W.B. Saunders, Philadelphia.

Usherwood, J., Wilson, A. 2005, Biomechanics: no force limit on greyhound sprint speed. *Nature* 438(7069):753–754.

Webster, E.L., Hudson, P.E., Channon, S.B. 2014, Comparative functional anatomy of the expaxial musculature of dogs (*Canis familiaris*) bred for sprinting vs. fighting. *J. Anat.* 225(3):317–327.

Wilke, H.J., Wolf, S., Claes, L.E. *et al.* 1995, Stability increase of the lumbar spine with different muscle groups. A biomechanical in vitro study. *Spine* 20(2):192–198.

Williams, G.N., Chmielewski, T., Rudolph, K. *et al.* 2001, Dynamic knee stability: current theory and implications for clinicians and scientists. *J. Orthop. Sports Phys. Ther.* 31:546–566.

Williams, G.N., Barrance, P.J., Snyder-Mackler, L. *et al.* 2004, Altered quadriceps control in people with anterior cruciate ligament deficiency. *Med. Sci. Sports Exerc.* 36:1089–1097.

Williams, S.B., Wilson, A.M., Rhodes, L. *et al.* 2008, Functional anatomy and muscle moment arms of the pelvic limb of an elite sprinting athlete: the racing greyhound (*Canis familiaris*). *J. Anat.* 213(4):361–372.

Wilson, A.M., Watson, J.C., Lichtwark, G.A. 2003, Biomechanics: a catapult action for rapid limb protraction. *Nature* 421: 35–36.

Winter, D. 2005, *Biomechanics and Motor Control of Human Movement*, 3rd edn. John Wiley & Sons, Hoboken, NJ.

Worth, D. 1995, Movements of the head and neck. In: Boyling, J., Palastanga, N. (eds), *Grieve's Modern Manual Therapy*, 2nd edn. Churchill Livingstone, Edinburgh.

Further reading

Bloomberg, M.S., Dee, J.F., Taylor, R.A. 1998, *Canine Sports Medicine and Surgery*. WB Saunders, Philadelphia.

Blythe, L.L., Gannon, J.R., Craig, A.M. 1994, *Care of the Racing Greyhound*. Graphic Arts Center, Portland, OR.

Brown, C. 1986, *Dog Locomotion and Gait Analysis*. Hoflin Publishing, Arvada, CO.

Elliott, R.P. 2009, *Dogsteps – A New Look*, 3rd edn. Fancy Publications, Los Angeles, CA.

Riegger-Krugh, C., Millis, D. 2007, Anatomy and biomechanics: forelimb. In: Wilmarth, M.A. (ed.), *Basic Science for Animal Physical Therapy: Canine*, 2nd edn. Independent Study Course 17.4.1, Orthopedic Section, APTA, Inc., LaCrosse, WI.

Riegger-Krugh, C., Weigel, J. 2007, Anatomy and biomechanics: hindlimb. In: Wilmarth, M.A. (ed.), *Basic Science for Animal Physical Therapy: Canine*, 2nd edn. Independent Study Course 17.4.2, Orthopedic Section, APTA, Inc., LaCrosse, WI.

Riegger-Krugh, C., Millis, D. 2007, Anatomy and biomechanics: spine. In: Wilmarth, M.A. (ed.), *Basic Science for Animal Physical Therapy: Canine*, 2nd edn. Independent Study Course 17.4.3, Orthopedic Section, APTA, Inc., LaCrosse, WI.

CHAPTER 5

Applied Equine Biomechanics*

Lesley Goff

Lecturer, Equine Science, School of Agriculture & Food Sciences, The University of Queensland, Gatton, Australia; Director, Active Animal Physiotherapy, Toowoomba, Australia

Summary

An understanding of concepts of neuromotor control, musculoskeletal physiotherapy and rehabilitation is vital to the application of physiotherapy for animals. The aim of this chapter is to introduce key concepts of applied biomechanics in the horse based on the limited research into animal functional biomechanics and kinematics.

5.1 Introduction

The aim of this chapter is to introduce key concepts of applied biomechanics in the horse based on the limited research into animal functional biomechanics and kinematics. This chapter does not address pure biomechanics, nor is it intended to replicate the theoretical basis of biomechanics or summarise current biomechanics literature and texts. The author's aim to direct the reader towards some of the applied principles of functional biomechanics in relation to animal physiotherapy assessment and treatment, based on evidence where possible.

An understanding of concepts of neuromotor control, musculoskeletal physiotherapy and rehabilitation is vital to the application of physiotherapy to animals. To enable the animal to achieve a complete functional sports-specific outcome through rehabilitation, the animal physiotherapist must be able to apply treatment techniques and management strategies based on an understanding of the mechanisms behind the cause of musculoskeletal injury in the cursorial mammal. Thus, animal physiotherapists require an understanding of each species' anatomy and biomechanics, as well as the requirements of the animal's sport. A working knowledge of the mechanical demands and constraints that animals operate under during locomotion is

---

*Adapted from the first edition chapter, which was written by Lesley Goff and Narelle Stubbs

Animal Physiotherapy: Assessment, Treatment and Rehabilitation of Animals, Second Edition. Edited by Catherine M. McGowan and Lesley Goff.
© 2016 John Wiley & Sons, Ltd. Published 2016 by John Wiley & Sons, Ltd.

essential to enable the clinician to assess the compensations, secondary neuromuscular and skeletal problems and pathology that ensue following failure of one or more elements. The reader is urged to review additional literature and texts referenced.

As outlined in Chapter 4, biomechanics refers to the application of mechanical principles in the study of living organisms. In that chapter, kinematics and locomotion are also described. This chapter will cover equine joint biomechanics and equine locomotion, and give examples of applied sports-specific biomechanics and biomechanics of the equine distal limb related to pathology.

5.2 Joint biomechanics

This section focuses on biomechanics related to individual joint motion in the horse, as joint movements indicate how the musculoskeletal system is working. Knowledge of the normal pattern and amount of movement allows the physiotherapist to detect abnormalities of movement (Lee 1995). The equine vertebral column joints will be addressed, followed by the equine peripheral joints.

The reader is encouraged to refer to the previous chapter's section 4.2 for a definition of movement of a joint and discussion of three-dimensional joint biomechanics. Definitions of joint stiffness and joint instability are covered in sections 4.2.1 and 4.2.2. Section 4.2.3 discusses clinical instability in the articular system and refers to research in the human, equine and canine fields.

5.3 Biomechanics of the equine vertebral joints

The aim of the section that follows is to summarise the functional anatomy of the articulations of the vertebral column in the horse, so that the physiotherapist may identify alterations in patterns of joint movement from the normal. In understanding the normal directions and planes of joint motion, the physiotherapist can apply passive movement tests during assessment, with a reasonable amount of accuracy. The reader is encouraged to refer to Chapter 4, section 4.2.1 for a description of the vertebral stabilising system and its subsystems; how the inclination of facet joints determines the movement at a given vertebral segment; how the relative thickness of intervertebral discs varies between species and may affect passive vertebral column mobility.

Knowledge regarding the morphology and kinematics of intervertebral joints or regions of joints has been determined in the horse via a series of *in vivo* research papers utilising reflective markers and Steinman pins implanted into vertebral levels to assess kinematics (Audigie *et al.* 1999; Faber *et al.* 2000; Zsoldos *et al.* 2010). A number of *in vitro* studies on kinematics have also provided some insight into equine vertebral and sacroiliac joint kinematics (Degueurce *et al.* 2004; Denoix 1999; Goff *et al.* 2006; Pagger *et al.* 2010; Townsend & Leach 1984). Studies using

dissection and imaging have documented some of the facet joint orientation in the vertebral column, and anatomical variations affecting vertebral bodies, articulations and spinous processes (Haussler *et al.* 1997; Stubbs *et al.* 2006).

5.3.1 Cervical spine (O/C1–7)
Atlantooccipital joint

This joint is a ginglymus formed by the concave articular surfaces of the atlas (C1) and the convex condyles of the occiput (Getty 1975). The main movement is flexion–extension, with small amounts of accessory axial rotation and lateral glide (Clayton & Townsend 1989; Getty 1975). The flexion–extension accounts for 32% of total dorsoventral movements of the cervical spine (Clayton & Townsend 1989). Clinical findings in the anaesthetised horse suggest that when the atlantooccipital joint is in extension, there may be a greater degree of accessory lateral flexion and rotation movements than when it is in flexion or neutral. This has not yet been documented.

Atlantoaxial joint

This joint is a pivot or trochoid joint formed between the articular surfaces of the atlas (C1) and corresponding saddle-shaped surfaces on the axis (C2), which extend upon the dens or odontoid process (Getty 1975). The main movement is rotation of the atlas and head upon the axis, with a small amount of accessory lateral flexion. Axial rotation here provides up to 73% of the total axial rotation of the cervical spine (Clayton & Townsend 1989).

C3–7

The articular surfaces of the cervical spine at these levels are planar, extensive and oval shaped, and oriented obliquely in the transverse plane. The orientation tends to be more transverse more caudally. The cranial articular processes face dorsomedially and the caudal articular processes face ventrolaterally (Mattoon *et al.* 2004) (Figure 5.1). Spinous process height increases caudally from C6. The main movements occurring

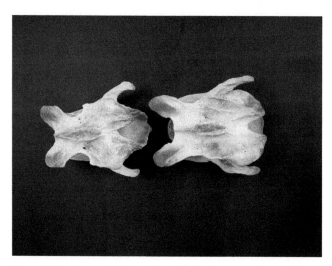

Figure 5.1 Equine cervical spine C3–4: dorsal view.

here are lateral flexion, with mean values of 25–45° for each joint except C1–2 which had mean lateral flexion of 3.9° (Clayton & Townsend 1989).

5.3.2 Cervicothoracic junction (C7–T1)

Due to the relative inaccessibility of the cervicothoracic junction, there is a paucity of information about kinematics of the articulation; however, this junction is a key area of neuromuscular and skeletal anatomy and function for locomotion. In a study by Clayton *et al.* (2012), which examined lateral bending movements of the horse's neck, performed via dynamic mobilisation exercises, the cranial and the caudal cervical spine were the areas of the horse's neck that shared most of the movement during lateral flexion. Santinelli *et al.* (2014) have identified anatomical variations at the equine cervicothoracic junction which are breed and sex dependent.

5.3.3 Thoracic spine (T1–18)

The caudal articular processes of the thoracic spine face ventrally and are placed at the base of the spinous process. The cranial articular processes are oval facets on the arch of the vertebra, which face dorsally. Each thoracic vertebra has a pair of costal facets on the dorsal body, except for the last thoracic vertebra, which only has cranial costal facets (Getty 1975) (Figure 5.2). The greatest amount of flexion in the thoracic spine occurs between T17 and T18 (and T18 and L1), with the least amount occurring in the region T3–9. The greatest extension occurs between T14 and T18, with the least between T2 and T9 (Denoix 1999).

Costovertebral and costotransverse joints

The head of the rib has two convex facets (cranial and caudal) that articulate with the two adjacent thoracic vertebrae. The first rib articulates with C7, T1 and the intervertebral disc. The tubercle of the rib articulates on the transverse process of the caudal vertebra of the adjacent thoracic pair. The movement at these

joints is rotation of the rib around an axis that connects the centre of the head and tubercle, and is greater in the caudal ribs (Getty 1975).

5.3.4 Lumbar spine (L1–6)

The cranial articular processes are fused with the mamillary processes and are concave dorsally, in a mostly sagittal alignment. The caudal articular processes are convex ventrally and correspond to the convexity of the cranial articular surfaces (Getty 1975). The main movements at the lumbar spine are flexion–extension, with lateral flexion and rotation almost non-existent, especially between L4–6, due to the presence of intertransverse joints (Denoix 1999).

Anatomical variation between equine thoracic and lumbar vertebrae

The bodies of thoracic vertebrae are short and are constricted in the middle (Getty 1975). The length of the tall, narrow thoracic spinous processes increases dramatically from T1 caudally to approximately T4 (the highest point of the withers), then diminishes gradually to approximately the anticlinal vertebrae, around T12–13. This is where the spinous processes become more vertically oriented before becoming angled in a cranial direction At T15, the spinous processes remain the same height. The transverse processes of the thoracic vertebrae are short and thick, and reduce in size and are placed more ventrally in the more caudal thoracic vertebrae (Dyce *et al.* 2002; Getty 1975).

The bodies of the lumbar vertebrae become wider and flatter caudally (Getty 1975). Lumbar transverse processes are dorsoventrally flattened and plate-like, and project the most laterally to L3, diminishing in lateral projection caudally (Figure 5.3) The two most caudal transverse processes curve cranially. L4, 5 and 6 (and S1) have articular facets on the transverse

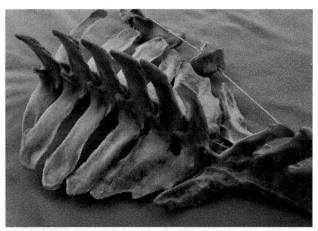

Figure 5.3 Equine lumbar vertebrae and lumbosacral junction showing the broad transverse processes of L1–6. There are fusions between the L5 and L6 transverse processes and pseudoarticulations at the transverse processes of L4 and L5, bilaterally. The lumbosacral divergence is at L6 and S1 in this specimen.

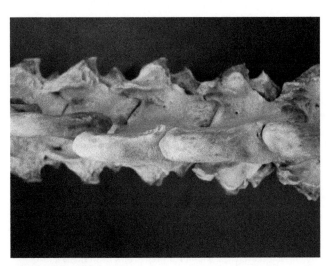

Figure 5.2 Orientation of equine thoracic spine articular facet: dorsal view.

processes – the intertransverse joints and these are thought to limit lateral flexion (Haussler *et al.* 1997). Haussler *et al.* (1997) have found that distribution of the intertransverse joints may be asymmetrical in some horses.

5.3.5 Lumbosacral and sacroiliac joint
Lumbosacral joint

The cranial articular processes of the first sacral vertebra are concave and face dorsomedially, for articulation with the caudal articular surfaces of the last lumbar vertebra (Getty 1975) (Figure 5.4). Few studies have investigated the control of intervertebral mobility in the horse. Due to instantaneous centre of rotation (ICR) location, lumbosacral (LS) dorsoventral motion is suggested to be an assimilated rotation around the centre of the more caudal vertebral body, as with the human (Denoix 1999; Panjabi *et al.* 1989). Lumbosacral dorsoventral motion is guided by intervertebral translation in the lateral part of the left and right intertransverse joints due to the cranial orientation of the L6–S1 transverse process (Denoix 1999). The vertebral body displacement is a result of coupled and accessory intervertebral motion, including translation and shearing movements within the intervertebral disc and greater tensile and compressive strain due to the thickness of the disc (Denoix 1987).

The largest motion in the equine thoracolumbar spine occurs at the LS junction in a sagittal plane (flexion–extension, *in vitro*) of up to 23.4° (Degueurce *et al.* 2004); however, Denoix (1987, 1999) reports measurements of ± 9–32° from L5 to S1 inclusive. This is thought to be due to the wide divergence of spinous processes; relative sagittal alignment of the facet joints; thickness and decreased height of the intervertebral disc compared with other vertebral levels (Denoix 1999); poorly developed interspinous ligament and absence of supraspinous ligament (Jeffcott & Dalin 1980); and the vertical orientation of the articular facets (Townsend & Leach 1984) (see Figure 5.3).

Variations in the numbers of thoracolumbar and lumbosacral vertebrae (vertebral formula) have been widely reported (Getty 1975; Haussler *et al.* 1997; Jeffcott 1979; Rooney 1969; Townsend 1987). In Thoroughbreds, it has been reported that only 61% have the normal vertebral formula (cervical 7, thoracic 18, lumbar 6, sacral 5, caudal vertebrae 15–21) (Haussler *et al.* 1997). Similarly, Stubbs *et al.* (2006) found that normal lumbosacral vertebral formula only existed in 67% of 120 horses examined. This occurred in 60% of Thoroughbreds (TB), 100% Standardbreds (SB) and 55% others (OB). In a study of 36 racehorses, Haussler *et al.* (1997) also reported that a transitional vertebra existed in over 20% of horses in the thoracolumbar region and in over a third of horses in the sacrocaudal region. The divergence of the spinous processes generally takes place between L6 and S1, but may occur between L5 and L6 (Denoix 1998; Haussler *et al.* 1997). A quantitative LS variation of the spinous process orientation relative to the vertebral body and relationship with breed in 120 horses has been reported by Stubbs *et al.* (2006). LS variations were found in a third of horses. In 8% of horses there were only five lumbar vertebrae and maximum dorsoventral motion was at L5–S1. Overall, 25% had the conventional L6–S1 formula, but with spinous process/vertebral orientation divergence of L5 cranially and L6 caudally, and interspinalis muscle between L5 and L6 (Figure 5.5). The divergence of the spinous processes between L5 and S1 may influence spinal mobility at the point of greatest dorsoventral motion and therefore affect performance and development of pathology in the LS region.

Lumbosacral movement is greater when the spine is in flexion rather than extension. Lateral flexion and rotation accessory movements are very small and are more likely to occur when the segment is in relative flexion (Denoix 1999). The high prevalence of L5–L6 spinal variations may have an effect on the

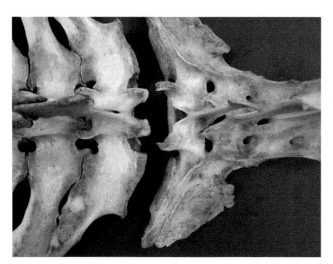

Figure 5.4 Equine caudal lumbar sacral spine disarticulated at the lumbosacral joint: dorsal view.

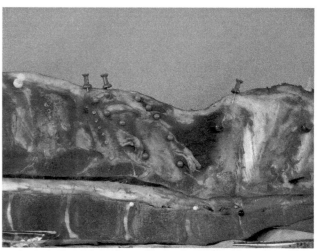

Figure 5.5 Variations in the number and orientation of the equine lumbar vertebrae exist, particularly at the lumbosacral junction. This horse demonstrates the common L5–6 divergence where L6 is orientated with the sacrum. Note the interspinalis muscle present only between the level of greatest divergence of spinous processes (here L5–6).

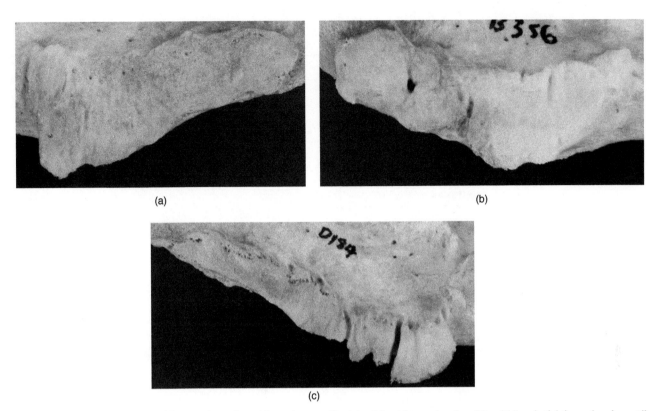

(a)

(b)

(c)

Figure 5.6 Variations in the shape of the articular surface of the equine sacroiliac joint: (a) a right sacral surface; (b) and (c) are both left sacral surfaces. All these joints were from Thoroughbred racehorses.

mobility in the LS region that may lead to altered function, performance and pathology.

Sacroiliac joint

As in the dog, the sacroiliac joint (SIJ) is responsible for transmission of forces from the hindlimb to the thoracolumbar vertebral column and forequarter. The equine SIJ has a synovial part and an interosseous part. The synovial part consists of 'L-shaped' articular surfaces on the ilium and the sacrum, although there are variations amongst horses in the shape of the joint (Figure 5.6) The interosseous part lies dorsocaudally to the synovial part and here the interosseous ligament connects the wings of the ilium to the sacrum. The plane of the synovial part of the joint is 30° to horizontal (Dalin & Jeffcott 1986).

Preliminary *in vitro* studies have revealed that the largest movement available at the equine SIJ is in the coronal plane, that is, a lateral movement of 2.56 ± 0.29° (Goff *et al.* 2006). This was measured during a lateral rotation, or movement of the pelvis on the fixed sacrum. Previously, Degueurce *et al.* (2004) had measured an average of just less than 1° of nutation at the sacrum, which is a rotational movement in the sagittal plane; however, these authors had not tested motion in lateral directions.

Note: rotation refers to the movement of the ventral aspect of the vertebral body, that is, left rotation involves movement of vertebral body to the left (relative movement of the spinous process to the right) (Denoix 1999).

5.3.6 Summary

There are many assumptions made regarding the contribution of facet joints, intervertebral discs and other structures to stability and/or movement of the vertebral column, based on morphology and observation. As some studies have shown, a given motion segment of the spine does not necessarily behave in the manner predicted by morphology. We can only be guided by the current knowledge of anatomy and morphology and the growing field of kinematics and motion analysis in the canine and equine vertebral columns.

5.4 Equine peripheral joints

Due to the interest in equine locomotion, there is a significantly larger bank of biomechanics research regarding the equine peripheral joints than for those of the canine, both relating to kinematics and forces about the joints during gait. Table 5.1 summarises the equine peripheral joints, but there are notes in the text, particularly regarding joint forces during gait. Two very comprehensive texts summarising a large portion of the current literature related to equine locomotion and biomechanics are Back & Clayton (2013) *Equine Locomotion*, and Hodgson *et al.* (2014) *The Athletic Horse*. These books may be a useful adjunct for those physiotherapists working with horses.

Table 5.1 A summary of the equine peripheral joints: joint type, articular surfaces, the primary motion of the joint and the accessory movements that occur at each complex

Joint	Joint type and articular surfaces	Main movement	Accessory movement
Glenohumeral	Spheroid, between the glenoid cavity of the scapula and the head of humerus, with the glenoid fossa on the scapula deepened by the glenoid labrum	Flexion and extension	Rotation and minimal ab/adduction
Elbow	Composite joint formed by the humeral condyle and the head of the radius (humeroradial joint) and the semilunar notch of the ulna (humeroulnar joint) – both simple hinge joints. Proximal radioulnar joint communicates with the main elbow joint – a simple pivot joint	Flexion–extension. No movement at proximal radioulnar joint	Minimal
Carpus	Composite joint made up of radiocarpal joint involving trochlea of radius and carpals (condylar); midcarpal joint involving proximal and distal carpal rows (condylar); carpometacarpal joint involving carpal bones II–IV and metacarpals II–IV (plane) and intercarpal joints involving carpals of the same row (plane)	Flexion–extension at radiocarpal (up to 90°); flexion–extension at midcarpal (up to 45°); carpometacarpal joint little planar motion; intercarpal joint little planar movement	Slight accessory rotation and lateral glide at radiocarpal joint
Metacarpophalangeal joint (fetlock)	Compound articulation between third metacarpal, proximal phalanx and proximal sesamoid bones – composite hinge joint	Flexion and extension	During flexion, small amounts of ab/adduction and axial rotation
Proximal interphalangeal joint (pastern)	Simple saddle joint between proximal and middle phalanx (forelimb and hindlimb)	Flexion and extension	Axial rotation and lateral movements
Distal interphalangeal joint (coffin joint)	Composite saddle joint between middle phalanx, distal phalanx, with hoof cartilage and navicular bone (forelimb and hindlimb)	Flexion and extension	Axial rotation and lateral movements
Coxofemoral joint (hip)	Composite spheroid joint, articulation between the femoral head and the acetabulum of the ilium, ischium and pubis. The acetabulum is deepened by a band of fibrocartilage on the rim of the acetabulum	Flexion and extension are the main movements	Multidirectional minimal abduction/adduction
Stifle	Complex joint, comprising the tibiofemoral joint (simple condylar) and the patellofemoral joint (simple, gliding joint). At the tibiofemoral joint, the convex femoral condyles articulate with the tibial condyles. The patellofemoral joint is between the patella and the trochlea of the femur	The main movements at the stifle are flexion–extension at the tibiofemoral joint, with the patella gliding in the trochlea during the movement	Tibiofemoral joint – at extreme extension there is accessory external rotation, and with flexion, accessory internal rotation
Tarsal joint (hock)	The hock complex includes the tarsocrural joint (simple cochlear joint), proximal and distal intertarsal joints, tarsometatarsal joint (composite plane joints) and intertarsal joints (perpendicular tight joints). The greatest amount of movement occurs at the tarsocrural joint	At the tarsocrural joint, flexion–extension. The intertarsal, proximal and distal tarsal (tarsometatarsal) joints undergo small amounts of translatory and rotatory movements during locomotion	At the tarsocrural joint, lateral and rotatory accessory movements
Metatarsophalangeal joint	See forelimb		
Proximal and distal interphalangeal joints	See forelimb		
Temporomandibular	A simple condylar joint which allows translatory movement, with an articular disc	Hinge – opening and closing	Lateromedial excursion; rostral glide of mandible with opening

Source: Adapted from Budras *et al.* 2001.

5.4.1 Scapulothoracic joint

The horse has no clavicle, so the thoracic limb is attached to the trunk via muscles – a *synsarcosis* (Budras *et al.* 2001), and also the dorsal scapular ligament. The movement of the shoulder on the thorax is rotation around a transverse axis passing through the scapula caudal to the dorsal part of the scapular spine (Getty 1975).

5.4.2 Glenohumeral joint

The glenohumeral articulation is formed between the distal end of the scapula (glenoid cavity) and the head of the humerus (Getty 1975). The main movement at the shoulder joint is flexion and extension. In stance, the angle between scapula and humerus is approximately 120°. There are some accessory rotatory movements, which have been noted when the stabilising muscles are removed. When the horse is not weight bearing on the limb, rotation can be achieved manually, but no motion measurements have been found in the literature (Getty 1975). This may implicate soft tissues such as the *lacertus fibrosus*, which may have a similar role to the dynamic stabilising muscles in the human.

The shoulder joint extends during most of the swing phase of walk, to ground contact and early stance phase (Hodson *et al.* 2000). During early stance phase, the shoulder flexes and then tends to maintain a constant angle during periods of bipedal support, and flexes slightly during tripedal support phase. At breakover, the shoulder flexes further. The shoulder has been described as acting as an energy damper during the stance phase of the walk, and also shows absorption of power during swing phase (Clayton *et al.* 2000).

5.4.3 Elbow

The elbow is a ginglymus between the distal trochlear surface of the humerus and the fovea of the proximal radius plus trochlear notch of the ulna (Getty 1975). The movements available are flexion and extension. In stance, the articular angle is 150°. There is little appreciable movement at the radioulnar joint, with the forearm being fixed in pronation (Getty 1975).

The elbow remains at a constant angle throughout the first 7% of walking stride, then, during breakover, which occurs between heel off (55% of stride) and lift off (64% of stride), it moves into flexion. The elbow shows a single flexion cycle during swing that elevates the distal limb during that phase. It reaches peak flexion at 84% of stride during swing phase (Hodson *et al.* 2000). The elbow shows net generation of energy to maintain the limb in extension during early stance phase and is the main joint of energy generation during walk gait in the forelimb (Clayton *et al.* 2000).

5.4.4 Carpus

There are three joints of the carpus:

- *antebrachiocarpal* (radiocarpal) joint (between the distal radius and ulna and proximal carpal row)

- *intercarpal* joint (between proximal and distal carpal rows)
- *carpometacarpal* joint (between distal carpal row and proximal ends of metacarpals).

The proximal and middle joints are ginglymi, but the distal joint is planar. The joints formed between the adjacent carpal bones of each row are also planar (Getty 1975). Main movement of the carpus as a whole is flexion–extension. With flexion, there is slight accessory rotation and lateral glide available. These movements occur mostly at the radiocarpal joint and intercarpal joints.

Just after initial ground contact during walking gait, the carpus rapidly assumes its close packed position between 7% and 12% of stride, to allow the limb to act like a propulsive strut through stance phase (Clayton *et al.* 2001; Hodson *et al.* 2000). The carpus then does not flex until breakover, with peak flexion occurring at 76% of stride. The carpus does not play an important role in energy absorption or generation during walking gait, but plays an active role in initiating breakover (Clayton *et al.* 2000).

5.4.5 Metacarpophalangeal joint

The fetlock, or metacarpophalangeal joint, is a ginglymus formed between the distal third metacarpal and the proximal end of the proximal phalanx. In stance, the joint is an extension angle of 140° (approximately 150° in the hind fetlock). The main movements at the fetlock are flexion–extension. During flexion, accessory movements of abduction, adduction and rotation can occur (Getty 1975).

The fetlock extends through the early stance phase of walk. Maximal extension occurs at around 34% of stride, when forces during gait change from braking to propulsive (Hodson *et al.* 2000). After this point, the fetlock flexes for the remainder of stance phase. It continues to flex during breakover, with peak flexion occurring at 82% of stride, during swing. The fetlock has been described as functioning elastically, as there is an initial absorption of energy during early stance and bursts of energy generation in late stance and during breakover. It shows bursts of energy absorption also during swing phase, at 86% of stride (Clayton *et al.* 2000).

5.4.6 Pastern joint and coffin joint (fore)

The pastern joint is the articulation of the proximal and middle phalanges and is classified as a ginglymus (Getty 1975). The joint is extended in stance. The main movement at the pastern joint is flexion–extension, which moves through 35° during the stance phase (Clayton *et al.* 2000). Accessory movements of medial and lateral flexion are available when the joint is flexed (Getty 1975).

The coffin joint is the articulation between the middle and distal phalanges and is in contact on the palmar aspect with the navicular (distal sesamoid) bone (Getty 1975). In stance, the joint is extended, and the main movements at the joint are flexion–extension. Accessory movements of lateral and medial flexion and rotation are available when the joint is in relative flexion (Getty 1975). Flexion–extension patterns in the pastern joint appear to mirror those of the coffin joint (Clayton *et al.* 2000). The pastern joint flexes for up to 10% of the stride (early stance) then reverses direction after this point. Flexion then occurs again during breakover and shows peak flexion during swing, at 84% of total stride (Hodson *et al.* 2000). The coffin joint has been described as an energy damper during stance, with a small amount of energy generation at the beginning of breakover (Clayton *et al.* 2000).

5.4.7 Coxofemoral (hip) joint

The coxofemoral joint is the articulation formed by the head of the femur and the deep ilial acetabulum bounded by a rim of fibrocartilage. Two ligaments, the ligament of the femoral head and the accessory ligament, limit internal rotation and abduction of the hip joint. Thus the main movements are primarily flexion and extension, which are responsible for protraction and retraction of the entire hindlimb during walking gait (Hodson *et al.* 2001). Maximal protraction occurs just before the end of swing phase and maximal retraction occurs at breakover. The hip joint is the main source of energy generation during stride, at the walk (Clayton 2001a).

5.4.8 Tibiofemoral and patellofemoral articulation (stifle)

The stifle is made up of the tibiofemoral and patellofemoral joints. The congruence of this tibiofemoral joint is enhanced by the menisci. The patella glides proximally and distally on the trochlea during tibiofemoral extension and flexion, respectively (Getty 1975).

In the standing position the articular angle is 150° (Getty 1975). The main movements at the tibiofemoral joint are flexion and extension, with the accessory translation of the tibia in a craniocaudal direction restricted by the cruciate ligaments (Clayton 2001a). At extreme extension, there is accessory external rotation, and with flexion, accessory internal rotation (Getty 1975).

At walk, during the initial 10% of stride, which is a period of rapid loading, the stifle joint flexes (Hodson *et al.* 2001). The stifle begins to flex further when the hindlimb is retracted beyond the midstance position, and flexion of stifle occurs with the swing phase and protraction of the limb, with the hock, which raises the distal limb. The stifle begins to extend in preparation for ground contact at about 80% of total stride.

The stifle joint absorbs equal amounts of energy in the stance and the swing phase of walk (Clayton 2001a).

5.4.9 Tarsocrural and tarsometatarsal joint (hock)

The hock is a composition of articulations, with most of the movement occurring at the most proximal joint, the tarsocrural joint, which is classified as a ginglymus (Getty 1975). In the standing position, the angle of the hock is approximately 150° (Getty 1975). The distal tibia rotates around the trochlea of the talus, allowing the main movement of flexion–extension

to occur, along with lateral and rotatory accessory movements. These articular surfaces are directed obliquely dorsal and laterally at an angle of 12–15° (Getty 1975).

The intertarsal and distal tarsal (tarsometatarsal) joints undergo small amounts of translatory and rotatory movements during locomotion. Clayton (2001b) presents some kinematic data on the movement at the distal tarsal joints, as this is most often the site of bone spavin. During the stance phase of walk, the cannon bone internally rotates at the distal joints and then slides cranially. This cranial slide becomes 'decoupled' in swing by the time the hock is flexed to 50°, and recouples later in swing as the joint reaches the same angle. During swing phase, at about 80% of stride, the hock reaches peak flexion along with the stifle (Hodson *et al.* 2001). After this, the hock extends in preparation for ground contact.

The hock joint assists the hips in generation of energy of stride during both stance and swing phases of walk (Clayton 2001b).

5.4.10 Metatarsophalangeal joint (hind)

During the initial 10% of walking stride, a period of rapid loading, the fetlock joint extends (Hodson *et al.* 2001).

5.4.11 Pastern joint/coffin joint (hind)

At 5% of stride (early stance phase), the coffin joint shows a peak in flexion. The coffin joint shows a peak in flexion at 80% of stride during swing phase. After this point, it extends in preparation for ground contact (Hodson *et al.* 2001).

The biomechanics of the fetlock, pastern and coffin joints in the hindlimb have been likened to those of the forelimb (Getty 1975).

5.4.12 Temporomandibular joint

The temporomandibular joint (TMJ) is a complex diarthrodial joint formed between the articular tubercles of the temporal bone and the condylar processes of the mandible. A fibrocartilagenous disc improves the congruency between the articular surfaces, and divides the joint into a dorsal and a ventral compartment (Baker 2002; Maierl *et al.* 2000; Moll & May 2002). The mandibular condyles are at an angle of 15° in a plane that runs laterocaudal to ventromedial and a plane that runs mediocaudal to laterorostral. TMJ movements are around a transverse axis. When the mouth opens, the mandibular condyle moves slightly in a rostral direction (Baker 2002).

5.4.13 Summary

Compared with the vertebral column, there has been little kinematic research carried out in the peripheral joints, particularly in the canine. In the equine, some data have been developed regarding forces and torques acting about the peripheral joints. As with the vertebral column, physiotherapists can only be guided by the current knowledge of anatomy and morphology and the growing field of kinematics and motion analysis in the canine and equine peripheral joints.

5.5 Biomechanics of equine locomotion

This section includes an overview of the equine anatomical and biomechanical adaptations which allow this animal to be energy efficient and travel at relatively high speeds over moderate distance, even though it is a large mass. The horse, like the dog, locates approximately 57% of body weight on the forelimbs at rest, with this load increasing during locomotion (Schamhardt 1998). However, the forelimbs of the horse have adapted to a primary support role, providing little propulsive force, while the hindlimb supports less weight but provides more propulsion (Wilson *et al.* 2000). To achieve this, the forelimbs act as energy-efficient springs, which store and release energy, decreasing the cost of locomotion. The structures that are biomechanically unique to equine locomotion are described below.

As the size of an animal doubles, the weight of the animal is cubed, yet the cross-sectional area of the limb musculature is only squared (Wilson *et al.* 2000). This means that in order to continue functioning, the animal must have grossly large muscle mass in the limbs to support the weight of the animal. To compensate for this, the horse has undergone many evolutionary adaptations to better meet the needs of a herbivorous quadruped while decreasing the cost of locomotion. These adaptations include an increase in the length of the limbs, restriction (via changed osteology) of the available range of movement in the limbs, and replacement of muscle tissue in the lower limbs with elastic tendons. This decreases the weight of the limb while increasing the capacity for energy storage, therefore decreasing the energy cost of locomotion. Muscles are located at the proximal end of the limb to reduce inertia, as the muscles are closer to joint centres of rotation (e.g. spinning ice skater extending his/her arms). This adaptation has also occurred in the Greyhound, which is bred to sprint. The Greyhound is a long-legged dog, with large proximal muscle mass and light distal limbs (Kemp *et al.* 2005).

There are mechanisms in the horse that increase the efficiency of locomotion as well as the efficiency of the horse's energy expenditure at rest. The unguligrade osseous formation of the limbs and the passive stay apparatus of the forelimbs and hindlimbs will be described here. The actions of these mechanisms during locomotion will be outlined further on in this section.

5.5.1 Biomechanical adaptions in equine anatomy
Distal limb adaptations
Due to the demand for faster, longer strides to enable the horse to survive as part of an effective protective flight response, the horse's distal limb has evolved from a digitigrade to an unguligrade osseous formation (Reilly *et al.* 2007). In unguligrade formation, there is one retained weight-bearing digit, which is the third metacarpal. Three metacarpals remain – the first and fifth have been lost. The elongated third metacarpal (or cannon bone) remains the sole weight-bearing metacarpal for the whole limb, with the vestigial second and fourth metacarpals (the medial and lateral splint bones respectively) functioning only to support the carpal bones. The long bone density of third metacarpal has a small spongy medullary cavity, leaving the slender shaft almost completely solid and more resistant to the compressive forces of locomotion. This provides maximal strength with minimal weight in the distal limb.

Proximal limb adaptations
The forelimbs of the horse lack a direct bony connection with the trunk. Instead, the forelimb/scapula complex and thorax are joined by an extensive composite of connective tissues (synsarcosis) rather than a bony articulation – the clavicle is absent and the coracoid process is fused to the scapula (Budras *et al.* 2001). The glenoid articulation faces cranioventrally rather than laterally due to the scapula being orientated in a lateral/vertical position. This scapular orientation is due to its position on the mediolaterally flattened thorax. This arrangement limits the range of shoulder motion due to its approximation with the trunk. In addition, the humerus has rotated medially, drawing the forearm into relative pronation, leaving the radius dominant in forearm weight bearing. These bony changes enable more efficient economy in locomotion in the forelimb, providing a more mechanically stable vertical limb alignment (Payne *et al.* 2004).

The trunk of the horse is suspended between the scapulae, cradled in a secure muscular sling (Goody 2011). This provides locomotive stability whilst allowing vertical and horizontal excursion of the thorax in relation to the limb, and providing absorption of vertical shock and horizontal propulsive forces The muscles that provide movement of the thorax in relation to the limb include the subclavius, serratus ventralis and rhomboid muscles (Goody 2011).

In the horse's limb, distal musculature has moved more proximally, reducing the forelimb moment of inertia. The proximal muscles have short fibres in a relatively short brachium providing proximal stability, while the antebrachium and distal arm have replaced muscle mass (weight) with long tendons spanning several joints and ligaments to minimise locomotive demand (Wilson *et al.* 2001a). Similar adaptations have occurred in the hindlimb.

The passive stay apparatus in the horse
The forelimb passive stay apparatus allows the horse to rest on its feet, and cope with the stance phase of locomotion, with minimal muscular effort. In the forelimb, it involves the synsarcosis and all the joints distal to the pastern joint, the suspensory apparatus and superficial and deep digital flexor tendons (SDFT and DDFT) (Budras *et al.* 2001). At the synsarcosis, the serratus ventralis is the principal weight-bearing connection and contains a large amount of tendinous tissue. The biceps tendon position relative to the cranial surface of the glenohumeral joint – in the intertubercular groove – has a stabilising role. The joint is further stabilised by the biceps tendon anchoring the muscle to the proximal radius, and via the lacertus fibrosus and extensor carpi

radialis (ECR), to the proximal third metatarsal. The weight of the trunk at the proximal scapula tenses the biceps–lacertus–ECR, causing relative extension at the elbow and the carpus.

The elbow is in turn further prevented from flexing by the carpal and digital flexors that arise from the epicondyles of the humerus. The carpus is stabilised by the ECR tendon. The attachment of flexor carpi ulnaris and ulnaris lateralis to the accessory carpal bone tends to keep the carpus extended. The fetlock is prevented from further extending by the suspensory apparatus that is associated with the interosseous tendon and the superficial and deep digital flexor tendons (SDFT and DDFT respectively).

The suspensory apparatus

The interosseous ligament arises from the carpus and the proximal third metacarpal and attaches to the proximal sesamoid bones. As it descends, it splits and sends extensor branches around the proximal phalanx to the common extensor tendon. Collateral ligaments attach the sesamoids to the metacarpal and proximal phalanx and a palmar ligament unites the sesamoids and forms a bearing surface for the flexor tendons. The tension in the interosseous ligament is carried distally by four sesamoidean ligaments.

The SDFT assists the suspensory apparatus via its accessory (check) ligament from the radius above the carpus to the proximal and middle phalanges. The DDFT and its check ligament provide additional support – this accessory ligament arises with the interosseous from the caudal aspect of the carpus and ends on the distal phalanx.

The suspensory apparatus acts to limit hyperextension at the metacarpophalangeal joint via the suspensory ligament, proximal sesamoidean ligaments, palmar ligaments and superior and inferior check ligaments. The deep and superficial flexor tendons act as high-tension cables to support the passive ligamentous restraints via a powerful flexion moment.

Specific hindlimb adaptations

The ability of the horse to prevent collapse of the hindlimb with minimal muscular effort involves the stifle-locking mechanism, the reciprocal apparatus/mechanism of stifle, hock and fetlock and the suspensory mechanism, which is similar to the forelimb.

Locking of the stifle is related to the larger medial ridge on the femoral trochlea, and its proximal tubercle, the patella and divergence of the intermediate and medial patellar ligaments. The medial trochlea sits in between these two patellar ligaments. The trochlear surface has two parts – the larger, gliding surface faces cranially and the smaller resting surface forms a narrow shelf above the gliding surface. Even in hindlimb weight bearing, the patella sits at the proximal end of the trochlea. When the horse rests a hindlimb, the patella on the supporting leg rotates medially about 15° and the medial patellar ligament slides caudally on the tubercle of the medial ridge, thus hooking the patella (via the parapatellar cartilage) on the tubercle, where it resists displacement. This converts the jointed column of the hindlimb

to a weight-bearing strut. A conscious contraction of the quadriceps is required to unlock the patella from the tubercle by laterally rotating the patella (Budras *et al.* 2001; Dyce *et al.* 2002).

The *reciprocal mechanism* is provided by the tendinous peroneus tertius and the SDFT. These pass between the distal end of the femur and the hock – the peroneus tertius arising from the lateral femoral condyle and passing cranially to the tibia to insert on tarsal bones and proximal metatarsal. the SDFT lying caudal to the tibia and connecting the caudal femur to the calcaneal tuber. This ensures that when flexion or extension of one joint occurs, it necessitates the same movement at the other (Budras *et al.* 2001; Dyce *et al.* 2002).

The fetlock and pastern joint are supported in a manner similar to the forelimb suspensory apparatus, but there are two differences in the arrangement. The accessory (check) ligament of the DDFT is thinner and the SDFT has no accessory ligament. The latter is compensated for by the tendon's strong attachment to the calcaneal tuber (Budras *et al.* 2001).

The legacy of adaptations

The lack of muscular protection and the weight-bearing demands on the distal limb create significant loads on the system of bone, tendon and ligament, with a narrow safety margin for tissue failure. Thus, the horse is predisposed to musculoskeletal injuries, especially in the distal forelimb. This is the most frequently injured site in horses of all types across all sports (Brown *et al.* 2003; Davies 2002; Dyson 2000). The extent and nature of compensation for injury reflect whether the injured structure is loaded more while absorbing energy and/or supporting the body or while actively moving the limb. Compensations become more difficult as the speed (racehorse) and vertical displacement (dressage horse) increase (Barrey & Biau 2002; Barrey *et al.* 2001; Clayton 1996) and the parameters that define superior performance in each case will show a measurable deficit.

5.6 Gait

Horses use and are trained to utilise many variations of the main gaits.

- At walk, the interlimb coordination changes with differing gaits, as defined by Wilson *et al.* (2000).
- Trot is a symmetrical, two-beat gait with the diagonal limb pairs moving synchronously and a short suspension phase between ground contacts of alternate diagonals.
- Pacing is a two-beat gait where unilateral forelimbs and hindlimbs move synchronously and there is a suspense phase between placements of the alternating pairs.
- Gallop is a four-beat asymmetrical gait where the forelimbs and hindlimbs work in two skipping pairs, with overlap between each limb contacting the ground. Therefore on a left lead, the foot placement would be right hind, left hind, right fore, left fore and suspension.

- Canter is a three-beat gait, with the same sequence of footfalls as the gallop but with the second hind and first fore leaving the ground at the same time.

The equine gait is manipulated by changing firstly the interlimb coordination, but also the timing of the phases of the gait cycle and the angulation of the joints. Weyland *et al.* (2000) showed that as the speed increases, from trot to gallop, the protraction or swing phase of the gait cycle actually remains the same. Instead, the time spent in stance decreases, and the force applied to the ground is larger; thus the time spent during stance can be represented as a fraction of the time for the stride of the limb, expressed as the duty factor. As the fraction gets smaller, that is, as the time in stance decreases, the force experienced by the limb increases. The maximum speed of the horse is limited by the minimum duty factor that can be sustained, that is, the maximum force that the legs can withstand. Start to relate these principles directly to the horse sports and therefore the type of lesion you would expect as you go through each applied biomechanical principle.

5.6.1 Stress and strain in gait

Training variables (e.g. gait, frequency, duration, surface type, hoof balance) load the limb in different ways (Clayton 2002). Stress is a measure of load per unit area. Strain is the length change due to the applied stress. The loading rate is determined by the speed and frequency of impact; thus gait is of primary importance in strain characteristics, and helps determine which structures are at maximum risk. Mechanisms are in place to cope with these different stressors, and improve the efficiency of locomotion. Impact forces are absorbed by the hoof, the suspensory apparatus, the digital flexor (DF) muscles and the shoulder synsarcosis (Payne *et al.* 2005b).

Sport-specific locomotion

The horse's ability to move at speed is not due to active muscle contraction alone (Brown *et al.* 2003; Wilson *et al.* 2003; Zarucco *et al.* 2004). The limbs rely on non-contractile structures to assist muscles by providing a passive role in joint stabilisation and elastic storage and release of energy. The biceps mechanism and suspensory apparatus of the distal forelimb, as described above, enable utilisation of stored elastic energy, reducing muscular energy expenditure and the weight of the distal limb (Dimery *et al.* 1986). The trade-off is a reduced capacity to make voluntary adjustments, thus placing tendons and passive soft tissues at risk (Schamhardt 1998). The superior check ligament, inferior check ligament and suspensory ligament combine to support more than 50% of the total moment developed about the metacarpophalangeal (MCP) joint in full extension in stance (Brown *et al.* 2003). These passive structures assist the superficial and deep digital flexor muscles to stabilise the MCP joint and provide assistance in propulsion into flexion of the joint at the completion of stance. The muscles themselves are relatively small and rely largely on a passive tendon and connective tissue contribution to support bodyweight. There is a linear relationship between speed and MCP joint angle (Brown *et al.* 2003), and passive structures are under greater load at higher speeds.

Wilson *et al.* (2003) described the biceps mechanism 'as a catapult that accelerates the protraction of the forelimb'. This is achieved by exploiting elastic potential energy, which is stored during stance phase as the biceps is stretched. This catapult action produces a peak power output of 2200 watts, rivalling a muscle 100 times the weight of the 0.4 kg biceps (Wilson *et al.* 2003). In a galloping horse, the biceps rapidly stretches up to 12 mm more than at the trot, releasing four times the energy.

Wilson *et al.* (2003) conclude that the biceps mechanism, through its substantial internal tendon elastic energy storage and release mechanism, is responsible for 80% of the shoulder extensor moment during limb protraction. The biceps internal tendon is stretched during limb retraction during stance, thus storing the energy required for the swing phase. The extension moment is dependent on energy storage and thus on speed, so is less effective in the slower paces. Thus, dressage horses are unable to recruit biceps in the same way to reduce the muscle demands of protraction.

Most of the length change in the distal forelimb muscle-tendon complex occurs passively as a result of the in-series arrangement and tissue properties of the elastic components, and not by concentric contraction of the DF muscles (Barrey *et al.* 2001). The DF muscles are 'tuned' by virtue of their short-fibred, deep heads to rapidly damp up to 88% of damaging vibrations (frequency 30–40 Hz) that transmit up the limb (Wilson *et al.* 2001a). Impact of this type is the most important factor in the development of degenerative joint disease, the most common cause of wastage in dressage horses (Clayton 1997).

The proximal spring, including the muscle-tendon units from the scapula to the elbow, has been shown to shorten by 12 mm during stance phase at gallop (McGuigan & Wilson 2003). The distal limb spring, from the elbow to the foot, in contrast shortens by 127 mm in stance at the gallop. These authors have sound evidence that the role of the proximal spring is to achieve a small tuning effect on the distal spring and to drive the distal spring. The role of the two units is to achieve shock absorption and energy storage and return to drive locomotion and, once again, is mainly a passive one.

The advantages of these passive stabilisation and propulsive mechanisms are two-fold during locomotion: (i) there is a reduced requirement for muscle contraction and therefore a significant energy saving; (ii) adjustments to higher speeds and thus higher loads can be done quickly and automatically without central nervous system input. It should be noted, however, that the efficiency of the passive mechanisms described reduces with decreasing speed to a point where at slow speed, e.g. walk and slow trot, the majority of moment production is performed actively by the muscles. Hence, there is a relatively greater energy demand at these slow gaits and while the passive structures are partly relieved of strain, the active muscle units and their associated structures are increasingly loaded. Consider the mechanisms involved in forelimb protraction as an example of the relationship between speed of gait and contributing mechanisms. Wilson *et al.* (2003) found that the catapult action of the biceps and internal tendon (passive action) contributed approximately 80% of the shoulder extensor moment at a 3 m/sec trot. The active concentric action of supraspinatus contributed the other 20%. The loss of the passive biceps catapult contribution would therefore have a huge impact on locomotion mechanics at slower speeds.

As previously stated, both Wilson *et al.* (2003) and Brown *et al.* (2003) report a linear relationship between speed of gait and MCP angle; as speed reduces, so does the angle of the MCP (preloading of passive structures), and the stance time increases. An increased stance time reduces peak ground reaction forces as the limb is loaded over a longer time period, thus reducing the stresses on the limb and reducing the likelihood of injury (Brown *et al.* 2003). A trot at 3 m/sec produces a forelimb stance time of 227 msec (milliseconds) (Holmstrom *et al.* 1995). The Piaffe movement of Grand Prix dressage horses, by comparison, has a speed of 0.09 m/sec and a forelimb stance time of 509 ms, more than twice the ground contact time at the trot (Holmstrom *et al.* 1995). Given the known linear relationship, it can be extrapolated that a significant quantity of passive elastic energy storage potential would be lost due to reduced elastic preloading and dampening of stored energy over time. Holmstrom *et al.* (1995) document the speed of the Passage movement at 1.7 m/sec with a forelimb stance time of 365 msec. This gait may also compromise passive mechanisms, and favour force production from active muscle contraction. Holmstrom *et al.* (1995) measured the hock extension angle during the Piaffe and concluded that due to reduced extension compared with other gaits, elastic strain energy may not be important in Piaffe.

At the quick end of the spectrum, a sprint horse may reach speeds of 20 m/sec, requiring very short stance time and greatly increasing peak limb force. McGuigan and Wilson (2003) report that it is stance time that drops with speed and that limb protraction time is relatively independent of the gait and speed of the horse. It is widely accepted (Batson *et al.* 2003; Brown *et al.* 2003; McGuigan & Wilson 2003) that it is due to high peak vertical forces producing hyperextension of the MCP joints that there is such a high rate of injury (50% of race horse injuries) to the superficial and deep flexor tendons, the superior and inferior check ligaments and the suspensory ligament, which are the predominant passive structures in the distal forelimb. Brown *et al.* (2003) calculated that the superior and inferior check ligaments and suspensory ligament combined supported more than 50% of the total isometric moment about the MCP joint at maximal extension. These are the soft tissue injuries of the galloper which obviously accompany the sequelae of bony injuries resulting from rapid overloading and overuse of unaccustomed structures.

5.7 Considerations in sport-specific pathology

5.7.1 Flat racing

Owing to the rapid protraction occurring repeatedly in the forelimbs in flat racing, there are large peak forces and extreme forelimb flexor tendon and ligament strains (Barrey *et al.* 2001; Wilson *et al.* 2003).

Racehorses utilise the passive energy output of the biceps catapult; therefore, owing to the high duty cycle, they are predisposed to the development of bicipital tendinitis and rupture. Musculotendinous injuries may first manifest as behavioural problems, refusal to stride out and slow training times, in addition to any of the classic signs of lameness such as unloading/head bobbing, altered gait parameters/asymmetry and inability to protract the limb. Latissimus dorsi and triceps brachii are required to contract from a lengthened position (Payne *et al.* 2004, 205a, b), producing powerful retraction to pull the body forward, and thus are at risk of injury.

Ground reaction forces on a single forelimb at gallop can reach 2.5 times the bodyweight, and MCP joint hyperextension can reach angles that almost parallel the ground (Schamhardt 1998). Stabilisation of the MCP joint is provided by the flexor tendons and ligaments (suspensory ligaments and superior and inferior check ligaments). The ligaments increase their contribution to stability as joint extension increases, up to a maximum of half of the total support at MCP joint maximum extension (Brown *et al.* 2003). Failure has been shown to occur *in vitro* at strains between 12% and 19.7%. Hyperextension of the fetlock at faster paces produces flexor tendon strains of between 5% and 10% (Barrey *et al.* 2001), with the SDFT experiencing double the strain of the DDFT (Brown *et al.* 2003; Dimery *et al.* 1986). Other investigators have measured tendon strains of 3% at walk, 6–8% at trot and 12–16% at gallop. Combined with surfaces that are too hard, too soft or too irregular, racehorses risk catastrophic tendon damage, and exhibit a high incidence of tendon, check and suspensory ligament injuries (Brown *et al.* 2003).

Davies (2002) studied the bones of maturing Thoroughbreds (2–3 years of age) whose bones undergo remodelling at a high rate. Remodelling alters the composition and lowers the mineral density (Davies 2002). Bone is a pseudoductile material with a relatively large elastic zone. Under ideal conditions, deformation is contained within the elastic zone and results in normal desirable adaptive hypertrophy. Galloping combines high stress (concussive load concentrated on a small surface area) applied at high rate (frequency with which the limb impacts the ground) (Davies 2002).

Flat racing imposes stress and strain of sufficient magnitude and rate to change the quality of bone from pseudoductile to brittle, increasing the risk of fatigue and catastrophic fractures (Davies 2002). Fast tracks and hard training surfaces have a high resistance and do not absorb impact forces well, increasing concussion and prolonging the attenuation time, and can lead to increased incidence of flexor tendinitis in racehorses.

Strain is defined as the change in length divided by the original length, and is measured at the dorsal mid-third of the forelimb cannon bone. Horses with third metacarpal pain will exhibit the signs of overtraining – loss of performance, appetite, behavioural problems, as well as palpable tenderness and swelling over the inflamed mid-third of the dorsal surface of the cannon bone.

Common racing injuries

- Concussive injuries – hoof/joint, flexor tendinitis, proximal suspensory desmitis
- Hyperextension of the fetlock – flexor tendon injuries/ rupture, suspensory ligament rupture
- Fractures – particularly of the carpus and third metacarpal (cannon)
- Shin soreness and fatigue fractures of the cannon
- Biceps tendinitis and rupture

Compensations

- Shin sore – refusal to stride out, slow training times
- Biceps tendinitis – reduced cranial phase; inability to protract the limb – increased recruitment of brachiocephalicus, asymmetry, head bobbing and leaning on the bit
- Suspensory apparatus – reduced weight-bearing phase and lateral unloading – unwillingness/refusal to lead on a particular leg, refusing to stride out, head bobbing/ crookedness

5.7.2 Dressage

Dressage training attempts to change the way horses carry themselves and interact with the ground, altering braking and propulsion characteristics, ultimately aiming to shift weight caudally to lighten and enable elevation of the forehand (Clayton 1996). Barrey & Biau (2002) analysed the characteristics of dressage as:

- exhibiting slow cadence-stride frequency and high regularity (similarity of acceleration patterns of each stride)
- large dorsoventral displacement (vertical movement)
- dorsoventral and longitudinal activity (power of the motion in vertical and longitudinal directions).

Thus dressage requires the horse to execute repetitive, controlled and powerful antigravity movement in all directions, forward, backward and lateral, and degrees of collection. Transitions between and within gaits require great muscular power, control and coordination (Barrey & Biau 2002) (Figure 5.7). The characteristics of dressage movement are as follows.

- Collection produces an increase in the upward acceleration and a decrease in the forward acceleration (Barrey & Biau 2002) – the hindlimbs apply a braking force to forward movement during Piaffe (Clayton 1996).
- There is a large range of motion at hock and at the elbow and carpus.
- Passage and Piaffe are characterised by a prolonged stride duration and slower stride frequency.
- Passage exhibits a higher longitudinal GRF in the hindlimb over the forelimb (Barrey & Biau 2002).
- There is repetitive concussive loading of limb joints.
- Front legs apply a braking force to forward movement during Piaffe.
- Circular and lateral movements are achieved by utilising the thoracic and pelvic muscular sling and adduction and abduction of the fore and hindlimb.

Vertical displacement at the trot is achieved through actively 'springing' off the ground via powerful concentric contractions of the propulsive muscles of the hindlimbs, flexors of the

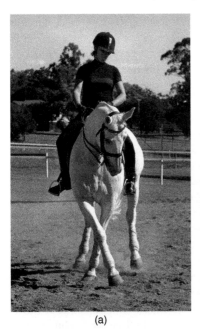 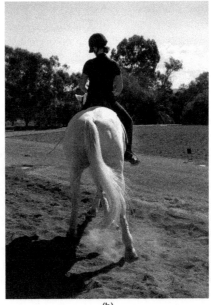 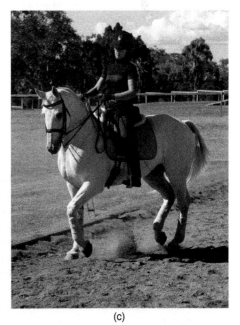

(a)   (b)   (c)

Figure 5.7 Dressage biomechanics.

distal forelimb, and utilising return of elastic energy in the flexor tendons. The increased impact loads apply repetitive concussive stresses to the joints of the fetlock, carpus, hock, stifle and pelvis (Barrey & Biau 2002) and place the flexor tendons and suspensory apparatus under strain. During slower versions of the trot, the reduced stretch on the flexor tendons (Robert et al. 2002) lessens their elastic energy storage and increases the antigravity workload, placing greater concentric demands on the muscles that move the forelimb. The muscles of the synsarcosis (e.g. serratus ventralis, pectorals) are required to dissipate repetitive ground reaction forces and more muscle activity is required to stabilise the spine (Robert et al. 2002).

Horses are trained to alter the temporal characteristics of the trot to produce the more collected variations of trot – the Passage and the Piaffe. Clayton has studied the temporal characteristics of the trot, Passage and Piaffe: the tempo remains the same but forward movement is converted into vertical motion, resulting in a longer period of suspension, greater ground reaction forces, increasing joint concussion. During the Passage, the hindlimb is primarily responsible for propulsion and the forelimbs act to brake forward motion and elevate the front end. The exception is Piaffe which requires the hindlimbs to 'brake' the forward movement while the front limbs propel (Clayton 1996).

Apart from the kinematic differences from the standard trot and gallop, dressage movements often require full collection (extreme flexion of the spine, in particular the upper cervical and lumbosacral spine), and exaggerated forelimb and hindlimb protraction, and flexion of the shoulder, elbow, carpus and fetlock joints, well beyond the normal locomotive functional range of these joints. The soft tissue structures commonly injured during galloping are mostly spared during this type of activity. Gibson et al. (1997) document the incidence of a galloper with a confirmed superficial digital flexor injury being unable to race but successfully competing injury free in dressage. The muscular physique of the top-level dressage athlete is a testament to the extreme muscle power and control requirements of the discipline.

The types of injuries experienced by the dressage athletes are expected to be in the proximal limbs and trunk due to the increased loading of unaccustomed muscles to somewhat unnatural movements. At the extremes of movement, e.g. at the height of forelimb protraction, the prime movers are working to produce slow-velocity movements with long, almost isometric holds at the end of range. Muscles prefer to work at a natural velocity within their most efficient length, which is usually close to their resting length. The brachiocephalicus becomes a prime mover in forelimb protraction in the Piaffe and Passage and it is forced to work in an extremely shortened position owing to collection of the neck and the extreme floating protraction of the forelimb. Working hard under these conditions is likely to cause muscle fatigue and strain. The isometric nature of the trunk postural muscles stabilising the spine while suspending the limbs in a slow temporal environment may cause local ischaemia and hasten fatigue, and cause compensations.

The repetitive nature of dressage training predisposes to overuse injuries, with acute traumatic injuries rare (Ross & Dyson 2003). Impact loading can induce fatigue fractures of the metacarpals and degenerative joint disease (Clayton 1996; Ross & Dyson 2003). There is an increased demand on range of motion at the elbow and carpal joints, and on antigravity and digital flexor muscle activity (dampening of vibration). Common soft tissue injuries involve the suspensory apparatus (e.g. proximal suspensory desmitis) and superficial digital flexor tendinitis (Clayton 2002).

Compensations

- Injured dressage horses lose rhythm, elevation and regularity, altering the swing phase of protraction and the flight path of the distal limb.
- Injury to the biceps mechanism compromises efficient shoulder extension and forelimb protraction – substitutes with increased activation of cervical trapezius/rhomboids, brachiocephalicus, brachialis and supraspinatus.
- Painful joints and inflamed flexor tendons and/or suspensory ligaments may cause the horse to shift weight to one side, lift the head, become unwilling to lead on a particular leg, or carry the rider on the affected diagonal in an attempt to reduce the vertical GRF (Clayton 1996; Ross & Dyson 2003).
- The horse reduces impulsion, and the digital flexors work harder to damp the shock of impact.
- Loss of range of motion at elbow and carpus reduces flexion of forelimb joints, altering the height and flight and destroying the expression of the movement.
- Back pain and appendicular joint injuries are adversely affected by torsion – the horse avoids performing lateral movements and moves asymmetrically (Ross & Dyson 2003).
- Back pain – the horse will hollow the back to avoid collecting and/or engaging the hindquarters.

Compensations to injury to the limbs are well documented. Wilson et al. (2001c) describe an early unloading of the heel onto the toe in early stance in horses with navicular pain. Weishaupt et al. (2004) measured a 15% reduction in vertical impulse in the lame limb by shifting load to the diagonal limb and by prolonging the stance time. Buchner et al. (2003) found a 34% reduction in vertical displacement and a 9 mm rearward shift of the body centre of mass in mid-stance in forelimb lameness. Buchner et al. (1996) found a significant reduction in fetlock extension in stance on the lame forelimb and increased shoulder flexion and retraction of the lame forelimb.

The common message from these studies is that the proximal joints act as load dampers to reduce peak forces in the lame forelimb, and compensations are made to avoid overloading of non-lame limbs. A well-recognised compensation for forelimb lameness is a rising of the head during the stance phase on the lame limb. This phenomenon tends to shift the centre of gravity caudally and thus relieves the weight from the forelimbs (Back et al. 1993). Perhaps the most obvious compensation to injury and pain is the refusal to perform for the rider, or uncharacteristic behavioural signs such as bucking, propping and running off. While these signs are indicative of a problem, the problem area may be anywhere from the spine to the foot.

Identification of an injury would involve the same assessment whether in a galloper or a dressage horse, but the fundamentals of the functional and biomechanical requirements of the individual disciplines are important as an adjunct to understanding the mechanisms of injury and how to prevent them from occurring. Further discussion of equine performance and sport injury management is provided in Chapter 21.

5.8 Biomechanics of the equine foot

It is beyond the scope of this chapter to describe equine hoof biomechanics and locomotive-related pathology in detail. But it is vital that physiotherapists have an in-depth knowledge of the equine foot and work closely with the treating veterinarian and farrier. Recognised as causing equine forelimb lameness for over a century, pathologies such as navicular disease and laminitis are complex acute–chronic conditions seen in riding and retired horses of all disciplines. On reviewing the vast amount of literature available, the necessity for understanding foot biomechanics and the pathogenesis both from a musculoskeletal and medicine perspective is evident. Gaining an accurate equine veterinarian differential diagnosis is essential as many other foot ailments have similar clinical signs, thus confusing the issue. Beneficial disease management includes farriery, once the possible aetiology or causations are understood.

Navicular disease is used here as an example. (This information is summarised from the following literature sources: Eliasher *et al.* 2002; McGuigan & Wilson 2001; Ostblom *et al.* 1982; Pardoe *et al.* 2001; Pool *et al.* 1989; Stashak 1987; Wilson *et al.* 2001b, c; Wright & Douglas 1993.)

Anatomically, the navicular or sesamoid bone at the back of the foot, beneath the frog, acts like a pulley, anchored/supported by the sesamoidean ligaments. Wrapping around it is the deep digital flexor tendon (DDFT) inserting into the pedal bone (distal phalanx), which is protected by the navicular bursa. The distal interphalangeal joint (coffin joint) also lies in close proximity. The navicular bone has two biomechanical functions and any alteration to these may predispose the animal to this multifactorial condition.

1 It provides a constant angle to maintain mechanical advantage for insertion of the DDFT like a fulcrum/pulley system.
2 It is an anticussion device, aiding shock absorption, with concussion being a definitive predisposing disease factor.

The navicular bone transmits a portion of the weight from proximal to the middle phalanx, with navicular pressure increasing further as it is forced against the DDFT/bursa as the bodyweight passes over the limb. Force alterations may be a vital factor in the disease process causing degenerative changes over time, along with bursitis, which in turn leads to hyperthermia and alteration of the flexor surface of the bone.

Research-based evidence now confirms that abnormal mechanical overload of the navicular bone results in gait changes and possibly the early or late disease stages; shifting leg lameness, shortened stride and the toe on the ground. The disease-associated gait is a vicious cycle resulting in a positive feedback loop, as the horse attempts to unload the heels and avoid pain by contraction of the deep digital flexor (DDF) muscle. Unfortunately, this increases the peak stress/force on the navicular (double compared with normal). Regional analgesia of the palmar digital nerves (nerve block) confirms this by causing a lowered compressive force.

A narrow, small, boxy, upright foot may not be the initial cause but further exacerbates the condition and may be a result of the disease. A flat foot, long toe, low collapsed heels, and broken back foot/hoof pastern axis is a proven predisposing factor, stretching the DDFT and hence increasing forces. The broken back foot pastern axis prolongs the breakover time, just before the heel leaves the ground (normal peak around 85% of stance) and increases toe-first contact, increasing forces through the navicular. The distal interphalangeal (DIP) joint position is then in permanent extension, causing greater tensile forces on the DDFT and ligaments and stress/concussive force on the navicular. Logically, then, poorly conformed and trimmed horses in work on hard surfaces are particularly liable to undergo mechanical changes.

As a result of the mechanical loading, there is an irreversible high rate of bone remodelling (turnover) and erosion of navicular fibrocartilage surface in contact with the DDFT in the central portion, reflecting ageing degeneration and adhesions of the DDFT. As a result, blood vessels in the navicular bone increase. Radiographs and bone scans in the advanced stages often show bony erosions, distal sesamoidean ligament ossification and arthritis of the coffin joint, with the DDFT becoming progressively destroyed. This identifies a possible endpoint for a variety of heel-related conditions.

Biomechanical corrective farriery attempts to normalise navicular forces at breakover, and reduce surrounding forces for pain relief and functional improvement. A reduction in the angle of deviation of the DDFT around the navicular bone can occur by elevating the heels, hence the heels leaving the ground earlier. Foot balancing reestablishes the correct anatomical relationship of the foot/pastern axis (ideally a straight line parallel to the hoof wall) and enables the foot to strike the ground level in relation to individual skeletal conformation, accurately assessed on X-ray. Also important is the medial/lateral hoof balance with hoof walls the same height and an imaginary line bisecting the frog–sole, with heels equidistant from the coronary band. Foot balancing ensures that the centre of rotation of the DIP joint falls on the midpoint of the bearing surface.

Other temporary remedial farriery includes raising the heel, shortening the toe or leaving the heels long. Increasing the thickness of the shoe from toe to heel by a tapered wedge with the bearing surface extending beyond the heels reduces DDFT tension and tensile navicular load, although it may delay the breakover and load the heels. But lowering the heels and allowing for the wedge (correct foot/pastern axis) encourages foot expansion, reducing vertical impact forces. Although more controversial (because of increased overall navicular pressure), a measure for horses with collapsed heels is the Eggbar shoe. This is often combined with a rolled toe or tapered wedge. Improved weight distribution can occur by extending the ground-contact surface, helping to reestablish a suitable heel for future support. Long-term use of heel wedges or Eggbar shoes is not advised as the vicious navicular cycle may recommence or it may be difficult to stop using them.

5.9 Conclusion

Knowledge of the concepts of functional biomechanics of animals from the orientation and movements available at individual joints, to the way in which movement differs between conformation breeds and between sports, will assist the animal physiotherapist in achieving the best outcome for performance in an animal.

References

Audigie, F., Pourcelot, P., Degueurce, C., *et al.* 1999, Kinematics of the equine back: flexion–extension movements in sound trotting horses. *Equine Vet. J.* 30(suppl): 210–213.

Back, W., Clayton, H. 2013, *Equine Locomotion*, 2nd edn. Saunders, Philadelphia, PA.

Back, W., Barneveld, A., van Weeren, P.R. 1993, Kinematic gait analysis in equine carpal lameness. *Acta Anatom.* 146(2/3): 86–89.

Baker, G. 2002, Equine temporomandibular joint (TMJ): morphology, function and clinical disease. *AAEP Proc.* 48, 442–447.

Barrey, E., Biau, S. 2002, Locomotion of dressage horses. In: Lindner, A. (ed.) *The Elite Dressage and Three Day Event Horse, Conference on Equine Sports Medicine and Science*, pp. 17–32.

Barrey, E., Evans, S.E., Evans, D.L., *et al.* 2001, Locomotion evaluation for racing in Thoroughbreds. *Equine Vet. J.* 33(suppl): 99–103.

Batson, E.L., Paramour, R.J., Smith, T.J., *et al.* 2003, Are the material properties and matrix composition of equine flexor and extensor tendons determined by their functions? *Equine Vet. J.* 35(3): 314–318.

Brown, N.A.T., Pandy, M.G., Kawcak, C.E., *et al.* 2003, Force- and moment generating capacities of muscles in the distal forelimb of the horse. *J. Anat.* 203, 101–113.

Buchner, H.H.F., Savelberg, H.H.C.M., Schamhardt, H., *et al.* 1996, Limb movement adaptations in horses with experimentally induced fore- or hindlimb lameness. *Equine Vet. J.* 28(1): 63–70.

Buchner, H.H.F., Obermuller, S., Scheidl, M. 2003, Load distribution in equine lameness: a centre of mass analysis at the walk and the trot. *Pferdeheilkunde* 19(5): 491–499.

Budras, K., Sack, W., Rock, S. 2001, In: *Anatomy of the Horse: An Illustrated Text*, 3rd edn. Iowa State University Press, Iowa City, IA.

Clayton, H. 2001a, Anatomy and biomechanics of the coxofemoral joint and stifle joints. Proceedings of the 7th Congress of Equine Medicine and Surgery, Geneva, Switzerland.

Clayton, H. 2001b, A new look at the hock. Proceedings of the 7th Congress of Equine Medicine and Surgery, Geneva, Switzerland.

Clayton, H., Townsend, H. 1989, Kinematics of the cervical spine of the adult horse. *Equine Vet. J.* 21(3): 189–192.

Clayton, H., Hodson, E., Lanovaz, J. 2000, The forelimb in walking horses: 2. Net joint moments and powers. *Equine Vet. J.* 32(4): 295–300.

Clayton, H., Hodson, E., Lanovaz, J., *et al.* 2001, The forelimb in walking horses: 2. Net joint moments and joint powers. *Equine Vet. J.* 33, 44–48.

Clayton, H., Kaiser, L., Lavagnino, M., *et al.* 2012, Evaluation of intersegmental vertebral motion during performance of dynamic mobilization exercises in cervical lateral bending in horses. *Am. J. Vet. Res.* 73(8): 1153–1159.

Clayton, H.M. 1996, Time-motion analysis in the sport of dressage. *Pferdeheilkunde* 12(4): 671–678.

Clayton, H.M. 1997, Biomechanics of the horse. McPhail Chair Presentations, USDF Convention, December 6.

Clayton, H.M. 2002, The optimal surface for training and competing. In: Lindner, A. (ed.), *The Elite Dressage and Three Day Event Horse, Conference on Equine Sports Medicine and Science*, pp. 33–42.

Dalin, G., Jeffcott, L. 1986, Sacroiliac joint of the horse 1. Gross morphology. *Anat. Hist. Embryol.* 15, 80–94.

Davies, H.M.S. 2002, Monitoring soundness in sport horses. In: Linder, A. (ed.) *The Elite Dressage and Three Day Event Horse, Conference on Equine Sports Medicine and Science*, pp. 109–114.

Degueurce, C., Chateau, H., Denoix, J-M. 2004, *In vitro* assessment of movements of the sacroiliac joint in the horse. *Equine Vet. J.* 36(8): 694–698.

Denoix, J.M. 1987, Kinematics of the thoracolumbar spine in the horse during dorsoventral movements, a preliminary report. *Equine Exercise Physiology 2*. ICEEP Publications, Davis, CA, pp. 607–614.

Denoix, J.M. 1998, Diagnosis of the cause of back pain in horses. *Conference on Equine Sports Medicine and Science*, pp. 97–110.

Denoix, J.M. 1999, Spinal biomechanics and functional anatomy. *Vet. Clin. North Am. Equine Pract.* 15(1): 27–60.

Dimery, N.J., Alexander, R.M., Ker, R.F. 1986, Elastic extension of leg tendons in the locomotion of horses (*Equus caballus*). *J. Zool. Lond.* 210, 415–425.

Dyce, K.M., Sack, W.O., Wensing, C.J.G. 2002, *Textbook of Veterinary Anatomy*, 3rd edn. Saunders, Philadelphia, PA.

Dyson, S. 2000, Lameness and poor performance in the sports horse: dressage, show jumping and horsetrials (eventing). *AAEP Proc* 46, 308–315.

Eliasher, E., McGuigan, M.P., Rogers, K.A., *et al.* 2002, The effect of shoe position to the toe on the kinetics of breakover during trot locomotion in sound horses. *Equine Vet. J.* 34, 184–190.

Faber, M., Schamhardt, H., van Weeren, R., *et al.* 2000, Basic threedimensional kinematics of the vertebral column of horses walking on a treadmill. *Am. J. Vet. Res.* 61(4): 399–406.

Getty, R. (ed.). 1975, *Sisson and Grossman's The Anatomy of the Domestic Animals*, vol. 1, 5th edn. WB Saunders, London, pp. 281–379.

Gibson, K.T., Burbidge, H.M., Anderson, B.H. 1997, Tendonitis of the branches of insertion of the superficial digital flexor tendon in horses. *Aust. Vet. J.* 75, 253–256.

Goff, L.M., Jasiewicz, J.M., Condie, P., *et al.* 2006, Preliminary studies to investigate *in vivo* and *in vitro* sacroiliac movement in the horse. *Equine Vet. J.* 36(suppl): 457–461.

Goody, P. 2011, *Horse Anatomy – A Pictorial Approach to Equine Structure*, 2nd edn. J.A. Allen, London, p. 44

Haussler, K., Stover, S., Willits, N. 1997, Developmental variation in lumbosacropelvic anatomy of Thoroughbred racehorses. *Am. J. Vet. Res.* 58(10): 1083–1091.

Hodgson, D.R., McGowan, C.M., McKeever, K. 2014, *The Athletic Horse*, 2nd edn. Saunders, Philadelphia, PA.

Hodson, E., Clayton, H., Lanovaz, J. 2000, The forelimb in walking horses: 1. Kinematics and ground reaction forces. *Equine Vet. J.* 32(4): 287–294.

Hodson, E., Clayton, H., Lanovaz, J. 2001, The hindlimb in walking horses: 1. Kinematics and ground reaction forces. *Equine Vet. J.* 33(1): 38–43.

Holmstrom, M., Fredricson, I., Drevemo, S. 1995, Biokinematic effects of collection on the trotting gaits in the elite dressage horse. *Equine Vet. J.* 27(4): 281–287.

Jeffcott, L.B. 1979, Back problems in the horse – a look at past, present and future progress. *Equine Vet. J.* 11(3): 129–136.

Jeffcott, L.B., Dalin, G. 1980, Natural rigidity of the horse's backbone. *Equine Vet. J.* 12, 101.

Kemp T.J., Bachus, K.N., Nairn, J.A., *et al.* 2005, Functional trade-offs in the limb bones of dogs selected for running versus fighting. *J. Exp. Biol.* 208(18): 3475–3482.

Lee, M. 1995, Biomechanics of joint movements. In: Refshauge, K., Gass, L. (eds), *Musculoskeletal Physiotherapy – Clinical Science and Practice*. Butterworth Heinemann, Oxford, pp. 19–23.

Maierl, J., Weller, R., Zechmeister, R., *et al.* 2000, Arthroscopic anatomy of the equine temporomandibular joint. *Pol. J. Vet. Sci.* 3(suppl): 28.

Mattoon, J., Drost, T., Grguruic, M., *et al.* 2004, Technique for equine cervical articular process joint injection. *Vet. Radiol. Ultrasound.* 45(3): 238–240.

McGuigan, M.P., Wilson, A.M. 2001, The effect of bilateral palmar digital nerve analgesia on the compressive force experienced by the navicular bone in horses with navicular syndrome. *Equine Vet. J.* 33, 166–171.

McGuigan, M.P., Wilson, A.M. 2003, The effect of gait and digital flexor muscle activation on limb compliance in the forelimb of the horse *Equus caballus. Eur. J. Morphol.* 206, 1325–1336.

Moll, H., May, K. 2002, A review of conditions of the equine temporomandibular joint. *AAEP Proc.* 48, 240–243.

Ostblom, L., Lund, C., Melsen, F. 1982, Histological study of navicular bone disease. *Equine Vet. J.* 14, 199–202.

Pagger, H., Schmidburg, I., Peham, C. *et al.* 2010, Determination of the stiffness of the equine cervical spine. *Vet. J.* 186 (3): 338–341.

Panjabi, M.M., Abumi, K., Duranceau, J., *et al.* 1989, Spinal stability and intersegmental muscle forces: a biomechanical model. *Spine* 14(2): 194–200.

Pardoe, C.H., McGuigan, M.P., Wilson, A.M. 2001, The effect of shoe material on the kinetics and kinematics of foot slip at impact using concrete topped forceplate. *Equine Vet. J.* 33(suppl): 70–73.

Payne R.C., Watson, J., Hutchinson, J.R., *et al.* 2004, Functional specialisation of the thoracic and pelvic limb in horses. *Integr. Comp. Biol.* 44(6): 736–736.

Payne, R.C., Hutchinson, J.R., Robilliard, J.J., *et al.* 2005a, Functional specialisation of pelvic limb anatomy in horses (*Equus caballus*). *J. Anat.* 206(6): 557–574.

Payne, R.C., Veenman, P., Wilson, A.M. 2005b, The role of the extrinsic thoracic limb muscles in equine locomotion. *J. Anat.* 206(2): 193–204.

Pool, P.R., Meagher, D.M., Stover, S.M. 1989, Pathophysiology of navicular syndrome. *Vet. Clin. North Am. Equine Pract.* 5, 109–129.

Reilly, S., McElroy, E., Biknevicius, A. 2007, Posture, gait and the ecological relevance of locomotor costs and energy-saving mechanisms in tetrapods. *Zoology* 110(40): 271–289.

Robert, C., Valette, J.P., Denoix, J.M. 2002, The effects of velocity on muscle activity at the trot. In: Lindner, A. (ed.) *The Elite Dressage and Three Day Event Horse, Conference on Equine Sports Medicine and Science*, pp. 189–198.

Rooney, J.R. 1969, Congenital equine scoliosis and lordosis. *Clin. Orthop.* 62, 25.

Ross, M.W., Dyson, S.J. (eds) 2003, Lameness in the sport horse. In: *Diagnosis and Management of Lameness in the Horse*. Elsevier Saunders, Philadelphia, PA.

Santinelli, I., Beccati, F., Arcelli, R., *et al.* 2014 Anatomical variation of the spinous and transvers processes in the caudal cervical vertebrae and the first thoracic vertebra in horses. *Equine Vet. J.* Dec 4. Doi: 10.1111/evj.12397

Schamhardt, H.C. 1998, The mechanics of quadruped locomotion. How is the body propelled by muscles? *Eur. J. Morphol.* 36, 270–271.

Stashak, T.S. 1987, Navicular disease. In: Stashak, T.S. (ed.), *Adams' Lameness in Horses*, 4th edn. Williams and Wilkins, Philadelphia, PA.

Stubbs, N.C., Hodges, P.W., Jeffcott, L.B., *et al.* 2006, Functional anatomy of the thoracolumbar and lumbosacral spine in the horse. *Equine Vet. J.* 36(suppl): 393–399.

Townsend, H. 1987, Pathogenesis of back pain in the horse. *Equine Sports Med.* 6, 29–32.

Townsend, H., Leach, D. 1984, Relationship between intervertebral joint morphology and mobility in the equine thoracolumbar spine. *Equine Vet. J.* 16(5): 461–465.

Weishaupt, M.A., Wiestener, T., Hogg, H.P., *et al.* 2004, Compensatory load redistribution of horses with induced weight bearing hindlimb lameness trotting on a treadmill. *Equine Vet. J.* 36(8): 727–733.

Weyland, P.G., Sternlight, D.B., Bellizzi, M.J., *et al.* 2000, Faster top running speeds are achieved with greater ground forces not more rapid leg movements. *J. Appl. Physiol.* 89, 1991–1999.

Wilson, A.M., van den Bogert, A.J., McGuigan, M.P. 2000, Optimisation of the muscle–tendon unit for economical locomotion in cursorial animals. In: Herzog, W. (ed.), *Skeletal Muscle Mechanics: From Mechanisms to Function*. Wiley, New York, pp. 517–547.

Wilson, A.M., McGuigan, M.P., Van den Bogert, S.A. 2001a, Horses damp the spring in their step. *Nature* 414, 895–898.

Wilson, A.M., McGuigan, M.P., Pardoe, C. 2001b, The biomechanical effect of wedged, eggbar and extension shoes in sound and lame horses. *AAEP Proc.* 47, 339–343.

Wilson, A.M., McGuigan, M.P., Fouracre, L., *et al.* 2001c, The force and contact stress on the navicular bone during trot locomotion in sound horses and horses with navicular disease. *Equine Vet. J.* 33, 159–165.

Wilson, A.M., Watson, J,C., Lichtwark, G.A. 2003, Biomechanics: a catapult action for rapid limb protraction. *Nature* 421, 35–36.

Wright, I.M., Douglas, J. 1993, Biomechanical considerations in the treatment of navicular disease. *Vet. Rec.* 135(5): 109–114.

Zarucco, L., Taylor, K.T., Stover, S.M. 2004, Determination of muscle architecture and fiber characteristics of the superficial and deep digital flexor muscles in the forelimbs of adult horses. *Am. J. Vet. Res.* 65(6): 819–828.

Zsoldos, R., Groesel, M, Kotschwar, A. *et al.* 2010, A preliminary modelling study on the equine cervical spine with inverse kinematics at the walk. *Equine Vet. J.* 38(suppl): 516–522.

Further reading

Back, W., Clayton, H.M. (eds) 2013, *Equine Locomotion*, 2nd edn. Saunders, Philadelphia, PA.

Hodgson, D.R., McGowan, C.M., McKeever, K. 2014, *The Athletic Horse: The Principles and Practice of Equine Sports Medicine*, 2nd edn. Saunders, Philadelphia, PA.

CHAPTER 6

Comparative exercise physiology

Catherine M. McGowan[1] and Brian Hampson[2]

[1] University of Liverpool, Liverpool, UK
[2] Sunshine Coast Equine Podiatry, Valdora, Australia

Summary

The aim of this chapter is to discuss principles of exercise physiology and to familiarise the physiotherapist with some of the sports their animal patients may undertake. The principles of training programmes in horses and athletic dogs are also covered.

6.1 Introduction

The aim of this chapter is to discuss principles of exercise physiology and to familiarise the physiotherapist with some of the sports their animal patients will be undertaking. The chapter presumes a basic understanding of the physiology of exercise in people, and aims to expand on knowledge of animal exercise physiology so that physiotherapists can more appropriately develop rehabilitation and exercise programmes for their animal patients.

The physiology of exercise in animals is similar in physiological principles to humans and much of the research work in man has been and is still carried out on animals for the purposes of enhancing knowledge for human exercise physiologists. However, certain differences clearly occur that can have clinical significance and may affect exercise potential. Of course, animals

Animal Physiotherapy: Assessment, Treatment and Rehabilitation of Animals, Second Edition. Edited by Catherine M. McGowan and Lesley Goff.

are quadrupeds, but other factors can be equally important, such as the inability of horses to mouth breathe and the fact that dogs only sweat in localised regions of their body.

For species-specific exercise physiology in animals, the greatest amount of research and knowledge has centred on the athletic horse, although this is gradually changing. Despite the advancements in research and clinical application of exercise physiology principles in animals, it may still surprise the physiotherapist used to working in a human sports setting to see how limited the translation of this knowledge is at the sporting industry level.

6.2 Principles of exercise physiology

6.2.1 Energy production for exercise

It is clearly the aim of trainers of performance animals to maximise the animal's capacity for exercise. In simplest terms, this means maximising the availability of energy for muscle contraction, in the form of adenosine triphosphate (ATP) and the fuels required to produce it.

There are limited stores of ATP within muscles for muscle contraction (either as ATP or high-energy phosphates like phosphocreatine) so energy is produced during exercise either aerobically or anaerobically, depending on the availability of oxygen (and substrate).

6.2.2 Aerobic energy production

Aerobic production of ATP occurs via a series of reactions within the mitochondria called aerobic or oxidative phosphorylation because of its requirement for oxygen, and the ultimate step is the phosphorylation of adenosine diphosphate (ADP) to make ATP. Aerobic energy production can occur using stored muscle glycogen or glucose from blood as an energy substrate. This involves glycogen or glucose undergoing glycolysis to produce pyruvate in the cell cytoplasm. Pyruvate can then be transported into the mitochondria where it is converted to acetyl coenzyme A (CoA) in the mitochondria, which enters the tricarboxylic acid (TCA) or Krebs cycle. The net result of the TCA cycle is the production of ATP and the production of the coenzymes nicotinamide adenine dinucleotide (NADH) and flavin adenine dinucleotide ($FADH_2$), which enter the electron transport chain producing ATP.

Complete aerobic metabolism of one glucose unit (entering as glucose-1-phosphate) from glycogen yields 39 molecules of ATP – three from glycolysis, two from the TCA cycle and 34 from the electron transport chain. If glucose from the bloodstream is used, it must first be converted to glucose-6-phosphate, requiring one molecule of ATP, so the net energy yield is only 38 molecules of ATP.

Fatty acids can also be used as substrate for oxidative phosphorylation via a process called beta-oxidation, producing acetyl CoA. Acetyl CoA then enters the TCA cycle producing NADH and $FADH_2$, which enter the electron transport chain as for carbohydrate substrates. Because fatty acids are composed of many carbon atoms and only two are required to produce acetyl CoA, the yield of energy from a typical fatty acid is very high. For example, the complete aerobic breakdown of palmitic acid (16-carbon fatty acid) yields 129 molecules of ATP.

6.2.3 Anaerobic energy production

Anaerobic energy production is reliant on the metabolism of stored muscle glycogen or glucose via glycolysis with the resultant production of pyruvate, but pyruvate remains in the cytoplasm and is converted to lactate. The amount of ATP produced via anaerobic glycolysis is much less than aerobic glycolysis and oxidative phosphorylation. If glycogen is the original substrate, there are three ATP molecules per glucose unit produced, while only two ATP molecules are produced if blood glucose was the original substrate.

6.2.4 Energy sources during exercise

During exercise in the healthy animal, the usual sources of energy are carbohydrates and fat. Glycogen is predominantly stored in the muscles and liver, and glucose is available in the blood. Fats are stored in the body as triglycerides but can be broken down to free fatty acids, which can circulate in the blood and be taken up by exercising muscle. Muscle also has triglyceride stores, which can be broken down within the muscle to release free fatty acids. In the horse, volatile fatty acids are produced as a result of their digestive process and these can also be directly used via beta-oxidation.

At the onset of exercise, when oxygen supply may be limiting, and during high-intensity exercise, when the requirement for ATP exceeds the rate of ATP production aerobically, substrates are predominantly utilised anaerobically. Anaerobic energy production is rapid and does not require the delivery of oxygen to the muscle, but the ATP yield is low compared with aerobic pathways and the production of lactate will decrease muscle pH. During low- to moderate-intensity exercise, aerobic metabolism predominates and will be a mixture of fatty acid and carbohydrate utilisation. Horses and dogs have both been shown to have the ability to utilise fatty acids for energy production, but this is probably limited to approximately 50% of the total energy and then only in exercise up to about 65% VO_{2max} as it is in humans (Hawley 2002). In most species, a greater ability to utilise aerobic energy sources during high-intensity exercise is beneficial for maximum performance and delaying fatigue (see VO_{2max} below).

In dogs and horses, the same principles apply. However, there are three important principles to consider that highlight the central role of energy production for exercise, especially aerobic energy production.

- Energy utilisation pathways are not all or nothing. At any moment during exercise, there are aerobic and anaerobic contributions to energy production.
- Energy partitioning of different species may vary enormously and whether an animal is working 'aerobically' or 'anaerobically' should not be extrapolated directly from humans, but

rather from research data pertinent to that species. This is explained in more detail in energy partitioning below.

- The intensity of exercise is used to describe many aspects of exercise, from substrate usage to specific training programmes. The intensity of exercise is often expressed as a proportion of maximal aerobic metabolic rate (VO_{2max}) (see both energy partitioning and VO_{2max} below), yet in animals with very high VO_{2max} this needs to be put into perspective. For example, extrapolating from research in humans, fat utilisation may only occur at intensities of <65% VO_{2max} (Hawley 2002). The same intensity in horses is a fast canter/working gallop and so fat usage may be important during a much greater proportion of exercise than in humans.

6.2.5 Energy partitioning

The relative contributions of aerobic and anaerobic energy sources during exercise is an important indicator of the type of exercise performed by an animal in a particular athletic pursuit and will be central to dictating training programmes and adaptations to training. For athletic events that are primarily aerobic in nature, much effort in a training programme will be on maximising the aerobic pathways. Athletic events that are anaerobic in nature may focus on increasing muscle strength and acceleration, but still require a foundation of aerobic training.

As mentioned above, there are considerable species differences in proportions of aerobic and anaerobic energy supply during exercise. In humans, short-term, high-intensity exercise such as a 60-second sprint to fatigue is a primarily anaerobic activity, yet the equivalent intensity sprint in a horse is primarily aerobic in nature (Table 6.1). This illustrates that the horse has a high reliance on aerobic energy supply, even in short-duration, high-intensity exercise. A 60-second horse race is only approximately 1000 m, and commonly termed a 'sprint', but is not predominantly anaerobic exercise.

Horses have evolved to gallop fast but to outrun predators, they must be able to sustain that speed. Hence the reliance on the more sustainable (aerobic) energy source during exercise. Horses do vary with breed, but even the Quarterhorse (bred to race over a quarter of a mile or 400 m or 2 furlongs) in a 400 m race would only have 60% of the energy supplied anaerobically. Of course, the Arabian has an even greater reliance on aerobic energy sources during exercise and during endurance riding will work about 96% aerobically (Eaton 1994). Similarly, an eventing horse relies primarily on aerobic energy sources, with anaerobic energy during jumping efforts (Marlin *et al.* 1995).

Table 6.1 Energy partitioning for equivalent intensity and duration exercise in human athletes and Thoroughbred horses

Duration of all-out exercise	Human (Hagerman 1992)	Horse (Eaton 1994)
60 sec	30% aerobic	70% aerobic
2 min	60% aerobic	80% aerobic

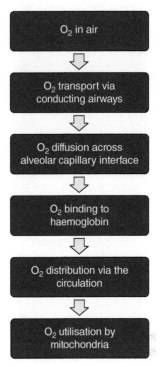

Figure 6.1 The oxygen transport chain.

Energy partitioning has not been well described for dogs. Despite the apparent variability in breeds that currently undergo sporting activities, wolves and dogs evolved to hunt in a pack over long distances and so have a greater reliance on aerobic energy sources during exercise. Trained sled dogs have been shown to have a VO_{2max} of approximately 200 mL/kg/min when trained (Banse *et al.* 2007). From the type of race and anecdotal information, it would seem logical that Greyhounds rely highly on anaerobic sources. However, this has not been tested and with evidence for a high VO_{2max} in Greyhounds (143 mL/kg/min; Staaden 1984), this assumption may need to be reevaluated.

6.3 The pathway of oxygen

The supply of oxygen to exercising muscle is vital to the performance ability of any animal, but particularly those that are relying on aerobic metabolism for sustaining energy, such as both the horse and dog. The pathway of oxygen is fundamental to an understanding of exercise physiology as it is the key to aerobic energy production. Limitations to oxygen supply anywhere along this pathway can seriously limit performance (Figure 6.1).

6.3.1 Maximal oxygen uptake (VO_{2max})

The key measure of the aerobic contribution to energy production during exercise is the oxygen uptake. As mentioned above, this can be used to determine the relative intensity of exercise. It is measured by measuring oxygen and carbon dioxide concentration in expired respiratory gasses.

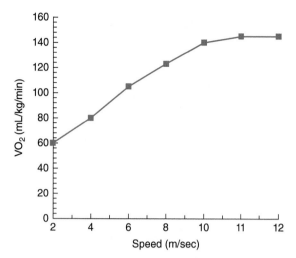

Figure 6.2 The relationship between VO_2 and speed in a horse during incrementally increasing speed.

Oxygen uptake or VO_2 is the overall use of oxygen by an animal. When measured during incrementally increasing exercise, VO_2 increases linearly, matched to demand during exercise (Figure 6.2), until it finally plateaus at a peak value called VO_{2max} = maximal aerobic metabolic rate. It has been measured in many different species including horses (Evans & Rose 1987) and dogs (Wagner *et al.* 1977) and is closely related to (endurance) performance ability. VO_{2max} is often used as an indicator of intensity of exercise, with 100% VO_{2max} usually indicating high-intensity exercise. However, it is important to note that 100% VO_{2max} is not 100% or maximal effort. One hundred per cent VO_{2max} is only the limit of the aerobic energy pathways, and the increased energy requirement at speeds/exercise intensities above VO_{2max} are supplied by anaerobic energy sources.

In the horse, there is a relatively small anaerobic contribution and a horse cannot reach speeds much greater than equivalent to about 120% VO_{2max} (Eaton *et al.* 1995) owing to its enormous ability to supply energy aerobically. Yet humans are capable of tests at 200% VO_{2max}.

6.3.2 Kinetics of oxygen uptake and effect of a warm-up

Animals with rapid oxygen kinetics have an advantage for performance because the faster the increase in aerobic energy production, the smaller the oxygen debt and lactate accumulation from anaerobic energy production at the beginning of intense exercise (Figure 6.3).

Horses have very rapid oxygen kinetics whereas humans have much slower oxygen kinetics. VO_{2max} can be reached in about 20 sec in a fit horse, while a human athlete would take over 2 min to reach VO_{2max} under the same conditions. More specifically, the time to reach 63% VO_{2max} in horses has been measured as 10 sec, in the dog it is approximately 20 sec and in a fit human about 30 sec (Poole *et al.* 2004).

In horses, oxygen kinetics have been shown to be improved by training (Bellenger *et al.* 1995). Oxygen kinetics are also generally improved by a warm-up before exercise (Geor *et al.* 2000; Tyler *et al.* 1996a). One study demonstrated a significant improvement in the aerobic contribution to energy demands during intense exercise shortly following 5 min of exercise at 50% VO_{2max} (Tyler *et al.* 1996a). Another study demonstrated similar effects irrespective of warm-up intensity (Geor *et al.* 2000). Physiological adaptations during the warm-up include cardiovascular and respiratory responses that ensure an adequate supply of oxygen to the working muscles where the working muscles receive a greater proportion of the blood flow at the expense of other organs such as the digestive system. The increased O_2 delivery to the muscles enhances their ability to work aerobically and reduces lactate build-up during exercise and delays the onset of fatigue due to lactate accumulation in high-intensity sports (McCutcheon *et al.* 1999). Warm-up in human athletes has been shown to increase VO_{2max} (Gray & Nimmo 2001). During the warm-up, the temperature of the working muscles rises by 1°C which is beneficial as warm muscles contract more powerfully and the fibres become more compliant, which reduces the risk of injury due to tearing of the fibres (Shellock & Prentice 1985). It is interesting to note that despite the evidence in horses for the physiological benefits of warm-up,

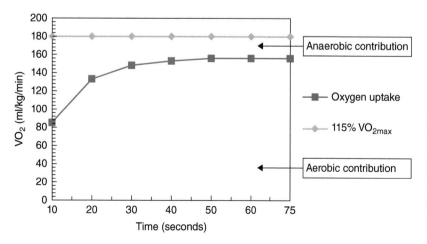

Figure 6.3 The relationship between VO_2 and time at a set speed (calculated to be 115% VO_{2max}) in a horse demonstrating energy partitioning during exercise as well as VO_2 kinetics. This figure shows the typical partitioning of energy in a horse performing supramaximal exercise (exercise >100% VO_{2max}). The area under the curve represents the aerobic contribution to exercise. Note the large anaerobic contribution in the first seconds of exercise. However, this horse reaches close to VO_{2max} by 20 sec into exercise.

there is limited warm-up performed before many equine competitions, especially Thoroughbred racing. Warm-up also has a potential role in injury prevention, although the current evidence for this is limited.

6.4 Cardiorespiratory function during exercise

Clearly, animals have adapted to increase respiratory gas exchange and transport during exercise – indeed, all components of the oxygen transport chain (see Figure 6.1) – in order to maximise the delivery of oxygen for energy production during exercise. During exercise there is:

- flaring of the nostrils and in some species mouth breathing to reduce upper respiratory tract resistance
- increased ventilation of the lungs (increases in minute ventilation from 80 L/min at rest to 1800 L/min in the horse)
- increased tidal volume (ventilation per minute) owing to frequency of respiratory cycles and decreased physiological dead space
- increased perfusion of alveoli – due to increased cardiac output and dilation of pulmonary blood vessels
- decreased transit time of pulmonary capillary blood flow – faster blood flow past the alveoli
- increased diffusion of O_2 and CO_2 from the alveoli into the capillaries perfusing the alveoli – due to increased gradient, increased blood flow
- increased haemoglobin concentration (in the horse) due to splenic contraction – increased oxygen-carrying capacity (the splenic reserve) and can increase the measured packed cell volume from around 35–40% to over 60%; increased red cell volume by one-third (Poole 2004)
- increased heart rate (HR) and stroke volume (SV) = increased cardiac output and overall transport of oxygen to the lungs and exercising muscle
- increased peripheral perfusion – capillaries in the periphery (muscles) are better perfused
- increased diffusion of O_2 and CO_2 from capillaries to or from exercising muscle due to increased gradient, temperature and blood flow and decreased pH.

During exercise, heart rate increases linearly to heart rate max with increasing intensity of exercise, similar to VO_2, and heart rate is a good indicator of VO_2 while maximal heart rate is directly proportional to VO_{2max} (Figure 6.4).

The higher the heart rate at a specific speed, the more 'stress' the horse is under. (This stress can be anything from excitement, through lack of fitness to cardiac insufficiency.)

6.5 The effect of training

Training results in improvements along the entire pathway of oxygen, reflected in increased VO_{2max} as a marker of overall aerobic metabolic rate. While this may be a major aim,

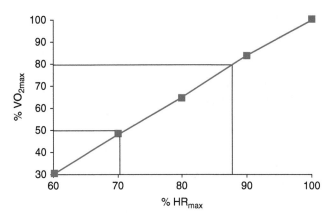

Figure 6.4 Schematic relationship between heart rate and VO_{2max} in the horse showing that 50% VO_{2max} is approximately 70% HR_{max} and 80% VO_{2max} is approximately 88% HR_{max}. *Source:* Data from Evans and Rose 1987.

training effects are not limited to cardiorespiratory system improvements, and improvements in components of anaerobic energy production, including muscle buffering capacity and resting muscle glycogen concentration, have been demonstrated in horses (McGowan *et al.* 2002).

As well as improvements in energy production during exercise, improvements in muscle size occur (Tyler *et al.* 1998), indicating increased muscle strength and considerable adaptation of bone, cartilage, tendon, ligaments and other connective tissue (Marlin & Nankervis 2002). More difficult to measure in the animal world, but well evidenced in human studies, are training improvements in skill acquisition, refinement in motor pathways and motor unit recruitment pattern and speed, as well as development of sports-specific proprioceptive and tactile feedback mechanisms. These training responses combine to improve performance and reduce error and injury rates and can be utilised in sports-specific training programmes to maximise adaptations and performance.

6.5.1 Cardiorespiratory responses to training

Increases of 30% in VO_{2max} from the detrained state have been recorded after 28 weeks' training in horses (Tyler *et al.* 1996b) and similar increases have been found in humans.

A few points to note regarding the effect of training in horses.

- VO_{2max} continues to increase over 28 weeks of training, and then tends to plateau.
- Half of the increase and the most rapid increase is in the first 7 weeks.
- Continual training stimulus will cause continual increases in VO_{2max} – important as many trainers keep a very even workload following initial training (Tyler *et al.* 1996b). In fact, there is a large increase in VO_{2max} with very little initial training. The potential effects of this on perhaps more slowly adapting musculoskeletal structures should be considered and this time period may be one of the danger periods for injury. Cardiovascular responses to training that have been shown to occur in horses (Poole 2004) in response to training include:

- heart rate decreases at the same speed – exercise at a lower proportion of heart rate max
- faster recovery
- stroke volume increases (heart size increases)
- increased plasma volume (heart preload)
- increased resting red cell volume (haemoglobin or Hb)
- increased capillary density in trained muscle.

These findings have been shown to occur to a greater or lesser extent in dogs, humans and horses. The horse appears to have a greater capacity to increase heart size and mass with training (Young 1999).

6.5.2 Skeletal muscle adaptations to training

There are significant adaptive responses in skeletal muscle in response to training in all species. In contrast to cardiorespiratory adaptations, these changes are slow to occur and slow to revert. Studies in horses have shown that it can take 16 weeks to detect most of the skeletal muscle adaptations and these changes did not revert during the 12-week period of detraining (Serrano et al. 2000; Tyler et al. 1998).

Interestingly, the major adaptive response in equine muscle is to improve aerobic energy supply via improvements in the pathway of oxygen, even when very high-intensity training exercise is used. This response includes (Tyler et al. 1998):

- increase in capillaries/mm^2
- decrease in diffusional index (area per capillary)
- no significant change in fibre types with training but significant increase in IIA to IIB ratio ($P<0.05$)
- increased mitochondrial volume
- increased activity of enzymes associated with aerobic muscle metabolism – both the TCA cycle (citrate synthase) and beta-oxidation of fatty acids (hydroxy acyl dehydrogenase) – but no increase in the activity of the muscle enzymes associated with anaerobic glycolysis (lactate dehydrogenase).

Other adaptations occur with high-intensity training and include increased fibre area in all fibres (I, IIA, IIB/IIX) (Tyler et al. 1998) and increased muscle buffering capacity and muscle glycogen concentration (McGowan et al. 2002). In humans, more exercise-specific adaptations to training have been achieved, but the genotype and phenotype variations between humans are far greater than in horses – compare the body type of a weight lifter with that of an endurance/marathon runner.

6.5.3 Muscle glycogen concentration

The horse has very high muscle glycogen stores compared with humans and while resting muscle glycogen concentration does increase with training, it is poorly responsive to 'glycogen loading' techniques used in humans. In short-duration, high-intensity exercise, muscle glycogen does not become depleted but in long-duration exercise, muscle glycogen depletion may occur, e.g. endurance riding. Of greater importance in horses are the slow glycogen repletion rates – it takes 48–72 h after glycogen depletion to replenish skeletal muscle glycogen stores. The effect of feeding post exercise is limited, with high-starch (grain) diets fed post glycogen depletion resulting in slightly higher glycogen concentrations in muscle at 48 and 72 h but not earlier (Lacombe et al. 2004). However, both carbohydrate loading and attempts to hasten glycogen repletion in horses are very dangerous and can induce laminitis. This is a good example of where extrapolation from the human literature can be perilous.

6.6 Detraining

The rate of loss of fitness primarily depends on the duration and level of training stimulus. In studies in horses, prolonged training resulted in prolonged maintenance of cardiorespiratory fitness. VO_{2max} decreased slowly with no change for 6 weeks and by 12 weeks, it was still 15% above pretraining values (Tyler et al. 1996b). Indices of cardiac function also did not change for 4 weeks and did not return to normal until 12 weeks of detraining (Kriz et al. 2000).

Another factor affecting detraining responses is the amount of exercise during the detraining period. This relates well to a forced rest because of injury. A small amount of daily exercise is effective in maintaining cardiovascular and musculoskeletal fitness. Human studies involving strict bedrest during the detraining period have evidenced the dramatic loss of cardiovascular fitness, bone density and muscle and ligament integrity. It is important to consider the rate of loss of fitness before commencing training, e.g. if cardiorespiratory fitness is maintained following an injury and 6 weeks' rest to heal the injury, the animal could reinjure itself by exercising at a greater capacity than the recently healed injury can withstand.

6.7 Applied exercise physiology

6.7.1 Principles of designing training programmes

As a physiotherapist, you will be designing training programmes predominantly to improve musculoskeletal and/or neurological function during treatment and rehabilitation. In many cases, you will be happy to restore function at a very low level of exercise intensity, yet in others you will be treating animals while they are actively competing. Therefore, when designing training programmes, it is important to consider the principles of exercise physiology and question what you are trying to achieve. These may be very different depending on the discipline and detailed sports-specific training programmes are outlined in the text, *The Athletic Horse* (Hodgson et al. 2014).

A major aim will always be to improve components of the oxygen transport chain (see Figure 6.1) through predominantly aerobic training. However, to be able to determine the intensity of training stimulus, exercise physiologists rely on use of heart rate and lactate measured during exercise. In horses, the major adaptive response to training is aerobic, irrespective of the intensity of training.

6.7.2 Use of heart rate in training programmes

Heart rate (HR) can be used to estimate VO_2 and is so used in training programmes to estimate the intensity of exercise performed. While heart rate during exercise in humans has been studied on a population basis, allowing calculations adjusted for age and gender, such information is not available in animals. The optimal method of determining the intensity of exercise using HR is by first finding out HR_{max}, as the intensity is most reflective of true VO_2 or exercise intensity, if expressed as a percentage of HR_{max} (see Figure 6.4).

Maximal heart rate varies considerably between species and breeds of animals. For example, the mongrel dog has a HR_{max} of approximately 300 beats per minute (Wagner *et al.* 1977) and the racing Greyhound 318 (Staaden 1984). The racing Thoroughbred or Standardbred horse can have a HR_{max} of 240–260 beats per minute (Tyler-McGowan *et al.* 1999). In horses, HR_{max} also decreases with age, with HR_{max} of horses over 20 <200 bpm compared with approximately 220 bpm in their younger and middle-aged counterparts (Betros *et al.* 2002).

HR_{max} does not increase with training (Evans 1985) so ideally, a horse could be assessed early in its training and the same HR_{max} used to tailor the training over time. However, in our experience, early in training a horse may not be fit enough to reach its HR_{max} before fatigue. Therefore, it may be better to delay measurement of HR_{max} until 2 weeks or more into the training programme.

Using heart rate in training without having obtained HR_{max} could produce very different relative intensities of training. For example, in one group of Standardbred racehorses of the same age (mean 4 years), HR_{max} varied from 215 bpm to 260 bpm. The relative intensity of exercise at 160 bpm then varied in these individuals from 74% to 62% of HR_{max}. Therefore, training intensity based on heart rate should be individualised for each animal.

Methods to monitor heart rate include telemetry heart rate monitors and global positioning satellite (GPS) monitors and these can be a valuable guide to training. In general, training heart rates are extrapolated from humans with early training heart rates or warm-up in the 70% HR_{max} (50% VO_{2max}) range (154 bpm for a horse with HR_{max} of 220 bpm); medium- or moderate-intensity training 80% HR_{max} (70% VO_{2max}) range (176 bpm for a horse with HR_{max} 220 bpm); high-intensity training 90–100% HR_{max} (80–100% VO_{2max}) range (>198 bpm).

6.7.3 Lactate and its use in exercise and training

Lactate production is a normal response to energy production and while increasing lactate concentration has a negative effect on muscle contraction and energy production in the horse, it is unlikely to be a limiting factor for short-term high-intensity exercise (racing). Horses have an enormous ability to generate lactate and after a race or maximal exertion will frequently have plasma or blood lactate concentrations of over 25–30 mmol/L (resting 0.5–1.0 mmol/L) (Harris *et al.* 1987).

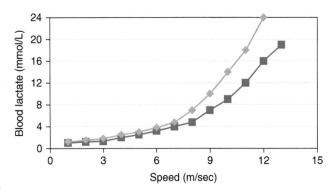

Figure 6.5 The typical relationship between blood lactate concentration and speed.

Lactate concentration increases when the speed increases above 7–9 m/sec (Eaton *et al.* 1999). The speed at which it begins to increase depends on gait, breed, horse, diet and state of training (Figure 6.5). Lactate threshold or onset of blood lactate accumulation (OBLA) can be used in training programmes with a higher speed at OBLA in fitter horses and those with greater ability to transport and use oxygen (higher VO_{2max}).

In reality, determination of the lactate curves of horses are hard to achieve practically in a training situation, so shortcuts have been developed and validated, e.g. vLa4 (speed when lactate reaches 4 mmol/L or approximately OBLA) or La10 (the lactate concentration at a speed of 10 m/sec). These derived values are comparable between horses and in the same horse over time and have been evaluated in field tests, with a number of different field tests developed and validated and correlated with performance (Davie & Evans 2000; Leleu *et al.* 2005).

It should be noted that OBLA corresponds in the horse and human, at least to around 80% VO_{2max}. This is moderate-intensity training and endurance athletes often use training at this intensity to maximise aerobic capacity or VO_{2max}. The racehorse at OBLA or about 80% VO_{2max} is travelling at 15 sec/furlong, or 13 m/sec, or 800 m/min (that is, a gallop) (Davie 2003). Typically, 'jogging' performed by Standardbred trainers and horsewalker exercise is quite low intensity. It is important to differentiate low-intensity exercise from moderate-intensity, and training programmes should incorporate moderate-intensity training as well as low- and high-intensity training.

6.8 High-altitude training

Current research for human athletes has demonstrated that living at high altitude and training at low altitude is superior to protocols involving high-altitude training, as the physiological benefits obtained by living and training at altitude are outweighed by the deficits produced in reduced VO_{2max} and total work output (Hahn & Gore 2001). This protocol remains untested in horses. Certainly, physiological changes occur in the horse in response to hypobaric hypoxia, and these changes may be beneficial to athletic performance if they occurred at sea level. These include (Wickler & Greene 2004):

- increased red blood cell number
- increased blood volume
- improved muscle capillarity
- improved metabolic capacity of muscle.

Unfortunately, these changes have not yet been linked directly to performance improvements at sea level. The limitations of high-altitude exposure and training must also be considered. Apart from the risk of altitude sickness, VO_2 reduces by 15–30% (Navot-Mintzer et al. 2003) and the capacity to train at high intensity is reduced.

6.9 Maximal performance and factors limiting maximal performance in the horse

Performance in horses may be described as dependent primarily on energy supply (respiratory and cardiovascular systems and the transport of oxygen) and the ability to use that energy efficiently in the form of locomotion (musculoskeletal system). The equine athlete is efficient and coordinated and has been selected for athletic performance. Horses have a large aerobic capacity (>160 mL/kg/min), well over double that recorded on a per kilogram basis in elite human endurance athletes (70 mL/kg/min). This reliance on aerobic energy and oxygen supply during exercise has helped the horse become a superior athlete, yet has implications for racehorse health because it leaves the racehorse highly susceptible to limitations in oxygen transport (see Figure 6.1) and despite all these adaptations, the horse appears to have a respiratory limitation to maximal exercise. This is evidenced by the development of arterial hypoxaemia and hypercapnia during intense exercise (galloping) (Art & Lekeux 1995). The horse has extremely high pulmonary vascular pressures to prevent rupture of the pulmonary capillaries under physiological conditions, so it has a relatively thick diffusion barrier, reducing the rate of diffusion, and this is the likely cause for much of the exercise-induced hypoxaemia (Christley et al. 1997).

6.9.1 Equine poor performance

Poor performance is an important area for the animal physiotherapist as many cases referred for physiotherapy have a veterinary diagnosis of poor performance. Yet it is important to determine what could be occurring in the horse with poor performance. It is vital to assess the nature of the performance problem: you should ascertain if the horse has never performed well, if there was a sudden decrease in performance, or if there was a decrease after improved class. When assessing horses for poor performance you should consider the following.

- What might have contributed to the poor performance, and remember to look beyond your own sphere of expertise.
- More than one problem can coexist.
- In horses performing maximally, subtle, subclinical problems may be the reason for poor performance.

The performance issue may be different for horses of different disciplines, e.g. for dressage horses, soundness, coordination and muscle control are essential while for endurance horses, fluid and temperature regulation are essential. In the poor-performing racehorse, poor performance resulting from disorders affecting oxygen transport or energy supply often presents similarly, despite the myriad causes and is generally described as 'stopping' at the end of a race. Examples of such disorders include upper and lower respiratory tract disorders, cardiac disease and disorders of the red blood cell oxygen-carrying capacity (anaemia) but can be any problem along the pathway of oxygen (see Figure 6.1). Other problems may be present such as respiratory stridor (noise), myopathy (tying up) or any musculoskeletal injury or disease (unsoundness). Muscle metabolic capacity is rarely limiting to performance, and anaerobic capacity is rarely routinely assessed (Martin et al. 2000).

A key point is that because racehorses exercise maximally, subtle or subclinical problems are enough to dramatically affect performance.

6.9.2 Upper respiratory tract disorders

Upper respiratory tract disorders affect oxygen transport by increasing the resistance of breathing and reducing air flow. This reduces the amount of oxygen available for the rest of the oxygen transport chain. The increased resistance to breathing is usually accompanied by a noise called respiratory stridor. The horse's unique anatomy and physiology only serve to compound any problems that exist. The horse is an obligate nasal breather so any anatomical narrowing of the nostrils or nasal passages will reduce performance. There is also a complicated relationship between the larynx and soft palate that makes this area particularly susceptible to disorders. Owing to the importance of the diameter of the airway passages to air flow and the airway resistance that develops even with 'normal' breathing during maximal exercise, very small alterations in the diameter of structures can seriously affect performance.

The most common disorder is the paralysis of the left side of the larynx called idiopathic laryngeal hemiplegia (ILH). The disease is caused by paralysis of the left recurrent laryngeal nerve that innervates the muscle of the larynx required for the opening and closing of the arytenoid cartilages. Other laryngeal problems include dorsal displacement of the soft palate and disorders of the epiglottis. Dorsal displacement of the soft palate is more common in Standardbred than Thoroughbred horses. It occurs when there is a loss of the seal between the soft palate and the larynx, resulting in a dorsal movement of the soft palate up in front of the larynx, obstructing air flow. Epiglottic and other disorders are less common.

6.9.3 Lower respiratory tract disorders

Lower respiratory tract disorders affect oxygen transport by reducing the diffusion of oxygen (and carbon dioxide) across the alveolar wall into the pulmonary capillaries, although some lower respiratory disorders also affect air flow through the smaller bronchioles (bronchoconstriction). It is postulated that the horse has evolved in such a way that its athletic capabilities are greater than the functional capacity of its respiratory system. Huge pulmonary vascular pressures are generated during maximal exercise and the diffusion membrane is as thick as it can be while still maintaining diffusion. While this means that the horse can withstand (in many cases) the enormous vascular pressures that other species would not be able to cope with, it leads to a diffusion limitation, evidenced by hypercapnia (high CO_2) and hypoxaemia (low O_2) during maximal exercise. What this means is that the healthy equine lung is at the limit of its capabilities during maximal exercise and any alteration to its function will reduce performance significantly.

The three main lower respiratory tract diseases are:
- inflammatory airway disease (IAD)
- exercise-induced pulmonary haemorrhage
- infectious disease.

Inflammatory airway disease (IAD) is a syndrome of small airway inflammation and resultant obstruction without infection that results in poor performance. Some people believe that it is an early form of the more severe clinical disease called recurrent airway obstruction (RAO), or heaves, that has some similarities with human asthma. In many cases it is clinically inapparent, although at other times it may result in coughing or nasal discharge. It is frequently associated with poor housing management, may be seasonal and may be associated with exercise-induced pulmonary haemorrhage.

Exercise-induced pulmonary haemorrhage (EIPH) is another significant lower airway disorder of racehorses. It is due to bleeding from the dorsocaudal lung lobes and can result in clinical epistaxis (nose bleeding). The pathogenesis of the disease is not clear but is likely to relate to the abnormally high pulmonary vascular pressures during exercise, causing rupture of capillaries into the alveoli (despite the relatively thick diffusion barrier). EIPH actually occurs to some degree in most (probably >90%) racehorses exercising maximally, detected by bronchoalveolar lavage. However, blood appearing at the nostrils (resulting in the horse being banned from racing in some countries, including Australia) occurs in considerably fewer than 1% of horses. It is not always associated with a reduction in performance, and performance is usually only reduced in those horses that have a severe episode.

6.9.4 Anaemia

Reduced circulating red blood cell volume, or anaemia, affects oxygen transport by reducing the binding of oxygen to haemoglobin because of reduced haemoglobin. Anaemia is, however, rare in the athletic horse. The horse has the unique ability to contract its spleen during exercise and as a result can release up to 12 L of extra blood into the circulation during exercise. Disease and possibly nutritional deficiencies could cause anaemia.

6.9.5 Cardiac disease

Cardiac disorders affect oxygen transport by reducing the transport of oxygen from the lungs to the muscle where it is required to produce energy. There is a high prevalence of cardiac murmurs in racehorses, many of which do not affect the horse at all, e.g. 16% of National Hunt racehorses have a right-sided murmur associated with tricuspid valve regurgitation (Patteson & Cripps 1993). Many murmurs simply represent turbulent blood flow and are called physiological murmurs. A number of murmurs, however, represent serious cardiac disease and limitations to performance through reduced cardiac output and cardiac failure. Horses may also suffer from arrhythmias reducing the cardiac output. If these are secondary to cardiac failure then they are always associated with a loss of athletic function. However, many are associated with abnormal electrical activity and may be treated effectively. The most common rhythm disturbance is atrial fibrillation and it is more common (in the uncomplicated form) in young Standardbred horses.

6.9.6 Musculoskeletal disorders

Musculoskeletal disorders are the most common cause of poor performance, either alone or in combination with other diseases. In the majority of cases, the horse will be clinically lame or unsound and a veterinary examination and/or physiotherapist's assessment will often reveal the source of the problem. However, in some cases there is a reduction in performance without obvious clinical signs and more sophisticated techniques like gamma scintigraphy and gait analysis may be needed to find the cause (see Chapter 7).

6.9.7 Other factors

A number of other factors are important for successful performance, including mental attitude or the 'will to win', and behavioural issues (particularly with overtraining or staleness – see later). The racehorse, like all horses, is dependent upon appropriate levels of nutrition. Also, abdominal disease, particularly gastric ulcers (see Chapter 3), can be an important problem in racehorse performance.

6.9.8 Overtraining syndrome in horses

Overtraining is simply an imbalance between training and recovery – either the training stimulus is too great or the recovery too short. Over time, this can result in a syndrome of fatigue and poor performance, usually accompanied by one or more other signs, e.g. weight loss, psychological changes and susceptibility to infections. Overtraining is a chronic syndrome that takes many weeks to months for recovery. It must be differentiated from overreaching which is an acute form of overtraining that only takes a few days for recovery.

In humans, overtraining can result from a training programme using the principles of overload training, but poorly regulated. Overload training techniques are commonly used in elite human athletes and are a fine tuning of training and maximising the recovery response – in fact, trainers aim to induce

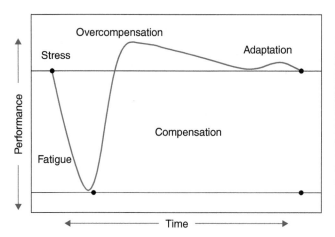

Figure 6.6 Schematic of the performance response to repeated stresses and the resultant adaptation or overload training principles.

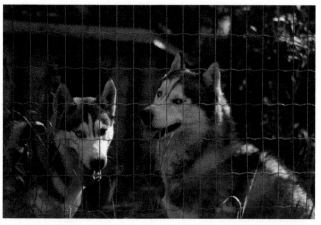

Figure 6.7 Siberian Huskies at rest. *Source:* Photo courtesy of Päivi Heino.

overreaching and time the 'supercompensation' or overcompensation for a competition (Figure 6.6).

Horse trainers certainly do not commonly use overload training principles, but similar principles, e.g. 'tapering' or reducing exercise just before racing, may cause similar responses. In humans, overload training is closely monitored by trainers and sports psychologists.

Signs of overtraining in horses include:

- poor performance (by definition)
- loss of bodyweight, loss of appetite
- muscle pain or increased muscle enzymes
- increased susceptibility to gastrointestinal or urinary infections
- incoordination
- increased rate of injury
- altered heart rates/lactates/VO_2
- unwillingness to train
- nervousness
- behaviour changes.

Diagnosis in human athletes relies heavily on mood profiling – behavioural changes in horses can also predominate. Diagnosis of overtraining in horses relies on identification of poor performance, exclusion of other major causes, identification of loss of bodyweight and behavioural changes. There may be subtle changes in blood tests, but these are frequently unrewarding. Human athletes tend to overtrain when social stresses are added to the stress of training and competition. Similar stresses in horses might be social stresses (e.g. stabled adjacent to a horse that is a bully), illness (e.g. viral respiratory disease), gastric ulcers, transport, boring routine, subtle lameness or musculoskeletal pain.

Ideal treatment of overtraining involves prolonged rest, decreased training load (especially high-intensity training) and addition of variety to the training and management routine. Examples might include hacking the horses if they are quiet, flat work, cavaletti work; turn the horse out into a paddock or

a change of yard. Also good husbandry to minimise external stresses, e.g. transport, illness and gastric ulcers, is important. Differentiation from overreaching is important; for example, a horse prepared too quickly that will have a response to short-term rest – this response is likely to be relatively quick and positive, i.e. supercompensation, so it would be ideal to be able to use the response to the trainer's advantage.

6.10 Training the sled dog (Husky)

The following sections outline some of the principles of how exercise physiology may be utilised to design training programmes in two extremes of dog sports – sled dog racing (Husky) and Greyhound racing.

6.10.1 Profile of the Husky as an athlete

The Husky was originally bred in Siberia under very cold and harsh conditions. The main purpose of the breed was to pull a load (a sled) to transport people and goods across snow and ice for very long distances. The Husky is therefore a thick-coated dog, of medium build and designed for strength and endurance (Figure 6.7). The dog is obviously very robust and tough and readily trainable, responding to verbal speed and directional cues. In former times, sled dogs were used for transport and although they have been largely superseded by mechanisation, they are still raced recreationally in both cold and more temperate zones on the globe. In warm conditions, overheating during training and racing is a major issue.

The aerobic capacity of the Husky is the highest recorded for any dog breed, with several dogs recording VO_{2max} of over 200 mL/min/kg (Banse *et al.* 2007). In comparison, VO_{2max} of 154 mL/min/kg was measured in a group of trained hunting foxhounds (Musch *et al.* 1985). This performance is impressive compared with human athletes (70 mL/min/kg) and elite athletic Thoroughbred horses (160–175 mL/min/kg). Van Citters & Franklin (1969) reported the working heart rate in Huskies at over 300 bpm for extended runs exceeding 1 h duration. Resting heart rate is typically between 40 and 60 bpm. Stepien *et al.* (1998) trained a group of 77 Huskies pulling a sled for an average of 20 km/day for 5 months. There was no dropout of dogs due to illness or injury during this 5-month period, attesting the natural durability of the Husky. However, this extreme lifestyle may not be without consequences. Human athletes who participate in sports in very cold weather, for example skaters and cross-country skiers, have an increased prevalence of lower airway disease that is hypothesised to result from repeated penetration of incompletely conditioned air into the lung periphery. It appears that canine winter athletes also suffer from increased prevalence of lower airway disease secondary to hyperpnoea with cold air (Davis *et al.* 2002).

Although the sled dog has very efficient aerobic energy utilisation, dogs may also have a significant anaerobic component of energy production during a sled run in comparison to the free run. Stepien *et al.* (1998) recorded oxygen uptake of 40% VO_{2max} at 4.4 m/sec. The majority of Husky training is performed approximately at this speed. Reynolds *et al.* (1995) reported anaerobic conditions in Huskies at 3 min into exercise at 6.7 m/sec on a 10° slope. Ready & Morgan (1984) investigated physiological responses in Siberian Husky dogs during a 90 sec sprint, a 7.5 km free run and a 6 km team sled run. Blood lactate levels of 1.74, 0.70 and 3.06 mmol respectively were reported 3 min after the run, with heart rates of 190, 211 and 166 bpm immediately on completion. This is probably due to the extra load requirements of pulling a sled and demands of challenging terrain.

6.10.2 Profile of a sled dog race

The Iditarod Sled Dog Race in the USA is an example of top-level competition at the extreme end of the performance spectrum. The race is run in snow and ice conditions and covers 1692 km in 12 days, averaging 141 km/day. The race has an energy demand for the human sled driver alone of 10,740 kJ/day (Cox *et al.* 2003).

Warm climates such as in Australia do not favour traditional sled dog racing as the window of opportunity for racing on snow is small, the terrain is limited, and conditions are generally too warm to allow long races. Therefore, the majority of sled dog races in warmer climates are over ground not snow, and races are generally limited to 20–25 km. They are often run in the early morning, as temperatures cannot exceed 10–12°C (Canberra Sled Dog Club 2005). A 25 km race in a warmer climate is generally run in 1 h at a speed of approximately 7 m/sec. A 30 km race is completed in 75 min at the same speed (Canberra Sled Dog Club 2005).

Summary of race profile in temperate climate
- 25–30 km race over variable terrain.
- 75 min duration.
- Average speed of 7 m/sec (25 km/h).
- 4.4 m/sec is equivalent to 40% VO_{2max}.

- Energy supply is predominantly aerobic but bouts of anaerobic metabolism are expected.
- Typical VO_{2max} for the sled dog can exceed 200 mL/min/kg.
- Blood lactate levels under race conditions are unknown.
- HR_{max} can exceed 300 bpm and can be sustained over long periods.

Components of a proposed sled training programme
- Fitness testing
- Play
- Cross-country course
- Dry treadmill – loaded and unloaded
- Wet treadmill
- Track work

Fitness testing
Fitness test data should form the basis of the exercise intensity prescription for elite athletes. Exercise prescription is best prepared for each individual dog. Evans (2000) reported significant differences in the response of physiological parameters to exercise between individual horses, and within individuals at different levels of training. A similar trend can be assumed for canine athletes. Fitness testing should include the following.
- Health and lameness assessment
- Determination of HR_{max} and VO_{2max} if possible
- Determination of blood lactate level versus speed
- Determination of heart rate vs. speed
  For health and lameness assessment see Chapter 8.

Determination of VO_{2max}
Maximum oxygen uptake defines the aerobic capacity of the horse (Evans 2000) and it has been used for many years as the measure of the aerobic capacity in humans. The ability of the sled dog to race over 30 km is largely dependent on the VO_{2max}. Similar to the adaptations in horses, training dogs for 8–12 weeks of treadmill running at 80% max heart rate, 5 days per week, improved VO_{2max} by 31% (Musch *et al.* 1985).

VO_{2max} should be used as one of the main indicators of the response of the dog to a training programme and the speed at which VO_{2max} is reached will determine training speed for interval training (Laursen & Jenkins 2002; Tyler-McGowan *et al.* 1999). Ideally, the velocity at VO_{2max} should be tested regularly during interval training periods so that the interval training speed can be adjusted with improvements in aerobic function. It is expected that the training velocity will require an increase of approximately 3% per week (Trilk *et al.* 2002).

Determination of blood lactate level versus speed
Blood lactate levels indicate the contribution of anaerobic metabolism to the energy supply. This curve is well known in horses and humans and has been investigated in the dog. Blood lactate levels in the horse rapidly rise during exercise speeds greater than 65–85% VO_{2max} (Evans 2000), and regularly

increase to 20–30 mmol. The only documented evidence of lactate levels in the trained Husky is at 3.06 mmol, 3 min after a 6 km sled run (Ready & Morgan 1984). Training in both humans and horses typically results in a shift of the curve to the right, indicative of an important training adaptation. Ready & Morgan (1984) observed no shift in the curve in response to a 12-week interval training programme in Huskies, perhaps as a result of insufficient intensity of exercise. Musch *et al.* (1987) observed significantly lower blood lactate levels at a given level of submaximal exercise following an aerobic training period.

Although exercise speeds can be calculated according to VO_{2max}, blood lactate levels can be taken for future reference. The speed at which a blood lactate level of 4 mmol (vLa4) is reached is significant as an interval training marker, as it is used widely in the horse industry, is repeatable, and reliably associated with racing success (Trilk *et al.* 2002). It is of interest that the same marker is used by elite human sprint and athletic trainers as a guide to training intensity (Steinacker 1993). Therefore, it is reasonable to assume that the same marker could be of value as a training tool for canine athletes.

Determination of heart rate versus speed

The heart rate to running speed relationship in humans (Steinacker 1993) and horses (Trilk *et al.* 2002) is linear at moderate-to-high workloads and is reproducible. There is a well-documented shift to the right of the curve with training in horses (Evans 2000) and humans. Musch *et al.* (1985) reported a lower heart rate at any level of submaximal exercise following an aerobic training programme in dogs. Heart rate is easily measured in the field situation and is a simple way to measure workload. Some degree of caution should be exercised, however, as heart rate tends to rise in dogs with anticipation of a stressor (Vincent *et al.* 1993) without an actual increase in workload. Heart rate can be monitored during testing and training sessions by a portable monitor. This information, along with speed and distance information from a portable GPS unit, gives valuable feedback on training performance and can be used for future reference (Hampson & McGowan 2007). If heart rate data are consistently reliable, and in line with VO_2 and blood lactate levels and adaptations, heart rate responses alone may be used to modify exercise intensity.

Play

Play is important to relieve training stress and for ongoing bonding between the trainer and dog. Play can also involve high-speed sprints (chasing a ball), jumps and swimming to add variety to the training programme. These sessions allow the trainer to include valuable suppling, balance and proprioception components to the programme design.

Cross-country course

The cross-country course is designed to give the dog long runs (10–15 km) in an interesting and stimulating environment, while challenging the dog with high work demands and variable terrain. The trainer will accompany the dog on the course on a wheeled sled or bicycle and monitor and control speed, workload and distance

Cross-country work forms a large part of basic training, to prepare the dog's musculoskeletal system for the training ahead, while providing a stimulus for aerobic work. Stepien *et al.* (1998) reported that 77 Huskies were trained for 5 months at 4.4 m/sec (40% VO_{2max}) for 20 km/day with no reported dropout. The proposed training goal of 120–150 km/week is therefore realistic, and given the robustness of the breed, is unlikely to lead to overtraining and injury under close monitoring. McKenzie *et al.* (2008) found that unconditioned dogs had significant differences in carbohydrate and fat metabolism during exercise, compared with aerobically conditioned dogs. Endurance training plays a critical role in optimising the dog's innate aerobic ability.

Dry treadmill – loaded and unloaded

The treadmill provides a secure environment for training at speed and incline while allowing the close monitoring of several physiological parameters (fitness test). Treadmill training provides a level surface with reduced injury risk. The dog can be loaded as per sled conditions by adding a harness and loaded at will, via a weight and pulley set-up. Overloading on the treadmill allows for accurate and measurable overload in a situation specific to the race conditions. Strength training is used extensively in human athletes and has been shown to improve the pattern of neural drive (Judge *et al.* 2003) and reduce muscle injury rate (Croisier *et al.* 2002) in track athletes. Gonyea & Sale (1982) describe the major features of muscle adaptation to weightlifting exercise as changes in contraction time, fibre size and fibre number. Similar adaptation could be expected with weight-loaded dog training.

The training effect of sled towing has been measured in humans, as this is a popular form of resistance training in sprinters. Lockie *et al.* (2003) found that a sled load of 12.6% of body mass had a performance benefit above a load of 32.2% body mass. Kinematics were also observed during this study. It is important to note that the 32.2% body mass load had an effect of reducing stride length by 24% and stride frequency by a lesser extent. In addition, sled towing increased ground contact time, trunk lean and hip flexion. These are important issues for training the sled dog. It is well established that training needs to be as specific as possible so that the right systems and muscle functions can adapt optimally. Training in a predominantly unloaded situation will not prepare the dog to race optimally in a loaded situation.

Stepien *et al.* (1998) support the idea of sled pulling in training as it applies a significant isometric load as well as the isotonic training of endurance running. These authors found training adaptations in excess of those found in non-pulling training, particularly with respect to cardiac function.

Wet treadmill

The wet treadmill allows the dog to exercise against the resistance of the water at belly level while walking, trotting and running at variable speed. This exercise in particular allows the loading of the limb protractors, which cannot be overloaded by pulling a sled. Human athletes benefit from weight training of these powerful forward flexors of the limbs, which are responsible for driving the limb forward to foot strike. The water environment also allows the Husky to be trained in a cool environment. Running in the water at the beach, dam or river is an obvious and practical alternative.

Track work

Track work can form the basis of the interval training and high-speed training programmes. Once again, work can be done under harness under the direction of the driver/trainer while monitoring speed and distance via GPS unit and heart rate monitor. The interval training programme should be split between the treadmill and track to relieve boredom and avoid staleness or overtraining.

6.10.3 Programme phases

An example is given of a 16-week programme, divided into four phases.
- *Basic training*: weeks 1–4
- *Substrenuous/resistance training*: weeks 5–8
- *Strenuous interval training*: weeks 9–14
- *Taper*: weeks 15–16

Basic training phase

Art & Lekeux (1995) found significant reductions in performance-related variables in horses with 2–6 weeks of rest. Rest in human athletes has more profound effects. Four weeks of rest in endurance-trained dogs is likely to have similar effects of reducing VO_{2max} by 15–20%. While allowing the musculoskeletal system recovery time, rest may leave the animal more vulnerable to injury under strenuous exercise conditions. The 4-week 'basic training' phase is designed to bring the dog gradually back into the training regime while allowing activities for skill development and 'fun'. During this period, the trainer should form a close and confident relationship with the dog, which will assist in accomplishing the more strenuous activities later in the programme.

Sinha *et al.* (1991) reported no difference between VO_{2max} following basic training of 40% and 80% VO_{2max}. Musch *et al.* (1985) reported a 31% gain in VO_{2max}, training at 80% maximum heart rate. It can be concluded that light exercise designed to prepare the musculoskeletal system is not conditional on intensity and that low- to moderate-intensity work is sufficient to stimulate some preparatory gain in VO_{2max}. It must be remembered, however, that the Husky is an endurance athlete, capable of pulling a load in excess of 140 km/day. A low-intensity 10 km walk/jog for a previously fit dog will not be physiologically demanding. Secondly, the endurance Husky, unlike the racehorse, is a mature animal. There are no age restrictions on races and no incentive to race at an early age. The incidence of injury due to an immature musculoskeletal system is, therefore, likely to be lower than observed in horses and racing Greyhounds.

During this period, the dog can be introduced to the various training venues and familiarised with the surroundings, regimes and equipment required in the training programme. It is best to familiarise the dog with a new procedure in a low-stress situation without time constraints. Attention should be given to address suppling, balance and proprioception tasks during this period to reduce incidence of training- and race-related musculoskeletal injuries.

Substrenuous/resistance training

The goals for this period are to:
- further improve aerobic performance in preparation for the next more intensive training phase
- progressively overload the musculoskeletal system in a way that is specific to the event situation to promote performance-enhancing adaptation and injury prevention
- further develop the training regimes and become expert with the training methods
- continue to work on suppling, balance and proprioception tasks for injury prevention.

High-intensity exercise must be gradually introduced and progressed to allow adequate stimulation and time for musculoskeletal and metabolic changes to occur. Significant changes in endurance performance-related variables will occur in the dog during a short endurance training programme (Musch *et al.* 1985), but evidence from human studies strongly suggests that further improvements will not occur unless the intensity is lifted. This period of training will gradually introduce the dog to the interval training protocol, which is used to obtain the required intensity of training. Training intensity should be based on velocity at VO_{2max} or HR_{max} obtained at the pre-phase fitness test and increased each week.

Resistance training forms a part of all human athletic endurance and strength training programmes, but is underutilised in the training of animals. This is no doubt partly due to difficulties in training design. Animals cannot be easily taught to lift heavy weights. Strength training allows the muscles to utilise more elastic energy and reduce the amount of energy wasted in braking forces (Saunders *et al.* 2004). Apart from improvements in performance with resistance training (Saunders *et al.* 2004), there are the benefits of injury prevention, particularly following previous muscle injury (Proske *et al.* 2004).

Strenuous interval training

Laursen & Jenkins (2002) reported that increases in volume of training in highly trained human endurance athletes do not further enhance either endurance performance or associated physiological variables. It seems that, for athletes who are already trained, improvements in endurance performance can only be achieved through high-intensity interval training.

The intensity of interval training in a previously fit athlete can be very high. Creer *et al.* (2004) reported for human athletes that a twice-weekly, 4-week sprint interval programme, consisting of 4 × 30-sec sprints, in addition to an endurance training programme, was superior to an endurance training programme alone. Significant gains in motor unit activation, total work output and increased blood lactate levels were reported.

Although some variety should be kept in the programme to relieve boredom and stress, this 6-week phase can focus on high-intensity interval training on the track and on the wet and dry treadmill. More rest intervals and longer recovery times (Laursen & Jenkins 2002) are essential as intensity of training is increased. The velocity at which VO_{2max} or HR_{max} is achieved may be selected as the goal interval speed. This intensity has been supported as the probable optimal training intensity for improving aerobic performance in both human studies (Laursen & Jenkins 2002) and horse studies (Tyler-McGowan *et al.* 1999). It should be noted that reassessment of aerobic capacity is required at regular intervals, as the intensity needs to increase with improvements in VO_{2max}. Overtraining is a risk at this period of training and signs should be closely monitored.

Velocity at VO_{2max} or HR_{max} can be determined on both wet and dry treadmills. Track training speed will be identical to the dry level treadmill speed. Ready & Morgan (1984) recorded high blood lactate levels with sled running (3.06 mmol) in Huskies compared with free running (0.70 mmol). It is expected also that the dog will exhibit high blood lactate levels and VO_2 at lower wet treadmill velocity than dry treadmill velocity. A study of interval training in agility competition dogs found that interval training did not require as much cardiovascular work as prolonged submaximal training and resulted in a lesser degree of training-induced cardiac hypertrophy (Rovira *et al.* 2010).

Taper

The aim of the taper is to reduce the physiological and psychological stress of daily training and optimise performance. There is little documented evidence of tapering methods in animals in the literature. However, tapering for human athletic events is a well-recognised practice and a well-researched topic. Tapering before a middle distance endurance event improves performance by 5–6%, due to positive changes in the cardiorespiratory, metabolic, haematological, hormonal, neuromuscular and psychological status of the athlete (Majika & Padilla 2003). It is widely agreed that tapering is best achieved by maintaining intensity of training while reducing training volume (to 60–90%) and slightly reducing training frequency (no more than 20%). Neary *et al.* (2003) reported that a 50% training volume reduction for 7 days prior to a performance was superior to 30% and 80% reductions, and documented a 5.4% performance improvement.

Dogs should be tapered progressively over a 2-week period before competition. Training volume can be reduced by 25% in week 1 and a further 25% in week 2. Training intensity should remain the same. The number of training sessions can reduce over the 2-week taper period.

6.10.4 Aims of the programme design
Cardiorespiratory responses
- Training-induced bradycardia and lower HR at a given velocity
- Increased VO_{2max} by 30–40%
- Increased maximum cardiac output by 30–35%
- Compensatory hypertrophy of the heart (up to 24% in Huskies)
- Reduced systemic vascular resistance by 25% during maximum exercise
- Increased velocity at which V4 is reached, goal of at least 20% increase

Musculoskeletal responses
- Increased muscle fibre area for both slow-twitch and fast-twitch muscle fibres
- Better utilisation of elastic energy due to strength training
- Increased muscle strength in both the propulsive and protracting musculature
- Increased muscle contraction time
- Increased resting intramuscular glycogen (15–20%) content
- Enhanced muscle oxidative capacity
- Increased motor unit activation/improved pattern of neural drive
- Increased tendon cross-sectional area
- Increased bone density

Injury prevention
- Low injury rate due to strength training and low-velocity long-distance training, in addition to improved flexibility, balance and proprioception through specifically targeted exercises.
- Avoidance of overtraining by varying training activities and regular fitness testing/health and lameness checks.

6.11 Training the racing Greyhound

6.11.1 Profile of the Greyhound as an athlete

The origins of the Greyhound are in recreational hunting. Dogs are bred to sprint and are very fast over a short distance and still have a strong hunting instinct. The dog typically weighs around 28–30 kg and has a very low percentage body fat (Schoning *et al.* 1995). The Greyhound is a long-legged dog, with large proximal muscle mass and light distal limbs (Figure 6.8).

The Greyhound is capable of running 500 m at 18 m/sec. In comparison, the Quarterhorse is just faster at 20 m/sec and humans are way behind at over 10 m/sec over 400 m. The Greyhound has a higher percentage of fast-twitch fibres than other dog breeds (Guy & Snow 1981) and can produce blood lactate levels of 27 mmol (Rose & Bloomberg 1989). Greyhounds have

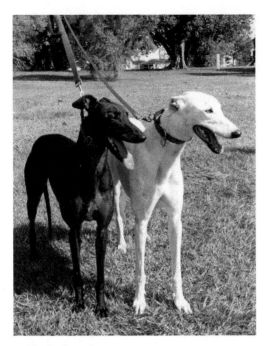

Figure 6.8 The Greyhound.

unique physiological characteristics such as high haematocrit, hemoglobin concentration, and whole blood viscosity in addition to low white blood cell count, neutrophil count, platelet count, and serum protein and globulin concentrations (Fayos *et al.* 2005). Greyhounds also have high glomerular filtration rate, functional murmurs of aortic stenosis, higher serum creatinine concentrations, and lower serum T_4 and fT_4 concentrations than other breeds of dog (Drost *et al.* 2006; Fabrizio *et al.* 2006; Feeman *et al.* 2003; Gaughan & Bruyette, 2001; Pape *et al.* 1986). Greyhounds have several physiological peculiarities, including high blood pressure, large left ventricle, high aortic velocity and high cardiac output, compared with non-Greyhound dogs (Vilar *et al.* 2008).

6.11.2 Profile of a Greyhound race

Greyhound races in Australia are typically over 297 m and are won at the elite level in about 17 sec. The race is run in an anticlockwise direction from a standing start. There are several dogs in the race and dogs regularly interfere with each other, risking injury.

The Greyhound relies predominantly on anaerobic metabolism during the 17 sec sprint race (Rose & Bloomberg 1989). A very high maximum heart rate with evidence for a high VO_{2max} of Greyhounds (143 mL/kg/min; Staaden 1984) suggests a higher aerobic capacity than expected for a sprint athlete with very little endurance training.

A dog is typically 'trained' by daily walks, some track work and the odd run on the bait to improve the 'desire'. It is generally thought that the dog has bred-in ability to run fast. However, research has shown that performance improvements can be achieved and that the dog has a similar metabolic reaction to training as the human sprinter.

Injuries on and off the racetrack are common in Greyhounds. The most common are right hindlimb gracilis muscle tears, fracture of the central metatarsal in the right hindlimb, fractured carpi in either forelimb (Schoning 1994) and shin splints on the left (railing) forelimb (Davis 1971). These bony injuries most likely result from training errors, either overtraining of young dogs leading to breakdown or underpreparation of the musculoskeletal system to cope with the rigors of sprint training and racing. The high injury rate requires special attention in training design. The selection of Greyhounds for high-speed running is associated with the evolution of relatively long, stiff, brittle limb bones with relatively low resistance to failure (Kemp 2005).

Speed, race distance and track design are significant factors that have been found to influence the injury rate of the racing Greyhound and should be areas to focus on for the prevention of injury (Sicard *et al.* 1999; Tharwat *et al.* 2014). Injuries are most likely to occur in the first turn of the race (Sicard *et al.* 1999) which may be exacerbated by poor attention to pre-race warm-up (Windred *et al.* 2007).

Cornering is a skill that requires learning at a slow speed and practising at increasing levels of difficulty until the dog is skill-competent and anatomically prepared at race speed. The dog cannot be expected to have the motor control at pace in cornering to avoid injury if it is not well rehearsed in the task (Helton 2009). Dogs' skill development shows marked improvement with increasing race experience (Helton 2009). Additional to motor control development is the importance of musculoskeletal development to withstand the angular forces sustained during cornering. Tissue is organised along the lines of stress. Therefore, there must be a significant amount of angular stress in the preparation and training programme to allow suitable bone, muscle, tendon and ligament adaptation. The issue of 'one-sidedness' then appears. In reality, the racing Greyhound is an athlete with a unilateral bias. Just like a right-handed tennis player, the dog should develop an acceptable asymmetry. Several authors (Bergh *et al.* 2012; Johnson *et al.* 2001; Thompson *et al.* 2012; Wernham *et al.* 2010) have reported specific asymmetrical and repeatable patterns of increased cortical thickness and geometric properties of distal limb bones in Greyhounds, suggesting site-specific adaptive responses associated with asymmetrical cyclical loading as a result of racing on circular tracks. Site-specific adaptive remodelling may be important in the aetiopathogenesis of fatigue fractures in racing Greyhounds and may be used to guide training regimens.

Summary of the race profile

- Approximately 300 m all-out sprint
- Run anticlockwise on circular track
- 17 sec race time
- Predominantly anaerobic metabolism
- Soft tissue and bony injuries are common

Programme components; evidence to support training methodology
- Fitness testing
- Skill development and basic training
- Track work under harness
- Wet treadmill
- Play/stretching/balance and proprioception training
- Sprint work
- Race track

Fitness testing

Regular health and lameness assessment will be important during the training programme. Particular care is required to assess for signs of lameness, palpable soreness and muscle injury.

VO_{2max} can be measured in the Greyhound, as in the Husky, as an indicator of improved aerobic capacity. In reality, HR is more commonly used as a training indicator, owing to the unavailability of VO_2 measurements in dogs.

As the athlete adapts to anaerobic-based training, the blood lactate level at a given velocity should reduce. This is an indication of efficiency (Creer *et al.* 2004). However, training adaptations should also allow the generation of higher blood lactate levels during maximal work. To measure these markers, the velocity must be controllable, thus the treadmill is ideal.

Skill development and basic training

The Greyhound has similar basic training requirements to the Husky in terms of musculoskeletal adaptations. Whereas the Husky is reliant on a large aerobic capacity to complete the 30 km race, the Greyhound requires aerobic fitness to endure the rigors of the pre-race training programme. Suppling, balance and proprioception training are important during this period.

Straight endurance work will be the main feature of this exercise but will be combined with skill development. The Greyhound must become very proficient at cornering left to cope with the race track situation. The trainer should regularly circle the dog left, first at a walk and later at a trot and run. The Greyhound will learn to balance itself during cornering and adapt neural mechanisms and tissues to suit the activity. This will start the grounding in injury prevention as well as performance enhancement. Dogs' skill development shows marked improvement with increasing training and race experience (Helton 2009).

Track work under harness

Even Greyhound dogs can be taught to pull a harness. Weighted sled towing is a common resisted sprint training technique in human athletes (Lockie *et al.* 2003). While this technique has the disadvantage of changing sprint kinematics (Lockie *et al.* 2003), it allows the trainer to adjust the velocity and load on the dog and regulate adequate rest breaks during interval training. It also allows further skill training and specific loading for cornering.

Wet treadmill

Lockie *et al.* (2003) and Judge *et al.* (2003) reported that resistance training is beneficial for both sprint performance and injury prevention. Resistance training has the effect of improving the pattern of neural drive, increasing muscle fibre size and speed of contraction and increasing power output in the activity specifically trained. The wet treadmill at belly depth provides a resistance for the limb protractors during the swing phase of gait. This is combined with a harness weight to provide a load to the propulsive muscles of gait. This activity closely matches fast running and fulfils some of the requirements for resistance training to be beneficial (Gonyea & Sale 1982).

Play/stretching/balance and proprioception training

This session provides a good bonding opportunity between dog and trainer and can allow some controlled sprint work, e.g. ball chasing and retrieval. A muscle-stretching session, particularly of the hindlimb hamstrings and adductors, should be incorporated. Balance and proprioception exercises can include a variety of terrain and obstacles to work over and around, to enrich the training environment.

Sprint work

The open field can be used. This session will form the basis of specific sprint speed development. A GPS unit secured to the Greyhound via a Lycra singlet can provide velocity feedback (Hampson & McGowan 2007). Attention should be paid to behavioural management in the starting cage to avoid bad habits developing during racing.

Race track

Specific sprint work on the race track is required towards the end of the programme to prepare the dog psychologically for racing and to provide more specificity in incorporating the particular musculoskeletal stresses of the race track. Further work on behaviour in the starting cage should be done to assist in relieving race stress and bad behaviour which may affect performance.

6.11.3 Aims of the programme design
Cardiorespiratory responses
- Training-induced bradycardia and lower HR at a given velocity
- Increased VO_{2max} by 30%
- Increased maximum cardiac output by 30–35%
- Compensatory hypertrophy of the heart (up to 24% in Huskies)
- Reduced systemic vascular resistance by 25% during maximum exercise
- Increased velocity at which V4 is reached, goal of at least 20% increase
- Increase exercising blood lactate levels

Musculoskeletal responses

- Increased muscle fibre area for both slow-twitch and fast-twitch muscle fibres
- Better utilisation of elastic energy due to strength training
- Increased muscle strength in both the propulsive and protracting musculature (24%)
- Decreased muscle contraction time
- Increased resting intramuscular glycogen (15–20%) content
- Enhanced muscle oxidative capacity
- Increased motor unit activation/improved pattern of neural drive
- Increased tendon cross-sectional area
- Increased bone density
- Selective musculoskeletal development to handle the stress of cornering left

Injury prevention

- Lower injury rate due to strength training and low-velocity, long-distance training
- Avoidance of overtraining by varying training activities and regular fitness testing/health and lameness checks
- Selective skill development and musculoskeletal development to handle the stresses of high race speeds and cornering left
- Correction of muscle tightness due to stretching programme, particularly in the hindlimb adductors and hamstring muscles
- Improved balance, coordination and proprioception

6.12 Conclusion

The principles of exercise physiology should be applied to rehabilitation programmes as well as the principles of reducing pain, improving movement and restoring normal muscle control for better motor performance and function. Optimal performance may vary depending on the species, breed and type of training. Training methods combine to optimise cardiorespiratory and muscular function (the pathway of oxygen) as well as the neuromotor control and skills training to perform optimally.

References

Art, T., Lekeux, P. 1995, Ventilatory and arterial blood gas tension adjustments to strenuous exercise in Standardbreds. *Am. J. Vet. Res.* 56(10): 1332–1337.

Banse, H.E., Sides, R.H., Ruby, B.C., Bayly, W.M. 2007, Effects of endurance training on VO2max and submaximal blood lactate concentrations of untrained sled dogs. *Equine Compr. Exerc. Physiol.* 4: 89–94.

Bellenger, S., Davie, A.J., Evans, D.L. *et al.* 1995, Effects of low intensity training on gas exchange at the start of exercise. *Equine Vet. J.* 18(suppl): 43–46.

Betros, C.L., McKeeve, R.K.H., Kearns, C.F. *et al.* 2002, Effects of ageing and training on maximal heart rate and VO₂max. *Equine Vet. J. Suppl.* (34): 100–105.

Bergh, M.S., Piras A., Samii, V.F., Weisbrode, S.E., Johnson, K.A. *et al.* 2012, Fractures in regions of adaptive modeling and remodeling of central tarsal bones in racing Greyhounds. *Am. J. Vet. Res.* 73(3): 375–380.

Canberra Sled Dog Club 2005, Available at: www.canberrasleddogclub.com.au/index.htm

Christley, R.M., Hodgson, D.R., Evans, D.L. *et al.* 1997, Effects of training on the development of exercise-induced arterial hypoxaemia in horses. *Am. J. Vet. Res.* 58(6): 653–657.

Cox, C., Gaskill, S., Ruby, B. *et al.* 2003, Case study of training, fitness and nourishment of a dog driver during the Iditarod 1049-mile dogsled race. *Int. J. Sport Nutr. Exerc. Metab.* 13(3): 286–293.

Creer, A.R., Ricard, M.D., Conlee, R.K., Hoyt, G.L., Parcell, A.C. 2004, Neural, metabolic and performance adaptations to four weeks of high intensity sprint interval training in trained cyclists. *Int. J. Sports Med.* 25(2): 92–98.

Croisier, J.L., Forthomme, B., Namurois, M.H. *et al.* 2002, Hamstring muscle strain recurrence and strength performance disorders. *Am. J. Sports Med.* 30(2): 199–203.

Davie, A. 2003, Principles of training. In: Davie, A. *Scientific Training of Thoroughbred Racehorses.* Northcoast Publishing, San Francisco, CA, pp. 31–38.

Davie, A.J., Evans, D.L. 2000, Blood lactate responses to submaximal field exercise tests in Thoroughbred horses. *Vet. J.* 159(3): 252–258.

Davis, P.E. 1971, Shin soreness in the racing greyhound. *Vet. Rec.* 89(23): 610–611.

Davis, M.S., McKiernan, B., McCullough, S. *et al.* 2002, Racing Alaskan sled dogs as a model of "ski asthma". *Am. J. Res. Crit. Care Med.* 166(6): 878–882.

Drost, W.T., Couto, C.G., Fischetti, A.J. *et al.* 2006, Comparison of glomerular filtration rate between Greyhounds and non-Greyhound dogs. *J. Vet. Intern. Med.* 20: 544–546.

Eaton, M.D. 1994, Energetics and performance. In: Hodgson, D.R., Rose R.J. (eds), *The Athletic Horse, Principles and Practice of Equine Sports Medicine.* W.B. Saunders, Philadelphia, PA, pp. 49–61.

Eaton, M.D., Evans, D.L., Hodgson, D.R. *et al.* 1995, Maximal accumulated oxygen deficit in Thoroughbred horses. *J. Appl. Physiol.* 78(4): 1564–1568.

Eaton, M.D., Hodgson, D.R., Evans, D.L. *et al.* 1999, Effects of low- and moderate-intensity training on metabolic responses to exercise in Thoroughbreds. *Equine Vet. J. Suppl.* 30: 521–527.

Evans, D.L. 1985, Cardiovascular adaptations to exercise and training. *Vet. Clin. North Am. Equine Pract.* 1(3): 513–531.

Evans, D.L. 2000, *Training and Fitness in Athletic Horses.* Report for Rural Industries Research and Development Corporation.

Evans, D.L., Rose, R.J. 1987, Maximum oxygen uptake in racehorses: changes with training state and prediction from submaximal cardiorespiratory measurements. In: Gillespie, J.R., Robinson, N.E. (eds), *Equine Exercise Physiology*, vol. 2. ICEEP Publications, Davis, CA. pp. 52–67.

Fabrizio, F., Baumwart, R., Iazbik, M.C. *et al.* 2006, Left basilar systolic murmur in retired racing Greyhounds. *J. Vet. Intern. Med.* 20: 78–82.

Fayos, M., Couto, C.G., Cline Iazbik, M.C., Wellman, M. 2005, Serum protein electrophoresis in retired racing Greyhounds. *Vet. Clin. Pathol.* 34: 397–400.

Feeman, W.E., Couto, C.G., Gray, T.L. 2003, Serum creatinine concentrations in retired racing Greyhounds. *Vet. Clin. Pathol.* 32: 40–42.

Gaughan, K.R., Bruyette, D.S. 2001, Thyroid function testing in Grey-hounds. *Am. J. Vet. Res.* 62: 1130–1133.

Geor, R.J., McCutcheon, L.J., Hinchcliff, K.W. 2000, Effects of warm-up intensity on kinetics of oxygen consumption and carbon dioxide production during high-intensity exercise in horses. *Am. J. Vet. Res.* 61(6): 638–645.

Gonyea, W.J., Sale, D. 1982, Physiology of weight lifting exercise. *Arch. Phys. Med. Rehabil.* 63(5): 235–237.

Grandjean, D., Mateo, R., Lefol, J.F. *et al.* 1983, Nutritional, physio-logical, biochemical and haematological controls in the racing grey-hound. *Rec. Med. Vet.* 159(9): 735–746.

Gray, S., Nimmo, M.J. 2001, Effects of active, passive or no warm-up on metabolism and performance during high-intensity exercise. *Sports Sci.* 19(9): 693–700.

Guy, P.S., Snow, D.H. 1981, Skeletal muscle fibre composition in the dog and its relationship to athletic ability. *Res. Vet. Sci.* 31(2): 244–248.

Hagerman, F.C. 1992, Energy metabolism and fuel utilization. *Med. Sci. Sports Exerc.* 24(9 suppl): S309–S314.

Hahn, A.G., Gore, C.J. 2001, The effect of altitude on cycling perfor-mance: a challenge to traditional concepts. *Sports Med.* 31(7): 533–557.

Hampson, B.A., McGowan, C.M. 2007, Physiological responses of the Australian cattle dog to mustering exercise. *Equine Compr. Exerc. Physiol.* 4(01): 37–41.

Harris, R.C., Marlin, D.J., Snow, D.H. 1987, Metabolic response to max-imal exercise of 800 and 2000 m. in the Thoroughbred horse. *J. Appl. Physiol.* 63(1): 12–19.

Hawley, J.A. 2002, Symposium: Limits to fat oxidation by skeletal muscle during exercise – Introduction. *Med. Sci. Sports Exerc.* 34(9): 1475–1476.

Helton, W.S. 2009, Exceptional running skill in dogs requires extensive experience. *J. Gen. Psychol.* 136(3): 323–336.

Hodgson, D.R., McGowan, C.M., McKeever, K.H. (eds), 2014, *The Ath-letic Horse, Principles and Practice of Equine Sports Medicine.* Elsevier, St Louis, MO.

Johnson, K.A., Skinner, G.A., Muir, P. 2001, Site-specific adaptive remodeling of Greyhound metacarpal cortical bone subjected to asymmetrical cyclic loading. *Am. J. Vet. Res.* 62(5): 787–793.

Judge, L.W., Moreau, C., Burke, J.R. 2003, Neural adaptations with sports-specific resistance training in highly skilled athletes. *J. Sports Sci.* 21(5): 419–427.

Kemp, T.J. 2005, Functional trade-offs in the limb bones of dogs selected for running versus fighting. *J. Exper. Biol.* 208(18): 3475–3482.

Kriz, N.G., Hodgson, D.R., Rose, R.J. 2000, Changes in cardiac dimen-sions and indices of cardiac function during deconditioning in horses. *Am. J. Vet. Res.* 61(12): 1553–1560.

Lacombe, V.A., Hinchcliff, K.W., Kohn, C.W. *et al.* 2004, Effects of feeding meals with various soluble-carbohydrate content on muscle glycogen synthesis after exercise in horses. *Am. J. Vet. Res.* 65: 916–923.

Laursen, P.B., Jenkins, D.G. 2002, The scientific basis of high-intensity interval training: optimising training programmes and maximising performance in highly trained endurance athletes. *Sports Med.* 32(1): 53–73.

Leleu, C., Cotrel, C., Courouce-Malblanc, A. 2005, Relationships between physiological variables and race performance in French stan-dardbred trotters. *Vet. Rec.* 156(11): 339–342.

Lockie, R.G., Murphy, A.J., Spinks, C.D. 2003, Effects of resisted sled towing on sprint kinematics in field-sport athletes. *J. Strength Cond. Res.* 17(4): 760–767.

Majika, I., Padilla, S. 2003, Scientific bases for precompetition tapering strategies. *Med. Sci. Sports Exerc.* 35(7): 1182–1187.

Marlin, D.J., Harris, P.A., Schroter, R.C. *et al.* 1995, Physiological, metabolic and biochemical responses of horses competing in the SE phase of a CCI**** three-day event. *Equine Vet. J.* 20(suppl): 37–46.

Marlin, D.J., Nankervis, K. 2002, Skeletal responses. In: Marlin, D. Nankervis K. (eds), *Equine Exercise Physiology*. Blackwell Science, Oxford, pp. 86–93.

Martin, B.B. Jr, Reef, V.B., Parente, E.J. *et al.* 2000, Causes of poor perfor-mance of horses during training, racing, or showing: 348 cases (1992–1996). *J. Am. Vet. Med. Assoc.* 216(4): 554–558.

McCutcheon, L.J., Geor, R.J., Hinchcliff, K.W. 1999, Effects of prior exer-cise on muscle metabolism during sprint exercise in horses. *J. Appl. Physiol.* 87(5): 1914–1922.

McGowan, C.M., Golland, L.C., Evans, D.L. 2002, Effects of prolonged training, overtraining and detraining on skeletal muscle metabolites and enzymes. *Equine Vet. J.* 34(suppl): 257–263.

McKenzie, E.C., Hinchcliff, K.W., Valberg, S.J., Williamson, K.K., Pay-ton, M.E., Davis, M.S. 2008, Assessment of alterations in triglyceride and glycogen concentrations in muscle tissue of Alaskan sled dogs during repetitive prolonged exercise. *Am. J. Vet. Res.* 69(8): 1097–1103.

Musch, T.I., Haidet, G.C., Ordway, G.A. *et al.* 1985, Dynamic exercise training in foxhounds. 1. Oxygen consumption and hemodynamic responses. *J. Appl. Physiol.* 59(1): 183–189.

Musch, T.I., Haidet, G.C., Ordway, G.A., Longhurst, J.C., Mitchell, J.H. 1987, Training effects on regional blood flow response to maximal exercise in foxhounds. *J. Appl. Physiol.* 62: 1724–1732.

Navot-Mintzer, D., Epstein, M., Constantini, N. 2003, Physical activity and training at high altitude. *Harefuah* 132(10): 704–709.

Neary, J.P., Bhambhani, Y.N., McKenzie, D.C. 2003, Effects of different stepwise reduction taper protocols on cycling performance. *Can. J. Appl. Physiol.* 28(4): 576–587.

Pape, L.A., Price, J.M., Alpert, J.S., Rippe, J.M. 1986, Hemodynamics and left ventricular function: A comparison between adult racing Grey-hounds and Greyhounds completely untrained from birth. *Basic Res. Cardiol.* 81: 417–424.

Patteson, M.W., Cripps, P.J. 1993, A survey of cardiac auscultatory find-ings in horses. *Equine Vet. J.* 25(5): 409–415.

Poole, D.C. 2004, Current concepts of oxygen transport during exercise. *Equine Compr. Exerc. Physiol.* 1: 5–22.

Poole, D.C., Kindig, C.A., Behnke, B.J., *et al.* 2004, Oxygen uptake (VO_2) kinetics in different species: a brief review. *Equine Compr. Exerc. Physiol.* 2(1): 1–15.

Proske, U., Morgan, D.L., Brockett, C.L. *et al.* 2004, Identifying athletes at risk of hamstring strains and how to protect them. *Clin. Exp. Phar-macol. Physiol.* 31(8): 546–550.

Ready, A.E., Morgan, G. 1984, The physiological response of Siberian Husky dogs to exercise: effect of interval training. *Can. Vet. J.* 25(2): 86–91.

Reynolds, A.J., Fuhrer, L., Dunlap, H.L., Finke, M., Kallfelz, F.A. 1995, Effect of diet and training on muscle glycogen storage and utilization in sled dogs. *J. Appl. Physiol.* 79: 1601–1607.

Rose, R.J., Bloomberg, M.S. 1989, Responses to sprint exercise in the Greyhound: effects on haematology, serum biochemistry and muscle metabolites. *Res. Vet. Sci.* 47(2): 212–218.

Rovira, S., Muñoz, A., Riber, C., Benito, M. 2010, Heart rate, electro-cardiographic parameters and arrhythmias during agility exercises in trained dogs. *Rev. Med. Vet.* 161: 307–313.

Saunders, P.U., Pyne, D.B., Telford, R.D. *et al.* 2004, Factors affecting running economy in trained distance runners. *Sports Med.* 34(7): 465–485.

Schoning, P. 1994, Gross pathological changes in Greyhounds: musculoskeletal system and skin, Part 1. *Canine Pract.* 19(4): 25–27.

Schoning, P., Erickson, H., Milliken, G.A. 1995, Body weight, heart weight and heart-to-body weight ratio in Greyhounds. *Am. J. Vet. Res.* 56(4): 420–422.

Serrano, A.L., Quiroz-Rothe, E., Rivero, J.L.L. 2000, Early and long-term changes of equine skeletal muscle in response to endurance training and detraining. *Pflugers Arch. Eur. J. Physiol.* 441: 263–274.

Shellock, F.G., Prentice, W.E. 1985, Warming-up and stretching for improved physical performance and prevention of sports-related injuries. *Sports Med.* 2(4): 267–278.

Sicard, G.K., Short, K., Manley, P.A. 1999, A survey of injuries at five greyhound racing tracks. *J. Small Anim. Pract.* 40(9): 428–432.

Sinha, A.K., Ray, S.P., Rose, R.J. 1991, Effect of training intensity and detraining on adaptations in different skeletal muscles. In: Persson, S.G.B., Lindholm, A., Jeffcott, L.B. (eds), *Equine Exercise Physiology 3*. ICEEP Publications, Davis, CA, pp. 223–230.

Staaden, R. (1984), *The Exercise Physiology of the Racing Greyhound*. PhD thesis, Murdoch University, Australia.

Steinacker, J.M. 1993, Physiological aspects of training in rowing. *Int. J. Sports Med.* 14(suppl 1): S3–S10.

Stepien, R.L., Hinchcliff, K.W., Constable, P.D. *et al.* 1998, Effect of endurance training on cardiac morphology in Alaskan sled dogs. *J. Appl. Physiol.* 85: 1368–1375.

Tharwat, M., Al-Sobayil, F., Buczinski, S. 2014, Influence of racing on the serum concentrations of acute-phase proteins and bone metabolism biomarkers in racing greyhounds. *Vet. J.* 202(2): 372–377.

Thompson, D.J., Cave, N.J., Bridges, J.P., Reuvers, K., Owen, M.C., Firth, E.C. 2012, Bone volume and regional density of the central tarsal bone detected using computed tomography in a cross-sectional study of adult racing greyhounds. *NZ Vet. J.* 60(5): 278–284.

Trilk, J.L., Lindner, A.J., Greene, H.M. *et al.* 2002, A lactate-guided conditioning programme to improve endurance performance. *Equine Vet. J.* 34(suppl): 122–125.

Tyler, C.M., Hodgson, D.R., Rose, R.J. 1996a, Effect of a warm-up on energy supply during high intensity exercise in horses. *Equine Vet. J.* 28(2): 117–120.

Tyler, C.M., Golland L.C., Evans D.L. *et al.* 1996b, Changes in maximum oxygen uptake during prolonged training, overtraining, and detraining in horses. *J. Appl. Physiol.* 81(5): 2244–2249.

Tyler, C.M., Golland L.C., Evans D.L. *et al.* 1998, Skeletal muscle adaptations to prolonged training, overtraining and detraining in horses. *Pflugers Arch. Eur. J. Physiol.* 436(3): 391–397.

Tyler-McGowan, C.M., Golland, L.C., Evans, D.L. *et al.* 1999, Haematological and biochemical responses to training and overtraining in Standard bred horses. *Equine Vet. J.* 30(suppl): 621–625.

Van Citters, R.L., Franklin, D.L. 1969, Cardiovascular performance of Alaska Sled Dogs during exercise. *Circ. Res.* 24(1): 33–42.

Vilar, P., Couto, C.G., Westendorf, N., Iazbik, C., Charske, J., Marin, L. 2008, Thromboelastographic tracings in retired racing Greyhounds and in non-Greyhound dogs. *J. Vet. Intern. Med.* 22(2): 374–379.

Vincent, I.C., Mitchell, A.R., Leahy, R.A. 1993, Non-invasive measurement of arterial blood pressure in dogs: a potential indicator for the identification of stress. *Res. Vet. Sci.* 54: 195–201.

Wagner, J.A., Horvath, S.M., Dahms, T.E. 1977, Cardiovascular, respiratory, and metabolic adjustments to exercise in dogs. *J. Appl. Physiol.* 42(3): 403–407.

Wernham, B.G.J., Roush, J.K. 2010, Metacarpal and metatarsal fractures in dogs. *Compend. Contin. Educ. Vet.* 29: E1–E7.

Wickler, S., Greene, H.M. 2004, High altitude acclimatization and athletic performance in horses. *Equine Comp. Exerc. Physiol.* 1(3): 167–170.

Windred, A.J., Osmotherly, P.G., McGowan, C.M. 2007, Pre-race warm-up practices in Greyhound racing: a pilot study. *Equine Compr. Exerc. Physiol.* 4(3-4): 119–122.

Young, L.E. 1999, Cardiac responses to training in 2-year-old Thoroughbreds: an echocardiographic study. *Equine Vet. J.* 30(suppl): 195–198.

CHAPTER 7

Equine lameness*

Chris Whitton

University of Melbourne, Melbourne, Australia

Summary

Equine lameness is an important area for the equine physiotherapist
to understand as many horses referred for physiotherapy, including
cases referred for undefined poor performance or behavioural
problems, will have an underlying lameness, which is often the
primary condition. However, in all cases to avoid the revolving door
of treatment and recurrence, it is essential to identify and treat the
lameness before you treat the animal either by referring back to the
veterinary surgeon or, ideally, working as a veterinary-physiotherapy
team.

7.1 Introduction

Orthopaedic disorders in horses occurring before and during
their performance careers represent a significant cost to the
equine industry and are the focus of considerable research.
Lameness is the most frequent reason for loss of performance

and interruption in training in racehorses (Bailey *et al.* 1997).
It is also common in non-racehorses with more than 50% of
horses examined during a prepurchase examination identified
as lame (van Hoogmoed *et al.* 2003), and 24% of dressage horses
reported to be lame in the preceding 2 years (Murray *et al.* 2010).
This chapter will focus on lameness problems related to bones,
joints, tendons and ligaments. For more information on muscle
disease see Chapter 10.

Lameness may be the result of direct trauma, tissue fatigue
due to repeated loading, congenital or acquired anomalies, infection, metabolic disturbances and circulatory disorders. Conformational faults and shoeing factors may contribute to the development of lameness by increasing loads on specific structures.
In addition, because the nervous system is intimately connected
to the musculoskeletal system, neurological disorders may sec-
ondarily result in gait deficits, unexplained lameness or muscle
atrophy. Examples include stringhalt, shivering and equine herpes virus 1 myeloencephalopathy (see Chapter 10).

Lameness is an abnormality in locomotion resulting in
unloading of one or more limbs. Because it is difficult to determine the precise cause of lameness based on the way the horse

---

*Adapted from the first edition chapter, which was written by Nicholas
Malikides

Animal Physiotherapy: Assessment, Treatment and Rehabilitation of Animals, Second Edition. Edited by Catherine M. McGowan and Lesley Goff.
© 2016 John Wiley & Sons, Ltd. Published 2016 by John Wiley & Sons, Ltd.

moves, it is essential for physiotherapists attending to lame horses to have an accurate diagnosis of the orthopaedic disorder made by a veterinary surgeon and to understand the pathoanatomical principles of this diagnosis. This will allow appropriate veterinary treatment, more specific physiotherapy treatment and an accurate prognosis to be made. For example, there is no advantage in treating trigger points in the scapular and pectoral region of a horse with an undiagnosed distal interphalangeal joint osteoarthritis. While such treatment may result in short-term improvements, the absence of a definitive diagnosis will result in a 'revolving door' of unsuccessful treatment, and ultimately client dissatisfaction. Further, due to the changeable nature of musculoskeletal problems in athletic animals, it is important to always include a lameness examination on each physiotherapy reexamination. Any new lameness problems that may have arisen should be referred back to the veterinary surgeon for pathoanatomical diagnosis and treatment. See also Chapter 11.

7.2 The lame horse

In this section, we will attempt to outline broadly the important anatomical, pathophysiological, mechanistic and therapeutic principles of equine orthopaedics with particular emphasis on the lame horse.

Veterinary surgeons and animal physiotherapists require a detailed knowledge of functional anatomy to assess orthopaedic disorders. For biomechanics see Chapter 5. Comprehensive anatomy texts are available (see Further reading). The benefits of becoming completely familiar with topographical anatomy cannot be overemphasised.

7.2.1 Conformational and clinical terms and definitions
Severe conformational abnormalities will predispose to lameness but the relationship between milder abnormalities and lameness is less certain. For example, carpal effusion and the incidence of carpal fracture were decreased in Thoroughbreds with carpal valgus (Anderson *et al.* 2004). Common conformational faults are presented in Table 7.1.

7.2.2 Approach to the lame horse
Lameness is by far the most common reason for performance and pleasure horses to be presented to a veterinary surgeon. Lameness is a manifestation of inflammation or degeneration resulting in varying degrees of pain in one or more limbs, or a mechanical defect, deformity or malformation that results in a gait abnormality.

Poor performance will also be a common presenting complaint for many equine orthopaedic problems. However, many horses can perform well despite mild lameness so other causes of poor performance need to be ruled out even if lameness is identified.

Veterinary surgeons focus on making a pathoanatomical diagnosis of the cause of lameness using a database of historical, clinical and diagnostic test information. In doing so, there are a number of first principles that should be followed.

1 Define and verify the problem. Is the problem primarily a gait abnormality or a swelling, or inflammation? Determine exactly what the horse demonstrates and the duration and character of the problem, e.g. if it is transient or intermittent.
2 Localise the problem. An attempt is made to localise the problem to a particular part of the body (ruling out neurological or other body system problems) by categorising the lameness, using manipulative tests and diagnostic analgesic techniques (see later).
3 Consider pathophysiological and pathological causes.
4 Establish an order of priority of the potential cause(s). Have a list of diagnostic possibilities *and* a plan of attack to rule in or out these options using the most informative tests (see section 7.5 Diagnostic imaging).

7.2.3 Components of the lameness examination
A lameness examination should follow a routine so that important steps are not left out and all appropriate information is collected. In some situations (e.g. financial and time constraints), the examination can change or be shortened. However, except for circumstances such as suspected stress fracture or unsuitable environment or temperament of the horse, it is always recommended to perform a full lameness examination and appropriate diagnostic tests before advising on a lame horse.

> **Key point**
>
> A complete examination is essential as many lameness problems involve multiple sites of pain and an obvious abnormality may not always be painful.

Components of the lameness examination include:
- a detailed clinical history, including the signalment of the horse
- a general physical examination
- examination from a distance, observing conformation, symmetry and posture
- examination of the horse at rest, including palpation and manipulation of each limb and use of hoof testers on all hooves (Figure 7.1)
- determination of the lame limbs or limbs and characterisation of the lameness. The severity of lameness is also graded. The horse should be observed walking and trotting on a hard surface in a straight line, trotting and cantering on a soft surface on the lunge, and trotting on a hard surface on the lunge. Some horses may need to be ridden if the lameness is most prominent with a rider on board
- perform flexion tests to exacerbate low-grade or undetected lameness
- localisation of the source of pain with nerve blocks

Table 7.1 Common faults in conformation

Common term	Synonym	Definition and details	Predisposes to:
Forelimbs			
Front perspective			
Base narrow		Standing with forelimbs inside 'plumb line'. Can be toe-in or toe-out. Found in large-chested horses	Depends on alignment of lower joints
Base wide		Standing with forelimbs outside 'plumb line'. Can be toe-in (rare) or toe-out. Found in narrow-chested horses	Depends on alignment of lower joints
Toe in	Pigeon-toed	Toes point toward one another; congenital and may involve limb from shoulder or fetlock down; common	Outward deviation of foot during flight (paddling or winging out)
Toe out	Splay-footed	Toes point away from each other; congenital, usually from shoulder down; uncommon	Inward arc when advancing; may result in interference with opposite forelimb especially if combined with base-narrow stance
Knock knees	Carpus valgus, knee narrowed (angular limb deformity)	Medial angular deviation of carpus with lateral deviation below carpus; common in foals; usually corrects itself with maturity	Outward rotation of cannon bone, fetlock and foot. May be protective for fetlock fracture or effusions in racing Thoroughbreds (McIlwraith *et al.* 2003)
Bow legs	Carpus varus, bandy-legged (angular limb deformity)	Lateral or outward deviation of carpus with medial deviation below carpus	Likely to result in increased compressive loads on medial aspect of the carpus
Bench knees	Offset knees	Cannon bones are offset (or deviate) laterally and don't follow a straight line from radius; congenital; often combined with carpus valgus	Increased stress on medial splint bone (splints) and suspensory ligament. Associated with increased risk of fetlock problems in racing Thoroughbreds (Anderson *et al.* 2004)
Side perspective			
Calf knees	Hyperextended knees, sheep knees, back at the knee	Backward deviation of carpus; increased weight/stress on carpal ligaments and front aspect of carpal bones	Unknown
Bucked knees	Knee sprung, goat knees, over in the knees	Forward deviation of carpus; knees knuckle forward so dangerous for rider; congenital form bilateral	Unknown
Open knees		Irregular carpal profile (side view) giving impression that joint not apposed; 1–3 year old often with physitis improves with age	Unknown
Standing under front		Entire limb below elbow placed too far under body; can occur with disease as well as being a conformational fault	Unknown
Camped in front		Entire forelimb from body to ground is too far forward	May be a result of navicular syndrome and laminitis
Short pastern		Often associated with base-narrow, toe-in conformation; in horses with short limbs and heavily muscled	Unknown
Long sloping pastern		Pastern bone too long with pastern angle normal or subnormal ($\leq 45°$)	Injury of flexor tendons, sesamoiditis, sesamoid fractures, suspensory desmitis
Hindlimbs			
Rear perspective			
Base wide		Distance between hooves greater than distance between centre of thighs; commonly associated with cow hocks; not as common as in forelimbs	Interference
Base narrow		Distance between hooves less than centre of the thighs; heavily muscled horses; often accompanied by 'bow legs' with hocks too far apart	Interference
Cow hocks	Tarsus valgus (medial deviation of hocks)	Hocks point toward each other (too close) and base-wide from hocks to feet; may be accompanied by 'sickle-hock' esp. Western performance horses	Osteoarthritis of the distal tarsal joints and increased risk of tarsal stress fracture in Thoroughbred racehorses

Table 7.1 (*Continued*)

Common term	Synonym	Definition and details	Predisposes to:
Side perspective			
Sickle hocks	Curby conformation, small hock angles	Excessive angulation of hock joints (≤53°)	Unknown
Straight behind		Excessively straight limbs (little angle between tibia, femur and hock)	Proximal suspensory desmitis
Camped behind		Entire limb too far back; often associated with upright pasterns	
Hooves			
Broken hoof/pastern axis	Broken back posture, run under heel	Low heel, long toe; hoof and pastern axis not in alignment	Heel bruising, navicular syndrome, hoof cracks, interference Increased risk of carpal problems in racing Thoroughbreds (Anderson *et al.* 2004)
Club footed	Broken forward posture	Too steep hoof angle, too low pastern angle; foot axis >pastern axis (short toe, high heel)	Extensor process of pedal bone injury, pedal osteitis, seedy toe
Lateromedial imbalance		One heel higher than other	Navicular syndrome, distal interphalangeal joint collateral ligament injury
Flat feet		Lacks natural concavity of sole; more common in fore hooves; heritable; normal in some draught breeds	Sole bruising and lameness
Contracted heels/foot		Hoof narrower than normal, especially back half; more common in front hooves; uni-or bilateral	Overly concave sole, recessed frog, chronic lameness; thrush
Buttress foot	Pyramidal disease	Swelling on the front of the hoof wall at the coronary band due to new bone growth from low ringbone, fracture of extensor process of pedal bone	Degenerative joint disease of coffin joint, low-grade lameness
Thin walls and sole		Hoof wall wears away too rapidly or doesn't grow fast enough to avoid effects of sole pressure; heritable	Low heel, which wears down; sole bruising and lameness after trimming

Plumb line = line drawn from point of shoulder or hip bisecting the forelimb or hindlimb respectively to the foot, when viewed from the front or back of the horse.

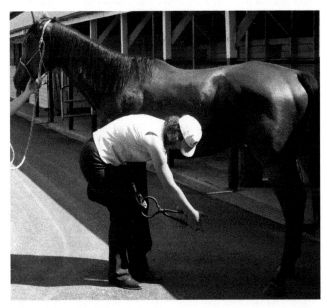

Figure 7.1 Application of hoof testers to determine if there is an area of pain within the hoof.

- selection of the most appropriate imaging technique(s) to attempt to confirm the diagnosis and identify pathology.

A detailed record of the examination, ideally using a standardised examination form, should be produced. Such forms ensure that steps are not missed and the records can be reviewed later for follow-up or repeat visits, especially in horses with more subtle lameness. For further reading on lameness, there are excellent veterinary texts available (see Further reading).

7.2.4 Signalment and history

1 What are the age, sex, breed and use (signalment) of the horse?
   - Some problems develop at specific ages, e.g.:
     a *neonates and foals*: developmental orthopaedic disease (DOD), rupture of the common digital flexor tendon and physeal fractures
     b *two-year-old racehorses* (skeletally immature): bucked shins
     c *adults*: osteoarthritis, navicular syndrome and tendinitis.
   - Certain breeds are predisposed to particular conditions, e.g. ponies with laminitis. Breed often determines the sporting

activity or use, which has an important impact on lameness distribution.

2 How long has the horse been lame?
 – Acute: may indicate fracture or infection.
 – Chronic: 1 month or more: permanent structural changes may have taken place that can prevent full recovery and prognosis is guarded.

3 Was the onset gradual or sudden?
 – Sudden, severe onset indicates trauma or infection.
 – Mild or insidious onset suggests degeneration.

4 Has the lameness worsened, stayed the same or improved?
 – Rapidly worsening lameness suggests infection.
 – No improvement even with rest and slowly worsening suggests degeneration (osteoarthritis).
 – Slow improvement with rest suggests fracture or mild-to-moderate soft tissue injuries.
 – Marked improvement in lameness generally indicates a better prognosis than horses that remain static or have worsened.

5 Does the horse 'warm into' (worsens with exercise) or 'out of' (improves with exercise) the lameness?
 – Lameness associated with stress fractures, tendon or ligament injuries, splints, curb and foot soreness may worsen with exercise.
 – Lameness associated with muscular or arthritic joint involvement often improves with exercise. Some horses can race or perform successfully despite the pain of joint degeneration and lameness can be difficult to detect.

6 Does the horse stumble?
 – May be due to a reluctance to flex during the swing phase of the stride.
 – Neurological disease, e.g. ataxia, proprioception deficits or weakness, may also be considered.

7 Is there a known cause such as trauma or foreign body?

8 Was any treatment given and was it helpful? Painful conditions should respond to an appropriate course of non-steroidal antiinflammatory drugs (NSAIDs) whereas mechanical causes of lameness may not.

9 Have there been any management changes recently?
 – *Shoeing*: hooves trimmed too short or trimmed aggressively, altered hoof balance, improper and irregular shoeing, or a nail driven into or near sensitive tissue may all predispose to lameness.
 – *Training and performance intensity*: a recent increase in training intensity or return to the same level after a rest may result in lameness related to stress-induced subchondral or cortical bone injury (e.g. bucked shins, stress fractures).
 – *Surface*: harder surfaces are associated with hoof lameness and a sudden change in racing surface may lead to episodic lameness in racehorses; soft or uneven surfaces may exacerbate ligament or tendon injuries.
 – *Diet and housing*: sudden changes in diet may result in excesses (e.g. grain) leading to laminitis or deficiencies (e.g. in calcium) leading to nutritional secondary hyperparathyroidism. Shipping to and from sales; foaling indoors; being turned out onto pasture with other horses; and exposure to weather all may be associated with soft tissue injuries, puncture or kick wounds and other trauma.

10 What health or lameness problems has the horse had in the past?

It is not always possible to obtain an entire history but recurrence of lameness, results of previous diagnostic tests and response to previous medication should be noted.

7.2.5 Examination at rest
Symmetry, posture and conformation

Careful visual examination with the horse standing squarely in a flat surface at rest is performed from all angles, first at a distance and then up close. Always compare with the opposite side (assuming that it is normal) during every stage of examination.

From a distance, the following should be observed.
- General body condition and symmetry of skeletal and soft tissues.
- Conformation of body, limbs and feet.
- Alterations in posture such as weight shifting (normally horses will not shift weight in forelimbs but will in hindlimbs), foot pointing or refusing to bear weight (resting a forelimb usually suggests a problem in that limb).
- Presence of any overt tissue injury.

At close observation, each limb and muscle group, particularly of the back and rump, is scrutinised and compared with its opposing member for symmetry. Hooves are checked for abnormal wear, cracks, imbalance, size and heel bulb contraction, whereas all joints and tendons and their sheaths are inspected for swelling. For example, the limb with the smaller hoof and higher heel is usually the (chronically) lame limb (see also Table 7.1). Gluteal muscle wastage usually indicates the lame hindlimb, while asymmetry of the position of the tuber coxae may accompany a pelvic fracture.

Basic abnormalities (in any segment of a limb or hoof) to observe include:
- change in size, shape, height and width of any structure (especially hooves)
- deformity (especially joints and hooves), skin wounds and muscle wasting
- swelling (tissue oedema or joint effusions) and thickening, indicative of inflammation
- draining (usually infected) sinus tracts from joints, bone or soft tissue
- old lesions or scars.

Palpation and hoof tester examination

Palpation and inspection of the hooves, limbs, back and neck should be performed methodically, starting at the hoof and moving up the limb. Comparison with the opposite 'normal' forelimb or hindlimb in the same horse, or in another sound horse if the problem is bilateral in the affected horse, is essential.

Examination of the hoof

- *Coronary band*: heat suggests laminitis; indented suggestive of pedal bone rotation; swelling ± discharging sinus suggests subsolar abscess (gravel) or necrosis/infection of lateral cartilages (quittor); effusion of the distal interphalangeal joint may be palpable at the dorsal aspect immediately proximal to the coronary band.
- *Bulbs of heels and above quarters*: swelling and pain ± discharge suggests subsolar abscess (Box 7.1).

Examination of the pastern (proximal interphalangeal joint)

- Structures that should be palpated for signs of inflammation (i.e. swelling, heat, pain) include the proximal and middle phalanges (fractures, ringbone), distal sesamoidean and collateral ligaments and superficial digital flexor (SDF) tendon branches and deep digital flexor (DDF) tendon (sprains and tenosynovitis common).
- Effusion in the proximal interphalangeal joint is rarely palpable. Osteoarthritis of the joint generally results in a firm swelling of the distal pastern due to periarticular fibrosis or new bone.
- Rotating and flexing pastern (fetlock, pastern and coffin joints) may elicit pain indicative of joint inflammation, injury or osteoarthritis (Figure 7.2).

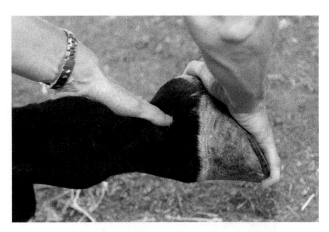

Figure 7.2 Palpation for rotation and shear of the distal interphalangeal (coffin, P2 P3) joint. It is important to stabilise the fetlock and pastern to isolate the movement.

Examination of the fetlock (metacarpophalangeal joint)

- Structures that should be palpated for swelling, effusion or pain include:
  - the dorsal pouch
  - the palmar pouch (between the suspensory ligament and cannon bone) of the fetlock joint (Figure 7.3)
  - SDF tendon, DDF tendon, proximal annular ligament and the digital sheath
  - suspensory ligament branches and sesamoid bones (desmitis, sesamoiditis, sesamoid fractures).

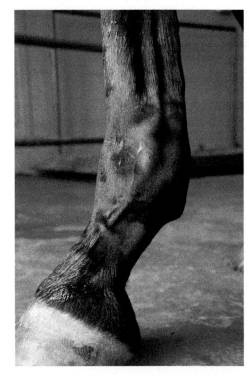

Figure 7.3 Swelling of the palmar pouch of the lateral aspect of the fetlock joint in a horse.

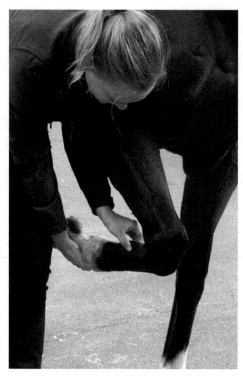

Figure 7.4 Palpation of the superficial and deep digital flexor tendons with the limb non-weight bearing.

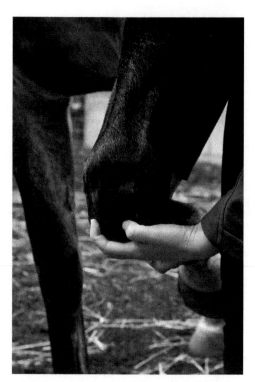

Figure 7.5 Evaluation of the carpus non-weight bearing with the carpus flexed to open up the antebrachiocarpal and midcarpal joints.

- Rotating and flexing fetlock to detect decreased range of motion (age or fetlock problem such as osteoarthritis, sprain or synovitis).

Examination of the metacarpus/metatarsus (MC/MT)

- The soft tissue structures of the metacarpus/metatarsus are palpated with the limb weight bearing first and then non-weight bearing in order to be able to separate the individual structures (Figure 7.4). The flexor tendons, SDF and DDF, lie within the digital sheath in the distal third of the metacarpus/metatarsus and effusion of the sheath may make palpation difficult. The inferior check ligament is palpated in the proximal third of the metacarpus between the DDF and the suspensory ligament. The body and branches of the suspensory ligament are easily palpated whereas the origin lies between the splint bones and is more difficult. The body of the suspensory ligament is normally painful when firmly palpated whereas pain on palpation of the flexor tendons and other areas of the suspensory ligament indicates injury.
- Pain, heat and swelling over the splint bones (MC/MT 2 and 4) indicate 'splints' or splint fractures, whereas these signs when palpating the dorsal middle third of the cannon (MC3) indicate 'bucked shins'.

Examination of the carpus

- Evaluation of the carpus should include examination weight bearing and non-weight bearing with the carpus flexed to

open up the antebrachiocarpal and midcarpal joints (Figure 7.5).
- Pain on carpal flexion is determined by pulling the pastern proximally lateral to the elbow and pushing down on the antebrachium (Figure 7.6).
- Effusion of the antebrachiocarpal or midcarpal joints is observed either side of the extensor carpi radialis tendon on the dorsal aspect of the carpus.
- In contrast, effusion of the extensor tendon sheaths extends proximally and distally in the case of the common digital flexor tendon.
- Fluid swelling on the lateral aspect of the carpus immediately caudal to the distal radius and proximal to the accessory carpal bone may be the palmar pouch of the antebrachiocarpal joint or the carpal sheath.

Examination of the antebrachium and elbow

The radius and ulnar are palpated for swelling or pain. The elbow can be flexed and extended but swelling of the joint is difficult to detect due to the overlying musculature.

Examination of the shoulder

- Palpate and visualise swelling or wastage of shoulder muscles (supraspinatus, infraspinatus muscles suggestive of nerve injury), and pain over greater trochanter, and bicipital tendon and bursa (bicipital bursitis, tendosynovitis) (Figure 7.7).
- Flex, adduct and abduct shoulder to detect pain indicative of scapula fractures and joint osteoarthritis.

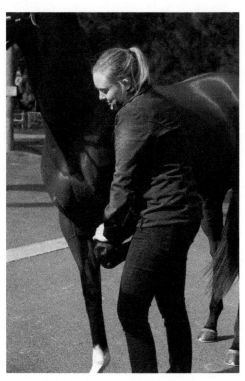

Figure 7.6 Pain on carpal flexion is determined by pulling the pastern proximally lateral to the elbow and pushing down on the antebrachium.

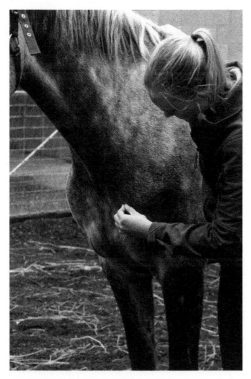

Figure 7.7 Palpation of the biceps tendon.

- Swelling of the shoulder joint and the bicipital bursa is difficult to detect due to the overlying musculature.

Examination of the hock (tarsus)

Major structures to palpate for swelling, effusion or pain include the following.

- Tarsocrural joint: effusion (*bog spavin*) is observed as large fluid-filled swellings dorsomedially and dorsolaterally either side of the complex of extensor tendons and laterally and medially between the calcaneus and the distal tibia (Figure 7.8) and suggests idiopathic synovitis, intraarticular fracture or osteochondritis dessicans (OCD) of tibia or talus. Periarticular swelling suggests chronic inflammation of the joint capsule associated with chronic fractures, capsule sprains and osteoarthritis.
- Distal intertarsal and tarsometatarsal joints: these are small joints where effusion is not detectable. In chronic cases of osteoarthritis, there may be a bony swelling on the medial aspect of these joints (*bone spavin*).
- Effusion of the tarsal sheath is observed between the calcaneus and distal tibia (*thoroughpin*) and is differentiated from tarsocrural swelling by a lack of dorsal swelling.
- A firm swelling on the plantar aspect of the calcaneus distal to the point of the hock (*curb*) may be due to injury of the plantar ligament or the SDF tendon.
- Point of hock: soft swelling/distension of subcutaneous bursa indicates acute calcaneal bursitis (*capped hock*); swelling becomes firm and fibrous with time.

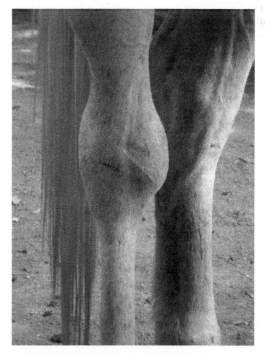

Figure 7.8 Tarsocrural joint effusion or bog spavin.

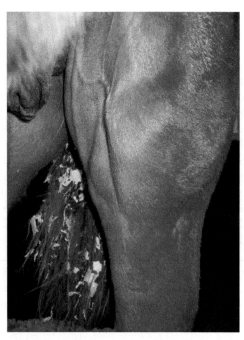

Figure 7.9 Examination of the stifle: marked medial femorotibial joint swelling.

Examination of the stifle

Relevant structures to palpate and test include the following.
- Wastage or swelling of surrounding muscles.
- Patella ligaments: medial, middle and lateral ligaments (desmitis); patella (displacement, fracture).
- Femoropatellar joint pouch: distension on either side of middle patella ligament suggests a problem in femoropatellar or medial femorotibial pouch as they often communicate (capsulitis, osteoarthritis, OCD, intraarticular fracture).
- Medial femorotibial joint swelling may occur without femoropatellar swelling and is palpable on the medial aspect of the joint medial to the medial patellar ligament and cranial to the medial collateral ligament when the horse is standing squarely on the hindlimbs (Figure 7.9). Lateral femorotibial swelling is rarely detectable due to the overlying musculature.

Examination of the upper limb and pelvis

- Abnormalities to inspect and palpate are asymmetry of the pelvis and upper limb muscles (fractures), signs of inflammation in muscles of the upper limb (particularly semimembranosus and semitendinosus muscles indicating myopathy), and crepitus of hip and pelvis suggestive of pelvic and femoral neck fracture.
- Vaginal and rectal examination by a veterinary surgeon is also useful to detect crepitus of a pelvic symphyseal fracture below the vagina (while manipulating the limb at the same time), and ileum and acetabular fractures of the pelvis.
- Pain on palpation of the tubera sacrale may be associated with desmitis of the dorsal sacroiliac ligament or a fracture of the

ilial wing. Asymmetry of the tubera sacrale is common and often of no significance.

Examination of the back and neck

Muscles of the back, thorax and neck should be palpated for tension, sensitivity and flinching (see also Chapter 11) as well as muscle wastage, asymmetry, swelling and heat.

Important palpation tests (looking for above abnormalities) include the following.
- Light and firm palpation (generally using a blunt instrument) along the back from withers to tail. Back pain may cause horses to resist ventroflexion (extension of the thoracolumbar spine), dorsiflexion (flexion of the lumbosacral region) and lateral flexion (when blunt instrument is run over the lateral sides of the back on both sides).
- Palpate tips of spinous processes looking for malalignment, depressions or protrusions indicating fracture.
- Excessive firmness of the musculature is an indicator of muscle spasm which is often secondary to other problems.
- Rectal examination by a veterinary surgeon to detect fractures of pelvis, sacrum and lumbar vertebrae as well as thrombosis of iliac artery.

7.2.6 Examination during movement
Confirmation and localisation of lameness

The primary purpose of examining a horse while in motion is to determine which limb(s) is (are) lame. Localisation of the source of the lameness is difficult based on observation of the gait but there may be some characteristics of the gait that are useful in some circumstances. For example, shortened cranial phase of stride is consistent with a source of pain proximally in the limb. The severity of the lameness should also be graded to allow assessment of improvement and appropriate communication with other professionals dealing with the horse (Table 7.2).

Requirements for a thorough gait evaluation
- A hard, level, non-slip surface and a soft surface, free from distractions and dangers. Lameness in the distal limb is often

Table 7.2 Lameness grade

Grades	Lameness is:
Grade 1	Difficult to observe, not consistently apparent when weight bearing or circling on inclines or hard surfaces
Grade 2	Difficult to observe at walk or trotting in straight line; consistently apparent when weight bearing or circling on inclines or hard surfaces
Grade 3	Consistently seen at trot under all circumstances
Grade 4	Obvious with marked head nodding or shortened stride
Grade 5	Obvious with minimal weight bearing in motion and/or at rest; inability to move

Source: AAEP 1991.

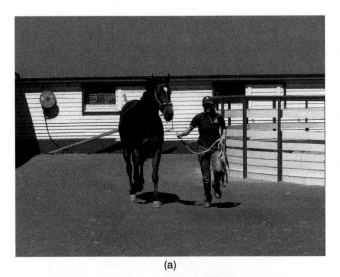

(a)

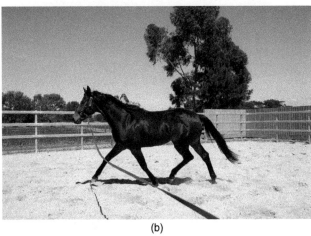

(b)

Figure 7.10 (a) Trotting on a hard surface in a straight line. (b) Lunging on a soft surface in both directions.

exacerbated on hard ground whereas proximal limb lameness may be worsened on soft ground.

- A competent handler and consideration of safety, particularly with difficult horses.
- The horse must be led with lead rope loose enough so it can move its head and neck freely but with enough control to prevent distracting movement. The horse must be moved at a consistent speed.
- The horse should be walked and slow trotted in a straight line (Figure 7.10a), in a circle, and in both directions, and should be observed from the front, the side and behind.
- Space for lunging in circles (in both directions) to help to demonstrate subtle lameness more clearly (Figure 7.10b).

Indicators of lameness (fore or hind)

- *Sound*: listen for regularity of rhythm and sound of footfall. A lame horse usually lands harder on the sound limb, resulting in a louder hoof contact with the ground. Horses with disparity of hoof size or loose shoes may confound interpretation. In

addition, horses that drag a hoof make a distinctive scraping noise.

- *Extension of fetlock*: generally, the fetlock joint of the sound limb drops down further when this limb is weight bearing *at the walk* than does the fetlock joint of the lame limb (which is being spared).
- *Drifting*: horses with hindlimb lameness generally drift or or turn their hindquarter away (moving on three tracks) from the lame limb, thus reducing weight bearing on that limb.
- *Abnormal limb movement*
  - *Reduced length of stride phase*: decreased cranial phase of stride in one limb may indicate lameness in the opposite limb. In normal horses, the length of stride of the paired forelimbs and hindlimbs, measured from hoof print to hoof print, is nearly identical from side to side. Also, the degree of extension and flexion of joints is similar.
  - *Altered limb and hoof flight*: for example, hoof travelling inwards (winging in) or outwards (winging out) or front hoof hitting the opposite forelimb or same side hindlimb; usually associated with conformational faults and may result in interference, self-trauma, pain and lameness.
  - *Altered arc and path of hoof*: lowering of the arc of the hoof during forward movement which can result in dragging of the toes.
  - *Reduced joint flexion*: particularly in hindlimbs and most observable in hocks; may be associated with alterations in hoof flight and reduced stride phase. This may be more apparent when the horse is lunged or ridden.
  - *Abnormal hoof placement*: if there is toe pain, weight will be placed on the heel and will land heel first. If pain is on the outside of the hoof sole then weight will be placed on the inside of the sole and the horse can be seen to land on the inside of the hoof first.

Forelimb lameness

- Forelimb lameness tends to be more common than hindlimb lameness but this may be partly because forelimb lameness is easier to identify.
- The majority (~95%) of lameness problems in the forelimb occur at the level of or distal to the knee (carpus).
- *Rules of thumb* for recognition of forelimb lameness
  - Best observed while the horse is trotted towards the examiner and when viewed from the side.
  - The head and forequarters drop down more when weight bearing on the sound limb and rise or move down less when weight bearing on the lame limb.
  - A bilateral forelimb lameness will result in a bilateral short stepping forelimb action.
  - Stride length characteristics, height of hoof flight, sound and fetlock drop (described above) also are helpful.

Hindlimb lameness

- Most lameness in the hindlimb is due to problems of the tarsus and below.

- Hindlimb lameness is best observed while the horse is trotted away from the examiner and if the examiner observes from the side of the lame limb.
- The hindquarters rise when the lame limb is weight bearing and drop when the contralateral limb is weight bearing. It is easier to see the rise as this movement is generally more rapid. It is easiest to look at the midline of the hindquarters, i.e. the base of the tail when the horse is moving away from the observer or the tubera sacrale when the horse is moving towards the observer.
- In more severe hindlimb lameness cases (grade 3 or higher), the head will drop when the lame hindlimb is weight bearing, giving the appearance of a forelimb lameness on the same side as the hindlimb lameness.
- Bilateral hindlimb lameness can present in many forms, including cantering rather than trotting, short striding and lack of impulsion.
- Stride length characteristics ('carrying' lame hindlimb when viewed from side), height of hoof flight, sound and fetlock drop (described above) are also helpful.

Multi-limb lameness

Multiple limb lameness is very common but one limb often predominates, making identification of other lame limbs challenging. Where a forelimb and hindlimb lameness are observed on the same side (ipsilateral), diagnostic analgesia (see later) starting with the hindlimb is essential to determine whether the forelimb lameness is real.

Inertial sensors

The use of inertial sensors as an aid in the identification of lameness is becoming more widespread (Keegan *et al.* 2011; Pfau *et al.* 2007). Sensors are attached to the poll and the pelvis to measure asymmetry of vertical movement (Figure 7.11) and one is placed on a distal limb to identify the timing of the stride. Like all diagnostic aids, inertial sensors are not a substitute for careful clinical examination. Rather, they are useful in allowing quantification of the degree of lameness and comparison of the gait before and after various interventions such as nerve blocks or therapy. And because they compare one side to another, they are less useful for the identification of bilateral lameness.

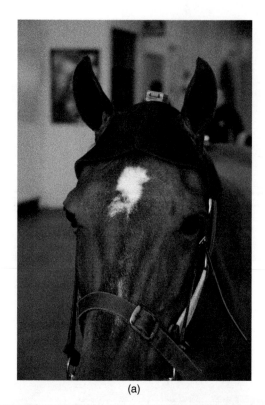

(a)

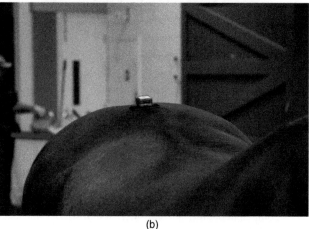

(b)

Figure 7.11 Inertial sensors attached to the poll (a) and the pelvis (b) to measure asymmetry of vertical movement when trotting.

7.3 Manipulative tests

After observing the horse at exercise and determining which limb (or limbs) is lame, the next step is to perform manipulative or provocative tests.

Provocative tests are not sensitive or specific and can lead to false-positive and false-negative results. Excessive force may 'create' lameness that may not have any clinical relevance to the lameness observed during movement examination. The results of provocative tests in the lame limb should be compared with the opposite, sound limb and interpreted in conjunction with

previously collected information and with the more specific results of diagnostic analgesia (Busschers & van Weeren 2001).

7.3.1 Flexion tests

Flexion tests should be performed in the least lame limb first as a marked response in the lame limb may mask a milder response in a non-lame limb. The joint under investigation is held in a firmly flexed position for 45–60 sec after which the horse is immediately trotted off for at least 12–15 metres and any worsening of gait noted. Because some joints and associated structures are inherently linked together in flexion or extension (e.g.

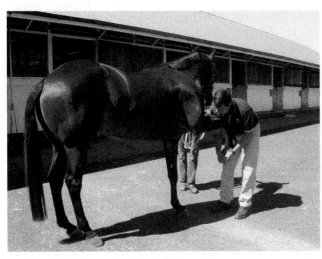

Figure 7.12 Flexion of the fetlock joint. Note this flexes all the phalangeal joints. It is important to ensure the carpus is not flexed at the same time.

hock and stifle, phalangeal joints and fetlock), the exact differentiation of pain responses between these joints and structures is not possible (Figure 7.12).

It is important to use a consistent technique (i.e. force applied, duration of test) and a 'positive' result is defined as obvious lameness or a 1–2 grade increase in lameness observed persistently for more than 5–8 strides while the horse trots in a straight line after flexion. Sound horses warm out of the normally mild response seen in the first few strides.

Flexion results in compressive or tension forces being applied to both articular structures within a joint as well as surrounding soft tissue. Therefore, a positive response to flexion of the lower limb (fetlock flexion test) can be observed with any disorder of the coffin, pastern and fetlock joints; navicular bone or bursa; other palmar heel structures; digital flexor tendon sheath; palmar pastern soft tissue; suspensory ligament branches or sesamoid bones.

7.3.2 Direct pressure tests
Response to localised pressure over any painful areas (limb or back), tendon swellings (suspensory branches or digital flexor tendons), splints, the front of the proximal phalanx and MC 3, and specific areas of the hoof (using hoof testers) can be as useful as flexion tests for localising the source of pain. Compression is usually maintained for approximately 30 sec and then the horse is trotted off and observed for exacerbation of lameness.

7.3.3 Wedge test
The wedge test is used specifically to stretch or compress the joints, subchondral bone, articular surfaces and associated soft tissues of the hoof, including the DDF tendon, SDF tendon, the suspensory ligament and collateral ligaments. A wedge with a 20° inclination is placed under the weight-bearing hoof to raise the toe (increased stress on DDF tendon, navicular bone and

associated ligaments and bursa) or the heel (increased stress on suspensory ligament). The horse is made to stand for 30–60 sec with the opposite limb elevated, after which the horse is trotted off in a straight line, observing for exacerbation of lameness. This test has relatively poor specificity and poor predictive value.

7.4 Diagnostic analgesia: nerves and joints

Although time consuming, invasive and sometimes hazardous to both horse and examiner, diagnostic analgesia ('nerve blocking') is the only objective means of determining the site of pain within a limb. Common local anaesthetic drugs used in horses – 2% solutions of lidocaine, mepivacaine and bupivacaine – block or inhibit nociceptive nerve conduction by preventing the increase in membrane permeability to sodium ions. Mepivacaine has become the agent of choice because it causes minimal tissue reaction and has a slightly longer duration of action (2–3 h).

Local analgesia may be used for:
- regional nerve block via perineural infiltration around specific nerves to desensitise the limb regions/structures supplied by that nerve distal to the site of the injection. (Therefore, if a horse becomes lame-free following the injection, one or more of these structures are the source of the pain and lameness.)
- Intrasynovial injection to block joints, tendon sheaths or bursae and surrounding structures.
- Direct local infiltration over suspect superficial lesions.
- Field analgesia, performed by circular injection around the suspected site of pathology, thereby blocking all nerve fibres entering the area.

Unless simply confirming a suspected lesion, use of local analgesia should start with the hoof and be continued sequentially up the limb, anaesthetising specific limb segments. After waiting an adequate time (at least 5–10 min for lower limbs and up to an hour for upper limb blocks), the block should be tested for its effect on removing superficial *and deep* pain using a blunt instrument or firm digital pressure. Improvement in degree of lameness >70–80% after regional or intraarticular analgesia may be considered to be a positive response.

While local analgesia is considered an objective test, there can be problems with interpretation owing to the effects of diffusion of local anaesthetic solution up the nerve, into communicating joints, or from joint pouches into surrounding tissues and nerves, which may result in unintended desensitisation of structures, so in general, horses should be reevaluated no more than 5–10 min after administration. Examples of diffusion and structural communications resulting in desensitisation of the structures after local analgesia include diffusion between coffin joint, navicular bursa, navicular and pedal bones.

Response to local analgesia can be complete where the lameness (mostly) resolves and the examination can be stopped, or the lameness switches to the opposite limb. Alternatively, the response can be incomplete owing to chronic or deep bone pain, which may remain resistant to analgesia. Individual variation in neuroanatomy and response to analgesia may also result in incomplete responses. Additionally, as a result of complex sensory innervation of joints, intraarticular analgesia inconsistently abolishes pain from many of the common articular problems, particularly subchondral bone pain (due to remodelling, cystic or erosive disorders, incomplete fractures and osteoarthritis). Because joint pain often arises from articular and periarticular tissues, regional analgesia more consistently abolishes pain from all aspects of the joint and surrounding soft tissue structures.

7.5 Diagnostic imaging

The number of imaging modalities has increased over recent years and, in addition to radiography, ultrasound and nuclear scintigraphy, the newer modalities of thermography, computed tomography and magnetic resonance imaging provide important means for more accurate and detailed orthopaedic diagnoses (McIlwraith 2003). Although the latter three modalities tend to be restricted to referral or university establishments, equine veterinary practitioners commonly use the other three. Imaging should ideally be used in conjunction with findings from the history, physical and lameness examinations.

7.5.1 Radiology/radiography

The choice of imaging modality depends on how well localised the source of pain is following a lameness examination and diagnostic analgesia, and on the tissues that require investigation.

Radiography and ultrasound are often the first choice due to their ready availability, with radiographs most useful for bony abnormalities and ultrasound most useful for soft tissue abnormalities. However, as only relatively small areas can be examined with these techniques efficiently and cost effectively, scintigraphy may be a better option if the lameness cannot be localised.

Most radiography of the lower limbs can be performed using a portable X-ray machine. However, larger radiographic machines found mostly at referral or university veterinary institutions allow better images of the proximal limbs and pelvis. A range of views has been developed for each individual segment of the forelimb and hindlimb (Park 2002).

It is common to radiograph yearlings during the yearling sale process. However, the association between radiographic findings and pain and dysfunction is not always clear cut and some lameness disorders are not correlated with radiographs at all (Kane *et al.* 2003).

7.5.2 Thermography

In thermography, a visual image is produced from infrared radiation emitted from the skin surface and detected using a photon detector connected to a computer. The image is displayed in colours (isotherms) which correspond to different skin temperatures, and which reflect changes in circulation, pain and temperature in deeper tissues. Although soft tissue and bony inflammation can be detected before clinical and radiographic changes by as much as 2 weeks, thermographic changes are non-specific and this technique should be complementary to other diagnostic modalities.

7.5.3 Ultrasonography

Ultrasonography has become an affordable and non-invasive diagnostic technique that enables repeated assessment of tissue lesions over time. Ultrasonography involves the use of high-frequency sound waves (>1 MHz) emitted from a transducer to image tissues of the body. Sound is reflected (or echoed) back to the transducer from interfaces between tissue of different physical characteristics or density (called acoustic impedance). Large differences in acoustic impedance between two tissues (e.g. bone versus fluid) result in greater amplitude of the reflected echo. Most sound is reflected at the interface of soft tissue with bone or air, leaving insufficient sound to penetrate deeper structures. Sound is additionally reflected or scattered when it meets small reflectors, representing internal architecture, within tissues.

Reflected sound is received by the transducer and converted back into electrical impulses to produce a grey-scale image. A loud or highly reflected echo is seen as a white image (hyperechoic, e.g. bone), weaker echoes as varying levels of grey (hypoechoic, e.g. soft tissue, tendons), and no echo (anechoic, e.g. fluid, blood) as a black region.

Ultrasonography is indicated for:

- diagnosis of soft tissue injuries, especially tendons, tendon sheath and ligaments but also muscular, vascular, joint capsule and bursal defects (including muscle size)
- monitoring the effect of training on soft tissue structures, especially tendons and ligaments, and prevention of potential injury in horses with subtle signs of tendon or ligament disease
- monitoring of healing of soft tissue injuries (correlates closely with histological changes)
- assessment of fluid accumulation (in joints, bursae, other soft tissues and masses)
- evaluation of bony surfaces (e.g. tubera coxae, metacarpus/metatarsus)
- investigation of wounds.

7.5.4 Nuclear medicine/scintigraphy

Nuclear scintigraphy involves the intravenous administration of technetium-99 m, a radioactive isotope, which emits gamma-radiation and, conjugated with methylene diphosphate or hydroxymethane, is preferentially taken up into the mineral lattice of bone at a level dependent on the rate of bone formation and the volume of blood flow to an area. Sites with a high rate of turnover or bone adaptation, as a result of physiological or pathological factors (i.e. disease), therefore accumulate more of the technetium than normal and this is reflected in increased gamma-radiation being emitted from a particular site ('hot spot'). The level of gamma emission is detected using an imaging system at a particular time after technetium administration.

The advent of scintigraphy over recent years, particularly in referral practice, has allowed early recognition of a range of subtle vascular (blood flow), soft tissue and especially bone lesions, such as inflammation (e.g. osteoarthritis, osteitis) and stress fractures, which in the past may have remained undiagnosed (Steyn 2002).

Scintigraphy is a highly sensitive technique that allows imaging of large areas of the body and is therefore often used in horses where diagnostic analgesia is not possible, contraindicated (possible incomplete fractures) or fails to localise the lameness.

7.5.5 Computed tomography

Computed tomography (CT) is an advanced imaging technique that involves radiography in three dimensions. Images are generated by an X-ray tube that rotates around the area of interest so general anaesthesia is required for imaging the limbs. The size of the tube limits scans to the limbs below the level of the mid-radius and tibia, and to the upper and mid-cervical spine and head. With modern CT equipment, image acquisition is very rapid, meaning it can be performed when a horse is being anaesthetised for another reason such as surgery and large areas of the limb can be imaged. Both soft tissue and bone can be imaged. Lesion identification can be enhanced with the use of intraarterial or intraarticular contrast agents (Figure 7.13).

7.5.6 Magnetic resonance imaging

Like CT, magnetic resonance imaging (MRI) allows imaging in multiple planes. A strong magnetic field is used to align the protons within tissues and radiofrequency is applied and then received in a coil wrapped around the area of interest. The strength of radiofrequency signal is dependent on the amount of water and fat in a tissue and the way the radiofrequency is applied.

The strength of the magnetic field determines the resolution of the images obtained and the size of the field of view. High-field systems consist of a large superconducting magnet. The size of these magnets limits access for equine imaging to the distal limb under general anaesthesia. Low-field systems have smaller magnets and this has allowed the development of MRI systems for imaging limbs of standing horses. Only small areas of the limb can be imaged at one time and the resolution is less than that achieved with high-field systems but for most applications, the images acquired are diagnostic.

Magnetic resonance imaging allows the imaging of soft tissues with high contrast. Although dense tissues like bone and tendon have very little signal, their outline can be seen due to contrast with the signal emitted by surrounding tissues and pathology does emit signal. It is most useful for imaging structures within the foot where the soft tissues are difficult to investigate with ultrasound due to the presence of the hoof capsule (Figure 7.14).

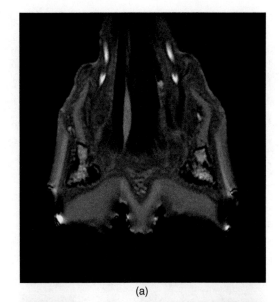

(a)

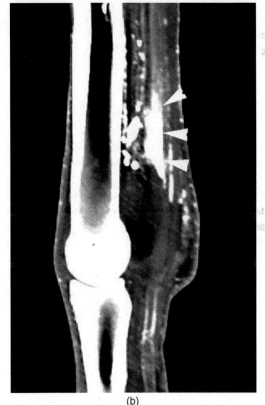

(b)

Figure 7.13 Magnetic resonance imaging (MRI) image of the flexor tendon region before (a) and after (b) intraarterial injection of contrast agent, showing a lesion within the deep digital flexor tendon that takes up contrast (*arrow heads*).

7.6 Selected orthopaedic diseases

7.6.1 Bone fracture

Fractures may be complete, resulting in loss of function of the limb, or incomplete, in which case lameness is the predominant

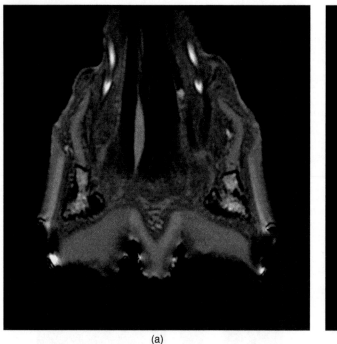
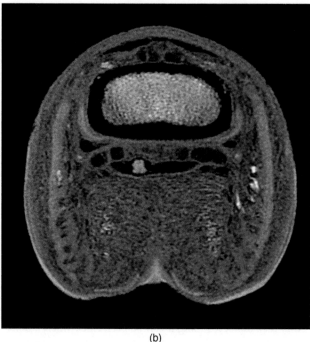

(a)   (b)

Figure 7.14 MRI image (T1 weighted) of the deep digital flexor tendon region from a dorsal (a) and transverse (b) plane with an area of increased signal in the medial lobe of the tendon (light grey area).

presenting problem and there may be few localising signs. Fractures may be due to a single load, often arising from falls or collisions, or the accumulation of fatigue damage from repeated loading, which is the most common cause of fracture in racehorses. Fatigue fractures or stress fractures occur most commonly in the metacarpus/metatarsus, proximal sesamoid bones, tibia, humerus and pelvis.

Most acute, complete fractures cause significant lameness regardless of their size and location. In every horse presented for acute non-weight-bearing lameness, a fracture should be high on the differential diagnosis list (which should also include bone, joint or tendon sheath infection or foot abscess). However, some fractures, such as an osteochondral chip fracture of a carpal bone, may only produce low-grade lameness.

Classification and prognosis

Fractures are broadly classified as complete or incomplete (stress), stable or unstable (non-displaced or displaced), and open or closed. Fractures also are categorised according to their configuration (oblique, transverse, spiral, multiple and comminuted), and their location and character (articular (through a joint), non-articular, diaphyseal, epiphyseal, Salter–Harris physeal, chip and slab) (Nunamaker 2002).

The prognosis for fracture repair depends on many factors. Incomplete fractures generally heal with confinement. For complete fractures, the horse needs to be able to bear weight on the affected limb otherwise there is a high risk of laminitis in the contralateral limb. Where there is substantial muscle

mass surrounding the affected bone such as the pelvis, healing can occur with conservative therapy. Complete fractures of the radius and tibia in adult horses carry a poor prognosis due to the difficulty in reconstructing these fractures with enough stability to withstand weight bearing. Some fractures of the lower limb can be reconstructed provided comminution is not excessive.

Fracture healing

During healing, bone reunites by either:

- primary remodelling without callus formation – this requires rigid fracture stabilisation and correct anatomical reduction of bone; or
- secondary fibrocartilage formation between fragments, which is later replaced by periosteal and endosteal new bone (callus).

Fractures heal via a series of sequential but overlapping processes.

- *Inflammatory phase*: crucial for vascular and bone repair and protection from infection.
- *Reparative phase*: depends on method of fracture fixation, stability and degree of displacement of fracture.
- *Remodelling phase*: to replace avascular and necrotic regions and realign bone.

As well as laminitis in the contralateral limb, some of the undesirable consequences of fracture healing include osteoarthritis of adjacent joints and flexural limb deformity. Joint stiffness, as occurs in humans, is rare. In young horses, increased laxity may occur following cast immobilisation in the affected limb and angular limb deformities in the contralateral limb.

7.6.2 Bone infection

It is worth summarising some important features of bone infection, which is commonly encountered in equine orthopaedics.

Osteitis and osteomyelitis describe inflammation of bone although the former term is applied to *inflammation* that begins in or involves the periosteum and outer bone cortex, whereas the latter term is used when *inflammation and infection* begins in or extends into the medullary cavity.

Osteitis

- Common in extremities (mostly cannon bones) owing to lack of soft tissue protection.
- Caused by trauma (kick with intact skin), break in skin or nearby infectious process.
- Damaged periosteum and outer cortex usually die from lack of blood which results in:
  - osteitis and bone sequestration if unexposed (i.e. skin still intact); or
  - osteitis, sequestrum formation plus contamination and infection if bone exposed – the development of a draining sinus tract and non-healing wound subsequently occurs.
- Pathogenic organisms (commonly *Staphylococcus*) reside within avascular necrotic bone and avoid immune defences. (Note: For this reason also, systemic antibiotics are of limited value unless there is associated cellulitis.)
- Lameness, swelling and a non-healing draining purulent wound are key signs (remains until sequestrum surgically removed).
- Radiographic evidence of a sequestrum is usually not visible until 2–3 weeks after the injury.

Osteomyelitis

- More extensive bone inflammation than osteitis and begins within or extends into the medullary cavity.
- Key signs are severe lameness, swelling (cellulitis) and a draining wound if trauma involved.

The three types of osteomyelitis are haematogenous, traumatic and iatrogenic.

Haematogenous

- Primarily in foals (often with immune system suppression due to failure of passive transfer of maternal immunoglobulins).
- Sluggish metaphyseal blood flow allows bacteria, spread from a primary site (e.g. umbilicus, gastrointestinal tract (GIT) or lung), to localise in the synovial membrane of joints (S-type), and/or the physis (P-type), and/or the epiphysis (E-type).
- Most common organisms isolated include *Escherichia coli*, *Salmonella* spp. and *Streptococcus* spp.
- Results in inflammation, blood vessel thrombosis and prostaglandin-induced bone necrosis and destruction.
- Frequently, foals that recover from an initial infection (umbilical or systemic) develop bone or joint infection several days later.

Traumatic

- As a result of a penetrating wound or open fracture, bacteria enter the medullary cavity through the open wound. Rarely, the skin is not broken but blood supply is compromised and necrotic tissue provides an ideal medium for bacteria that arrive from a haematogenous route.
- Many types of Gram-negative and Gram-positive organisms may be isolated.
- Open fractures in which bone fragments lose their blood supply are particularly prone to osteomyelitis.

Iatrogenic

- Develops as a result of contamination during internal fixation (using metal plates) of open or closed fractures.
- Fracture haematoma, lack of blood supply at fracture site and the implantation of foreign pins, screws and plates provide favourable conditions for bacterial colonisation and growth.
- Highly resistant bacteria such as methicillin-resistant *Staphylococcus aureus* and Gram-negative bacteria may be involved.

7.6.3 Injury and repair of tendons and ligaments

In a galloping Thoroughbred at maximal speed, the SDF tendon operates close to its physiological mechanical limits with a relatively narrow safety margin. The majority of tendon strains occur as a cumulative subclinical process, with fatigue of collagen resulting in degeneration of the tendon core followed by tearing of groups of fibrils and eventually complete tendon rupture if training is not ceased.

Remember: the major *acute* pathological endpoints of strain are degeneration (initially subclinical) and inflammation of tendon components resulting in pain, oedema, heat, swelling and consequently lameness.

In contrast to muscle and bone (in which increasing mechanical demand with age and exercise results in both tissues undergoing an increase in mass and architectural change), tendons appear to have little ability to adapt after skeletal maturity (≥2 years) and cumulative micro-damage weakens the tendon matrix.

The healing of tendon and ligament follows a sequence of haemorrhage, oedema, acute inflammation, fibroblastic proliferation, collagen production and chronic remodelling.

- Unchecked inflammation in the early stages of tendinitis may result in release of proteolytic enzymes, which, although directed at removing necrotic collagen, also digest relatively intact tendon collagen, causing progression of the lesion.
- Tendon tissue is not regenerated. Rather, scar tissue (produced by paratendon and endotendon cells), characterised by haphazardly arranged collagen (predominantly type III), is laid down. This scar tissue:
  - is *weaker* than normal tendon tissue, but the tendon is usually thicker at the scar, compensating for this
  - is less elastic than the adjacent normal tendon, resulting in strain concentration at the junction between normal tendon and scar tissue

– is slowly remodelled over many *months* (usually >6) into type I collagen, although the tissue never becomes normal tendon. Controlled exercise during this phase may encourage this remodelling, with improved alignment of collagen fibrils and mechanical properties of the scar tissue.

Strain of tendons and ligaments

Tendinitis is inflammation of tendon and tendon muscle attachments caused by excessive strain and commonly affects flexor tendons of the lower limbs (particularly the SDF tendon). In contrast, desmitis is inflammation of a ligament. Disorders range from minor tearing to complete rupture or avulsion from bony attachments.

- Flexor tendons of the forelimbs are more commonly affected than those in the hindlimbs, and the SDF tendon is more often affected than the DDF tendon in forelimbs.
- Lesions are generally localised to the core of the mid-metacarpal region of the SDF tendon in the forelimb (where cross-sectional area is smallest), but may also occur within the SDF tendon branches on the palmar aspect of the pastern.
- Suspensory ligament (SL) desmitis may occur in its origin, body or branches. Injury of the suspensory ligament origin occurs commonly in both forelimbs and hindlimbs whereas body and branch lesions are more common in forelimbs.

The initial signs of tendon and suspensory ligament injury are pain on palpation and localised swelling (Figure 7.15). If a tendon injury occurs within a tendon sheath, effusion of the sheath may be the first sign. Initially there will be no or only mild lameness. More severe lameness indicates severe tendon injury or another cause of lameness. The exception is proximal suspensory desmitis which first presents as lameness. Ultrasound is used to differentiate peritendinous swelling from a tendon injury and to document the extent of injury in order to monitor the healing process.

Principles of management of tendon injury

> **Key point**
>
> The key tendon injury management is a controlled exercise programme monitored with serial ultrasound examination.

Medical therapy

Veterinary surgeons presented with an acute severe tendon injury will usually:

- stop training and initiate complete stall rest, initially for 4–6 weeks, followed by controlled exercise for a minimum of 6–10 months (see later)
- control inflammation (decrease oedema, swelling and pain) and progression of damage
- minimise excessive scar tissue and encourage normal repair
- recommend controlled exercise and rehabilitation, which involves an initial programme of hand-walking/swimming for 3 months followed by increasing strength exercise for a further 3–4 months. Progress is monitored via ultrasound.

Note: Although clinical signs of lameness are usually resolved after a short period of rest, *much longer is needed before substantial healing of the tendon has occurred.*

A number of therapies have been used for tendon injury but there is limited evidence supporting their efficacy.

Stem cell implantation

Stem cell therapy is now widely used for the treatment of tendon injuries. Although no direct comparison has been made between treated horses and untreated controls, injury rates following stem cell treatment in National Hunt horses in the UK are lower than those reported for other treatments (Godwin *et al.* 2012). Stem cells are derived from bone marrow or fat and are injected directly into tendon core lesions under ultrasound guidance once the acute inflammation has subsided. There does not appear to be any decrease in recovery time and treatment should be combined with a controlled exercise programme.

Surgical therapy

Surgical treatments that have been proposed for tendon injury include the following.

- *Accessory ligament desmotomy.* Transection of the accessory ligament of the SDF tendon to increase involvement of the SDF muscle and reduce load on the tendon itself when

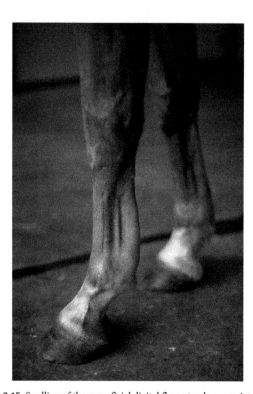

Figure 7.15 Swelling of the superficial digital flexor tendon associated with tendon strain.

the horse returns to work. Although there are some data suggesting a reduced reinjury rate, increased suspensory ligament injury rates have been documented in horses undergoing this procedure.

- *Percutaneous tendon splitting*. For acute tendinitis where the intratendinous haematoma and oedema are relieved from a core lesion using scalpel stabs or needle sticks. There is no evidence that this procedure improves long-term outcomes.

> **Key point**
>
> Synthetic tendon implants and counter-irritation (via application of topical 'blister ointments' or 'pin-firing') are now considered to be inappropriate therapies for tendinitis (although there is still support for them in some countries). As with many treatments for tendinitis in the horse, conclusive proof of the effectiveness of these controversial therapies is lacking.

The tendon sheath

Synovial effusion of a tendon sheath (tenosynovitis) is common in all types of horses. Damage to any of the structures within a sheath will result in effusion so careful examination of the contents of the sheath is required. In many cases, no obvious injury to the tendons within the sheath is identified and if there is no lameness then no treatment may be required.

Causes of tenonsysnovitis include tendonitis within the sheath, annular ligament constriction, direct trauma to the sheath, manica flexoria tears, impingement by osteochondromas or bone projections, inflammation of adjacent tissues and tendon sheath infection.

Septic tenosynovitis

- Marked synovial effusion with swelling, heat, pain and severe lameness – an emergency (and red flag)! Infection most commonly is introduced via a penetrating wound, which frequently goes undetected, particularly in the pastern region. Infection may also occur after contaminated intrasheath injection or rarely via the haematogenous route. The pathogenesis, signs, diagnosis and treatment are similar to septic arthritis.
- Septic tenosynovitis is a critical condition because of the:
  - severity of lameness
  - difficulty in eliminating infection and propensity to become chronic
  - high risk of long-term complications resulting in chronic lameness, e.g. adhesion formation, rupture of tendon (digested by inflammatory cell enzymes if progressed enough), extension of infection and laminitis in opposite limb.
- Major sites affected are the digital flexor sheath over fetlock (88%), digital extensor tendon sheath and tarsal sheath.
- Diagnosis:
  - marked lameness unless sheath open and draining from wound or tract
  - synovial fluid analysis (Ross & Dyson 2003)

- confirmation of penetrating tract
- culture of offending organisms (usually mixed bacteria, *Streptococcus*, Enterobacteriaceae, *Staphylococcus aureus* and *Klebsiella* most common)
- ultrasonography to identify adhesions, complicating injuries of tendons and involvement of the annular ligament (in digital flexor tenosynovitis).

> **Key point**
>
> Treatment for septic tenosynovitis involves aggressive intrasynovial and systemic broad-spectrum antibiosis, with copious lavage of the sheath. Usually these cases should be referred and hospitalised. However, adhesion formation may result in failure of the horse to return to athletic activity.

Principles of management of tenosynovitis

Treatment varies depending on the cause and different clinical manifestations. Where there is no lameness and no evidence of tendon injury, treatment is not necessary. Key principles include the following.

- Stall rest the horse (not really necessary in idiopathic cases).
- Control inflammation (although in idiopathic cases no treatment is necessary).
- Reduce effusion and adhesion formation and return to previous function.
- Control infection in septic tenosynovitis.
- Surgery.
  Arthroscopy may be used to:
- inspect the surface of the tendons and the sheath as an additional diagnostic aid
- debride torn tendons and associated structures
- break down adhesions
- perform debridement, removal of foreign material and lavage
- place an in-dwelling drain in infected cases to allow further irrigation and local therapy. Regional IV perfusion of antibiotics, slow-release antibiotic depot systems and antibiotic infusion pumps may be placed at this time
- transect the annular ligament where there is evidence of constriction of the tendons
- debride any tissues impinging on the tendons.

7.6.4 Osteoarthritis

Osteoarthritis is the endstage of a number of joint conditions. These include trauma, either a single injury or more commonly repeated loading resulting in fatigue injury to the subchondral bone, cartilage or supporting ligaments, sepsis, osteochondrosis and immune-mediated arthritis.

Osteoarthritis is characterised by degeneration and loss of articular cartilage (splitting and fragmentation) and the development of new bone on joint surfaces and margins (Figure 7.16). Loss of joint congruity results in changes in joint surface loading which contribute to joint surface injury.

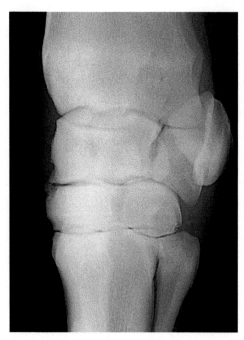

Figure 7.16 Severe osteoarthritis of the carpus with periarticular bone modelling.

Septic (infective) arthritis

Septic arthritis, or bacterial infection of a joint, is the most severe joint problem in horses (Figure 7.17) and is a common cause of death in foals.

Bacterial colonisation of the synovial membrane results in:

- mild-to-severe inflammation with necrosis of the synovial membrane and formation of fibrinopurulent exudation

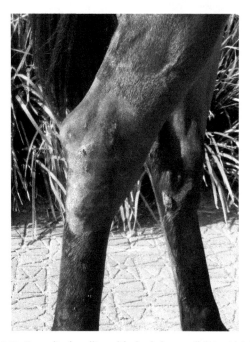

Figure 7.17 Generalised swelling of the hock due to cellulitis with joint sepsis.

- release of a diverse range of inflammatory mediators, which potentially cause rapid loss of glycosaminoglycans, proteoglycans and collagen and eventually cartilage degradation.

Bacteria enter joints via:

- haematogenous spread from umbilical, respiratory or gastrointestinal infections in foals (especially *Actinobacillus* spp., *Escherichia coli*, *Streptococcus* spp. and *Salmonella* spp.)
- local penetration or direct trauma in adults (especially *Streptococcus* spp., *E. coli* and anaerobes)
- iatrogenic routes associated with intraarticular injection of steroids or joint surgery (especially *Staphylococcus* spp.).

Risk factors for development of septic arthritis include foal factors, such as failure of passive transfer of maternal immunoglobulins and septicaemia (high sepsis score), and trauma in poorly managed environments. The tarsocrural (tibiotarsal) joint of the hock is the most commonly affected, followed by the fetlock, carpus and stifle.

Principles of management of joint disease
Medical therapy

- Maintain regular moderate exercise unless this is contraindicated; for example immediately post surgery.
- Reduce the magnitude of loads on the joint.
- Control pain, inflammation and eliminate production of inflammatory mediators.
- Antibiotic therapy for septic arthritis.

Surgical therapy

- To treat primary causes of osteoarthritis such as osteochondrosis, intraarticular fracture and chips and meniscal tears. Arthroscopic surgery is the most common technique.
- Arthroscopy for lavage and debridement in septic arthritis to remove fibrin proliferative synovium, necrotic bone or foreign material.
- Surgical arthrodesis for joint luxation and endstage osteoarthritis, particularly for low-motion joints (e.g. pastern and distal tarsal joints).
- Surgical curettage of full- and partial-thickness defects in cartilage and bone.

7.6.5 The vertebral column/back

The back of the horse is most commonly defined as the thoracolumbar spine and sacrococcygeal spine supported and maintained under tension by a complex arrangement of soft tissue structures (i.e. muscles and ligaments). Pathology of the spine is highly prevalent so it is easy for clinicians and owners to blame the back as a cause of clinical problems. Determining the significance of back pathology involves ruling out other causes of the clinical presentation such as lameness and local treatment of analgesia of the suspected problem followed by reassessment of the presenting complaint.

A wide range of conditions can be mistaken for back pain by owners, including:

- hindlimb lameness
- hypersensitivity of the back ('thin skinned')
- initial stiffness and hypersensitivity to saddling and mounting ('cold backed')
- ill-fitting saddle
- poor schooling or riding
- temperament problems
- lack of ability of horse to perform to owner's expectations
- cervical or thoracolumbar spinal cord compression presenting with weakness or stiffness behind.

Assessment of the equine back is covered in detail in Chapter 11.

References

Anderson, T.M., Mcilwraith, C.W., Douay, P. 2004, The role of conformation in musculoskeletal problems in the racing thoroughbred. *Equine Vet. J.* 36:571–575.

Bailey, C.J., Rose, R.J., Reid, S.W., Hodgson, D.R. 1997, Wastage in the Australian thoroughbred racing industry: a survey of Sydney trainers. *Aust. Vet. J.* 75:64–66.

Busschers, E., van Weeren, P.R. 2001, Use of the flexion test of the distal forelimb in the sound horse: repeatability and effect of age, gender, weight, height and fetlock joint range of motion. *J. Vet. Med. A Physiol. Pathol. Clin. Med.* 48:413–427.

Godwin, E.E., Young, N.J., Dudhia, J., Beamish, I.C., Smith, R.K. 2012, Implantation of bone marrow-derived mesenchymal stem cells demonstrates improved outcome in horses with overstrain injury of the superficial digital flexor tendon. *Equine Vet. J.* 44:25–32.

Kane, A.J., Mcilwraith, C.W., Park, R.D. *et al.* 2003, Radiographic changes in thoroughbred yearlings. Part 2: associations with racing performance. *Equine Vet. J.* 35(4):366–374.

Keegan, K.G., Kramer, J., Yonezawa, Y. *et al.* 2011, Assessment Of repeatability of a wireless, inertial sensor-based lameness evaluation system for horses. *Am. J. Vet. Res.* 72:1156–1163.

Mcilwraith, CW. 2003, *Advanced techniques in the diagnosis of bone disease*. Kentucky Equine Research Nutrition Conference, pp.1–11.

Murray, R.C., Walters, J.M., Snart, H., Dyson, S.J., Parkin, T.D. 2010, Identification of risk factors for lameness in dressage horses. *Vet. J.* 184:27–36.

Nunamaker, D.M. 2002, *On bone and fracture treatment in the horse.* Milne Lecture, American Association of Equine Practitioners, pp. 90–102.

Park, R.D. 2002, Radiology. In: Stashak, T.S. (ed.), *Adams' Lameness in Horses*, 5th edn. Lippincott, Williams & Wilkins, Philadelphia, PA, pp. 185–312.

Pfau, T., Robilliard, J.J., Weller, R., Jespers, K., Eliashar, E., Wilson, A.M. 2007, Assessment of mild hindlimb lameness during over ground locomotion using linear discriminant analysis of inertial sensor data. *Equine Vet. J.* 39:407–413.

Ross, M.W., Dyson, S.J. (eds) 2003, *Diagnosis and Management of Lameness in the Horse.* Saunders, Philadelphia, PA.

Steyn, P.F. 2002, Nuclear medicine. In: Stashak, T.S. (ed.), *Adams' Lameness in Horses*, 5th edn. Lippincott, Williams & Wilkins, Philadelphia, PA, pp. 347–375.

Van Hoogmoed, L.M., Snyder, J.R., Thomas, H.L., Harmon, F.A. 2003, Retrospective evaluation of equine prepurchase examinations performed 1991–2000. *Equine Vet. J.* 35:375–381.

Further reading

Dyce, K.M., Sack, W.O., Wensing, C.J.G. 2002, *Textbook of Veterinary Anatomy*, 3rd edn. WB Saunders, Philadelphia, PA.

Fossum, T.W. (ed.) 2002, *Small Animal Surgery*, 2nd edn. Mosby, St Louis, MO.

Getty, R. (ed.) 1975, *Sisson and Grossman's The Anatomy of the Domestic Animals*, 5th edn. WB Saunders, Philadelphia, PA.

Nickel, R., Schummer, A., Seiferle, E. 1973–1986, *The Anatomy of the Domestic Animal*, trans. W.G. Siller *et al.* Paul Parey, Berlin/Springer Verlag, New York.

Ross, M.W., Dyson, S.J. (eds) 2011, *Diagnosis and Management of Lameness in the Horse*, 2nd edn. WB Saunders, Philadelphia, PA.

Stashak, T.S. (ed.) 2011, *Adams' Lameness in Horses*, 6th edn. Lippincott, Williams & Wilkins, Philadelphia, PA.

CHAPTER 8

Canine lameness*

Lance Wilson and Bruce Smith

University of Queensland, Brisbane, Australia

Summary

The dog is an athletic species and lameness is commonly encountered. The speed and complexity of movement combined with the limited ability of animal patients to communicate their condition pose specific challenges in diagnosis. Diagnosis is best performed by or in conjunction with a veterinarian using a systematic approach to consider signalment, history, observation of movement, physical examination and appropriate application of diagnostic testing. Correct diagnosis relies on a detailed understanding of musculoskeletal anatomy and physiology as well as the range of differential diagnostic possibilities.

8.1 Introduction

The aim of this section is to provide an overview of the veterinary orthopaedic examination, placing particular emphasis on the more commonly encountered conditions and those more relevant to the role of a veterinary physiotherapist. Diagnostic investigations of these conditions are limited only to physical findings, while therapy, including any potential surgical and rehabilitation options, is not discussed in any detail.

*Adapted from the first edition chapter, which was written by Tom McGowan

A comprehensive orthopaedic examination can be divided into three main areas.
- Conformation
- Gait
- Clinical examination

The importance of a thorough knowledge of normal canine anatomy in the diagnosis and treatment of canine lameness conditions cannot be overemphasised. While a suitable 'normal' reference, in the form of the contralateral limb, is often available, canine developmental and degenerative conditions are frequently bilateral. Awareness of normal physical findings will allow the examiner to be alert to the more subtle conditions when they present. The reader is referred to three excellent canine anatomy reference texts (Done *et al.* 2009; Evans & de Lahunta 2012; Schaller & Thieme 2007).

The procurement of a full history is also very important in lameness work-up. Knowledge of when the lameness commenced, whether any inciting cause was noted by the owner, the progression of the lameness, findings of any diagnostic procedures and response to any therapy administered is vital in the characterisation of the lameness and development of a therapeutic plan. Often, the knowledge of what activity exacerbates the lameness can be very important. For example, although generalising somewhat, a joint-based lameness often improves with

Animal Physiotherapy: Assessment, Treatment and Rehabilitation of Animals, Second Edition. Edited by Catherine M. McGowan and Lesley Goff.

exercise, but worsens after a period of rest following the activity. Conversely, a lameness with a soft tissue aetiology will tend to worsen with further activity and improve with rest.

It must be noted that the role of an animal physiotherapist is not to make a pathoanatomical diagnosis and, indeed, this may be illegal in some regions. An orthopaedic referral for specialist diagnostics and surgical intervention may be required for a number of diseases discussed herein to obtain a definitive diagnosis and ensure optimal patient outcome.

8.2 Examination

8.2.1 Conformation

Conformation in a veterinary sense is defined as the shape or structure of the animal. Variables to assess include the alignment of bones and joints and the standing angle of joints. Angular deformities in all planes, including medial-lateral (valgus and varus), cranial-caudal (procurvatum/recurvatum) and torsion (internal/external rotation), must be recognised, along with any length discrepancies between limbs and bones.

It must be noted that substantial variability in conformation can exist between dog breeds. Examples include the relatively extended pelvic limb of a mastiff breed compared to a more flexed conformation in a German shepherd dog. Similarly, chondrodystrophoid breeds such as the dachshund possess angular deformities of their antebrachii that in a non-chondrodystrophoid dog would likely induce lameness.

Pathological conditions can alter the conformation of a limb, while abnormal conformation can induce pathology. Such an example is seen in the case of tarsal hyperextension, where the pathology is not typically present at the level of the tarsus. Instead, an orthopaedic condition of the proximal limb, generally the stifle, causes the dog to hyperextend the tarsus in an effort to alter the biomechanics of the diseased joint. Conversely, a pathological tibial plateau slope of greater than 32° has been shown to predispose a dog to cranial cruciate ligament rupture (Morris & Lipowitz 2001).

8.2.2 Gait assessment

If possible, the dog should always be examined while ambulating. This is important both in the initial diagnostic work-up and later on as a means of evaluating response to therapy. Gait assessment should be performed on a flat, regular, non-slip surface. Examination should entail walking the dog in a controlled, systematic manner on a lead, going away from, coming towards and passing by the examiner. This should then be repeated with the patient at a trot.

The lame limb(s) should be identified, typically by noting a 'head bob' when the affected thoracic limb contacts the ground, and a 'hip hitch' when the lame pelvic limb is loaded. This arises as the dog is more reluctant to place weight on the painful limb, leading to a decreased stance time. As the affected limb has less chance to drop down with pressure, it will subsequently ride higher than the non-affected limb. Additionally, the stance time of the individual limb can be assessed, while circumduction of the limb will often indicate pathology due to reluctance to fully flex a joint as the dog ambulates.

A lameness score can then be assigned to the limb, based on the examiner's chosen system. The authors prefer a 0–10 lameness scoring system, whereby 0 is assigned to a sound limb and 10 is a non-weight-bearing lameness (Johnson 2013).

In the case of a subtle lameness, gait assessment can be performed after physical manipulation, which may serve to make the lameness more apparent. Similarly, evaluation of a transient lameness may be better performed immediately after completion of an activity known to exacerbate the lameness. Occasionally. a dog will not display overt lameness when ambulating but will weight shift when standing. This can sometimes be detected by gently attempting to raise the limb while the dog is standing and comparing the amount of force required to do so with the contralateral limb.

Unfortunately, the subjective nature of visual gait assessment leads to poor sensitivity, especially in the detection of mild lameness. Computer-assisted gait analysis techniques such as pressure platforms and pressure walkways are objective, reliable, more sensitive and less prone to variation than visual analysis. However, at this point in time the cost, analysis time required and cumbersome nature of gait analysis systems have constrained their use to large referral institutions and the research setting.

8.2.3 Clinical examination

Clinical examination in lameness work-up involves visualisation, palpation and manipulation of the bones, joints and overlying soft tissues of the dog's limbs. A systematic, repeatable routine should be developed by the examiner to allow an accurate, thorough and expedient investigation in a lameness case.

Visualisation and palpation are employed to identify features such as pain, soft tissue swelling and hypertrophy, muscle wastage, joint effusion, crepitus, instability and heat. Manipulation of joints is utilised to measure range of motion, instability, crepitus and pain. A pain response is one of the most important findings in the work-up of lameness. However, the examiner must remember that individual animals may respond differently to the same level of stimulus. Certain stoic individuals may not respond when an obviously painful stimulus is applied, and in some instances (for example, the iliopsoas stretch test), while the stimulus will often generate pain, it is the level of discomfort that is the measureable response.

When examining a patient with an obvious region of discomfort, it is typically prudent to leave evaluation of that region until last. This may allow a more thorough examination to be performed as the animal is less likely to guard or overreact when other sites are scrutinised.

The examination technique described herein is a 'distal to proximal' system that commences at the animal's toes and finishes at the proximal aspect of the limb. The examination is

Box 8.1 DAMN IT system

D	Degenerative
	Developmental
A	Autoimmune
	Anomalous
M	Metabolic
	Mechanical
	Mental
N	Nutritional
	Neoplastic
I	Inflammatory
	Infectious
	Ischaemic
	Immune
	Inherited
	Iatrogenic
	Idiopathic
T	Traumatic
	Toxic

divided into multiple regions based on major anatomical structures, but it is important to note that often a single disease process can affect multiple sites, while multiple independent issues can also arise in different regions. Within each section, a differential diagnosis list is provided based on the DAMN IT system (http://medical-dictionary.thefreedictionary.com/DAMN+IT) (Box 8.1). While this list is not exhaustive, it covers the more frequent causes of canine lameness likely to be seen by a veterinary physiotherapist.

Examination of the bones and joints should be performed with the animal standing and then in lateral recumbency if possible. The former will provide information about when the limb is loaded and greater freedom of examination is allowed when the animal is in recumbency.

The anatomical nomenclature for directions and locations in quadrupeds differs somewhat from humans and should be utilised to allow accurate communication between veterinary professionals (see Chapter 4, Figure 4.1).

8.3 Thoracic limb

8.3.1 Phalanges/metacarpals

Each of the four weight-bearing digits II–V is composed of three bones: the first (P1), second (P2) and third (P3) phalanx. The articulations of P1/2 and P2/3 represent the proximal and distal interphalangeal joints respectively. These are saddle-type joints with most motion in flexion and extension. Stability is provided by the joint capsule, the collateral ligaments and the dorsal extensor and palmar flexor tendons respectively. The nail is attached to the ungual process of P3.

The proximal end or base of P1 articulates with the distal end or head of the respective metacarpal, forming the metacarpophalangeal joint. The metacarpophalangeal joints are saddle

joints with two sesamoids on the palmar aspect and a single smaller dorsal sesamoid. The palmar sesamoids are numbered 1–8 from the medial-most sesamoid of the metacarpophalangeal joint of digit II. Stability is provided by the joint capsule, dorsal extensor tendons and a small dorsal ligament, collateral ligaments medially and laterally and the palmar, lateral and medial collateral sesamoidean, cruciate and short sesamoidean ligaments on the palmar aspect.

Most dogs will possess a first digit, referred to as the dew claw. This non-weight-bearing digit contains the first metacarpal, and only two phalanges.

On the end of each digit is a digital pad, which consists of specialised thickened skin covering the digital cushion, a thickened region of subcutaneous adipose tissue interspersed with bundles of collagen and elastin. Above the digital pads resides the large metacarpal pad, which is responsible for the majority of weight bearing in the limb.

Visual assessment of the paw is first performed to evaluate for generic causes of the lameness such as traumatic nail injuries, lacerations, neoplasia and infection. The digits should be aligned in the sagittal plane, with the digital pads contacting the ground. Normal positioning of the canine digit is facilitated by a balance between the superficial and deep digital flexor tendons located on the palmar surface and the dorsal elastic ligaments. Rupture of the superficial digital flexor, which inserts on the base of P2 of digits II–V, will result in slight elevation of the nail and flaccid extension of the digit, due to loss of flexion between P1 and P2. Rupture of the deep digital flexor tendon, which inserts on P3 of digits II–V, will lead to a more noticeable elevation of the nail.

The nail beds should be evaluated for swelling or discharge. A chronic nail bed infection that is partially or non-responsive to antibiotics could represent underlying neoplasia or deep infection such as osteomyelitis, and should be investigated further. In lighter haired dog breeds, discolouration of the digital hair can often be appreciated if the animal has been licking the region excessively. The discolouration is a result of staining from porphyrins in the animal's saliva.

Tactile assessment and manipulation can now follow. The digits and pads can be palpated for any firm, painful regions that may reveal a corn, foreign body or neoplastic process. Corns are wart-like lesions of the pad seen as circular, firm, raised, hyperkeratotic masses, typically in the centre of the digital pads of digits III or IV of the thoracic limb, although often multiple digits are affected. The Greyhound is the breed most commonly affected and a mechanical cause is suspected.

Digits should be manipulated in flexion, extension, rotation and medial and lateral stress at each joint level. Rupture of a collateral ligament will often reveal pain and instability upon opening stress of the joint.

The palmar sesamoids are a well-recognised source of lameness in young dogs. Termed sesamoid disease or sesamoid fracture/fragmentation, this condition is most commonly seen in young Rottweilers, with an average age of 2 years. Sesamoids II and IV are overrepresented. The aetiology is unknown but theories include trauma, congenital disorders of ossification, degenerative joint disease and avascular osteonecrosis. Pain is typically elicited on direct palpation of the affected sesamoid bone and manipulation of the metacarpophalangeal joint. It is important to note that although radiographic evidence of sesamoid disease is relatively common, clinical signs are often not present.

Effusion, thickening, pain and instability can also be noted at the metacarpophalangeal joints with metacarpophalangeal osteoarthritis. This condition has an unknown cause, and joints IV and V are predisposed.

The metacarpal bones should be firmly palpated along their length. Although traumatic fractures are often easily noticed, non-displaced stress fractures can also be seen in racing Greyhounds, with digit V of the left thoracic limb and digit II of the right thoracic most commonly affected.

A differential diagnosis list for musculoskeletal conditions of the canine metacarpophalangeal region is as follows.

- Corns
- Paronychia
- Sesamoid disease
- Collateral ligament sprain
- MCP/P disease
- Fracture
- Syndactyly/ecrodactyly
- Neoplasia
- Laceration

8.3.2 Carpus

The carpal joint is a series of complex articulations involving seven carpal bones. These bones include the radial, ulna and accessory carpal bones and the numbered carpal bones C1–C4. The carpus is divided into three main joint levels. In a proximal to distal direction, these are the antebrachiocarpal joint, the middle carpal joint and the carpometacarpal joint. The antebrachiocarpal joint is formed by the articulation between the distal radius and ulna proximally and the radial and ulna carpal bone distally. The middle carpal joint consists of the articulation between the radial and ulna carpal bones and C1–C4 while the carpometacarpal joint is formed by C1–C4 and the bases of metacarpals I–V. Joints between the individual carpal bones of each row are known as the intercarpal joints. The accessory carpal bone is located at the palmarolateral aspect of the carpus and acts as a fulcrum for the insertion of flexor tendons and supportive ligaments.

The carpus is largely a hinge joint but does allow some medial to lateral movement. Greatest movement occurs at the antebrachiocarpal joint, followed by the middle carpal and carpometacarpal joints. Stability is achieved by a relatively thickened joint capsule and a complex array of ligamentous, fibrocartilaginous and musculotendinous structures. The most noteworthy of these include the short medial and lateral collateral ligaments which prevent valgus and varus instability respectively; the palmar carpal fibrocartilage located at the level of the

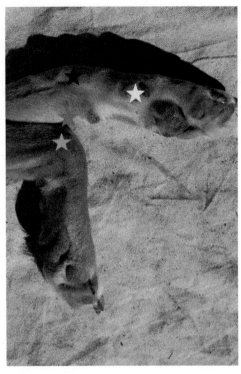

Figure 8.1 Surface anatomy of the carpus showing medial aspect of left limb and lateral aspect of right limb. The black star is over the radial styloid process, blue star over the ulnar styloid process, yellow star over the dew claw and red star denotes the accessory carpal bone, with the carpal pad overlying slightly distally.

palmar carpometacarpal joint; and multiple short palmar ligaments that provide palmar stability with weight bearing. Importantly, there are no continuous ligaments that traverse all three carpal joints. The reader is referred to an anatomy text for a more thorough description of this complex joint.

Anatomical landmarks for examination of the carpus include the medially located styloid process of the distal radius, the laterally located styloid process of the distal ulna, the accessory carpal bone, the carpal pad and the lateral base of metacarpal V (Figure 8.1).

The carpus should be inspected visually for evidence of hyperextension when the dog is weight bearing and ambulating. The normal weight-bearing angle of the carpal joint as a whole ranges between 10° and 47° of extension, depending on the time within the stance phase.

Palpation and manipulation can follow. Effusion is typically appreciated over the dorsal and medial aspects of the carpus; any effusion detected on palpation is typically suggestive of a pathological process. Flexion of the carpus should be well tolerated with the digital pads able to be brought in contact with the caudal antebrachium. Extension should be beyond 0° but note that this is typically much less than the dog will achieve on its own when loading the limb. A small amount of varus and valgus motion will be achieved but the operator should feel the relevant collateral ligament tighten under a finger when stress is applied.

Rupture of the ligamentous supporting structures is a common cause of lameness in dogs. Causes range from trauma in athletic and working dogs to degenerative and inflammatory aetiologies. Carpal hyperextension results from loss of some or all of the palmar supporting structures. The dog will generally present with a hyperextended carpus if weight bearing, and effusion and pain are normally noted. The joint level involved differs between reports, with one study documenting 31%, 22% and 47% at the antebrachiocarpal, middle carpal and carpometacarpal joints respectively, while another reported 10%, 50% and 40% for the same joint levels (Parker *et al.* 1981).

It is important to recognise carpal hyperextension injuries when they are present. Given the location on the tension side of the joint and the amount of load placed through the limb when ambulating (108% of body weight at a trot), conservative management with coaptation is generally unrewarding, and either surgical treatment via partial or pancarpal arthrodesis or long-term application of a custom carpal splint is typically required.

Collie-type breeds appear to be affected by an idiopathic degenerative condition that involves the ligamentous stabilisers of the small joints. A history of insidious lameness is present and the joints will palpate markedly thickened and fibrosed, with decreased range of motion.

Young large breed puppies can be affected by a condition known as carpal laxity syndrome. The condition can manifest as hyperextension of the carpus or, more commonly, as hypoextension of the carpus, whereby the limb will be seen to buckle forward under loading. Puppies tend to present between 2 and 5 months of age and the condition can be unilateral or bilateral. No pain can be elicited and a normal range of motion is present. The cause is unknown, although various husbandry, nutrition, environmental and inherited causes have been proposed, while the pathophysiology seems to imply an imbalance between the flexor and extensor muscles. Generally, this condition will resolve within 2–4 weeks untreated although the provision of a well-balanced diet and a controlled exercise regime on natural flooring is typically recommended. Temporary splinting can be required in the more severe cases, although this should be changed regularly.

Differential diagnosis includes the following.
- Carpal hyperextension
- Fracture
- Medial/lateral instability
- Carpal luxation
- Primary osteoarthritis
- Immune-mediated polyarthritis
- Septic arthritis
- Neoplasia
- Juvenile carpal laxity syndrome

8.3.3 Radius/ulna

The canine antebrachium is composed of the craniomedially located radius and the caudolaterally positioned ulna. The radius is primarily a weight-bearing bone while the ulna functions both in weight bearing and as a lever arm.

The antebrachium is the most common site for an angular limb deformity in the dog. This often arises due to premature closure of a physis in a young animal, most commonly the distal ulna physis, although other causes have been described. Because the radius and ulna grow independently from separate physes, any inhibition in the growth of one bone will cause it to tie down growth of the limb. The other bone will attempt to continue growth, but this 'bow-string' effect from the shortened bone will result in angulation, bowing and torsion of the limb, and potential incongruency at adjacent joints.

The bones should be palpated for any pain. The distal radial metaphysis is the second most common site for osteosarcoma which is typically seen in middle-aged to older large to giant breed dogs. Lameness is often initially insidious as a result of bone microfracture and/or periosteal disruption. Later in the disease process, swelling can be appreciated and occasionally a gross pathological fracture will propagate through the diseased bone.

Two other well-recognised causes of bone pain that are recognised in young, large breed dogs are panosteitis and metaphyseal osteopathy. Panosteitis is the most common cause of lameness in young, large breed dogs (Bohning *et al.* 1970). It is a self-limiting disease of unknown aetiology that is characterised by osseous proliferation and excessive bone remodelling. Classic signs include insidious lameness with pain on bone palpation, typically starting at the site of the nutrient foramen. Most cases present between 5 and 12 months of age, and males are overrepresented, while it is well recognised to recur episodically, resulting in 'shifting leg lameness'. The ulna is the most common bone affected in one study, followed by the radius, although multiple bones can be affected at the same time. Treatment is generally supportive and the long-term prognosis is excellent.

Metaphyseal osteopathy is a less commonly seen disease of large to giant breed juveniles. Characterised by severe inflammation of the metaphyseal bone adjacent to the physis, presentation is generally at 3–5 months of age and signs include severe lameness, anorexia, malaise, fever and swelling over the affected area. The distal radius and ulna are most commonly affected. Treatment is systemic administration of corticosteroids and supportive care, and unless a limb deformity develops, prognosis is typically good (Grondalen 1976).

Differential diagnosis includes the following.
- Panosteitis
- Hypertrophic osteodystrophy (HOD)
- Angular limb deformity
- Fracture
- Neoplasia

8.3.4 Elbow

The elbow is a common site for pathology that can create lameness, especially in the young dog. It is a complex composite joint, with articulation between the capitulum of the humeral condyle and the radial head, called the humeroradial joint, and the trochlea of the humeral condyle and the trochlea notch and coronoid of the ulna, termed the humeroulnar joint. Together, the humeroradial and humeroulnar joints are strictly a hinge joint. The humeroradial joint functions largely as a weight-bearing joint, while the humeroulnar joint has weight-bearing function in addition to its role as a lever arm and stabiliser. Historically, it has been thought that the humeroradial joint was responsible for the majority of weight transfer to the elbow, but a study has shown that the humeroradial and humeroulnar joints support approximately 52% and 48% of the respective forces through cadaveric limbs (Mason *et al.* 2005). A joint also exists between the proximal radius and ulna, called the radioulnar joint, that allows rotation of the radius within the radial notch of the ulna, permitting a small amount of pronation and a larger amount of supination.

The normal range of motion of the elbow joint as measured in awake adult Labrador Retrievers is approximately 130°, ranging from 36° in flexion to 165° in extension. Like many of the large joints in a dog, 135° is considered to be the approximate standing angle of the elbow. Stability of the elbow is provided by the joint capsule, the locking mechanism of the anconeal process of the ulna into the olecranon fossa and the collateral ligaments. At a standing angle, the anconeal process provides stability in pronation while the lateral collateral is the main stabiliser in supination. However, when the elbow is flexed to 90°, the medial collateral ligament is responsible for torsional stability.

Anatomical landmarks for manipulation of the elbow include the medial and lateral epicondyles, which are the attachment sites of the flexor and extensor muscles respectively, the olecranon of the ulna, upon which the triceps muscles insert, and the radial head, at the craniolateral extent of the elbow (Figure 8.2).

The elbow should be inspected visually. If significant effusion is present, this can typically be visualised as a swelling on the lateral aspect of the joint, between the olecranon and lateral

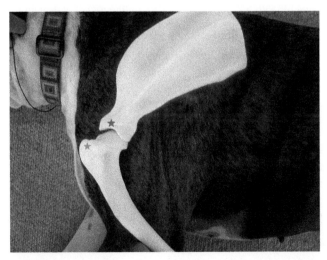

Figure 8.2 Surface anatomy of the shoulder. The red star is over the acromion and blue star denotes the greater tubercle.

epicondylar ridge. Dogs with elbow pain will often sit with their elbows slightly abducted and extended, in an effort to reduce the pain of elbow flexion. Similarly, if medial compartment disease is present, they will often stand with their elbows slightly adducted to transfer weight through the less diseased lateral compartment of the joint.

Palpation should be performed to detect joint capsule thickening and more subtle effusion, while a full range of motion should be performed to evaluate range and a pain response. In cases of elbow disease, flexion will often be decreased due to the restriction of periarticular fibrosis, while pain will be detected on end-range extension. The radial head should be in the same frontal and sagittal plane as the lateral epicondyle, sitting directly proximal to it. The medial epicondyle especially should be palpated for pain if flexor enthesiopathy is suspected.

Campbell's test evaluates the integrity of the medial collateral ligament. Here, the elbow is flexed to 90° and pronation and supination are performed to measure stability. However, studies have shown a large variation in the degree of rotation between dogs, so a comparison with the contralateral joint is likely more beneficial if medial collateral instability is suspected. Campbell's test can also be utilised to evaluate for a pain response in cases of elbow dysplasia.

Elbow dysplasia (ED) is an umbrella term that pertains to a number of separate yet often concomitant heritable, developmental conditions of the canine elbow. These conditions include medial coronoid disease (MCD, previously referred to as fragmented coronoid process or FCP), osteochondrosis dissecans (OCD) of the medial humeral condyle, ununited anconeal process (UAP) and elbow incongruency (EI). A full discussion of ED is beyond the scope of this chapter, but the typical signalment is that of a large or giant breed dog, presenting with an insidious-onset thoracic limb lameness between 5 and 12 months of age. Male dogs are approximately twice as affected as female dogs, bilateral disease is common (20–80%, depending on the study) and common breeds affected include the Labrador Retriever, Bernese Mountain Dog, German Shepherd Dog, Rottweiler, Newfoundland and the Mastiff breeds (Cook 2001; Janutta *et al.* 2006). Typical signs elicited on orthopaedic examination, dependent on the type of ED and severity of disease, include a weight-bearing lameness that is worse in the morning or after exercise, pain on elbow extension and Campbell's test and joint effusion and thickening.

Incomplete ossification of the humeral condyle (IOHC) is a developmental disease of the elbow that is typically seen in Spaniel breeds and Labrador Retrievers. Most common in the United Kingdom, it arises from failure of fusion of the two ossification centres on the humeral condyle. Cases can present after catastrophic fracture, generally involving the lateral condyle, but a history of insidious thoracic limb lameness may also be present. Pain on elbow manipulation is the most common finding, and effusion is generally not appreciated.

Septic arthritis of the elbow arising from either haematogenous spread or via local extension from a deep pyoderma is well recognised, especially in mature dogs with preexisting elbow degenerative joint disease. Suspicions should be raised in cases of severe acute-on-chronic lameness with significant joint effusion, heat and pain.

The elbow is also one of the most common sites for joint tumours such as synovial sarcoma. An acute to chronic history of progressive lameness in a middle-aged to older dog with periarticular soft tissue thickening and pain on manipulation and palpation is suggestive.

Differential diagnosis includes the following.
- ED:
    - MCD
    - OCD
    - UAP
    - EI
- Flexor enthesiopathy
- IOHC
- Congenital elbow luxation
- Traumatic elbow (sub)luxation
- Ununited medial epicondyle
- Septic arthritis
- Neoplasia

8.3.5 Humerus

The humerus should be palpated for any pain that may indicate pathology such as panosteitis or osteosarcoma. The proximal humeral metaphysis is the most common site for canine appendicular osteosarcoma.

The triceps and biceps/brachialis muscles can be palpated at the caudal and cranial extent of the brachium respectively. Dogs with chronic thoracic limb lameness will frequently demonstrate wasting of the triceps and myofascial trigger points can often be detected in the triceps muscle bellies.

Differential diagnosis includes the following.
- Panosteitis
- Fracture
- Neoplasia

8.3.6 Shoulder

Termed the glenohumeral joint, the shoulder is formed by the articulation between the shallow glenoid cavity of the scapula and the large humeral head and is the most mobile of all canine appendicular joints. It is a ball-and-socket joint that allows movement in all directions; however, the primary direction is in flexion and extension, with a recognised range between 57° and 165° degrees.

Shoulder stability is provided by both static and dynamic stabilisers. Static stabilisers include the shallow ball-and-socket structure of the joint, the adhesion-cohesion effect of the synovial fluid, the medial and lateral collateral ligaments, the joint capsule and the joint labrum. Active stabilisers include the 'rotator cuff' muscles of human anatomy, namely the subscapularis and coracobrachialis medially, the supraspinatus craniolaterally

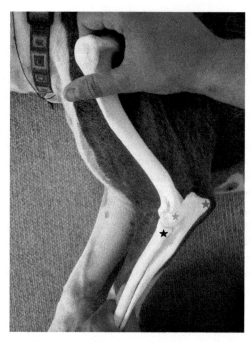

Figure 8.3 Surface anatomy of the elbow. The red star is over the olecranon; blue star over the humeral epicondyle and black star over the radial head.

and the infraspinatus and teres minor laterally. Other less important active stabilisers include the biceps brachii, long head of the triceps, the deltoideus and the teres major muscles.

Anatomical features to recognise include the greater tubercle on the cranioproximal border of the humerus and the acromion at the distal extent of the scapula spine (Figure 8.3).

The shoulder is commonly implicated as the site of canine thoracic limb lameness. However, an excellent grasp of the complex regional musculotendinous anatomy and accurate examination technique are required to arrive at the correct clinical diagnosis. This is further complicated by the difficulty in examining the shoulder in isolation, without manipulating the elbow, and the propensity for concomitant shoulder and elbow disease in veterinary patients.

Given the muscle bulk surrounding the shoulder joint, joint effusion is generally very difficult to detect. Wasting of the supraspinatus and infraspinatus muscles is often noticeable as a prominence of the spine of scapula, in more chronic lameness cases.

Range of motion should be tested and pain evaluated. The abduction angles can also be assessed in many awake dogs. This involves lying the dog on its side with the affected limb uppermost. The limb is placed at a standing angle and the scapula is stabilised with one hand while the other is used to abduct the distal limb. The angle formed by the shaft of the humerus and spine of the scapula is measured: the normal abduction angle for a large breed dog is approximately 30°. Mediolateral and craniocaudal stability should be assessed. Mediolateral stability is tested by stabilising the scapula with one hand while the other grasps the brachium and manipulates the limb in a medial to lateral plane. Similarly, craniocaudal stability is assessed by manipulation of the brachium in a caudal to cranial direction. This test is known as the shoulder draw test.

Shoulder instability can be seen in both large and small breed dogs. In small breed dogs, it is generally associated with a congenital dysplasia of the glenoid or soft tissue laxity and hence is often seen in young animals. In large breed dogs, it is typically a result of trauma – either the more common cause of repetitive microtrauma or occasionally with acute traumatic overload. Instability is most common in the mediolateral plane, although craniocaudal and multidirectional instability are also seen. Shoulder instability is generally seen in middle-aged, male, large breed dogs with a history of chronic lameness that is minimally responsive to antiinflammatories and rest. In clinical cases of medial instability, the average abduction angle measures 50°, and pain is typically noted on shoulder abduction.

Pain on shoulder manipulation, especially flexion, extension and internal/external rotation at mid-flexion is seen in many conditions. In young dogs, a common cause of thoracic limb lameness and shoulder pain is osteochondrosis dissecans (OCD), a developmental condition of the canine shoulder involving an articular cartilage flap or defect of the humeral head. Large to giant breed males are overrepresented, with 27–68% of animals having bilateral lesions, and the average age of presentation is between 4 and 8 months of age (Berzon 1979).

Palpation of the insertion of the supraspinatus muscle on the greater tubercle should be performed. Just medial to the supraspinatus insertion lies the biceps brachii tendon of origin in the intertubecular groove. This region should also be palpated for a pain response. The bicipital stretch test involves testing the biceps muscle and its tendinous insertions for pain. The shoulder is maximally flexed and the elbow maximally extended. The other hand is then used to place pressure on the biceps tendon of insertion near the cranial aspect of the elbow, thus maximally stressing the bicipital musculotendinous unit.

Supraspinatus tendinopathy is a common cause of insidious-onset, chronic lameness seen in middle-aged dogs. Labradors are overrepresented and the disease appears to respond best to prolonged periods of rest. A repetitive strain injury of the supraspinatus tendon of insertion with healing prevented by a relative hypovascularity and ongoing activity is postulated to cause the condition. Lameness is typically worse after exercise and pain is commonly elicited on direct palpation of the tendinous insertion, the shoulder draw test and shoulder hyperflexion with and without rotation.

Likewise, biceps brachii tendinopathy is a well-recognised cause of lameness in dogs. Signalment, history and disease aetiology are similar to those of supraspinatus tendinopathy. Clinical findings are also similar, with pain on direct palpation of the tendon, shoulder flexion and the bicipital stretch test.

Differential diagnosis includes the following.
- OCD
- Shoulder instability:
  - Glenoid dysplasia
  - Congenital soft tissue
  - Traumatic
  - Degenerative
  - Accessory ossification centre of the caudal glenoid?
- Synovial chondrometaplasia
- Fracture
- Septic arthritis
- Soft tissue:
  - Bicipital tendinopathy
  - Supraspinatus tendinopathy
  - Teres minor myopathy
  - Infraspinatus contracture
- Neoplasia

8.3.7 Scapula

The scapula is infrequently a source of lameness in the canine. The position of the scapula and acromion process should be evaluated. Palpation of the spinatus muscles can be performed to evaluate for atrophy, while the bone can be palpated for any pain response that may indicate a fracture or neoplastic process.

Differential diagnosis includes the following.
- Fracture
- Ununited supraglenoid tuberosity
- Osteosarcoma
- Scapula luxation
- Neoplasia

8.4 Pelvic limb

8.4.1 Phalanges/metatarsals

Examination is performed as per the thoracic limb.

8.4.2 Tarsus

The tarsus is a complex composite joint consisting of seven tarsal bones functioning purely as a hinge joint, articulating in flexion and extension. In a proximal to distal direction, these bones are the talus, calcaneus, central tarsal bone and the numbered tarsal bones T1–T4. These bones form three irregular rows and as such, six main articulations with four distinct joint levels are recognised. The articulations are the tarsocrural, formed by the distal tibia and the talus, the talocalcaneal, the talocalcaneocentral, the calcaneoquartal, formed by the calcaneus and T4, the centrodistal, formed by the central tarsal and T1–T3 and the tarsometatarsal of T1–T4 and metatarsals II–V. The talocalcaneocentral and the calcaneoquartal joints form the proximal intertarsal joint while the centrodistal joint is known as the distal intertarsal joint. As per the carpus, small vertical intertarsal joints are present between the tarsal bones in each row.

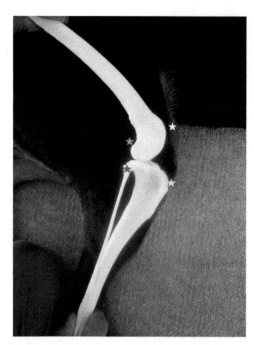

Figure 8.4 Bony anatomy of the hock. The red star is the calcaneal tuber of the left hindlimb; yellow stars are the lateral (left hind) and medial (right hind) malleoli; green star is the base of fifth metatarsal; blue star is head of fifth metatarsal.

Standard tarsal joint range of motion in the dog is from approximately 40° in flexion to 165° in extension, with a normal standing angle of 135–145°; 90% of this range is provided by the tarsocrucral joint. The tarsocrural joint is oriented at a 25° lateral deviation to allow the pelvic limb paw to swing past the ipsilateral thoracic limb paw as the dog ambulates.

Anatomical landmarks utilised in examination of the tarsus include the lateral malleolus of the distal fibula, the medial malleolus of the distal tibia, the caudolaterally located calcaneus and the lateral base of metatarsal V (Figure 8.4). The joint should be palpated for any pain, crepitus or effusion. Joint effusion is typically best appreciated at the proximocaudal aspect of the joint between the distal tibia and the calcaneus. Range of motion should be evaluated and stability tested.

Tarsal stability is provided largely by the strong collateral and plantar ligamentous support structures. The reader is referred to a veterinary anatomy text for a more in-depth description of hock anatomy. Unlike the carpus, the collateral ligaments of the tarsus are quite complex, with elements that span the entire joint length. Each collateral ligament originates on the distal aspect of its respective malleolus and has a short and long component. The long component is oriented somewhat parallel with the long axis of the joint and provides stability in joint extension, while the short components are largely at 90° to the joint and provide rotational stability in flexion. This is important as isolated traumatic rupture of the short collateral ligaments is well described but can be easily missed unless specifically evaluated. Testing of the collaterals involves varus and valgus stress applied to the distal limb with the tarsus at a standing angle to evaluate the long components. The hock is then flexed to 90° and varus and valgus stress imparted on the distal limb to create a rotational force at the tarsus. Critically, as the short collaterals run caudally from each malleolus, torsion towards the lateral aspect of the hock tests the short component of the lateral collateral, while medial stress evaluates the short component of the medial collateral.

Collateral ligamentous injury can occur acutely as a result of trauma and result in joint luxation or subluxation. A repetitive sprain injury to the medial collateral is well recognised in Collie-type breeds that present with a chronic lameness often exacerbated by exuberant exercise. A firm, often spectacular soft tissue swelling is appreciated over the medial aspect of the hock, and although some pain can be elicited with valgus stress, instability is generally not noted.

Plantar support is provided by a complex arrangement of strong ligaments and the tarsal fibrocartilage. Plantar stability is assessed by grasping the distal tibia and proximal calcaneus in one hand while applying dorsal force to the paw with the other hand. Trauma can induce plantar instability that will result in significant lameness and a plantigrade stance. A degenerative condition of unknown aetiology is known to affect the plantar ligamentous structures of the proximal intertarsal joint in Collie breeds. Middle-aged overweight dogs appear overrepresented and bilateral disease is common. A plantigrade stance is present and although marked instability is appreciated, minimal pain response is typically seen.

Tarsal bone fractures are well recognised in the racing Greyhound. Typically seen in the right limb due to the severe compressive forces imparted on the outside limb as the dog races, fractures of the central tarsal bone predominate; however, fracture of the other numbered tarsal bones and the calcaneus can also be seen. Although a severe acute-onset lameness is characteristic of most fractures, occasionally small slab fractures will result in a lower-grade chronic lameness. Direct palpation over such a slab fracture will generally reveal subtle thickening of the joint capsule and a pain response.

The superficial digital flexor tendon runs over the plantar aspect of the calcaneus. A condition seen almost exclusively in Shetland sheep dogs is luxation of the tendon, whereby degeneration of the medial retinaculum over the calcaneus leads to lateral displacement of the tendon. Medial luxation is occasionally seen. Presentation is typically variable due to intermittent luxation and reduction while diagnosis is typically straightforward. The tendon is normally swollen and bulbous over the tip of the calcaneus and can be readily luxated with digital pressure or via medial rotation of the paw with the tarsus in flexion.

Osteochondrosis dissecans of the medial or lateral talar ridge is a debilitating developmental disease of young dogs that typically results in severe progressive lameness. Labrador Retriever and Rottweiler breeds are overrepresented and affected dogs tend to present between 4 and 8 months of age. Severe joint effusion, muscle wasting, crepitus and pain on manipulation are found and in cases of medial talar ridge OCD, the deficit can occasionally be palpated with the hock in flexion. Bilateral disease is common.

Differential diagnosis includes the following.

- Plantar instability
- Fracture
- Medial/lateral instability
- Chronic medial collateral sprain
- Osteochondrosis dissecans
- SDFT luxation
- Primary osteoarthritis
- Immune-mediated polyarthritis
- Neoplasia
- Septic arthritis

8.4.3 Tibia/fibula

The larger tibia is the main weight-bearing bone of the crus, while the much smaller, laterally located fibula has its main role as the attachment for the lateral collateral ligaments of the stifle and tarsus.

The cranial tibial muscle is located on the craniolateral aspect of the proximal tibia. It is often the first muscle to undergo neurogenic atrophy in cases of sciatic neuropathy.

Located at the caudal aspect of the crus are the paired gastrocnemius muscles and the superficial digital flexor muscle deep to them. The tendons from these muscles join with the common tendon of the biceps femoris, semitendinosus and gracilis muscles to form the calcaneal tendon (CT), also known as the Achilles tendon, which inserts on the proximal aspect of the calcaneus. The calcaneal tendon should be palpated for any thickening, loss of definition, focal deficits or pain. Disruption to the CT mechanism can occur at three levels: the musculotendinous junction of the gastrocnemius tendon, the mid-substance of the tendon and at the tendinous insertion on the calcaneus. Rupture can involve part or all of the CT components, and is typically either a result of trauma or an isolated chronic, degenerative insertionopathy of the gastrocnemius tendon, seen classically in middle-aged to older Doberman Pinscher and Labrador Retriever breeds. Complete rupture of the CT will result in a plantigrade stance, where the dog's tarsus is contacting the ground, while rupture of the gastrocnemius mechanism alone will create a characteristic stance where the hock is moderately plantigrade while the toes are in a clawed position due to the pull of the intact superficial digital flexor tendon.

The tibia and fibula should be examined for normal alignment and palpated for pain. The proximal and distal tibial metaphyses are well-recognised common regions for primary osteosarcoma.

Differential diagnosis includes the following.

- Fracture
- Panosteitis
- Neoplasia
- Angular limb deformity
- Calcaneal tendon rupture:
  - Complete rupture
  - Gastrocnemeus tendon insertionopathy

8.4.4 Stifle

The stifle is defined as a complex condylar synovial joint. Relevant structures include the medial and lateral femoral condyles, the tibial plateau and the medial and lateral menisci stationed between them. The patella is the largest sesamoid in the canine body and runs in the trochlea groove located at the cranial extent of the distal femur. Thus the two main joints in the stifle are the femorotibial joint and the femoropatellar joint. The menisci are semilunar fibrocartilaginous discs that enhance femorotibial congruency and stability, dispel compressive forces across the joint, reduce friction via hydrostatic lubrication and provide sensation.

The primary function of the stifle is in flexion and extension, but some internal rotation is also allowed. Normal range of motion in Labrador Retrievers has been reported at 41° of flexion and 162° of extension and the normal standing angle of the stifle has been described as 130–140° (Jaegger *et al.* 2002).

Anatomical reference points for the stifle include the patella, the straight patella ligament, inserting on the tibial tuberosity, the lateral fabella and the fibular head (Figure 8.5).

Given its inherently unstable osseous anatomy, the stifle relies on a number of important soft tissue structures to provide support. These include both static and dynamic stabilisers. Static stabilisers include the cruciate (cranial and caudal) and collateral (medial and lateral) ligaments, the paired menisci and the straight patellar ligament. The cranial cruciate ligament (CrCL)

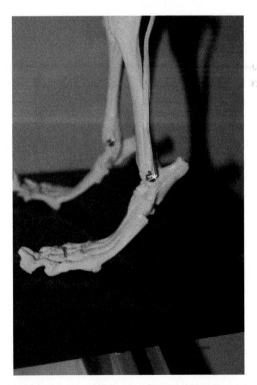

Figure 8.5 Surface anatomy of the stifle. The white star indicates the patella; yellow star indicates tibial tubercle; blue star the fabella; and red star the head of fibula.

originates at the caudal aspect of the intercondylar notch on the medial aspect of the lateral condyle and runs in a craniomediodistal direction to insert on the cranial tibial plateau. The caudal cruciate ligament (CaCL) originates at the cranial aspect of the intercondylar notch on the lateral aspect of the medial condyle and runs in a caudolaterodistal direction to insert on the caudal aspect of the tibial plateau. The medial and lateral collaterals originate on the medial and lateral epicondyles and insert on the medial tibia and fibula head respectively. Dynamic stabilisers include muscles such as the biceps femoris, semitendinosus, semimembranosus and gastrocnemius that cross the stifle joint and provide additional active stability if required.

The stifle should first be examined with the dog standing. The examiner should bend or kneel behind the dog and palpate the stifle for effusion or thickening. This is best performed by using a finger just medial to the straight patellar ligament to assess the sharpness to the edge of the ligament. Any joint effusion or capsular thickening will cause the joint capsule to bulge out, making the edge of the ligament less distinct. In cases of chronic stifle instability, florid firm capsular thickening will develop at the medial aspect of the joint over time; this is colloquially termed a medial buttress. Palpation of the medial joint line with a firm thumb has been shown to be very sensitive and moderately specific for the detection of damage to the caudal pole of the medial meniscus, the common site for meniscal tears. The medial joint line is palpated from a cranial to caudal direction and the dog is assessed for a pain response.

The stifle should be placed throughout its range of motion and discomfort and crepitus assessed. A 'meniscal click' has been reported as a measure determining meniscal pathology, whereby a slight clicking sound is heard as the damaged meniscus is displaced throughout stifle range of motion. However, this has been shown to be poorly sensitive in detecting meniscal disease, and should not be relied upon. The patella should be evaluated to ensure it is well located throughout its range and is unable to be medially or laterally luxated.

Cranial cruciate ligament disease is the most common orthopaedic condition seen in dogs. There are four main presentations for the disease:

- acute traumatic rupture
- chronic degeneration in small dogs, often linked to chronic medial patella luxation
- progressive degeneration in young, large to giant breed dogs often associated with anatomical abnormalities
- progressive degeneration in older large breed dogs.

In the large and giant breed dogs with progressive degeneration, a repetitive strain aetiology is suspected, although a primary inflammatory cause has not been disproved. Factors such as obesity, conformation and lack of fitness have been associated with the disease, while a heritable cause has been proven in Newfoundlands and is suspected in other breeds. The condition is most prevalent in female dogs and desexing has been strongly linked to an increased disease prevalence. It is extremely rare to

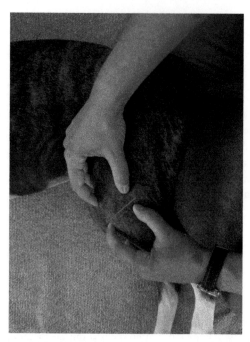

Figure 8.6 Cranial draw test. The arrow denotes cranial drawer direction of the tibia relative to the femur.

see CrCL disease in dogs younger than 1 year while, depending on the study, approximately 50% of dogs will rupture their contralateral CrCL within 6–12 months of the first injury (Buote *et al.* 2009; Doverspike *et al.* 1993).

A diagnosis of CrCL rupture can typically be strongly suspected based on clinical examination findings. The often mentioned 'gold standard' test for determination of CrCL disease is known as the cranial draw test. To perform this test, the dog is best placed in lateral recumbency with the tested stifle uppermost positioned at a standing angle of approximately 135°. From the caudal aspect of the stifle, one hand is placed over the distal femur with the index finger on the cranial aspect of the patella and the thumb caudal to the lateral fabella while the other hand is placed over the proximal tibia with the index finger on the cranial aspect of the tibial tuberosity and the thumb caudal to the head of the fibula (Figure 8.6). The hand on the tibia then attempts to move the proximal tibia cranially in the sagittal plane, being mindful not to exert any internal rotation on the tibia. Any degree of motion in an adult dog is considered abnormal, but in juvenile dogs some degree of movement is anticipated. The movement should be differentiated from a pathological finding by the presence of a firm stop or 'endpoint' as the CrCL is activated.

A second test of CrCL integrity is the tibial compression test. Here the examiner's proximal hand is positioned at the distal femur, similar to the cranial draw test, while the other hand is placed over the metatarsus. While the stifle is firmly stabilised at a standing angle, the tarsus is flexed (Figure 8.7). Abnormal cranial displacement of the tibial tuberosity indicates failure of the CrCL.

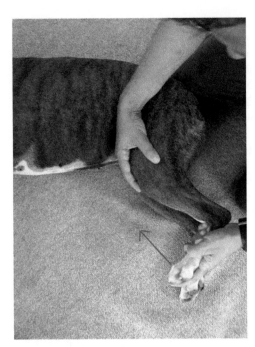

Figure 8.7 Tibial compression test. The arrow denotes direction of thrust.

While a positive result on these tests is highly correlated with CrCL insufficiency, a negative test does not rule out CrCL disease. Instability can be obtunded by severe stifle effusion or periarticular fibrosis and masked by activation of the periarticular active stabilisers, especially in well-muscled, painful or anxious animals. However, the main shortcoming of these tests is in the case of partial CrCL rupture. While sometimes a pain response will be elicited with the draw test in partial CrCL tearing, and mild instability may be detected in cases of selective rupture of the craniomedial band of the CrCL if the draw test is performed at mid-flexion, these tests are insensitive at detecting partial CrCL tears.

In the authors' opinion, the first sign of CrCL degeneration is a pain response on hyperextension of the stifle. The three functions of the CrCL are to prevent cranial translation of the tibia, internal rotation of the tibia and hyperextension of the stifle. Manual hyperextension places a large amount of strain through the CrCL, causing pain as the degenerating CrCL fibres are stretched. The next most sensitive sign is detection of joint effusion, followed by pain on the cranial draw test. Another 'test' often utilised in the diagnosis of CrCL disease is the sit test. Basically, a non-specific indicator of stifle pain, it is demonstrated when a dog is sitting down. Instead of sitting square with its stifles flexed underneath, the dog will hold the affected leg out to the side due to its reluctance to flex the painful joint. Although commonly seen in cases of CrCL disease, other causes of stifle pathology can also cause sit test failure.

The importance of early detection of CrCL degeneration is realised by the proactive institution of surgical and/or non-surgical interventions that may serve to halt CrCL degeneration or, more importantly, preserve meniscal integrity. However, the high incidence of bilateral concurrent disease can make diagnosis more difficult due to the lack of a normal reference. For these reasons, the reader is strongly encouraged to critically refine their examination of the stifle in an attempt to elucidate the subtle signs of early CrCL disease.

Although partial CrCL rupture creates lameness via the stretching of diseased CrCL fibres and the presence of progressive synovitis, and complete CrCL rupture creates more severe inflammatory disease, haemarthrosis and instability, the major determinant of lameness severity is the status of the meniscus. A recent study in CrCL-deficit dogs demonstrated that those with meniscal tears had significantly higher lameness scores than those without meniscal pathology, while a long-term study demonstrated that dogs undergoing meniscal resection due to a meniscal tear had significantly more osteoarthritis at a mean of 3 years follow-up. Depending on the study, somewhere from 30% to 70% of dogs with CrCL disease will have meniscal pathology; however, it is rare to see a meniscal tear in a stable joint, even in the presence of a partial CrCL tear (Bennett & May 1991).

Rupture of the CaCL is typically seen as part of a multiligamentous injury in cases of severe trauma, although it can occasionally occur independently as a result of a caudally directed force imparted on the tibial tuberosity. Although lameness is often not severe with CaCL injury, it must be differentiated from a CrCL rupture as the prognosis and treatment differ substantially. Joint effusion will typically be observed, with mild pain on stifle manipulation. The stifle is examined for the spatial relationship between the patella and the tibial tuberosity. By holding the limb with the cranial aspect of the stifle pointing dorsally, the limb is held by the hock with the stifle unsupported. A subtle 'sag' of the tibial tuberosity may be noted as the tibia caudally subluxates in the absence of an intact CaCL. The caudal draw test can also be performed. Basically the opposite of the cranial draw test, the operator must be alert to a firm endpoint with cranial motion of the tibia and a comparatively soft endpoint as the tibia is subluxated caudally.

Similarly, tearing of the collateral ligaments is rarely seen in isolation and is generally seen in conjunction with acute traumatic CrCL rupture. The medial collateral is taut throughout the entire range of the stifle and is tested with the dog in lateral recumbency by applying valgus stress to the distal limb with one hand while the other stabilises the distal femur. A thumb can be placed over the ligament where it crosses the joint line and utilised to feel the ligament tightening as stress is placed. In cases of suspected grade I or II ligament sprain where ligament functional integrity is largely retained, the dog should be observed for a pain response as stress is applied. Conversely, the lateral collateral is only tight in extension, so is tested by varus stress at a standing angle.

Osteochondrosis dissecans of the lateral and occasionally medial femoral condyle is a well-recognised condition in dogs. Large breed, male dogs appear overrepresented and commonly present between 5 and 9 months of age. Lameness can be severe and physical examination findings include joint effusion, pain and crepitus on manipulation and muscle wasting.

Another common condition affecting the canine stifle is patella luxation (PL). Patella luxation can be medial (MPL) or lateral (LPL). Although LPL is seen mostly in large breed dogs, MPL is the most common form of PL across all breeds, constituting over 90% of all patella luxation cases in most studies. Although the aetiology of PL is unclear (Hayes *et al.* 1994), it appears that multiple anatomical anomalies are present that cause the patella to escape its normal position in the trochlea groove. Lameness ensues from a mechanical standpoint due to loss of the efficiency of the extensor mechanism and an inflammatory perspective as increased cartilage wear occurs on both the articular surface of the patella and the trochlea ridge.

A grading scheme for MPL is widely used, whereby grade 1 denotes a patella that can be manually luxated with the stifle at full extension but will spontaneously reduce; grade 2 represents patellae that will luxate on stifle flexion without manual force and will stay luxated until stifle extension or manual reduction; grade 3 signifies cases where the patella is luxated continuously but can be manually reduced; and in grade 4 cases the patella is permanently luxated and cannot be reduced.

Evaluation for MPL is best performed with the dog in lateral recumbency with the affected leg uppermost. The patella is initially palpated to detect if it is already luxated, and manual pressure is used to assess stability. The stifle is then positioned at a standing angle and one hand is placed over the distal femur with the thumb resting on the lateral aspect of the patella and the remaining fingers on the medial aspect of the distal femur. The other hand is placed over the metatarsus and used to simultaneously internally rotate the proximal tibia and flex the stifle while the thumb from the proximal hand provides medially directed pressure.

Differential diagnosis includes the following.
- Cranial cruciate ligament disease
- Medial patella luxation
- Lateral patella luxation
- Collateral ligament rupture
- Stifle luxation
- Long digital extensor avulsion/luxation
- Osteochondrosis dissecans
- Fracture
- Straight patellar ligament tendinitis/rupture
- Neoplasia
- Septic arthritis

8.4.5 Femur

The femur is a relatively straight bone with a typically large muscle bulk surrounding it. In situations of chronic ipsilateral limb lameness, muscle wasting will typically manifest as a noticeable crease in the lateral thigh between the lateral vastus of the quadriceps and the biceps femoris of the hamstring group. With chronic pelvic limb lameness, myofascial trigger points will commonly be detected in the hip flexor muscles, most notably the tensor fascia lata.

The distal femur is a well-recognised site for primary bone neoplasia, with the proximal femur less commonly implicated.

Differential diagnosis includes the following.
- Myofascial trigger points
- Neoplasia
- Panosteitis
- Fracture

8.4.6 Hip

The coxofemoral joint is a ball-and-socket joint formed by the head of the femur and the acetabulum of the pelvis. The cotyloid nature of the joint allows substantial range of motion in all planes, although the major direction is in flexion and extension. The hip is typically held in approximately 5° of extension in a weight-bearing position.

Stability of the hip joint is provided by a number of mechanisms. These include the primary stabilisers: the ligament of the head of the femur or round ligament which runs from the fovea capitis of the femoral head to the acetabular fossa, the joint capsule and the dorsal acetabular rim. Secondary stabilisers include the acetabular labrum that extends from the acetabular rim, the hydrostatic pressure provided by the adhesion/cohesion effect of minimal synovial fluid and the periarticular muscles of the gluteal complex that insert on or near the greater trochanter.

Anatomical landmarks for the hip include the greater trochanter at the most proximolateral aspect of the limb, the ischiatic tuberosity and the ilial wing of the pelvis (Figure 8.8). In a fully reduced hip, the greater trochanter should sit ventral to an imaginary line drawn from the ischiatic tuberosity to the ilial wing.

Given the deep location of the hip joint, effusion is typically impossible to detect. The hip should be manipulated through its full range of motion, including flexion/extension, abduction/adduction and internal/external rotation, assessing for restriction in range, crepitus and pain.

Hip dysplasia is a common inherited developmental condition seen in large to giant breed dogs, characterised by initial joint laxity that leads to joint subluxation and osteoarthritic change. Dogs will often exhibit a biphasic distribution for clinical signs with hip dysplasia. Initial lameness at 5–9 months of age is generally attributed to initial capsular stretching/tearing, round ligament degeneration, synovial fluid overproduction, subchondral bone microfracture and the resultant synovitis initiated by the aforementioned processes. Stability typically ensues with synovial fluid reduction, joint capsule hyperplasia and bone remodelling, but adult-onset lameness then tends to appear due to the consequences of osteoarthritis and cartilage loss. It is important to recognise that although hip dysplasia is a common condition, it is a disease of varying levels of severity and in many cases is subclinical. Dogs at risk for hip dysplasia are often overrepresented for other orthopaedic conditions such as osteochondrosis dissecans or panosteitis at an early age and cranial cruciate

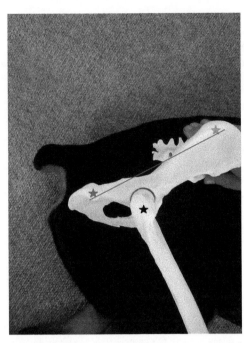

Figure 8.8 Surface anatomy of the pelvis. The blue star is over the ilial wing; red star denotes ischial spine; black star denotes greater trochanter. Hip joint should fall ventral to an imaginary line drawn between the iliac wing and ischial spine (in red).

ligament rupture or osteosarcoma later in life. Indeed, one study found that 32% of dogs referred to a veterinary teaching hospital with a presumptive diagnosis of hip dysplasia were instead suspected to have cranial cruciate ligament disease (Powers *et al.* 2005). In the authors' opinion, it is unusual for dogs to present after 1 year of age with severe lameness resulting from hip dysplasia, and that when compared to other joints, coxofemoral osteoarthritis appears to be a condition better tolerated by dogs.

Hip dysplasia is commonly a bilateral disease. Dogs may present with slightly abducted limbs in an attempt to increase acetabular coverage and a pelvic swaying gait used in an attempt to reduce hip flexion. A short-striding pelvic limb gait and weight shifting to the thoracic limbs may be noted and a 'bunny-hopping' gait is often reported, whereby both pelvic limbs are loading simultaneously to reduce individual loading. Pelvic limb muscle wasting may be noted and pain on coxofemoral extension is a consistent finding. However, pain on extension is not pathognomic for hip dysplasia and can be elicited with multiple other conditions, such as stifle, lumbosacral and muscular disease. Dogs affected by hip dysplasia should also demonstrate pain on hip abduction and rotation. As the dog ages and the condition progresses, the range of motion is typically markedly reduced and crepitus is appreciated.

Two manipulative tests are used to assess coxofemoral instability. The first is the Ortolani test, which can be performed on both limbs simultaneously with the dog in dorsal recumbency or on individual limbs with the dog in lateral recumbency. The authors consider the lateral position easiest in sedated or anaesthetised animals. Here the hip is positioned in neutral while one hand is placed distal to the flexed stifle and the other is placed over the rump to stabilise the animal. Axial pressure is then directed along the femur towards the dorsum of the dog via the hand grasping the stifle. In animals with hip laxity, this will induce coxofemoral subluxation, noted as a mild clunk. The limb is then abducted slowly and with maintenance of the axial force until a louder clunk is detected as the femoral head reduces into the acetabulum. The Bardens test or hip lift is also performed with the animal in lateral recumbency. With the femur in a neutral position, one hand is used to grasp the mid-femur while the other rests on the pelvis and greater trochanter. Direct lateral pressure is applied to the femur in an effort to lift the femoral head out of the acetabulum. Any movement greater than 5 mm is suggestive of hip laxity. The operator must bear in mind when performing the Bardens test that manual pressure on the medial thigh alone will often induce a pain response in a dog, while the subluxation produced by the hip lift is almost universally painful.

Young, small to toy breed dogs are known to develop a disease known as avascular necrosis of the femoral head, or Legg–Calvé–Perthes disease. This condition is characterised by a transient, non-inflammatory local ischaemia that leads to necrosis of the femoral head trabeculae. Such necrosis results in collapse of the femoral head, with revascularisation and remodelling resulting in a deformed, osteoarthritic joint. Dogs are typically between 4 and 11 months of age, with varying degrees of lameness.

Injury to the iliopsoas muscle-tendon unit is a relatively recently reported condition in the veterinary literature (Nielsen & Pluhar 2005). Dogs can be any age or breed but have a typical history of strenuous activity. Agility dogs appear overrepresented in the authors' opinion. Dogs with chronic iliopsoas strain have a long history of intermittent or progressive pelvic limb lameness that is improved with rest and worsened with exercise. Iliopsoas strain is presumptively an acute muscle tear, typically at the musculotendinous junction, that progresses to chronic fibrosis, mineralisation and atrophy.

A characteristic hitching pelvic limb gait may be displayed and pain is typically induced on hip extension and palpation of the lumbar hypaxial muscles. This pain response is significantly worsened with internal rotation of the hip and direct palpation of the musculotendinous region. To perform an iliopsoas stretch test, have the dog in a standing position with a second handler securing the head. Extend the hip fully and internally rotate the limb by placing torsional force with one hand on the lateral stifle. The other hand can be used to palpate the musculotendinous region, at the medial aspect of the hip approximately 10 mm cranial to the insertion of the muscle on the lesser trochanter.

Differential diagnosis includes the following.
- Hip dysplasia
- Iliopsoas strain
- Avascular necrosis of the femoral head
- Coxofemoral luxation

- Fracture
- Inflammatory joint disease?

References

Bennett, D. & May, C. 1991, Meniscal damage associated with cruciate disease in the dog. *J. Small Anim. Pract.* 32(3):111–117.

Berzon, J. 1979, Osteochondritis dissecans in the dog: diagnosis and therapy. *J. Am. Vet. Med. Assoc.* 175(8):796–799.

Bohning, R. Suter, P., Hohn, R., Marshall, J. 1970, Clinical and radiologic survey of canine panosteitis. *J. Am. Vet. Med. Assoc.* 156: 870–883.

Buote, N., Fusco, J., Radasch, R. 2009, Age, tibial plateau angle, sex, and weight as risk factors for contralateral rupture of the cranial cruciate ligament in Labradors. *Vet. Surg.* 38(4):481–489.

Cook, J. 2001, Forelimb lameness in the young patient. *Vet. Clin. North Am.* 31(1):55–83.

Done, S.H., Goody, P.C., Stickland, N.C., Evans, S.A. (eds) 2009, *Color Atlas of Veterinary Anatomy*, vol 3, The Dog and Cat, 2nd edn. Mosby, St Louis, MO.

Doverspike, M., Vasseur, P., Harb, M., Walls, C. 1993 Contralateral cranial cruciate ligament rupture: incidence in 114 dogs. *J. Am. Anim. Hosp. Assoc.* 29(2):167–170.

Evans, H.E., de Lahunta, A. (eds) 2012, *Miller's Anatomy of the Dog*, 4th edn. Saunders, Philadelphia, PA.

Grondalen, J. 1976, Metaphyseal osteopathy (hypertrophic osteodystrophy) in growing dogs: a clinical study. *J. Small Anim. Pract.* 17(11):721–735.

Hayes, A., Boudrieau, R., Hungerford, L. 1994 Frequency and distribution of medial and lateral patellar luxation in dogs: 124 cases (1982–1992). *J. Am. Vet. Med. Assoc.* 205(5):716–720.

Jaegger, G., Marcellin-Little, D., Levine, D. 2002, Reliability of goniometry in Labrador retrievers. *Am. J. Vet. Res.* 63(7):979–986.

Janutta, V., Hamann, H., Klein, S. *et al.* 2006, Genetic analysis of 3 different classification protocols for the evaluation of elbow dysplasia in German shepherd dogs. *J. Small Anim. Pract.* 47(2): 75–82.

Johnson, K. 2013, Lameness grading, worthwhile or futile? *Vet. Comp. Orthop. Traumatol.* 26(2):V.

Mason, D., Schulz, K., Fujita, Y. *et al.* 2005, In vitro mapping of normal canine humeroradial and humeroulnar joints. *Am. J. Vet. Res.* 66(1):132–135.

Morris, E., Lipowitz, J. 2001, Comparison of tibial plateau angles in dogs with and without cranial cruciate ligament injuries. *J. Am. Vet. Med. Assoc.* 218(3):363–366.

Nielsen, G., Pluhar, G. 2005, Diagnosis and treatment of hind limb muscle strain injuries in 22 dogs. *Vet. Comp. Orthop. Traumatol.* 18(4):247–253.

Parker, R., Brown, S.G., Wind, A.L. 1981, Pancarpal arthrodesis in the dog: a review of forty-five cases. *Vet. Surg.* 10:35–43.

Powers, M., Martinez, S., Lincoln, J. *et al.* 2005, Prevalence of cranial cruciate ligament rupture in a population of dogs with lameness previously attributed to hip dysplasia: 369 cases (1994–2003). *J. Am. Vet. Med. Assoc.* 227(7):1109–1111.

Schaller, O. (ed.) 2007, *Illustrated Veterinary Anatomical Nomenclature*, 2nd edn. Thieme Verlag, Stuttgart.

CHAPTER 9
Small animal neurological and muscular conditions

Philip A. Moses[1] and Rita Gonçalves[2]

[1] University of Queensland, Gatton, Australia
[2] University of Liverpool, Liverpool, UK

Summary

Neurological disease in animals is an area where physiotherapy is frequently required. However, many neurological diseases are acutely life threatening and an accurate veterinary diagnosis following thorough and appropriate investigation must be sought prior to any physiotherapy intervention. Physiotherapists should draw on their human training and work with veterinary surgeons to apply their knowledge most appropriately. This chapter outlines the principles of the veterinary diagnosis and neurological conditions that may be encountered by the animal physiotherapist.

9.1 Introduction

Animal neurology follows the same principles as human neurology, yet clearly there will be major differences in the neurological examination of animals and humans, particularly where verbalisation and comprehension are important in differentiating lesions in man. The aim of this chapter is to familiarise the reader with some differences in neuroanatomy between humans and animals, to describe the process of the neurological examination in small animals and to identify and explain some commonly encountered neurological and muscular conditions in small animals.

9.1.1 Definitions
- CNS – central nervous system; composed of the brain and spinal cord
- UMN – upper motor neuron: brain and spinal neurons that initiate and control movement
- LMN – lower motor neuron: neurons with cell bodies located in the ventral horn of the spinal cord and brainstem; fibres (axons) travel outside the CNS, connecting it to muscles and producing movement
- Plegia and paralysis – complete loss of motor function
- Paresis – partial loss of motor function; weakness
- Tetraparesis or plegia – paresis/plegia involving all four limbs
- Paraparesis or plegia – paresis/plegia involving both pelvic limbs

Animal Physiotherapy: Assessment, Treatment and Rehabilitation of Animals, Second Edition. Edited by Catherine M. McGowan and Lesley Goff.
© 2016 John Wiley & Sons, Ltd. Published 2016 by John Wiley & Sons, Ltd.

Table 9.1 Vertebrae in the dog and cat

Usual number of vertebrae	Dog and cat
Cervical (C)	7
Thoracic (T)	13
Lumbar (L)	7
Sacral (S)	3
Caudal (Ca)	Varies with tail length

- Hemiparesis or plegia – paresis/plegia involving thoracic and pelvic limbs on one side
- Monoparesis or plegia – paresis/plegia involving one limb

9.2 Neuroanatomy

9.2.1 The spinal cord

The spinal cord is contained within the vertebral canal; there is a larger epidural space in the cervical region compared to caudally. The spinal cord extends from the brainstem and terminates at L5–6 (dogs) and L6–7 (cats) but there is both intra- and interbreed variation (Tables 9.1 and 9.2).

Spinal cord segments generally correspond to their respective vertebral segments from C1 to L1 or L2; caudal to this, spinal cord segments become shorter relative to the vertebral bodies.

The cord widens in two regions called the intumescences, a cervical (C6–T2) and a lumbar (L4–S3). The lower motor neurons (LMN) of the thoracic and pelvic limbs arise from these segments respectively. LMNs are the efferent neurons for muscle contraction and are part of the simple reflex pathway. LMN reflex pathways are controlled for voluntary movement by higher motor centres – the upper motor neurons (UMN). UMN pathways tend to have a calming effect on reflexes, but their major role is in directing the various LMNs in voluntary movement. Major descending UMN pathways include the rubrospinal, reticulospinal and vestibulospinal tracts. As well as descending influences from the higher CNS centres (cerebral cortex, brainstem and cerebellum), ascending pathways carry sensory information. These pathways include (from most superficial to deepest within the spinal cord) conscious proprioceptive, unconscious proprioceptive and nociceptive/pain pathways (de Lahunta 2009).

Table 9.2 The relationship between spinal cord segments and vertebral bodies in small animals

Vertebral segment	Spinal cord segments contained
L2	L2–3
L3	L3–4
L4	L4, 5, 6 (7)
L5	L7, S1, 2, 3

Descending UMN pathways can be divided into pyramidal and extrapyramidal systems. The pyramidal system is mostly involved in controlling finely adjusted movements, and the extrapyramidal, coarser movements, particularly in stereotypic locomotor patterns. The pyramidal system is of great importance in man, but significantly less so in domestic animals. In dogs, pyramidal fibres reach all levels of the cord, though fibre numbers decrease by 50% at the cervical cord. This explains the decreased importance of corticospinal motor pathways in animals and why large lesions destroying the cerebrocortical motor centres do not cause permanent abnormality in gait, except for deficits in postural reaction testing in the contralateral limbs (de Lahunta 2009).

The blood supply to the spinal cord is from the paired spinal arteries. These give rise to the dorsal and ventral radicular arteries. The arterial supply in the dog and cat is more consistent with that present in man, with each spinal segment well supplied. There appears to be good capacity for collateral supply as well. Venous drainage is from small spinal veins, which drain into the large internal vertebral venous plexus that lies on the floor of the vertebral canal.

9.2.2 Vertebral anatomy of small animals

The cervical vertebrae numbered C1–7 contain spinal cord segments C1–8. The first vertebral body is the atlas, C1, a ring-shaped structure with prominent lateral wings. The axis, C2, has two smaller, caudally projecting transverse processes and a large dorsal spinous process. A strong dorsal atlantoaxial ligament joins C1–2 while ventrally, the prominent dens on C2 articulates with C1 and has strong ligamentous attachments. There is no intervertebral disc between C1 and C2. Vertebrae C3–7 have similar morphology with a block-shaped vertebral body beneath an arched neural canal. There is a dorsal spinous process as well as transverse processes extending ventrolaterally.

The thoracic vertebrae are basically similar in structure to the caudal cervical vertebrae. The ribs arise from the costal fovea of the transverse processes laterally. There is a strong intercapital ligament between left and right rib heads from T1 to T9 and for this reason, intervertebral disc disease is uncommon in this area. There are large dorsal spinous processes that tilt caudally on T1–10. T11 is termed the anticlinal vertebra, as the dorsal process is more vertical. T12 and T13 have dorsal processes that tilt cranially.

The lumbar vertebrae have larger, block-shaped vertebral bodies; the transverse processes are small and extend caudally. These transverse processes become larger more caudally and the dorsal processes become smaller more caudally.

The three sacral vertebrae are fused and articulate with the two ilial bodies via a C-shaped cartilaginous auricular surface. The dorsal spinous processes are small and the dorsal lamina is thin. There is an average of 20 caudal vertebrae although the number may vary from six to 23. Cats have less variation.

9.2.3 The intervertebral discs and intervertebral disc disease (IVDD) in small animals

Intervertebral discs separate all vertebral bodies with the exception of C1–2. The discs provide flexibility between vertebrae and act to absorb shock along the spinal column. The discs have an external annulus fibrosus composed of collagen fibres arranged in lamellae. Collagen comprises 70–80% of the annulus. There are also elastic fibres arranged circularly, longitudinally and obliquely. The lamellae are separate to allow gliding movement during loading. The lamellae can form complete or incomplete rings. There may be some sensory (pain) fibres in the outer lamellae of the intervertebral disc. The annulus fibrosus may be weaker dorsolaterally as the lamellae are often incomplete in this region. This eccentric loading of the annulus fibrosus explains the propensity for the intervertebral disc to extrude dorsally. Only the outer layers of the annulus have blood vessels, with the rest of the intervertebral disc receiving nutrition by diffusion (Bergknut *et al.* 2013).

The nucleus pulposus forms the inner portion of the intervertebral disc. It is an embryonic remnant of the notochord and is located slightly eccentrically. The nucleus pulposus is composed of an unorganised matrix of collagen and proteoglycans and is bound in 80–88% water. The nucleus pulposus is avascular and aneural. With age, it desiccates and undergoes degeneration. These changes occur very early in the chondrodystrophic breeds and may be complete by 2 years of age.

There are two distinct types of disc degeneration described by Hansen in his seminal work in 1952, known as 'Hansen type I' and 'Hansen type II'. In Hansen type I disc disease, more commonly seen in the chondrodysplastic breeds, the intervertebral disc undergoes chondroid metaplasia. Type I disc disease usually leads to extrusion of the nucleus pulposus through the annular fibres into the vertebral canal and results in acute clinical signs. It is characterised by increased collagen content, an alteration in the glycosaminoglycan concentration, a loss of water and an alteration of the proteoglycan content of the intervertebral disc. The disc becomes more cartilaginous and the nucleus more granular. There is a lack of gross distinction between the nucleus pulposus and the annulus fibrosus. The nucleus pulposus may undergo dystrophic calcification, resulting in a loss of shock-absorbing qualities. Calcified intervertebral discs have been observed in Dachshund puppies as young as 5 months of age. Type I disc disease may affect multiple discs within the vertebral column.

In Hansen type II disc disease, more commonly seen in mature non-chondrodysplastic dogs, the disc undergoes fibroid metaplasia. Type II disc disease typically results in bulging or protrusion of the annulus fibrosus and is slow and insidious in onset. Water and proteoglycans are lost from the intervertebral disc, resulting in its narrowing. The nucleus pulposus is particularly affected and becomes indistinguishable from the inner lamellae of the annulus fibrosus. There is a reduction of glycosaminoglycans in the nucleus and annulus. The nucleus pulposus becomes fibroid in nature but rarely mineralises.

Ventral herniations have also been reported and are thought to be associated with the formation of osteophytes and spondylosis deformans.

IVDD is rare in the cat but both disc extrusions and protrusions have been reported.

Note: There may be a blurring between Hansen type I and II disc disease and both processes may often occur simultaneously.

9.2.4 The brain

The major intracranial structures include the:
- forebrain (including the cerebral cortex and the diencephalon)
- brainstem (including the midbrain, pons and medulla oblongata)
- cerebellum.

The forebrain is the most rostral region of the brain and is the area that consciously perceives all information collected throughout the body (such as vision, hearing, proprioception, pain, etc.). It is important for behaviour and decision making.

The brainstem links the forebrain to the spinal cord and 10 of the 12 pairs of cranial nerves have their nuclei in here. The largest portion of the centres for consciousness (the ascending reticular activating system – ARAS) is located here along with important regulatory centres for the cardiovascular and respiratory systems. Part of the vestibular system (the vestibular nuclei) is also located here.

The cerebellum is in charge of controlling the rate, range and force of movement. It cannot initiate movement, but rather it smoothes the movement which is induced by the UMN system. The cerebellum also has a role in maintaining balance by inhibiting the vestibular nuclei in the brainstem.

The vestibular system, in charge of maintaining balance and orientation against gravity, is scattered throughout different regions. The sensory receptors are located in the inner ear and the information collected by these is transmitted to the brain through the vestibulocochlear nerve (CN VIII); this is the peripheral part of the vestibular system. The central part of the vestibular system (inside the brain) is located partly in the brainstem and in the cerebellum. A lesion in any of the above-mentioned structures can result in vestibular deficits.

9.3 Neurological examination

While the neurological diagnosis is clearly the realm of the veterinary surgeon, an animal physiotherapist should be able to perform a neurological examination, including localisation and grading of the findings as part of the assessment process. Recording and monitoring of these findings will allow an objective assessment of the patient's response to treatment. Physiotherapists may be involved in treating and rehabilitating postsurgical neurological cases or may be the clinicians in charge of long-term follow-up of many chronic neurological problems. *Many neurological cases require the team effort of both the veterinary surgeon and physiotherapist.*

9.3.1 Preliminary examination and history

Initial collection of data, as for any other area, is important and should include:

- patient signalment – age, sex, breed and use
- a veterinary physical examination
- clinical history (of this and other problems).

A thorough veterinary physical examination will help differentiate neurological from metabolic, cardiovascular and musculoskeletal disorders.

Signalment is important to develop differential diagnoses, as there are breed and age predispositions. More useful still to help narrow down the differential diagnoses list is to characterise disorders as:

- acute or chronic onset
- progressive, static or improving
- painful or not painful
- persistent or intermittent.

9.3.2 From a distance

The aim of the neurological examination is to establish the presence of neurological disease and determine the neuroanatomical location. A consistent, complete and methodical approach is essential.

A neurological examination form can be helpful to ensure the examination is carried out in a thorough and methodical manner. Repeated/serial neurological examinations should be performed to assess for any changes or progression of the signs.

The first step of the neurological examination is based on observation, as there is a lot of important information that can only be gathered this way. There are four parameters that should be assessed.

- Mentation
- Behaviour
- Posture
- Gait

Mentation

When abnormal, mentation can be a sign of forebrain or brainstem dysfunction (where the ARAS is located). Mentation can be classified in different states:

- alert – normal response to environmental stimuli
- disorientated/confused – abnormal response to environment
- depressed/obtunded – inattentive, less responsive to environment
- stuporous – unconscious but can be roused by painful stimuli
- comatose – unconscious and unresponsive to any (including painful) stimuli.

Behaviour

Behaviour abnormalities are always a sign of forebrain dysfunction, as this part of the brain modulates the animal's 'personality'. Common abnormalities that can be identified include aggression, compulsive walking or circling, loss of learnt behaviour (such as toilet training) and excessive vocalisation.

Posture

There are several abnormal postures that can be easily identified when the animal is at rest. Common abnormalities found include a head tilt (rotation of the median plane of the head, with one ear lower than the other) or a head turn (nose is turned to the side with the head still perpendicular to the ground) amongst others (Figure 9.1). Searching for postural abnormalities can be very useful as they provide important information for lesion localisation; for example, the head tilt is a sign of vestibular dysfunction whilst the head turn is a sign of forebrain disease. Once

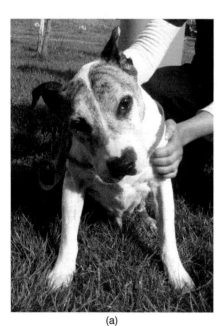

(a)

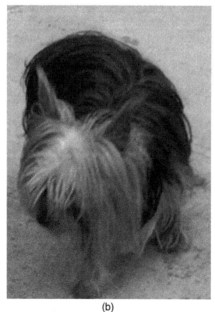

(b)

Figure 9.1 (a) A 5-year-old crossbreed presented with a right-sided head tilt due to idiopathic vestibular disease. (b) A 3-year-old Yorkshire terrier presented with a right-sided head turn due to meningoencephalitis of unknown origin.

the clinician has this information, they already have a strong suspicion of where the lesion should be so they can use the hands as part of the neurological examination to confirm this and hopefully narrow it down even further.

A posture that is often seen with spinal cord lesions is the Schiff-Sherrington posture. This phenomenon is usually an indication of severe thoracic or cranial lumbar spinal cord injury. It is caused by loss of ascending inhibition from pelvic limbs resulting in thoracic limb and neck hypertonicity. In these cases, the thoracic limbs maintain voluntary movement and normal postural reactions but there is paralysis of the pelvic limbs.

Gait

Especially pertinent to the physiotherapist is gait assessment. The gait may be affected secondary to lesions in several areas of the CNS and abnormalities are usually classified as follows.

- Ataxia – uncoordinated gait. Can be seen with cerebellar lesions (cerebellum coordinates movement); vestibular disease (loss of balance); spinal disease (due to decreased sensory information arriving from the limbs to tell the CNS where they are in space at any given time).
- Paresis – weakness, reduced voluntary movement. Should be further specified as ambulatory if the dog can still walk unaided or non-ambulatory if voluntary movement is still present but the patient requires support to move (such as from a sling).
- Paralysis or plegia – complete loss of voluntary movement.

Paresis and plegia are in most cases secondary to spinal cord disease, when there is interference with the motor tracts that arise in the brain and travel down the spinal cord to eventually synapse in LMNs to the limbs. Mild paresis can also be seen with lesions in the brainstem (where most of the motor tracts start) but in those cases, several other signs suggestive of brainstem disease (such as cranial nerve deficits and abnormal mentation) should also be obvious.

It is essential that physiotherapists are comfortable evaluating the gait of dogs and cats in order to be able to assess for signs of improvement or deterioration during treatment.

9.3.3 Hands-on examination

Following the observation phase, a hands-on neurological examination should be undertaken. This is usually divided into four stages.

- Postural reaction testing
- Spinal reflexes
- Evaluating for spinal pain
- Cranial nerve assessment

Postural reaction testing

This part of the neurological examination is aimed at testing awareness of the precise position and movement of the body (especially limbs). There are proprioceptors located in muscles, tendons and joints and they transmit information to the cerebral cortex, where it is consciously perceived. There are also

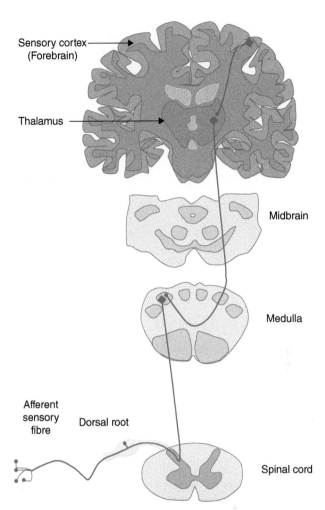

Figure 9.2 General proprioception pathway to the cerebral cortex.

special receptors in the inner ear that collect information regarding movement of the head; this is called special proprioception.

When testing proprioception, the pathway involved in the responses is very complex and includes a large part of the nervous system. For example, when testing paw position, the information of the position of the foot is received by the proprioceptors in that limb and transmitted to the sensory peripheral nerve, ascends through the sensory tracts in the spinal cord and eventually is acknowledged by the contralateral cerebral cortex, after passing through the brainstem (Figure 9.2). For the foot to be corrected, the cortex 'makes that decision' and then transmits it down to the foot by the descending motor tracts in the spinal cord and peripheral motor nerve and eventually this action is undertaken by the skeletal muscle. So this test is very sensitive to pick up lesions in the nervous system but poorly specific to localise them as it tests so many areas.

The information postural reaction testing provides is invaluable but in order to interpret it, one needs to add information from the rest of the neurological examination. Neurolocalisation should be seen as a mathematical exercise; once all the information gathered is recorded, it should be added up so that

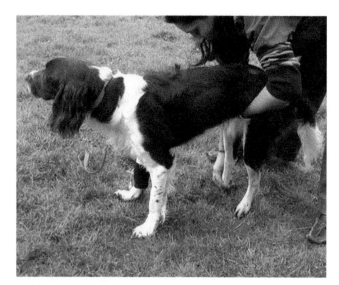

Figure 9.3 Proprioceptive positioning being tested in the right pelvic limb.

it can only be explained by a lesion in one region of the nervous system.

There are many tests that can be used to test proprioception but the most reliable are the paw position, hopping and placing. Other tests that can be used but that are more complex and therefore harder to interpret are wheelbarrowing, hemiwalking, hip sway and extensor postural thrust.

Proprioceptive positioning (paw position)
If the dorsum of the paw is placed on the floor, the paw should be immediately returned to a normal position (Figure 9.3). It is important to support the weight of the patient whilst performing this test. Delayed or absent responses indicate neurological disease.

Hopping
The animal is supported under the abdomen and allowed to bear weight on one leg and is then moved laterally (Figure 9.4). Poor initiation of movement suggests a postural reaction deficit.

Placing reactions
The animal is supported under the thorax and is then moved towards a table until the tested limb touches the edge of the table. A normal response is to immediately place the feet on the table for positional support. This test is only appropriate for small breed dogs and cats.

Spinal reflexes
The spinal reflexes test the integrity of sensory and motor components of the reflex arc and the influence of the descending motor pathways on this arc. They are essential to localise lesions within the spinal cord and the peripheral nervous system.

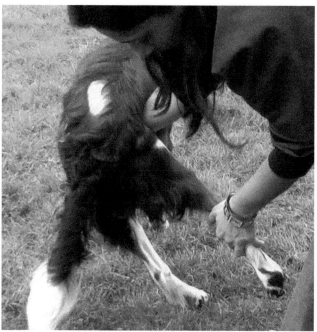

Figure 9.4 Hopping response being tested on the left pelvic limb.

There are three possible responses.
- Absent or depressed reflex due to complete or partial loss of either sensory or motor component of the reflex arc; this is described as a LMN response
- Normal reflex
- Exaggerated reflex due to an abnormality in the descending pathway from brain to spinal cord; this is described as a UMN response

Thoracic limb reflexes
Thoracic limb withdrawal reflex
The animal is placed in lateral recumbency and mild noxious stimuli inflicted on the foot. A normal response is flexion of the entire limb. Thoracic limb withdrawal reflex primarily involves the spinal cord segment C6–T2. Absent or depressed responses indicate a lesion of either this spinal cord segment or the peripheral nerves in this region. This reflex is the most reliable in the thoracic limb with the following three sometimes not being able to be elicited in normal animals.

Extensor carpi radialis reflex
The animal is placed in lateral recumbency with the elbow supported and flexed and carpus flexed. The proximal belly of the extensor carpi radialis muscle is tapped with the tendon hammer. A normal response is mild extension of the carpus. The extensor carpi radialis reflex is innervated by the radial nerve and the spinal cord segment C7–T2.

Triceps reflex
The animal is placed in lateral recumbency with the uppermost leg supported under the elbow. The triceps tendon is struck

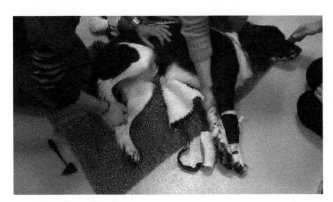

Figure 9.5 Withdrawal reflex being tested in the right pelvic limb.

with a reflex hammer just proximal to the olecranon. A normal response is slight extension of the elbow. The triceps reflex is innervated by the radial nerve and the spinal cord segment C7–T1.

Biceps reflex

The animal is placed in lateral recumbency with the elbow slightly extended. A reflex hammer is struck on a finger placed over biceps tendon just proximal to the elbow. A normal response is slight flexion of the elbow. The biceps reflex is innervated by the musculocutaneous nerve and the spinal cord segment C6–8.

Pelvic limb reflexes

Pelvic withdrawal reflex

The animal is placed in lateral recumbency and mild noxious stimuli inflicted on the foot. A normal response is flexion of the entire limb (Figure 9.5). Pelvic limb withdrawal reflex primarily involves the spinal cord segment L6–S2. Absent or depressed responses indicate a lesion of either this spinal cord segment or peripheral nerves in this region (such as the sciatic nerve).

Patellar reflex

The animal is placed in lateral recumbency with the affected leg uppermost and supported underneath the limb. The patella tendon is struck with a reflex hammer (Figure 9.6). A normal

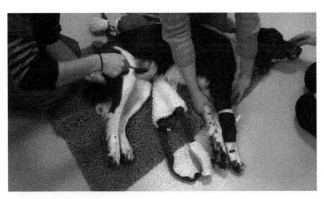

Figure 9.6 Patellar reflex being tested in the right pelvic limb.

response is a single, quick extension of the stifle. The patellar reflex is innervated by the femoral nerve and the spinal cord segment L4–6. Absent or depressed responses indicate a lesion of either this spinal cord segment or femoral nerve.

Gastrocnemius reflex

The animal is placed in lateral recumbency and the tendon of insertion of the gastrocnemius is struck dorsal to the hock. A normal response is extension of the hock. The gastrocnemius reflex is innervated by the tibial nerve and L7–S1 spinal cord segment.

Crossed extensor reflex

This reflex can observed during withdrawal reflexes of either the pelvic or thoracic limbs. Toe pinching of one limb results in flexion of that limb and extension of the contralateral limb. A crossed extensor reflex is caused by a lesion affecting descending inhibitory pathways UMN and therefore suggests a lesion cranial to the limb being tested; it only develops in animals with chronic lesions.

Perineal reflex

Gentle stimulation is applied to the perineal area with the tip of forceps. A normal response is contraction of the anal sphincter. The sensory and motor innervation is via the pudendal nerve and spinal cord segment S1–Cd5. An absent or depressed response indicates a lesion in the sacral spinal cord or pudendal nerve.

Cutaneous trunci reflex (sometimes called panniculus reflex)

A pinprick stimulus (with fingers or forceps) is applied to the skin at the level of L5 and subsequently moved cranially. A normal response is bilateral contraction of the cutaneous trunci muscle, which causes twitching of the skin in the back. An absent cutaneous trunci reflex suggests a lesion slightly cranial to the point of stimulation so this test is most useful to narrow down thoracolumbar spinal cord lesions. This reflex is affected mainly in patients with severe or chronic lesions.

Urinary bladder innervation

The bladder is innervated by both autonomic (hypogastric and pelvic) and somatic (pudendal) nerves and associated spinal cord segments (L1–4 and S1–3). The pudendal nerve innervates the striated muscle (external sphincter) and the hypogastric nerve innervates the smooth muscle (internal sphincter) of the urethra. The hypogastric and pelvic nerves coordinate bladder filling and emptying by controlling detrusor muscle (bladder wall) function. A lesion above L7 will generally cause spasm of bladder outflow and difficulty in expression of the bladder. A lesion at the level of the sacral segment will cause lack of sphincter tone and an easily expressible bladder.

Table 9.3 Cranial nerve functions, available tests to evaluate each nerve and resulting deficits in case of dysfunction

Cranial nerve	Function	Evaluation	Dysfunction
I Olfactory	Olfaction	Difficult, subjective	Reduced or absent smell
II Optic	Vision	Menace response PLR	Partial or complete blindness
III Oculomotor	Pupil size, eyelid movement	PLR Physiological nystagmus Eye position at rest	Ventrolateral strabismus, inability to move eye, dilated unresponsive pupil, ptosis upper lid
IV Trochlear	Contralateral dorsal oblique m.	Physiological nystagmus	Dorsolateral strabismus (on fundic examination)
V Trigeminal	Sensory innervation of face and motor to MM	Size and symmetry of MM, sensory function (corneal, palpebral, nasal)	MM atrophy and jaw weakness; facial hypo/anaesthesia; neurotrophic keratitis
VI Abducens	Ipsilateral lateral rectus and retractor bulbi m.	Physiological nystagmus Corneal reflex	Medial strabismus, inability to move eye laterally and retract eyeball
VII Facial	Motor innervation of facial muscles, taste for rostral tongue	Palpebral reflex Corneal reflex	Drooping, inability to move ear and lip, absent blink, KCC
VIII Vestibulocochlear	Hearing, vestibular function	BAER Lifting head	Deafness, vestibular disease
IX Glossopharyngeal	Motor innervation of pharynx and palate, sensory to caudal tongue and pharynx	Gag	Dysphagia, absent gag
X Vagus	Motor innervation of larynx, pharynx and oesophagus; parasympathetic innervation of all thoracic and abdominal viscera	Gag	Dysphagia, inspiratory dyspnoea, dysphonia, regurgitation, absent gag
XI Accessory	Motor innervation of trapezius and part of sternocephalicus m.		Trapezius atrophy
XII Hypoglossus	Motor innervation of tongue		Tongue atrophy, prehension problems

BAER, brainstem auditory evoked responses; KCC, keratoconjunctivitis sicca; m., muscle; MM, masticatory muscles; PLR, pupillary light reflex.

Pain perception

Pain perception provides crucial prognostic information and although it is not a spinal reflex, it is usually tested whilst evaluating the reflexes as the animal is in the appropriate position for this. In most cases, it is only worth performing this test in patients that have lost the ability to move as most dogs that have motor function will still retain pain perception. The only exceptions are patients with sensory neuropathies or certain cases with very central lesions in the spinal cord (such as ischaemic myelopathies) that may primarily affect the pain pathways whilst sparing some of the motor tracts which run more peripherally in the cord.

A painful stimulus is applied to each foot and the tail; progressively stronger painful stimuli may be applied in an attempt to elicit a response if necessary. Perception of pain is indicated by a significant behavioural response (i.e. turns and looks, vocalises or attempts to bite). Demonstrating the presence of pain perception may be affected by temperament, drugs, pain threshold and experience. The absence of pain perception is a poor prognostic sign.

Evaluating for spinal pain

Pressure is applied to the spinous processes and paraspinal muscles of the thoracic and lumbar region and transverse processes and paraspinal muscles of the cervical region; the neck should also be moved in all directions to look for signs of resistance or pain. Increased sensitivity may occur at the level of spinal cord disease.

Cranial nerve examination

There are 12 pairs of cranial nerves and each has different functions. Cranial nerves can be sensory, motor or both and some have autonomic functions such as lacrimation and salivation. The main functions of each nerve are summarised in Table 9.3, along with the resulting deficits in case of a lesion affecting a specific nerve.

Understading the functions of each nerve has guided development of different tests that can be used to assess different combinations of nerves (Table 9.4). Finding cranial nerve deficits should point to brainstem or peripheral nerve disease (generalised or affecting a single nerve only).

A common abnormality seen in cases with cervical or brachial plexus pathology is Horner's syndrome secondary to lesions affecting the sympathetic supply to the eye (Figure 9.7). The sympathetic pathway to the eye is long and complex, starting in the midbrain, passing through the cervical spinal cord, T1–3 nerves, vagosympathetic trunk in the neck, tympanic bulla and finally reaching the eye; a lesion anywhere in this pathway can result in Horner's syndrome.

Table 9.4 Tests used in the assessment of cranial nerves

Tests	Afferent	Intermediate	Efferent	Effect
Palpebral reflex	V	Brainstem	VII	Blink after touching medial or lateral canthus of eye
Corneal reflex	V	Brainstem	VII and VI	Blink and globe retraction after touching cornea
Physiological nystagmus	VIII	Brainstem	III, IV and VI	Nystagmus evoked by moving head
Menace response	II	Forebrain Cerebellum Brainstem	VII	Blink after menacing gesture
Pupillary light response	II	Brainstem	III	Pupillary constriction after shining light in the eye
Gag reflex	IX and X	Brainstem	IX and X	Pharyngeal contraction after touch

9.4 Gait, proprioception and reflexes – spinal lesions

The first step when localising spinal lesions is gait observation. This allows the examiner to grade the severity of the lesion and to determine which limbs appear affected. Postural reaction testing then confirms which limbs are abnormal as these should display delayed reactions. With this information, the clinician can narrow down a lesion to cranial or caudal to T3 (remember the cervical intumescence which contains the LMNs to the thoracic limbs ends at T2). So, if all four limbs are affected, the lesion must be cranial to T3 as a problem caudal to this would spare the thoracic limbs. If only the pelvic limbs are affected, then the lesion must be caudal to the areas of the spinal cord that possess tracts or LMNs to the thoracic limbs; it therefore must be caudal to the cervical intumescence. The spinal reflexes then allow us to classify the condition as UMN or LMN and therefore narrow down the localisation further (Table 9.5). It is important to take into account that in patients with polyneuropathies, all limbs will be affected too; these patients can present tetraparetic but the spinal reflexes allow differentiation from a cervical lesion.

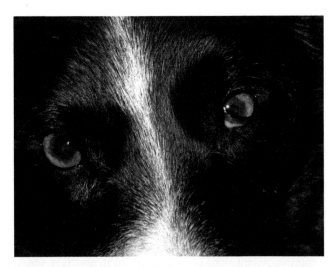

Figure 9.7 Horner's syndrome in the left eye. This syndrome describes the following ophthalmic changes: miosis (constricted pupil), enophthalmos (sinking of the eyeball), protrusion of the third eyelid and ptosis (drooping) of the upper eyelid.

Spinal cord injury in most cases results in loss of function in the following order.
1 Conscious proprioception
2 Voluntary motor function
3 Pain perception

Return of function following spinal cord injury happens in the reverse order. The timeframe in which recovery occurs also depends on the duration of the clinical signs. For example, a Dachshund with a disc extrusion that loses motor function in a few hours should walk quicker after surgery than a German Shepherd with a 6-month history of weakness due to a chronic disc protrusion before becoming non-ambulatory.

Aetiology of spinal cord lesions may be assessed on the basis of history and presence or not of pain.
- Acute and static/improving
  - Vascular (e.g. fibrocartilaginous embolism or infarction)
  - Trauma (e.g. acute non-compressive nucleus pulposus extrusion)
  - Degenerative (e.g. type I IVDD)
- Acute and progressive
  - Degenerative (e.g. type I IVDD)
  - Inflammatory (e.g. discospondylitis or meningomyelitis)
  - Trauma (e.g. fracture–luxation)
  - Anomalous (e.g. atlantoaxial subluxation)
- Chronic and progressive
  - Degenerative (e.g. type I and II IVDD, lumbosacral degenerative stenosis, cervical spondylomyelopathy or degenerative myelopathy)
  - Inflammatory (e.g. discospondylitis and meningomyelitis)
  - Neoplasia (e.g. intra- or extradural spinal tumours)

Table 9.5 Spinal cord lesions may be localised according to the neurological status of the limbs

Lesion	Thoracic limbs	Pelvic limbs
C1–5	UMN or normal	UMN or normal
C6–T2	LMN	UMN or normal
T3–L3	Normal	UMN or normal
L4–S3	Normal	LMN
Polyneuropathies	LMN	LMN

LMN, lower motor neuron (absent or reduced reflex); UMN, upper motor neuron (exaggerated reflex).

9.5 Diagnostic techniques

9.5.1 Survey radiographs

General anaesthesia is essential for accurate positioning of small animals. Although the spinal cord cannot be seen on plain films, they are essential to assess vertebral body shape for abnormalities. Assessment of vertebral alignment is important, particularly post trauma. Alignment should always be assessed in two planes. Spinal deviation may also occur with developmental anomalies such as hemivertebrae but as plain radiography is incapable of assessing spinal cord compression, its significance will remain questionable.

There are some characteristic radiographic changes associated with IVDD, although these are just suggestive of this condition and further imaging is required for diagnosis. Collapse of the intervertebral disc space and narrowing of the articular process joint space and foramen may be seen. Mineralised IVDs, while not diagnostic alone, are characteristic of type I IVDD. Occasionally, extruded disc material may be seen in the spinal canal.

Vertebral shape should be assessed for anomalies, fracture or pathology so knowledge of normal anatomy and variations is important. Vertebral osteomyelitis or discospondylitis causes bone lysis and sclerosis of vertebral bodies and endplates respectively.

9.5.2 Myelography

Myelography can be used for assessment of spinal cord compression but with the widespread availability of advanced imaging such as CT and MRI, it is nowadays less used although still more commonly than in human medicine. Myelography can differentiate between extradural and intradural-extramedullary lesions although it cannot visualise the spinal cord itself or soft tissues around it. It can be useful for cases with IVDD, certain neoplasias, vertebral body abnormalities, traumatic injuries and many other conditions.

9.5.3 Computed tomography and magnetic resonance imaging

These diagnostic modalities have become increasingly available within veterinary medicine over the previous decade. CT offers better contrast resolution than radiography and is superior at identifying the cause of extradural compression, vertebral body neoplasia, presence of spinal cord swelling and subtle abnormalities in vertebral shape and structure.

Magnetic resonance imaging nonetheless is the imaging modality of choice. It allows direct assessment of neural tissue parenchyma, which none of the other modalities can achieve. There are several MRI sequences that can be used (T2WI are often the most useful) and combining the information acquired by each one can provide important information on the nature of different lesions. It also allows acquisition of images in all three planes (dorsal, sagittal and transverse) which is essential to allow better lesion localisation and demarcation (Figure 9.8).

9.5.4 Cerebrospinal fluid analysis

Cerebrospinal fluid (CSF) analysis is recommended in order to gather further information about intracranial and spinal lesions. It rarely allows for a definitive diagnosis but alongside advanced imaging, it provides useful information about the most likely cause for the lesion identified. Several parameters are usually analysed, including the total nucleated cell count, red blood cell count and protein concentration. CSF analysis is most useful in cases with inflammatory disease as these tend to present with high total nucleated cell counts; note that the severity of the disease does not correlate with the severity of the CSF findings.

9.6 Neurological disease in small animals

9.6.1 Intracranial disease

There are multiple conditions that will result in intracranial disease. Most can affect any of the different regions of the brain; for example, tumours or strokes can cause signs of forebrain, brainstem or cerebellar disease depending on where the lesion is located in that specific case. Other conditions typically only affect one area of the brain; for example, metabolic conditions such as hypoglycaemia or hepatic encephalopathy classically cause signs of forebrain dysfunction as this is the part of the brain that is most likely to suffer from metabolite deficiency or toxicity.

Forebrain disease is a major red flag for physiotherapists and any case that develops or shows signs of forebrain disease that has not been diagnosed and treated by a veterinary surgeon should be immediately referred back.

Brainstem disease can affect the gait, causing paresis, so it is important that physiotherapists are aware of how to localise lesions to this area as different investigations and treatment are indicated (Table 9.6). These cases are often considered emergencies as the brainstem contains important cardiovascular and respiratory centres and pathology in this region can be life threatening.

Vestibular dysfunction, independent of the underlying cause, has been shown to improve significantly quicker in humans with the use of specific physiotherapy exercises. Typical signs of vestibular dysfunction include a head tilt, nystagmus and ataxia with falling and rolling to one side. A modified testing and repositioning postural manoeuvre has been proposed for use in dogs following acute vestibular signs but its value has not yet been proven (Kraeling 2014).

Examples of common intracranial disease include the following.
- Cerebrovascular accidents (strokes) – can happen anywhere in the brain but more common in the cerebellum. In general, animals present signs of peracute brain dysfunction which improves with time.
- Inflammatory disease – can be infectious (e.g. *Neospora caninum* or distemper virus) but most commonly is immune

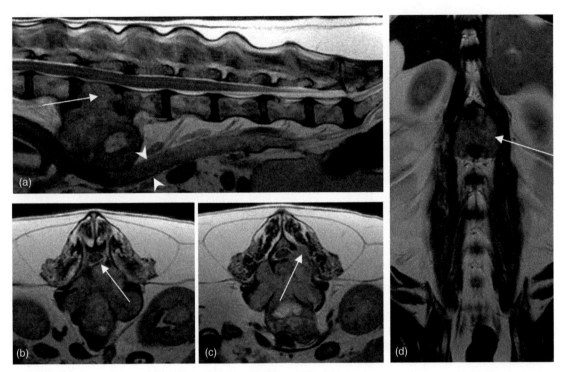

Figure 9.8 MR images of a dog with a vertebral body tumour. (a) Sagittal T2WI showing the large mass arising from the vertebral body of L2, causing marked ventral displacement of the aorta (*arrowheads*). (b, c) Transverse T2WI through the region of the mass allowing identification of invasion of the vertebral canal and spinal cord compression (b) as well as extension of the mass to the dorsal lamina of L2 (c). (d) Dorsal T2WI; this view is most important for localisation of the lesion and assessment of nerve roots.

mediated. Meningoencephalitis of unknown origin (MUO) is a common immune-mediated condition that affects young to middle-aged small breed dogs. Typically, dogs present with acute and often multifocal signs of brain disease that progress over hours to days. MUOs are life-threatening so treatment should be started as soon as possible.

- Brain malformations (such as hydrocephalus) with clinical signs starting at a young age.
- Brain tumours – typically cause signs of focal, lateralised brain dysfunction that progresses over weeks to months. As dogs and cats live longer, brain tumours are diagnosed with increased frequency.

- Idiopathic conditions – there are many conditions of unknown underlying cause that result in temporary neurological deficits in dogs and cats. A typical example is idiopathic vestibular disease, which is very common in dogs. In affected cases, severe vestibular signs such as falling and rolling, marked ataxia and a head tilt appear acutely and most owners believe their dogs have suffered a stroke. The cause for this condition is unknown but there are signs of inflammation of the vestibulocochlear nerve on MRI. Affected dogs improve over a few days with the signs resolving in most cases after 3–4 weeks.

Table 9.6 Localisation of intracranial lesions

	Forebrain	Brainstem	Cerebellum
Mentation	Disorientation, depression	Depression, stupor, coma	Normal
Cranial nerve deficits	Contralateral blindness (with normal pupillary light response)	Several cranial nerve deficits (III–XII) vestibular signs	Ipsilateral menace response deficit with normal vision, vestibular signs
Gait	Normal gait	Paresis of all or ipsilateral limbs	Ataxia, hypermetria, intention tremors
Posture	Head turn, head pressing	Possibly decerebrate rigidity	Possibly decerebellate rigidity
Postural responses	Decreased in contralateral limbs	Decreased in all limbs or ipsilateral limbs	Delayed and often hypermetric in ipsilateral limbs
Spinal reflexes and muscle tone	Normal to increased	Normal to increased	Normal
Other findings	Seizures, behavioural changes, circling, pacing	Respiratory or cardiac abnormalities	Rarely increased urinary frequency

9.6.2 Spinal conditions affecting small animals

The most commonly encountered spinal conditions affecting small animals are as follows.

- Vertebral body anomalies
- IVDD types I and II
- Spinal fractures
- Atlantoaxial luxation/subluxation
- Cervical spondylomyelopathy (wobbler syndrome)
- Lumbosacral degenerative stenosis
- Fibrocartilaginous embolism
- Discospondylitis
- Degenerative myelopathy

Vertebral body abnormalities

There are many malformations affecting the vertebrae that are commonly seen in dogs and cats (Westworth & Sturges 2010). Despite this, these are most frequently incidental findings and are not associated with clinical signs.

Diagnosis of many simple vertebral deformities can be readily made with radiographs of the vertebral column in orthogonal projections. However, CT myelography or MRI is required to identify the degree of spinal cord involvement and therefore its clinical significance. MRI provides visualisation of the spinal cord parenchyma, allowing identification of possible associated anomalies such as cysts, syringomyelia, oedema, etc. CT, on the other hand, provides better bony detail and can prove superior at identifying the degree of bony malformation in complex or multiple malformations. When identified, if such anomalies are determined to be significant, surgical options should be explored whenever possible.

The most common vertebral body abnormalities seen in small animals are:

- hemivertebrae
- transitional vertebrae
- block vertebrae
- spina bifida.

Hemivertebrae are most commonly seen in the screwtail breeds, i.e. Boston Terrier, Pug, English and French Bulldogs. It is an extremely common anomaly but most dogs that have these malformations are not significantly affected by it (Figure 9.9). There

is a failure of ossification of part of the vertebral body, unilateral, dorsal or ventral. Clinical signs are secondary to cord compression (which is why diagnosis usually relies on MRI rather than radiography alone) and may be chronic or acute in onset; most dogs in which it becomes clinically significant are under 1 year of age. Decompressive and/or stabilisation surgery may be indicated in cases with progressive neurological deficits. Animals with vertebral body abnormalities should not be used for breeding.

Transitional vertebrae may be seen at any level of the spinal column. The main area of clinical significance is at the lumbosacral junction where transitional vertebrae may result in instability and nerve root compression, causing significant pain and reluctance to exercise.

Block vertebrae result from improper separation of the vertebrae during development. Block vertebrae are inherently stable and are not usually clinically significant.

Spina bifida is characterised by an incomplete dorsal lamina and may not be of clinical significance in mild cases; however, in more severe cases with meningeal involvement, neurological abnormalities are often evident and corrective surgery may be required. Spina bifida is more commonly seen in the screwtail breeds and in Manx cats.

IVDD types I and II

Due to the blurring between type I and II IVDD, these will be discussed together and within spinal cord regions.

Cervical disc disease

Cervical disc extrusions often cause severe pain in the absence of other clinical signs. Nerve root signs are common (mainly thoracic limb lameness) and Horner's syndrome may also be seen (as the sympathetic supply to the eye passes through the cervical spinal cord). In more severe or chronic lesions, tetraparesis can become evident.

Diagnosis is based on clinical signs and imaging. Plain spinal films will help rule out possible differential diagnosis and myelography or MRI are essential prior to treatment.

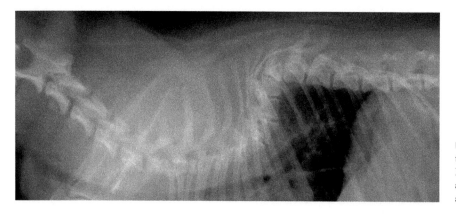

Figure 9.9 Lateral projection radiograph of the thoracolumbar spine of an English Bulldog. Note the obvious vertebral anomalies at T7 and T8 causing marked spinal kyphosis at that level.

In general, the animal's collar should be removed and not replaced. Use of a harness for the remainder of the animal's life is advised.

Medical management of cervical disc disease may be attempted. Absolute rest and the judicious use of analgesia may be beneficial. However, if severe pain is present, this condition is best treated surgically.

The most common site for cervical disc disease in small breed dogs is C2–3 whilst C5–6 and C6–7 are the most commonly affected discs when all breeds are considered together (Brisson 2010). Cervical IVDD in large breeds is usually associated with type II IVDD and most commonly occurs between C5 and C7 associated with cervical spondylomyelopathy and is discussed later.

Surgical options

Common surgical treatments include:
- ventral slot
- dorsal laminectomy
- dorsolateral hemilaminectomy.

The ventral slot is the most commonly performed technique for surgical management of cervical IVDD. The advantages include minimal muscle dissection and easier access to the intervertebral discs.

A ventral approach is made to the cervical spine, the relevant disc space identified and a slot-shaped laminectomy is performed commencing ventrally and extending into the neural canal. Disc material is removed from the canal. Closure is then undertaken. Fusion between vertebral bodies occurs approximately 8–12 weeks postoperatively.

Disadvantages include occasional severe intraoperative haemorrhage due to laceration of the venous sinus, incomplete removal of disc material, difficulty in performing the procedure on more than one vertebra due to the risk of instability and, very rarely, postoperative vertebral body fracture or collapse.

Prognosis is dependent on the degree of neurological deficits as well as location of IVDD but in general, it is good as the spinal canal is wider in the cervical region and most dogs are ambulatory on presentation. Long-standing tetraparetic animals have a significantly worse prognosis. Rarely, a C2–3 lesion will cause progression of neurological signs leading to brainstem swelling and respiratory and cardiac arrest. Following surgery, many dogs will either be normal or have mild cervical discomfort within 2 weeks of surgery. Recurrence of pain occasionally occurs within 1–2 weeks, usually because of incomplete disc removal or vertebral collapse, and should be investigated. Physiotherapy plays a vital role in recovery following spinal surgery and is increasingly becoming an invaluable component of therapy (see Chapter 17).

Thoracolumbar disc disease

This is the most common form of disc disease in small animals, accounting for 66–87% of all cases (Brisson 2010).

In type I disc disease, animals present acutely due to extrusion of disc material into the vertebral canal; clinical signs can vary from spinal pain to paraplegia. Type I IVDD usually occurs in chondrodysplastic breeds of young age or mature non-chondrodysplastic dogs. T12–13 and T13–L1 are the most commonly affected sites with incidence decreasing caudally in chondrodystrophic breeds (Figure 9.10).

In type II disc disease, animals present with a chronic and insidious history of paraparesis that deteriorates slowly over weeks to months. It usually affects older non-chondrodysplastic animals; L1–2 is the most common site affected (Figure 9.11).

Grading of these cases is important in deciding treatment options and prognosis. The following grades are generally used although other systems are available.
- Grade I – presence of spinal pain with no proprioception deficits or motor weakness. Prognosis is good with both medical management or surgery.
- Grade II – ambulatory paraparesis. Prognosis is good with both medical management and decompressive surgery.
- Grade III – non-ambulatory paraparesis. Prognosis is good with decompressive surgery and fair with medical management.
- Grade IV – paraplegia with intact pain perception. Prognosis is good with decompressive surgery; recovery is still likely with medical management but recurrence of signs or persistence of neurological deficits is probable. Reported recovery rates for non-ambulatory small breed dogs that retain pain sensation

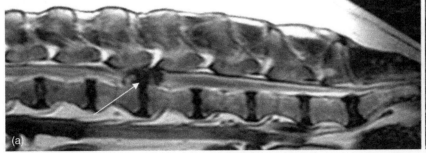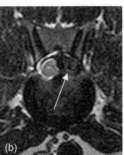

Figure 9.10 MR images of type I disc disease. (a) Sagittal T2WI showing a large disc extrusion between L3 and L4; note that the degenerate (*black*) disc material is inside the vertebral canal. (b) Transverse image through the disc extrusion; the disc material is occupying approximately 50% of the vertebral canal and is on the left side of the spinal cord; this information is essential for surgical planning.

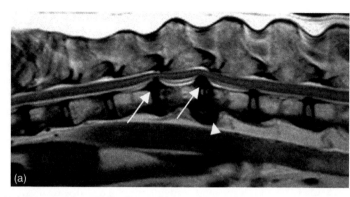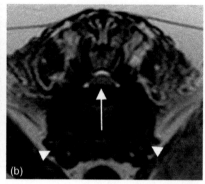

Figure 9.11 MR images of type II disc disease. (a) Sagittal T2WI showing intervertebral disc protrusions at T13–L1 and L1–2. (b) Transverse image through L1–2 showing moderate spinal cord compression due to bulging of the disc; also, note the presence of marked spondylosis ventral to the disc (*arrowheads*).

are around 90% whilst for large breed dogs they are slightly lower at around 80%.

- Grade V – paraplegia with absence of pain perception. Prognosis is grave with medical management, with recovery being extremely unlikely. Prognosis improves with decompressive surgery (approximately 50–60% for small breed dogs and around 25% for large breeds) if performed early in the course of disease.

Treatment options – conservative or surgical

Many animals will respond to conservative management, but recurrence of clinical signs is likely (between 30–50%). Conservative management involves strict rest and pain relief.

Which animals are good candidates for medical management? Mainly grade I and II animals which have a similar prognosis with medical versus surgical management. It is important nonetheless to take into account that the recurrence rate is significantly higher for medically managed animals.

For non-ambulatory animals, those with uncontrollable or recurrent pain and those deteriorating despite initiation of medical treatment, surgical intervention is indicated. The commonly practised surgical options include:

- hemilaminectomy
- pediculectomy
- corpectomy.

Dorsolateral hemilaminectomy   With the animal positioned in sternal recumbency, a dorsal incision is made. The fascial attachments in the midline are incised and the epaxial musculature elevated from the dorsal spinous process. The muscular attachments onto the articular facets are sharply dissected. The articular facets are removed with rongeurs and the dorsolateral pedicles removed with a high-speed bur. Once the spinal cord is exposed, the extruded disc material can be removed and the canal lavaged to remove remaining debris. The affected disc and, often, adjacent discs are fenestrated (removal of part of the remaining nucleus pulposus) at the same time in an attempt to prevent recurrence of disc herniation. Closure is routine.

Advantages of hemilaminectomy are removal of the majority of the intervertebral disc, retrieval of disc material with minimal

spinal cord trauma, ability to extend laminectomy cranially and caudally to improve retrieval of disc material and minimal effect of hemilaminectomy on torsional stability of the thoracolumbar spine.

Physiotherapy plays a vital role in recovery following spinal surgery and is increasingly becoming an invaluable component of therapy (see Chapter 17).

Factors affecting neurological recovery

As expected, the severity of neurological disease significantly affects recovery, with the prognosis deteriorating with increasing neurological grade.

The time interval between the onset of neurological disease and surgical decompression is a major influencing factor. The recovery rate is far more rapid in dogs undergoing decompressive surgery within 48 hours of onset of clinical signs than those surgically treated after that. This delay has more profound effect on the prognosis of more severely affected animals and is especially important in dogs that have lost pain perception; in these cases, prognosis for recovery after surgery performed within the first 24 h is 50–60%. If surgery is performed after 72 h of losing pain perception, functional recovery is still possible but very rare (Brisson 2010).

The presence or absence of pain sensation is the major prognostic factor. The pain fibres are located in the dorsal aspect of the ventral commissure of the spinal cord so severe spinal cord injury is required for animals to lose pain sensation.

Addition of physiotherapy post surgery hastens neurological recovery.

Spinal trauma

Vertebral fractures and luxations are most commonly associated with severe external trauma such as road traffic accidents or falls. They will typically result in pain and variable neurological deficits, depending on the severity and location of the lesion within the vertebral column. Up to 10% of animals have a second spinal fracture-luxation, making it is essential to image the entire spine and ensure orthogonal views are obtained.

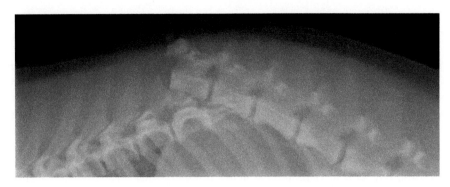

Figure 9.12 Lateral projection radiograph of a fracture-luxation at the level of T13–L1 causing marked vertebral displacement.

Cervical fractures

Cervical fractures are uncommon. They can be associated with trauma or developmental weakness of a pathological nature. Overall, 50% of cervical fractures occur at C2 (Hawthorne *et al.* 1999). Any animals with severe neck pain following trauma must be managed very carefully, especially if anaesthetised for radiography, as severe vertebral displacement in the cervical region is often fatal due to respiratory distress.

Thoracolumbar fractures

The level of the thoracolumbar junction (T10–L2) is the most common site of spinal fracture-luxation in the dog and cat (Figure 9.12). This is most likely due to its location between T1–10 (where the intercapital ligment provides added rigidity) and the well-muscled lumbar spine. Most are traumatic, usually with severe concurrent soft tissue and orthopaedic injuries, and multiple fractures are not uncommon in these cases.

Lumbosacral and coccygeal fractures

Lumbosacral and coccygeal fractures are not uncommon in small animals. Animals subject to trauma from behind, usually in car accidents, often have fractures in this area. A major problem, along with loss of locomotion, is the loss of bladder control and anal tone. Bladder management in particular is vital both short and long term. Tail pull injuries are commonly seen in cats and often result in sacrococcygeal luxation and traction of the nerve roots at that level. Although no change in gait will be seen in these cases, urinary and faecal incontinence are common and

may be permanent if the damage to the nerve roots is severe (neurotmesis).

Diagnosis

In most cases, radiography is sufficient to diagnose fracture-luxation. It is prudent to radiograph the entire spine due to the possibility of multiple trauma and orthogonal views should be obtained. Care must be taken, especially in animals under general anaesthesia with reduced muscle tone, not to displace luxations further. In certain cases, advanced imaging with CT and/or MRI may be indicated for surgical planning or to assess the integrity of the spinal cord.

Treatment

Treatment options are non-surgical or surgical management. Conservative management may be attempted for minimally displaced, stable fractures in the absence of severe neurological signs. The presence of instability is difficult to determine in many cases. This is often assessed using the 'three-column system' adapted from human patients, which divides the length of the vertebral column into three sections and if two or more are disrupted, then the fracture-luxation is considered to be unstable (Jeffery 2010). In this system, the dorsal column consists of the laminae, spinous processes and their associated ligaments. The middle column consists of the dorsal longitudinal ligament, dorsal annulus and dorsal cortex of the vertebral bodies. The ventral column consists of the ventral longitudinal ligament, ventral annulus and ventral cortex of the vertebral bodies (Figure 9.13).

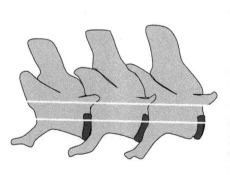
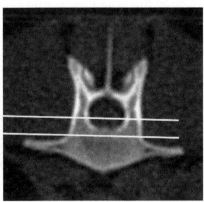

Figure 9.13 'Three-column system'.

Whether conservative or surgical management is used, physiotherapy should speed and aid recovery.

Non-surgical management

Conservative management typically involves strict cage confinement (for 4–6 weeks), use of a neck brace or back splint and appropriate analgesia. Splints aim to immobilise the vertebral segments cranial and caudal to fracture-luxation but can be difficult to apply and maintain in place in small animals. They can result in several complications such as loosening, skin abrasions and pain. Bladder management, if the animal is not urinating voluntarily, is vital. If there is any deterioration in neurological status, the animal should immediately be reassessed.

Surgical management

Surgical management is indicated in unstable fracture-luxations or if conservative therapy is unsuccessful. Surgical management allows for decompression of the spinal cord, if appropriate, as well as vertebral stabilisation.

A variety of surgical techniques have been described, mainly adapting to the shape of the different vertebrae and adjacent anatomic structures (Jeffery 2010). Some of the most commonly used include the use of Steinmann or threaded pins and polymethyl methacrylate (PMMA), locking plates (such as SOP plates) and modified segmental spinal fixation (spinal stapling).

Postoperative management involves appropriate anagesia and cage rest for 4–6 weeks. Prevention of complications of recumbency with adequate nursing care and bladder management are also very important. Serial neurological examination is advised and any deterioration in neurological status should be thoroughly assessed.

Prognosis

Prognosis depends on neurological status before surgery, method of repair and response to postoperative management. There is a poor correlation between degree of vertebral displacement and neurological deficits.

Poor prognostic factors include severe neurological status, deteriorating neurological status and an interval of more than 5 days before treatment. Most importantly, the absence of pain perception after spinal trauma carries a guarded prognosis. The likelihood of recovery in such cases is less than 5% if the vertebrae are displaced and around 25% if there is no vertebral displacement (Olby *et al.* 2003).

In general, animals undergoing conservative management tend to have milder neurological injury, a slower improvement but reduced hospital stay times, while those managed with surgery tend to have more severe neurological injury, more rapid improvement but increased hospital stay times.

Physiotherapy plays a vital role in recovery following spinal surgery and is increasingly becoming an invaluable component of therapy (see Chapter 17).

Atlantoaxial instability

Atlantoaxial (AA) instability may be either congenital or acquired.

Congenital subluxations occur with little or no trauma and are secondary to failure of normal development of the dens (most common) but can also be seen with congenital absence of the transverse ligament or incomplete ossification of the atlas. This condition has been reported in many different breeds but it is typical of toy breeds such as the Yorkshire Terrier, Lhasa Apso, Chihuahua, Pekinese, Toy Poodle and Pomeranian. AA subluxation can also happen following trauma, often associated with fracture of the dens (Westworth & Sturges 2010).

Clinical signs

Clinical signs include abnormal low head carriage, progressive tetraparesis and ataxia associated with neck pain. In the cases associated with congenital malformations, there may be an acute presentation after very minor trauma and the animal may dislike its head being touched. Usually it occurs in young animals, less than 12 months of age.

Luxation may be due to axial fracture at the synostosis between the dens and body of the axis or luxation with an intact dens. The transverse ligaments and often the apical ligaments must rupture for AA luxation.

Diagnosis

Diagnosis is usually achieved using plain radiography; CT may be of benefit in planning surgical reconstruction.

Treatment
Conservative management

Conservative management includes strict cage rest (6–12 weeks), a neck brace and appropriate analgesia (Figure 9.14). Although conservative management often results in clinical

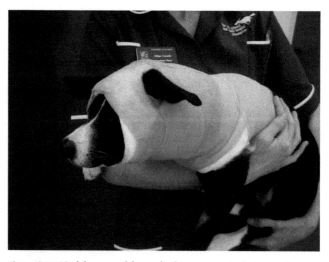

Figure 9.14 Neck brace used for medical management of a traumatic atlantoaxial subluxation in a young crossbreed.

improvement, recurrence is common, as only limited soft tissue fibrosis appears to occur between the atlas and the axis. Medical treatment is more successful in traumatic cases than in dogs with congenital malformations.

Surgical management

Surgical management is more common. Indications include severe neck pain, severe or progressive neurological signs or if conservative management is not successful.

Either ventral or dorsal stabilisation may be undertaken. Ventral stabilisation is most commonly used as it has a better success rate and less implant failure; it involves reduction of luxation and fusion of the articular joints with bone graft and screws.

Prognosis

The prognosis depends on the severity of neurological signs and therapeutic management. Conservative management has a worse prognosis due to recurrence. Surgical management has a good to excellent prognosis although it can be associated with high perioperative morbidity and mortality. Physiotherapy plays a vital role in recovery following spinal surgery and is increasingly becoming an invaluable component of therapy (see Chapter 17).

Cervical spondylomyelopathy

Cervical spondylomyelopathy (CSM) is a degenerative and progressive disorder affecting the cervical vertebrae and associated soft tissue structures (including the intervertebral discs and ligaments), resulting in mechanical compression of the spinal cord and nerve roots (de Decker *et al.* 2012). It is a multifactorial, complex and poorly understood neurological syndrome. It is often classified as disc associated (DACSM) or osseous associated (OACSM). The first form is more common and tends to affect middle-aged to older large breed dogs whilst OACSM is more common in younger giant breed dogs (Gasper *et al.* 2014). The caudal cervical region (C5–6 and C6–7) is most commonly affected and in around 50% of dogs, more than one site is abnormal (up to 80% in giant breeds). As the names suggest, DACSM is mainly associated with IVDD type II whilst in OACSM, vertebral canal stenosis is secondary to vertebral malformations and osteoarthritic changes of the articular facets. The underlying pathogenesis of CSM is still not understood but congenital, genetic, nutritional and conformational aetiologies have been proposed (de Decker *et al.* 2012).

Clinical signs

Regardless of aetiology and classification type, CSM may be divided by functional appearance into static or dynamic compressive lesions. This is based on the myelographic or MRI appearance of the compression under traction and helps decide on the most adequate treatment modality. When imaging of the spine is undertaken, mild traction is applied to the neck and if the compression is unchanged, the lesion is termed static but if the lesion improves with traction, it is termed dynamic.

Any breed can be affected by CSM but the breeds most commonly associated with CSM are the Doberman and the Great Dane. The clinical signs generally become evident at a young age (<2 years) in the OACSM cases whilst DACSM dogs present at an older age (>7 years).

The typical clinical history is of general ataxia and progressive tetraparesis over a period of weeks to months. The thoracic and pelvic limbs are affected but signs begin earlier and are more pronounced in the pelvic limbs. Dogs may also present acutely after minor trauma. There is cervical pain in only around 50% of cases.

Neurological examination reveals stiff, short-strided and choppy gait, generalised ataxia and tetraparesis in the more severe cases. Muscle atrophy in the thoracic limbs may be evident and neck pain may be noted with manipulation in some cases. Most dogs will show proprioceptive deficits in all limbs and in cases with more caudal lesions, the spinal reflexes in the thoracic limbs will be reduced.

Diagnosis

Diagnosis is based on clinical and neurological examination and imaging findings. Myelography allows for easier evaluation of how traction responsive lesions are but MRI allows visualisation of the spinal cord, providing important information on severity, chronicity and therefore prognosis of lesions. As transverse images can be obtained, it is also very useful to evaluate compression of nerve roots or dorsolateral compression arising from overgrown articular processes, which may be underestimated in myelography alone (Figure 9.15).

Treatment

Conservative management

Conservative management may provide short-term relief. Results of conservative management are controversial, with different studies suggesting variable results. It seems likely that around 50% of dogs will improve or remain stable with medical management comprising exercise restriction and low-dose corticosteroid therapy but many dogs are euthanased within a year of diagnosis.

Surgical management

The plethora of surgical techniques described (over 20) highlights the disagreement among surgeons as to the best course of treatment (Jeffery & McKee 2001). Like surgical management of cranial cruciate ligament disease, it would seem that each surgeon has their own technique.

The aims of surgery are to relieve spinal cord compression and in some cases also attempt to distract and stabilise the affected spinal segment. The mechanism by which this is achieved will depend on the underlying cause of the compression, number of lesions and affected sites and in some cases also presence or absence of a dynamic lesion. The most commonly used techniques for DACSM include the ventral slot, numerous different ventral techniques attempting to distract (using bone grafts,

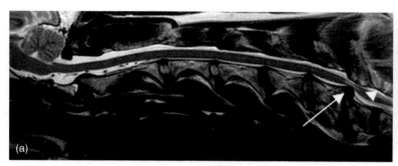 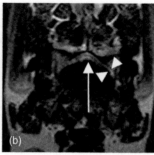

Figure 9.15 MR images of a Doberman with cervical spondylomyelopathy. (a) Sagittal T2WI showing significant spinal cord compression secondary to an intervertebral disc protrusion at C6–7. Note the associated spinal cord atrophy at that level and the presence of hyperintensity (brightness) inside the spinal cord (*arrowhead*); this is thought to represent ischaemic damage. (b) Transverse T2WI through the protruded disc showing the marked spinal cord compression and associated nerve root compression (*arrowheads*).

cages or disc replacements) and stabilise (with screws and bone cement or locking plates) the affected spinal segment or multi-level dorsal laminectomy in cases with multiple lesions.

In OACSM, the main aim of surgery is decompression, with the technique chosen guided by the affected site; dorsal laminectomy or hemilaminectomy are most commonly used. In cases with several affected sites, distraction-stabilisation techniques may also be considered. Independent of which technique is used, the success rate of surgical treatment is reported to be around 80%.

Many Dobermans have von Willebrand's disease and coagulation profile is highly recommended before surgery.

Prognosis

Cervical spondylomyelopathy is a difficult condition to deal with but in view of the reported success rates previously mentioned, surgical treatment appears most likely to result in improvement of the clinical signs. Physiotherapy plays a vital role both in dogs receiving medical management and in dogs recovering from surgery and is increasingly becoming an invaluable component of therapy (see Chapter 17).

Lumbosacral degenerative stenosis

Lumbosacral degenerative stenosis (LSDS) is a multifactorial disorder in which a combination of bony and soft tissue structures causes progressive stenosis of the lumbosacral (LS) region with compression of the cauda equina and associated nerve roots. LSDS is a common condition and generally affects mature large breed dogs. Vertebral canal and intervertebral foraminal stenosis can be secondary to one or more abnormalities: intervertebral disc protrusion, ligamentous and articular process hypertrophy, osteophyte formation and vertebral misalignment or instability (Meij & Bergknut 2010).

Clinical signs

Clinical signs are related to compression of the cauda equina and/or nerve roots and may be intermittent. Pain at the LS region, lameness (which may worsen with exercise), urinary and/or faecal incontinence, self-mutilation of the tail, perineum, genitals or extremities may all be seen. Reluctance to jump or sit and reluctance to exercise are very common complaints, along with intermittent claudication. In more severe or chronic cases, clinical findings may also include neurological deficits such as weakness (evident through scuffing of pelvic limb toenails) and a dropped hock, abnormal tail carriage and pelvic limb muscle atrophy.

Diagnosis

Diagnosis may be difficult as the condition is often dynamic, at least in part, and clinical signs may be intermittent.

Plain radiographs may reveal degenerative changes but the significance of this is always difficult to interpret as they are very common and in most cases not associated with clinical signs. These would be most useful in cases where the compression is associated with malformations such as transitional vertebrae, although once more, the significance of these finding can only be confirmed with advanced imaging. Myelography is usually pointless, as the epidural sac of the spinal cord often does not cross the LS joint and epidurography is very difficult to interpret. MRI is undoubtedly the method of choice to image the LS region as it allows visualisation of the cauda equina and the nerve roots. It allows easy identification of intervertebral disc degeneration, protrusion and/or extrusion as well as evaluation of the intervertebral foramina where there may be compression of the L7 nerve roots by osteophytes; the latter is impossible to assess by other imaging modalities (Figure 9.16).

Treatment

Conservative management

Conservative management is associated with a fair prognosis and its success often depends on the main underlying cause of the clinical signs. It relies on initial strict rest (6–8 weeks) and analgesia followed by a slow and gradual return to controlled exercise. The use of repeated epidural infiltrations with methylprednisolone acetate has also been reported to result in improvement of the clinical signs and may be the treatment of choice in older patients where surgery is less desirable (Janssens *et al.* 2009).

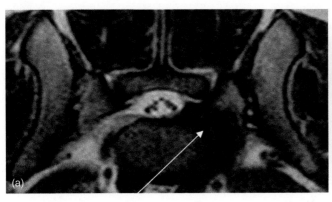 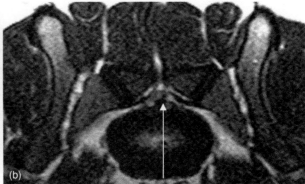

Figure 9.16 MR images of lumbosacral degenerative stenosis. (a) Transverse T2WI showing foraminal stenosis causing marked compression of the left L7 nerve root. (b) Transverse T2WI showing an intervertebral disc protrusion at the level of the LS junction causing compression of the cauda equina.

Surgical management

Surgical management is advised if pain is severe or there is no improvement following conservative management.

The most common procedure is the dorsal laminectomy. A dorsal approach is made to the LS joint and the dorsal lamina removed. The cauda equina/nerve roots are carefully retracted and disc material removed from the neural canal. If nerve root impingement is evident at the level of the intervertebral foramina, a foraminotomy procedure may also be performed.

An alternativee technique is the distraction fusion procedure, which involves distraction of LS space, which is maintained by screws across the facet joints and the addition of an autogenous cancellous graft. A dorsal laminectomy may also be undertaken.

Exercise restriction for 8–12 weeks after surgery is essential as excessive postoperative activity may result in a poor outcome.

Prognosis

The recovery rate for dogs managed medically is thought to be around 50% (de Decker *et al.* 2014). For cases managed surgically, the prognosis is fair to good with reported short- to medium-term rates of improvement between 50% and 95% (Meij & Bergknut 2010). Urinary and faecal incontinence rarely resolve if present before surgery although some animals improve. Physiotherapy plays a vital role in recovery following spinal surgery and is increasingly becoming an invaluable component of therapy. It is also pivotal in patients managed medically as often these dogs have mild but persistent clinical signs that can be controlled with a combination of analgesia and physiotherapy (see Chapter 17).

Fibrocartilaginous embolism (FCE)

Fibrocartilaginous embolism occurs when fibrocartilaginous material histologically identical to the nucleus pulposus of the intervertebral disc occludes a spinal vessel, causing ischaemic necrosis of the spinal cord.

Neurological deficits are peracute in onset; the exact signs and severity depend on the site and extent of the spinal cord infarction but are asymmetrical in more than 50% of dogs (due to asymmetrical branching of the spinal vasculature). These deficits usually stabilise within 24 h, and subsequently remain static or improve and are typically not associated with pain. FCE is most commonly seen in large breed dogs and often the signs start during exercise; at that time, sudden and transient hyperalgesia (such as yelping in pain) is described after which time no further signs of pain are identified (de Risio *et al.* 2008).

Another condition that is very similar to FCE is the acute non-compressive nucleus pulposus extrusion (ANNPE). In these cases, the presentation and clinical signs are very similar and, in certain cases, even indistinguishable on MRI. In ANNPE, it is thought that there is a peracute extrusion of a non-degenerate, 'healthy' disc that is placed under supraphysiological mechanical stress during athletic activity; a portion of the nucleus is explosively expelled, causing negligible spinal cord compression but significant contusion and subsequent ischaemia (de Risio *et al.* 2009).

Diagnosis

The diagnosis of FCE is based on the typical clinical presentation and exclusion of other causes through diagnostic imaging and CSF analysis. Myelography can exclude compressive lesions whilst MRI usually allows visualisation of a focal, relatively sharply demarcated and often asymmetrical lesion inside the spinal cord, representing oedematous infarcted tissue (Figure 9.17). MRI can also be normal in cases with very mild deficits or imaged very close to the time of injury (within 24–48 h); these patients tend to have a quicker recovery.

Treatment

Treatment for both FCE and ANNPE mainly involves nursing care (regular turning, skin care to prevent decubital ulcers and urine scalding, bladder and bowel management, adequate nutrition) and physiotherapy to stimulate neuronal plasticity and minimise disuse and immobilisation changes such as muscle atrophy and muscle and joint contractures (see Chapter 17).

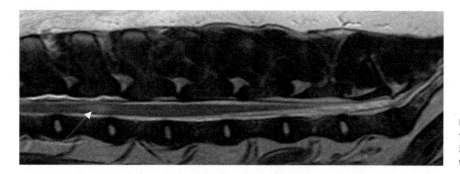

Figure 9.17 Sagittal MR image (T2W) of a dog with a fibrocartilaginous embolism. Note the intramedullary hyperintense (bright) lesion at the level of L2.

Prognosis

The prognosis depends on the severity and extent of the ischaemic injury but it is generally good. Negative prognostic indicators include severity of the neurological signs at presentation, with symmetrical deficits carrying a worse prognosis, loss of pain perception and presence of lower motor neuron signs. Time for maximum recovery is usually about 3–4 months but time to ambulation is much shorter at around 2 weeks.

Discospondylitis

Discospondylitis refers to infection of the intervertebral disc and osteomyelitis of the adjacent vertebral endplates and bodies. These infections are relatively common in dogs but not in cats. Discospondylitis tends to affect large breed dogs and the most commonly affected area is the LS junction; the caudal cervical, midthoracic and thoracolumbar spine are also common sites for infection (Burkert et al. 2005). Males outnumber females by 2:1 except for fungal discospondylitis, which is more common in females.

Clinical signs

The clinical signs are variable but often include spinal pain, pyrexia and lethargy. With time and proliferation of the inflammatory tissue, compression of the neural structures can occur and therefore result in neurological deficits (such as proprioceptive deficits and paresis).

Diagnosis

Radiography of the spine will generally confirm the diagnosis by demonstrating collapse of the disc space with lysis of the adjacent vertebral endplates and vertebral body osteolysis, proliferative sclerosis and osseous bridging in later stages (Figure 9.18). It can take up to 4–6 weeks for radiographic changes to develop though so, in some cases, MRI can be used for early diagnosis. MRI can show bone oedema and typically reveals contrast enhancement of the intervertebral disc and endplates, as well as of the epidural space in many instances.

Treatment

Treatment requires a minimum of 2 months of antibiotics. Ideally, the causative agent should be identified. Blood and urine cultures should be collected; this usually identifies positive results in 50–75% of cases. Surgery may be indicated if spinal instability is present or if the neurological deterioration occurs despite appropriate antimicrobial therapy. Fungal discospondylitis is not cured but it may be managed with medication for some time.

Prognosis

Prognosis is dependent on early diagnosis and treatment, the pathogen involved and sensitivity to antibiotic therapy and the degree and severity of neurological involvement. Physiotherapy plays a vital role in recovery following spinal injury and is increasingly becoming an invaluable component of therapy (see Chapter 17).

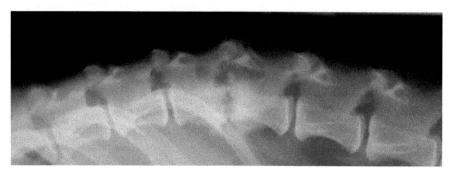

Figure 9.18 Lateral projection radiograph of a dog presented with thoracolumbar pain. Note the irregular bone lysis and sclerosis of the vertebral endplates of L1 and L2 and mild spondylosis at that level; these findings are compatible with discospondylitis.

Degenerative myelopathy

The name degenerative myelopathy (DM) was chosen due to the histopathological nature of this condition, which is a non-specific degeneration of spinal cord tissue of undetermined cause. Immunological, metabolic or nutritional factors, oxidative stress, excitotoxic and genetic mechanisms have been hypothesised and studied as possible underlying causes of DM (Coates & Wininger 2010).

Although most commonly associated with German Shepherd Dogs (GSD), DM has been recognised as a common problem in several breeds, with an overall prevalence of 0.19%. Age of onset of neurological signs is usually at 8 years or older (mean age of 9 years). Histopathologically confirmed cases of DM have been identified in the following dog breeds: GSD, Siberian Husky, Miniature Poodle, Boxer, Pembroke Welsh Corgi (PWC), Chesapeake Bay Retriever, Rhodesian Ridgeback, Bernese Mountain Dog, Standard Poodle, Kerry Blue Terrier, Cardigan Welsh Corgi, Golden Retriever, Wire Fox Terrier, American Eskimo Dog, Soft-coated Wheaten Terrier and Pug.

Clinical signs

The typical clinical signs include progressive, asymmetrical paraparesis and pelvic limb ataxia, without associated spinal pain. The clinical picture is complex at times as many of these larger breed older dogs can also have concurrent IVDD type II and osteoarthritis.

The clinical course of DM varies, with a mean time for disease duration of 6 months in larger dog breeds and a median disease duration in the PWC of around 18 months; this was thought to possibly be related to the ease of nursing for a smaller sized dog. Most large dogs progress to non-ambulatory paraparesis within 6–9 months from onset of clinical signs.

Diagnosis

Diagnosis is based on the relentlessly progressive clinical signs in the absence of any findings on diagnostic investigation (diagnosis of exclusion). Most importantly, it relies on the absence of compressive lesions on myelography or MRI of the spine. A DNA test based on the SOD1 (superoxide dismutase – free radical scavenger) mutation is also commercially available. The test is useful for supporting or helping exclude the condition but on its own, the results are insufficient for diagnosis.

Treatment and prognosis

There is no treatment for DM and long-term prognosis is grave. Several treatments have been proposed in the past but none has resulted in long-term benefits (including corticosteroids, aminocaproic acid, N-acetylcysteine, vitamins B, C, E or tocopherol). Physiotherapy has been shown to improve survival times and quality of life so it is currently the recommended treatment for DM (Kathmann *et al.* 2006). Prognosis is poor as the condition will eventually result in LMN paraplegia and affect the thoracic limbs so most patients are euthanased within 6–18 months.

9.7 Neuromuscular disease

The neuromuscular system is composed of the peripheral nerves, muscles and neuromuscular junction. Lesions affecting this system may be localised (for example, a peripheral nerve sheath tumour affecting one or a group of nerves such as the brachial plexus) or may be generalised and affect most nerves or muscles.

9.7.1 Peripheral neuropathies

The peripheral nerves may be damaged anywhere along their pathway, from the cell body to the peripheral nerve ending on the effector organ. Abnormality of function will depend on the nerve(s) affected and the location of damage or disease. Peripheral neuropathy may be sensory or motor. Sensory neuropathy alone is uncommon but can result in severe clinical signs such as generalised ataxia and self-mutilation. Motor neuropathy results in weakness, muscle atrophy and loss of reflexes.

Peripheral neuropathies may be acquired or congenital.

Acquired peripheral neuropathies

- *Trauma.* This may be due to fractures, bite wounds or penetrating injuries (including injections). A common injury is brachial plexus avulsion secondary to trauma. Damage to the nerve can be classified as neuropraxia (temporary interruption of function without structural damage), axonotmesis (partial damage to the nerve but with possibility to regenerate) or neurotmesis (complete severance of the nerve).
- *Metabolic.* Peripheral neuropathies may occur secondary to hypoglycaemia or hyperlipidaemia and to several endocrine conditions such as diabetes mellitus and hypothyroidism.
- *Paraneoplastic syndromes.* Several paraneoplastic syndromes can cause peripheral neuropathies.
- *Infections.* Infection by *Toxoplasma gondii* and *Neospora caninum* have both been associated with peripheral neuropathies, usually in young animals.
- *Immune-mediated disease.* The most common manifestation is idiopathic polyradiculoneuritis (called Coonhound paralysis in the USA and very similar to Guillain–Barré syndrome in people); this condition often results in non-ambulatory tetraparesis with severe generalised muscle atrophy so the use of physiotherapy in these cases is of paramount importance during the recovery period (from 4 to 12 weeks). Other conditions include distal denervating disease and chronic inflammatory demyelinating polyneuropathy.
- *Toxins.* Toxicity from lead, organophosphates or mercury as well as chemotherapeutic drugs such as vincristine.

Congenital peripheral neuropathies

There are numerous hereditary conditions affecting different breeds; genetic testing is available for some conditions. They are mostly found in young dogs and are generally progressive in nature. For further reading on peripheral neuropathies, see Granger (2011).

9.7.2 Junctionopathies

The neuromuscular junction includes the axon terminal of the peripheral nerve, the synaptic cleft and the endplate of the skeletal muscle. Diseases affecting the neuromuscular junction can disturb transmission of the electrical impulse at any of these structures and are subsequently classified as presynaptic, postsynaptic or enzymatic; the clinical signs can therefore vary. Junctionopathies in small animals are rare except for myasthenia gravis. Animals with presynaptic disorders present with LMN-type weakness affecting all limbs, with reduced spinal reflexes and obvious loss of muscle tone. Patients with postsynaptic disorders present with exercise-induced weakness that improves following rest.

Possible causes include:

- myasthenia gravis (postsynaptic) – usually an immune-mediated acquired disease due to antibodies directed against muscle acetylcholine receptors
- botulism (presynaptic)
- tick paralysis (presynaptic) – the tick responsible inhabits Australia and USA.

9.7.3 Myopathies

In most patients with intrinsic muscle disease, the neurological examination is normal. In cases with generalised myopathies, the main complaints tend to be exercise intolerance, generalised weakness with a stiff and stilted gait that generally worsens with exercise, ventroflexion of the neck (mainly in cats due to absence of a nuchal ligament in this species) and possibly muscle atrophy. In very severe cases, there may be proprioceptive deficits and reduced reflexes if there is so much muscle loss that the patient does not have the strength to replace the foot or withdraw the limb, but this is less common. In focal myopathies, the clinical signs vary significantly but can result in very mild clinical signs such as lameness.

Delayed-onset muscle soreness and muscle strain injury

Delayed-onset muscle soreness (DOMS) is virtually unreported in the veterinary literature but is likely to occur in animals, especially animals used for athletic activities, as it does in man (Cheung *et al.* 2003; Connolly *et al.* 2003).

Muscle strain injury occurs as a result of overstretching of muscle leading to disruption of fibres, which can subsequently lead to inflammation and healing with fibrosis. While it certainly can be a cause of lameness in dogs, it can be difficult to diagnose or is sometimes even overlooked as a cause of lameness. Muscle strain injury is quite common in athletic dogs. It occurs particularly in those muscles that cross two or more joints, especially near the musculotendinous junction but also at the origin and insertion of the muscle (Steiss 2002).

Based on the system in humans there are four grades.

1 Tearing of a few fibres
2 Pain
3 Local spasm
4 Complete muscle rupture

Recovery is rapid with low-grade injuries, but fibrous tissue may predispose to reinjury or contracture.

Diagnosis

Muscle injury should be a differential as a cause of lameness. Palpation may reveal pain or even a defect. Ultrasonography is probably the most appropriate imaging technique for muscle injuries themselves, although if the injury occurs at the origin or insertion of a muscle, radiography is important to determine if there has been an avulsion fracture at the site. Nuclear scintigraphy and other imaging techniques may reveal the inflammation.

Common sites of muscle strain injuries in the dog are:

- *thoracic limb*: rhomboideus, serratus ventralis, pectorals, triceps, biceps and flexor carpi ulnaris
- *pelvic limb*: iliopsoas, tensor fascia lata, sartorius, pectineus, gracilis and Achilles mechanism.

Treatment of muscle strain injury

Low-grade injuries should be treated with conservative physiotherapy, using the principles you would use in man; see also Chapter 18. High-grade injuries may be amenable to surgical treatment (dogs), including surgical debridement, repair or tenomyectomy.

Ossifying/fibrotic myopathies in dogs
Semitendinosus fibrotic myopathy

Occurs in German Shepherds, uncommon, poorly responsive to surgery. Presents with a characteristic gait pattern due to the tethering of the forward phase of limb flight.

Myositis ossificans

Usually secondary to trauma (there have been some reported cases in Dobermans secondary to clotting disorders). Sites of predilection include the hip (Dobermans), shoulder, quadriceps and cervical regions, and it occurs in large, middle-aged, active dogs and presents as lameness from mechanical interference. Surgical debulking is the preferred treatment.

Contractures
Infraspinatous contracture

Occurs in large, active, middle-aged dogs, with tethering of normal shoulder motion and circumduction of the limb. There is palpable atrophy of the muscle. Proposed to be secondary to injury causing fibrosis and functional shortening of the muscle. Treatment is surgical – infraspinatous tenotomy.

Quadriceps contracture

Occurs in actively growing dogs <6 months old following fracture of the distal femur with voluntary or enforced immobilisation. The result is prolonged hyperextension of stifle muscle contracture and adhesions. It is best prevented but if it occurs, early recognition is essential as prognosis once advanced is poor. Physiotherapy responses have been good (see Chapter 18).

Gracilis contracture

Occurs in active, middle-aged, large dogs, secondary to injury such as infraspinatous contracture. Affected dogs can maintain normal function but have a characteristic jerky gait and shortened stride. Affected dogs tend to have a guarded long-term outlook owing to recurrence after surgery.

References

Bergknut, N., Smolders, L.A., Grinwis, G.C. *et al.* 2013, Intervertebral disc degeneration in the dog. Part 1: Anatomy and physiology of the intervertebral disc and characteristics of intervertebral disc degeneration. *Vet. J.* 195(3): 282–291.

Brisson, B.A. 2010, Intervertebral disc disease in dogs. *Vet. Clin. North Am. Small Anim. Pract.* 40(5): 829–858.

Burkert, B.A., Kerwin, S.C., Hosgood, G.L., Pechman, R.D., Fontenelle, J.P. 2005, Signalment and clinical features of diskospondylitis in dogs: 513 cases (1980–2001). *J. Am. Vet. Med. Assoc.* 227(2): 268–275.

Cheung, K., Hume, P., Maxwell, L. 2003, Delayed onset muscle soreness: treatment strategies and performance factors. *Sports Med.* 33(2): 145–164.

Coates, J.R., Wininger, F.A. 2010, Canine degenerative myelopathy. *Vet. Clin. North Am. Small Anim. Pract.* 40(5): 929–950.

Connolly, D.A., Sayers, S.P., McHugh, M.P. 2003, Treatment and prevention of delayed onset muscle soreness. *J. Strength Cond. Res.* 17(1): 197–208.

De Decker, S., da Costa, R.C., Volk, H.A., van Ham, L.M. 2012, Current insights and controversies in the pathogenesis and diagnosis of disc-associated cervical spondylomyelopathy in dogs. *Vet. Rec.* 171(21): 531–537.

De Decker, S., Wawrzenski, L.A., Volk, H.A. 2014, Clinical signs and outcome of dogs treated medically for degenerative lumbosacral stenosis: 98 cases (2004–2012). *J. Am. Vet. Med. Assoc.* 245(4): 408–413.

De Lahunta, A. 2009, Upper motor neuron. In: de Lahunta, A., Glass, E. (eds), *Veterinary Neuroanatomy and Clinical Neurology*, 3rd edn. WB Saunders, Philadelphia, PA.

De Risio, L., Adams, V., Dennis, R., McConnell, F.J., Platt, S.R. 2008, Association of clinical and magnetic resonance imaging findings with outcome in dogs suspected to have ischemic myelopathy: 50 cases (2000–2006). *J. Am. Vet. Med. Assoc.* 233(1): 129–135.

De Risio, L., Adams, V., Dennis, R., McConnell, F.J. 2009, Association of clinical and magnetic resonance imaging findings with outcome in dogs with presumptive acute noncompressive nucleus pulposus extrusion: 42 cases (2000–2007). *J. Am. Vet. Med. Assoc.* 234(4): 495–504.

Gasper, J.A., Rylander, H., Stenglein, J.L., Waller, K.R. 2014, Osseous-associated cervical spondylomyelopathy in dogs: 27 cases (2000–2012). *J. Am. Vet. Med. Assoc.* 244(11): 1309–1318.

Granger, N. 2011, Canine inherited motor and sensory neuropathies: an updated classification in 22 breeds and comparison to Charcot-Marie-Tooth disease. *Vet. J.* 188(3): 274–285.

Hansen, H.J. 1952, A pathologic-anatomical study on disc degeneration in dogs. *Acta Orthop. Scand.* 11: 1–117.

Hawthorne, J.C., Blevins, W.E., Wallace, L.J., Glickman, N., Waters, D.J. 1999, Cervical vertebral fractures in 56 dogs: a retrospective study. *J. Am. Anim. Hosp. Assoc.* 35(2): 135–146.

Janssens, L., Beosier, Y., Daems, R. 2009, Lumbosacral degenerative stenosis in the dog. The results of epidural infiltration with methylprednisolone acetate: a retrospective study. *Vet. Comp. Orthop. Traumatol.* 22(6): 486–491.

Jeffery, N.D. 2010, Vertebral fracture and luxation in small animals. *Vet. Clin. North Am. Small Anim. Pract.* 40(5): 809–828.

Jeffery, N.D., McKee, W.M. 2001, Surgery for disc associated wobbler syndrome in the dog – an examination of the controversy. *J. Small Anim. Pract.* 42(12): 574–581.

Kathmann, I., Cizinauskas, S., Doherr, M.G., Steffen, F., Jaggy, A. 2006, Daily controlled physiotherapy increases survival time in dogs with suspected degenerative myelopathy. *J. Vet. Intern. Med.* 20(4): 927–932.

Kraeling, M. 2014, Proposed treatment for geriatric vestibular disease in dogs. *Top. Compan. Anim. Med.* 29(10): 6–9.

Meij, B.P., Bergknut, N. 2010, Degenerative lumbosacral stenosis in dogs. *Vet. Clin. North Am. Small Anim. Pract.* 40(5): 983–1009.

Olby, N., Levine, J., Harris, T., Muñana, K., Skeen, T., Sharp, N. 2003, Long-term functional outcome of dogs with severe injuries of the thoracolumbar spinal cord: 87 cases (1996–2001). *J. Am. Vet. Med. Assoc.* 222(6): 762–769.

Steiss, J.E. 2002, Muscle disorders and rehabilitation in canine athletes, *Vet. Clin. North Am. Small Anim. Pract.* 32(1): 267–285

Westworth, D.R., Sturges, B.K. 2010, Congenital spinal malformations in small animals. *Vet. Clin. North Am. Small Anim. Pract.* 40(5): 951–981.

CHAPTER 10

Equine neurological and muscular conditions*

Harry Carslake

University of Liverpool, Liverpool, UK

Summary

The aim of this chapter is to furnish animal physiotherapists with the essential information needed to recognise and contribute to the management of common neurological and muscular disorders of the horse. A protocol for the complete equine neurological examination is described, including interpretation of abnormal findings, neuroanatomical localisation and further diagnostic techniques such as radiology. The diagnosis and treatment of the major neuromuscular conditions of the horse, with an indication of where physiotherapy is appropriate, is also included. It should be read in conjunction with Chapter 9, which covers neuroanatomy and physiology common to both the dog and the horse.

10.1 Introduction

The horse presents some unique challenges in both the examination and management of the neuromuscular system, which are mostly related to the size and temperament of the patient. The aim of this chapter is to outline the differences in neuroanatomy between small animals and horses, to describe neurological assessment of the horse and to review some of the more commonly encountered neurological and muscular conditions in horses. It should be read in conjunction with Chapter 9, which covers basic neuroanatomy, physiology and pathology and gives some definitions of commonly used terms.

10.2 Neuroanatomy

The neuroanatomy of all mammals follows the same basic pattern, and the horse is similar to that described for dogs and cats in Chapter 9. There are some differences which are clinically significant, however, and these are described below.

10.2.1 The spinal cord

The horse's vertebral column consists of seven cervical, 18 thoracic, six lumbar (although variations do occur – see later),

---

*Adapted from the first edition chapter, which was written by Catherine M. McGowan

Animal Physiotherapy: Assessment, Treatment and Rehabilitation of Animals, Second Edition. Edited by Catherine M. McGowan and Lesley Goff.
© 2016 John Wiley & Sons, Ltd. Published 2016 by John Wiley & Sons, Ltd.

five fused sacral and approximately 20 caudal vertebrae. As in other species, the spinal cord is divided into spinal segments, which correspond to the intervertebral space from which the spinal nerves exit the vertebral canal. The shortening of the spinal segments towards the caudal end of the cord is less pronounced in horses compared to cats and dogs. Segments of the spinal cord terminate at approximately S2 (de Lahunta & Glass 2009). The subarachnoid space also runs further caudally in horses compared to small animals, allowing reliable collection of cerebrospinal fluid from the lumbosacral space (Dyce *et al.* 2010a).

Upper motor neurons (UMN) and lower motor neurons (LMN) are described in Chapter 9. The descending UMN pathways can be divided into the pyramidal (controlling finely adjusted movements) and the extrapyramidal (controlling coarser movements such as stereotyped locomotor patterns) (Dyce *et al.* 2010b). The pyramidal system is highly developed in primates, but less so in domestic species. Division of the descending motor pathways into the pyramidal and extrapyramidal systems is described in Chapter 9. Horses have poorly developed pyramidal tracts compared to dogs and cats, with virtually no input caudal to the brachial plexus. The most developed area is that responsible for movement of the lips and muzzle, suggesting that this is the most finely controlled activity that the horse performs (de Lahunta & Glass 2009). The extrapyramidal system is of much greater importance in controlling locomotion. Even quite extensive lesions of the cerebrocortical motor centres in horses will only result in minor alterations in gait, demonstrating the minor role the pyramidal system plays in locomotion (Mayhew 2009).

10.2.2 Vertebral anatomy

Horses' cervical vertebrae are similar to those in small animals, although relatively longer and with large transverse processes palpable to C5 or C6 (Figure 10.1). The thoracic

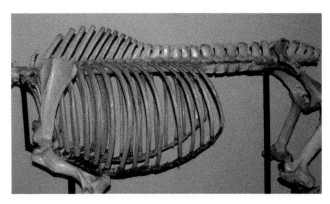

Figure 10.2 Lateral view of the 18 thoracic, six lumbar and five fused sacral vertebrae.

vertebrae have very long dorsal spinous processes (DSPs) with the exception of T1, and T2 is usually deep to the scapulae, therefore T3 is usually the first palpable DSP and forms the start of the withers. The lumbar vertebrae have very long horizontal transverse processes, with synovial joints frequently developing between the L4–L5 or L5–L6 transverse processes, sometimes eventually resulting in fusion (Figure 10.2). Variation of the lumbosacral junction is common, with variations occuring in around a third of horses, including sacralisation of the sixth lumbar vertebra or only five lumbar vertebrae (more common in Arabs) (Dyce *et al.* 2010a; Stubbs *et al.* 2006). The five sacral vertebrae are fused and S1 articulates with the ilium at the sacroiliac joint. The intervertebral discs in the horse are relatively thin, with a less distinct boundary between the nucleus pulposus and annulus fibrosis than in other species.

10.3 Neurological examination

There is increasing recognition of the role that animal physiotherapists can play in the treatment and rehabilitation of horses with neurological conditions, although it is less common than in small animal neurology. As for small animals, though, the veterinary-physiotherapy team approach is ideal. The diagnosis is obviously the realm of the veterinary surgeon, but physiotherapists should be able to recognise neurological signs and perform a neurological examination to localise or grade a lesion for reassessment if treatment is an option. Because of their size and temperament, horses with neurological disease can be particularly dangerous to people and themselves, especially if they are disorientated, ataxic or recumbent. Forebrain disease is often accompanied by blindness which adds to the horse's unpredictable behaviour. In some circumstances, such as encephalopathies or recumbency, only a reduced examination is possible. These conditions must be considered 'red flags' for physiotherapy assessment or treatment with prompt referral to the veterinary surgeon essential.

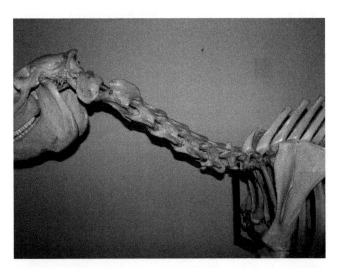

Figure 10.1 Lateral view of the cervical vertebrae of the horse. Vertebrae C1 (the 'atlas') and C2 (the 'axis') are different shapes from C2–7.

The primary aim of the neurological examination is to determine whether a neurological abnormality exists, and if it does then where it is located. Only when this has been achieved can a diagnosis be reached. The examiner should be careful not to rush in with a diagnosis or interpretation, but initially just describe the abnormality they see (e.g. unpredictable foot placement), and then interpret those findings (e.g. ataxia) once the examination is complete. Musculoskeletal and neurological diseases are sometimes challenging to tell apart, and can occur concurrently. For example, determining whether a gait abnormality is due to weakness, pain or both can often be difficult. It is essential that a physiotherapist is able to recognise neurological signs. It is not uncommon to have been asked to assess or treat a horse for what was thought to be a musculoskeletal condition when it was actually neurological, which should prompt immediate referral back to the veterinary surgeon.

10.3.1 Signalment and history
Initial collection of data, as for any other body system, is important and should include:

- patient signalment – age, sex, breed, use and sometimes value
- history of the presenting and any other medical conditions.

Signalment can help rule in or out some breed- or age-associated diseases. A complete general medical history is essential to ascertain the onset, progression and exact nature of the problem experienced by the owner. Some diseases affecting other body systems can have secondary neurological effects, and a complete history and physical examination are required to detect these. Once a diagnosis is reached, the use of the horse will often have a significant impact on the prognosis.

10.3.2 General physical examination
Prior to the neurological examination, a thorough general physical examination should be performed. Before entering the stable, the horse should be observed over the door and its mentation, posture and behaviour observed from a distance. Frequently, this is a neglected part of the examination which can yield useful information. Some neurological clinical signs (e.g. weakness, obtundation) are seen secondary to a wide range of diseases affecting other body systems. A thorough veterinary physical examination will help differentiate neurological from metabolic, cardiovascular and musculoskeletal disorders.

10.3.3 The neurological examination procedure
A consistent, complete and methodical approach to the neurological examination is essential. The most commonly adopted is the head-to-tail approach as described by Mayhew (2009).

A neurological examination form is essential to ensure that the examination is carried out in a thorough and methodical manner and that a full record of the examination is created. The examination should be performed in a quiet area free from distractions and initially in a space where low ambient light can be provided. An area of flat, hard ground with good footing for the horse, a soft area (field or manège) and ideally a slope are required for the dynamic examination.

10.3.4 Examination of the head
The procedure for examination of the head is outlined here and expanded upon under the individual cranial nerves below.

Examination of the head starts with observation of behaviour, mentation and posture from a distance. Obtundation, abnormal behaviour, seizure activity or a head tilt or turn can all be consistent with brain dysfunction. A closer examination of the head is performed next, which is best done standing directly in front of the horse so any asymmetry can easily be appreciated. The head and neck should be held in line with the rest of the vertebral column, and observed for a head tilt, which is rotation of the poll around the axis of the vertebral column. Symmetry of the shape and movement of the face should be observed. Olfactory function is difficult to assess in the horse, but offering two closed hands, one containing a mint and one without, can give an indication of bilateral loss of function. Unilateral loss of olfactory function is not normally detectable. Response to a noise with no visual stimulus (such as a hidden hand clap or a horse walking nearby) allows assessment of hearing, but again, unilateral loss of function is difficult to detect. The eyes are then examined for abnormal/asymmetrical eyelid or globe position and pupil size. The menace response from a temporal and nasal direction, dazzle reflex and pupillary light reflexes are all performed. The head is elevated to observe for abnormal eye position (strabismus) and then moved from side to side to look for normal, physiological nystagmus with the fast phase in the same direction as the head is moving.

Facial sensation is assessed using a blunt probe such as a ball point pen, and usually gentle stimulation is sufficient to gain a subtle response without annoying your patient. In severely obtunded horses, stimulation of the nasal septum and ear canal are most likely to elicit a response, and haemostats can be used for skin sensation. Tongue tone is tested by grasping the tongue via the interdental space (Figure 10.3), when muscle atrophy can also be assessed. Offering the horse a small feed allows any dysphagia to be recognised, and coughing and difficulty swallowing can indicate pharyngeal or laryngeal dysfunction.

The thoracolaryngeal response ('slap test') is performed by palpating the dorsolateral larynx with one hand and administering a firm slap over the contralateral withers with the other, during exhalation. If intact, the response will cause contraction of the abductor muscles of the arytenoids contralateral to the slap, which can be palpated with the fingers as a flick. The cervicofacial reflex is then performed by gently prodding the skin over the region of lateral C2–7 and observing for a twitching of the ipsilateral commisure of the lips.

Cranial nerve examination
There are only minor differences in cranial nerve anatomy and function between horses and other domestic species, and the

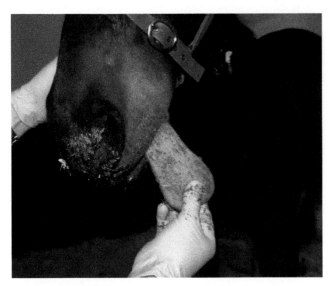

Figure 10.3 Tongue tone is assessed by pulling the tongue out of the interdental space, which the horse should replace easily. The horse in this image presented for dysphagia, and had markedly reduced tongue tone.

reader is referred to Chapter 9 for a full description of the cranial nerves. Assessment of the cranial nerves varies between species, however, and Table 10.1 lists how the major function of each cranial nerve can be assessed in the horse.

The head is entirely innervated by peripheral nerves branching directly from the brain, with the exception of the sympathic nervous system which exits the spinal cord at T1–3 and ascends the neck as the cervical sympathetic trunk. Further details of the clinical signs associated with loss of sympathetic innervation (Horner's syndrome) can be found later in this chapter.

10.3.5 Examination of the neck, trunk, limbs, tail and perineum

The horse is stood square and observed from all angles for posture and any asymmetry or muscle atrophy. The muscles and bony prominences of the neck, back and pelvis should be palpated for any pain or asymmetry. With the examiner standing to the side of the horse, cutaneous sensation is assessed along the neck at the level of each vertebra, dorsal and ventral to the transverse process using a blunt probe and assessing local skin reflexes and conscious awareness by the patient. In a very obtunded or stoical patient, pinching with haemostats might be required to elicit a response. From the withers to the tail head, skin sensation is tested over the paravertebral muscles, in the same manner. Caudally from the level of the elbow, the cutaneous trunci reflex is then assessed. Firm stimulation of the skin with a blunt probe (e.g. a finger tip) should elicit contraction of the cutaneous trunci muscle locally over the lateral thorax. The sensory branch of this reflex enters the spinal cord at the level of the cutaneous

Table 10.1 Assessment of cranial nerves in the horse

Cranial nerve		Principal function	Test of function
Olfactory	I	Smell	Response to smell
Optic	II	Sensory from retina to brain	Menace response, pupillary light reflex, dazzle response. Pupil dilation. Obstacle course
Oculomotor	III	Eye position and pupil constriction	Pupil size and symmetry Pupillary light reflex Eye position/movement
Trochlear	IV	Eye positon	Abnormal/asymmetrical eye position
Trigeminal	V	Sensory to head/face	Skin sensation over face, nasal cavity, eye
		Motor to muscle of mastication	Observe for dysphagia, jaw tone, atrophy of muscles of mastication
Abducens	VI	Eye position	Abnormal/asymmetrical eye position
Facial	VII	Muscles of facial expression	Facial symmetry – drooping ear/eyelid/lip, muzzle deviation, muscle tone. Facial reflexes, menace response. Feed packing in cheeks
		Lacrimation	Dry eye +/- corneal ulceration
Vestibulocochlear	VIII	Sensory to balance apparatus	Observe for head tilt, circling, ventral deviation of eye, abnormal nystagmus and ataxia Signs exacerbated by blindfolding (care as horse can fall over)
		Hearing	Response to sound
Glossopharyngeal	IX	Sensory and motor to pharynx	Swallowing feed/gag reflex with stomach tube. Endoscopy
Vagus	X	Sensory and motor to larynx	Swallowing feed, gag reflex, endoscopy. Upper respiratory sounds. Slap test
		Parasympathetic to thoracic and abdominal organs	Swallowing, heart rate, gastrointestinal motility
Accessory	XI	Motor to muscles in neck	Unclear, possibly cervical scoliosis or muscle atrophy
Hypoglossal	XII	Motor to tongue	Grasp tongue, assess tone and atrophy. Observe eating

stimulation, travels cranially to C8–T1 where the motor branch exits the spinal cord and innervates the cutaneous trunci muscle. The limbs are examined for muscle atrophy, and then skin sensation is tested (with care in the pelvic limbs).

A normal horse has good tail tone, which is assessed by grasping the dock at the base and moving it up and down. With the tail elevated, skin sensation around the perineum and anal reflexes can be assessed. Gentle stroking of the perineal skin usually causes the tail to lift, firmer stroking causes it to clamp down ventrally. Gentle prodding of the anus results in contraction of the anal sphincter and allows assessment of anal tone. Loss of these reflexes indicates damage to the sacrococcygeal spinal cord segments, nerves or the muscles they innervate. If such a lesion is suspected then a veterinary surgeon should perform a rectal examination to assess urinary and faecal incontinence.

10.3.6 Posture and gait examination in horses

Assessment of brainstem, spinal cord, peripheral nerve and muscle function in horses relies primarily on observation of movement and posture during normal gaits and in response to specific manoeuvres. The type of case most likely to be presented to an animal physiotherapist for examination or treatment is that in which the neurological abnormality affects gait rather than cranial nerves or mentation. The physical size of the horse precludes many of the tests for dogs outlined in Chapter 9, and care must be taken to ensure the safety of the handler and examiner.

The order of the examination will vary between individuals, but a complete examination with a consistent approach should be adopted for every patient. A full examination includes the following.

1 Walk and trot in a straight line observed from the back, front and side.
2 Walk in a straight line with the head elevated.
3 Back up for several paces.
4 Turn in tight circles in both directions. Lead the horse forward into a large (approximately 5 m diameter) circle initially and then gradually make tighter. Don't circle more than 4–5 times to avoid the horse becoming dizzy.
5 With the horse stood square, sharply pull on the tail to the side in both directions, then push on the shoulder in both directions.
6 While the horse is being walked forward in a straight line, pull on the tail to the side for 2–3 steps and then abruptly release (Figure 10.4).
7 Lead the horse forwards in a serpentine path by the examiner walking backwards so the thoracic limbs can be observed. Try and abruptly change direction during the swing phase.
8 Taking the lead rope and tail, simultaneously circle the horse tightly, assessing resistance to lateral pull, and then stop abruptly and observe recovery.
9 Walk the horse up and down a slope with a neutral head position (Figure 10.5). Repeat walking down the slope with the head raised.

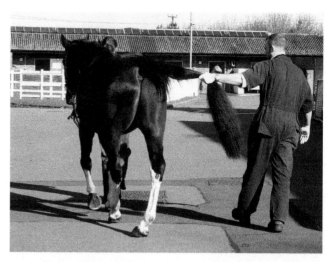

Figure 10.4 Pulling a horse's tail to the side while it walks as a test for UMN weakness and ataxia. The resistance to lateral pull and its recovery on releasing the tail are both assessed.

On a softer surface with good footing (grass paddock is ideal), perform the following.

1 Light each limb in turn, assess range of movement, and observe the contralateral limb during increased weight bearing.
2 While lifting each thoracic limb, push the horse away from the limb, causing the horse to hop on the contralateral limb (Figure 10.6).
3 In cases where visually compensated gait is suspected, gradually place a blindfold (e.g. towel around the head collar) and observe for any exacerbation of a head tilt or abnormal gait. Care should be taken as horses can fall over or behave unpredictably during this test.

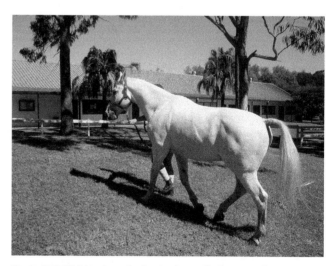

Figure 10.5 Walking down (and up) a slope will often exacerbate abnormalities in conscious proprioception (especially if the head is concurrently raised), weakness and gait abnormalities (hypermetria or hypometria).

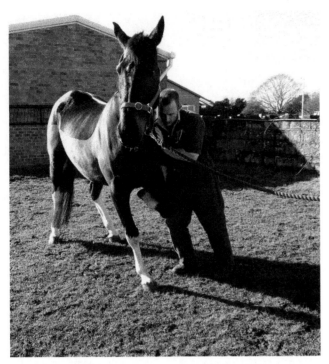

Figure 10.6 Picking up one forelimb results in increased weight bearing on the contralateral limb, causing exacerbation of signs associated with extensor weakness such as trembling. If the horse is not overtly weak then the examiner pushes the horse away, eliciting a hop.

10.4 Interpretation of the gait and posture examination

10.4.1 Lameness

'Lameness' is a term generally reserved for a gait abnormality caused by pain. As a general rule, lameness is a consistent and predictable gait abnormality, the same with every step, whereas neurological disease is generally inconsistent and less predictable (Table 10.2). Often they are difficult to tell apart and can occur concurrently. Assessing response to analgesia (nonsteroidal antiinflammatory trial) can determine the contribution

Table 10.2 Gait abnormalities are graded on a 0–4 scale similar to that originally proposed by Mayhew *et al.* (1978)

Grade	Classification of deficits
0	No neurological gait deficits detected; normal strength and coordination
1	Subtle – deficits just barely detected at normal gait, occur during backing, stopping, turning, swaying, neck extension, etc.
2	Mild – detected at normal gait, exaggerated by more complex manoeuvres
3	Moderate – prominent at normal gait, tend to buckle and fall with above techniques
4	Severe – tripping or falling spontaneously at normal gait

of pain, but objectively assessing the gait before and during analgesia can be difficult.

10.4.2 Weakness (paresis)

Weakness can be associated with dysfunction of UMN, LMN, neuromuscular junction or muscles. UMN weakness is almost always accompanied by proprioceptive deficits (ataxia) in the same limb, due to the proximity of the two spinal tracts. If there is marked weakness without ataxia evident in the same limb, then LMN or 'neuromuscular disease' may be suspected. LMN weakness causes more marked muscle atrophy than UMN. Neuromuscular weakness can be generalised (e.g. botulism) or localised to a single peripheral nerve (e.g. femoral nerve paralysis).

Specific tests for weakness (paresis) include the following.
- Look for hoof wear – dragging toes, low arc of flight of the hoof (more indicative of LMN weakness, low muscle tone).
- Tail pull – at rest (if unable to fix limb in extension more likely to be LMN) and during walking. With UMN weakness, horses are able to reflexly resist while standing still, but due to combination of ataxia and paresis, weakness in response to pulling the tail is more pronounced at the walk.
- Difficulty hopping, circling and walking on a slope, trembling and buckling of weak limb, knuckling over during walk/trot.
- Often simply picking up one leg will be all that is required to elicit trembling and buckling of the weight-bearing limb in a very weak horse.
- Note: horses with generalised weakness often 'walk better than they stand', i.e. they can't fix themselves in standing.

Interpretation
- If there is generalised weakness, with no ataxia and spasticity, neuromuscular disease should be suspected.
- If there is localised weakness, LMN or peripheral nerve disease should be suspected.
- If weakness and ataxia are both present, a UMN lesion affecting the descending motor pathway and ascending proprioceptive pathways is suspected.
- There can be apparent 'weakness' associated with vestibular disease as horses tend to fall or collapse towards the side of the lesion.

10.4.3 Ataxia

Ataxia is a lack of coordination of general body and limb movements. It normally presents as irregular and mostly unpredictable placement of the limbs, trunk, neck and head, especially during more complex manoeuvres. There are three types of ataxia: general proprioceptive, cerebellar and vestibular, according to the system affected and the presenting signs.

Specific tests for ataxia
- Observe for poor coordination, swaying, limb moving excessively during the swing phase – weaving, abduction, adduction, crossing of limbs and stepping on their own feet.

Table 10.3 Abnormalities versus region – once each limb has been assessed for the presence of ataxia, weakness and gait changes, this information can be used to localise the lesion

Region affected	Predominant signs
Brainstem/spinal cord white matter (UMN)	Ataxia, paresis, hypermetria (usually pelvic limbs), spastic hypometria (usually thoracic limbs)
Vestibular system	Ataxia, hypometria in all limbs
Cerebellum	Ataxia, hypermetria in all limbs, especially thoracic
Ventral grey matter or motor nerves (LMN)	Paresis, atrophy
Muscular system	Paresis, (hypometria)

LMN, lower motor neuron; UMN, upper motor neuron.

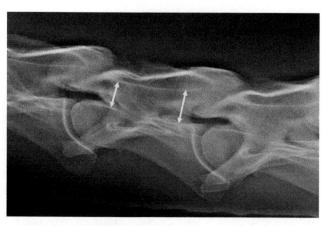

Figure 10.7 A lateral radiograph of cervical vertebrae C3–5. Note the vertebral canal, marked by double arrows.

- Abnormalities exaggerated by tight circles (pivoting, circumduction), serpentine walking, sudden stopping, backing, walking up or down a slope and raising the head.
- 'If on asking the question "Does this horse know where its limbs are relative to its body?" the answer is "No", then it is likely to be displaying general proprioceptive ataxia' (de Lahunta & Glass 2009).

10.4.4 Other gait abnormalities (Table 10.3)
- Hypermetria refers to increased range of limb flight, usually associated with increased muscle tone and hyperreflexia, and may be accentuated by ataxia.
- Hypometria refers to decreased range of limb flight. If a horse is hypometric, it may be due to either low muscle tone/weakness (LMN) or increased muscle tone and spasticity (UMN).
- Dysmetria refers to either hyper- or hypometria or a combination, i.e. an abnormal range of limb flight.

10.5 Further diagnostic techniques

10.5.1 Radiographs
When compared to smaller animals, the horse's vertebral canal does not lend itself well to radiography, due to the large mass of soft tissue surrounding it. In all but the smallest equids, the vertebral canal can only be imaged in lateral or lateral oblique projections from C1 to T1 or T2 (Figure 10.7). Using high-output equipment, dorsoventral views can be obtained from C1 to C5 (Butler *et al.* 2008). However, in the standing horse this is normally too dangerous for the horse and equipment. Lateral, dorsoventral and oblique radiographs of the head can be obtained for assessment of the bony structures associated with the nervous system. In foals and small ponies, diagnostic radiographs of the thoracolumbar and sacral vertebral canal are sometimes possible, but are often low quality with superimposition of other structures (Figure 10.8).

Cervical radiographs are most commonly indicated when stenosis of the vertebral canal is suspected. Sometimes radiographical lesions are obviously associated with neurological signs, (e.g. some fractures/subluxation), but in many cases the stenosis will be due to more subtle developmental or acquired radiographic abnormalities.

10.5.2 Myelography
Myelography involves the injection of positive contrast agent into the vertebral canal, usually in order to detect sites of compression (Figure 10.9). In the horse, myelography is generally performed under general anaesthesia. The technique does,

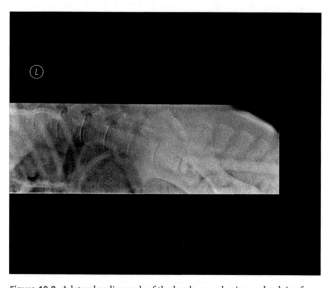

Figure 10.8 A lateral radiograph of the lumbosacral spine and pelvis of a foal. Note the superimposition of the abdominal contents on the vertebrae. This foal presented with neurological signs in the hindlimbs. There is a radiolucency in the cranial vertebral body of the first sacral vertebra, caused by a septic physitis.

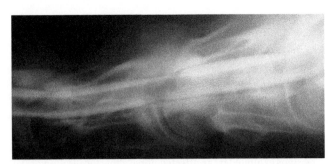

Figure 10.9 A lateral myelogram of C5–6 of a yearling Thoroughbred showing narrowing of the vertebral canal at C5–6.

however, have limitations for the detection of cervical stenosis (van Biervliet *et al.* 2004).

10.5.3 Computed tomography (CT) and magnetic resonance imaging (MRI)

Both these advanced imaging techniques allow three-dimensional imaging of the head and cervical spine – the caudal limit depending on the size of the horse, whether it is under general anaesthesia and the equipment available. With specialist equipment, CT images of the entire cervical spine have been obtained in horses up to 670 kg (Kristoffersen *et al.* 2014). Generally speaking, CT gives the best detail for bony structures (Figure 10.10) and MRI for soft tissue (such as brain).

10.5.4 Routine blood analysis

This can be useful for the investigation of some neurological conditions, especially infectious or inflammatory conditions, and metabolic diseases affecting the neurological system such as hepatic encephalopathy and electrolyte disturbances. Analysis of muscle enzymes (e.g. creatine kinase (CK) and aspartate transaminase (AST)) and urinalysis for myoglobinuria are particularly useful for investigation of myopathies.

10.5.5 Cerebrospinal fluid (CSF) analysis

Cerebrospinal fluid is a clear, colourless fluid which bathes the central nervous system. Collection and analysis are indicated in undiagnosed neurological disease localised to the central nervous system. It is collected from the subarachoid space, usually from the lumbosacral space in the standing horse (Figure 10.11) or from the atlantooccipital space in the anaesthetised horse. The procedure is technically demanding and not without risk to the horse. CSF analysis may also be a useful indicator of inflammatory or haemorrhagic CNS conditions, and detection of specific antibodies or infectious agents can help support an infectious diagnosis.

10.6 Equine neurological diseases

10.6.1 Forebrain disease

As for small animals, forebrain disease in horses is a big red flag for physiotherapists and veterinary attention should be sought

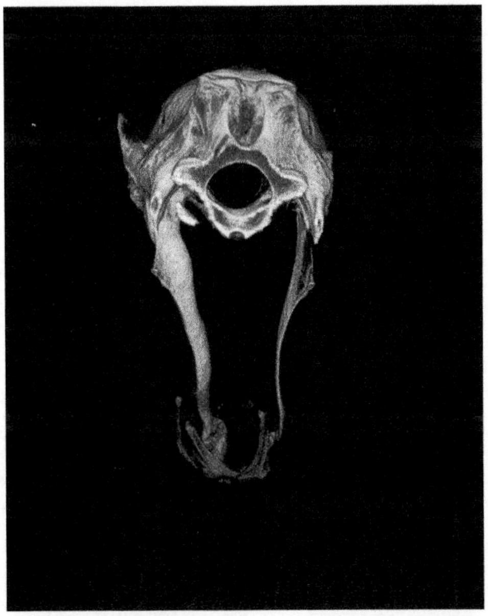

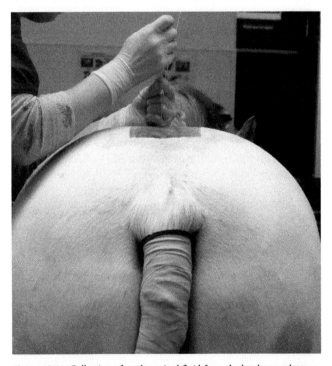

Figure 10.10 A caudal view of a volume-rendered, 3D CT reconstruction of the skull and hyoid apparatus in a horse which presented for left-sided facial nerve paralysis and vestibular signs. The left stylohyoid bone is markedly thickened, consistent with a diagnosis of left-sided temporohyoid osteoarthropathy.

Figure 10.11 Collection of cerebrospinal fluid from the lumbosacral space in a standing, sedated horse.

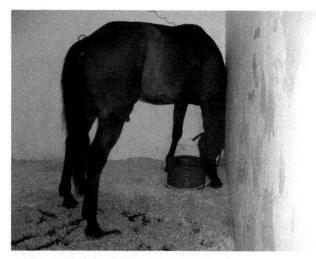

Figure 10.12 A horse with severe forebrain signs, demonstrating head pressing. The horse had forebrain dysfunction secondary to liver disease (hepatic encephalopathy). Thirty minutes before head pressing, the horse was only mildly obtunded.

immediately for any characteristic signs of abnormal mentation or depression (Figure 10.12). Some horses might start by appearing quiet and depressed but suddenly develop maniacal behaviour or seizures.

10.6.2 Brainstem and cranial nerve disease

Several brainstem/cranial nerve disorders occurring in horses may well be amenable to physiotherapy in their treatment. This section will focus on facial nerve paralysis and vestibular disease, which occur reasonably frequently. Clinical signs of dysfunction of other cranial nerves are described above.

Brainstem lesions are most commonly caused by trauma, but some infectious neurological diseases such as equine herpes virus-1 (EHV-1) or equine protozoal myeloencephalitis (EPM) can be causative. A common traumatic injury to the brainstem is caused by a horse rearing, going over backwards and striking its poll on the ground, causing a basilar skull fracture.

Horner's syndrome will also be discussed in this section, as, although it is a deficit of the sympathetic nerve supply to the head and not a specific cranial nerve or brainstem lesion, anatomically its signs manifest in the same region and it needs to be differentiated from eye abnormalities caused by specific cranial nerve deficits.

Facial nerve paralysis

Injury to this cranial nerve is relatively common in horses. The peripheral nerve initially passes through the petrous temporal bone, making it susceptible to fractures of this bone or coexisting middle ear disease. The distal nerve has branches which are superficial and can be injured by external trauma. General anaesthesia in lateral recumbency without removal of the head collar is a common cause of facial nerve paralysis, owing to the position of the buckle directly over buccal branches of the nerve.

The vestibulocochlear nerve and proximal part of the facial nerve share a close anatomical relationship and so are often affected by the same lesion. They arise close together in the brainstem and both traverse the petrous temporal bone. Injuries to this area may cause injury and clinical signs involving both nerves.

Clinical signs of facial nerve dysfunction

The signs exhibited by an affected horse allow localisation of the lesion, which is important when determining the aetiology and prognosis. Deficits are only seen distal to the site of the lesion.

1 Facial nerve lesions on the side of the face/mandible cause deviation of nares and muzzle away from the lesion, and drooping of lower lip and feed packing in the cheeks on the same side.
2 Lesions between stylomastoid foramen (exit from skull) and mandible – cause signs in (1) above with ear and eyelid droop (Figure 10.13).
3 Petrous temporal bone lesions (within skull) – cause signs in (2) above, loss of lacrimation +/- vestibular nerve signs.
4 Brainstem lesions – cause signs in (3) above, usually accompanied by other cranial nerve deficits, ataxia and obtundation.

Horses with facial nerve paralysis with prolonged/permanent deficits can have serious complications including:

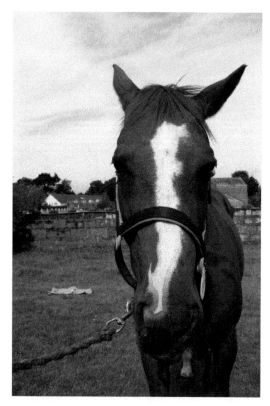

Figure 10.13 A horse with left-sided facial nerve paralysis. Note the drooping left ear and upper eyelid and muzzle deviation to the right.

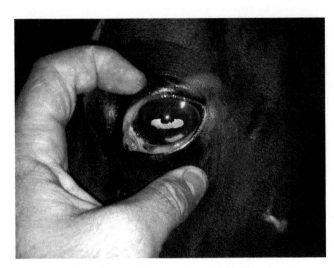

Figure 10.14 The left eye of the horse in Figure 10.13. There is a fluorescein-positive corneal ulcer with secondary anterior uveitis, caused by the facial nerve paralysis. This horse had left-sided temporohyoid osteoarthropathy.

- eye injury, dry eye, causing ulceration +/- secondary uveitis (due to loss of lacrimation and eyelid paralysis) (Figure 10.14)
- dysphagia and feed packing in cheeks
- poor performance – due to nostril collapse
- severe eye disease and nostril collapse may cause the end of an athletic career for some horses.

Treatment

Limiting further damage to the nerve is the first priority, by stabilising bony fractures and/or administering antiinflammatory medication or antimicrobials. With a proximal lesion, the effects of reduced lacrimation and upper eyelid dysfunction are ameliorated by frequent application of artificial tears and sometimes a temporary tarsorrhaphy (suturing the eyelid closed). Massaging impacted feed from the cheeks helps avoid putrid feed building up and periodontal disease. Longer term treatment is focused on limiting neurogenic atrophy and fibrous contracture of the affected muscle groups, and consultation with a veterianry physiotherapist is recommended.

Prognosis

There are three categories of peripheral nerve injury which apply to all peripheral nerves, including the cranial nerves, which are described later in this chapter (10.6.5). Prognosis depends on which of these is present.

Vestibular disease

As for small animals, vestibular disease is classified as peripheral if the lesion affects the nerve after it leaves the brainstem, or central if it affects the brainstem. Central vestibular disease is normally accompanied by other signs of brainstem dysfunction such as obtundation, other cranial nerve deficits and ataxia.

Trauma, otitis media and interna and ankyloses of the temporohyoid joint with subsequent fracture of the petrous temporal bone (temporohyoid osteoarthropathy – THO) are the most common causes of vestibular dysfunction in horses. Unlike in small animals, it rarely occurs as an extension from external ear infections (otitis externa). Part of the cerebellum and the cranial cervical dorsal nerve roots have input to the vestibular nucleus and so lesions in these structures can also result in vestibular signs.

Clinical signs and treatment

Clinical signs can vary from subtle to very severe. In milder dysfunction, horses have the ability to compensate visually, particularly in chronic/long-standing cases. Vestibular disease should be considered in horses that are reported to be 'one-sided' when ridden, and has also been associated with head shaking (Blythe 1997a). Other signs of unilateral vestibular dysfunction are a head tilt (Figure 10.15), ataxia, with a tendency to circle or drift towards the side of the lesion, ventral deviation of the eyeball and nystagmus, although this usually only lasts for 24–48 hours. Blindfolding (or moving from light to dark) is an important part of the neurological examination, but should be performed cautiously as the horse can fall over. If vestibular disease is suspected, look for evidence of facial nerve paralysis as well.

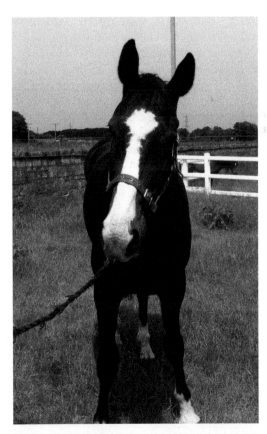

Figure 10.15 A horse with left-sided peripheral vestibular dysfunction. Note rotation to the left of the poll around the spine (left-sided head tilt), and the wide-based stance.

To evaluate the area further, endoscopy of the guttural pouches (to visualise the stylohyoid bone and temporohyoid joint), and radiography or CT of the head are advised. Physiotherapy could be considered in vestibular cases to maintain extensor strength in the limbs of the affected side.

Prognosis

Prognosis depends on the degree of initial and ongoing damage to the vestibular apparatus and vestibulocochlear nerve. In general, cases caused by infection or THO have a worse prognosis than those caused by trauma (Mayhew 2009). As mentioned before, horses can visually accommodate mild non-progressive vestibular dysfunction very well, and some cases can return to ridden work.

10.6.3 Horner's syndrome

Loss of sympathetic innervation to the head and neck is termed Horner's syndrome. Sympathetic innervation of the head and neck exits the spinal cord at T1–3. The close anatomical association between the cranial cervical ganglion and the guttural pouch means that they can be affected by the same lesion.

Clinical signs of unilateral Horner's syndrome in horses are ipsilateral miosis (abnormal constriction of the pupil), ptosis (drooping of the upper eyelid), mild enophthalmos and protrusion of the third eyelid and unilateral cutaneous vasodilation and sweating (Figure 10.16). Swelling of the nasal mucosa can cause reduced air flow through the nostril on the affected side. The caudal extent of the sweating depends on the location of the lesion. Sweating from the midline of the face to the level of C2 (Figure 10.17) is consistent with a lesion anywhere along the cervical trunk, whereas sweating with its caudal extent at the base of the neck indicates that the spinal nerves and/or cervicothoracic ganglion is affected. Lesions in the descending sympathetic tracts in the spinal cord very rarely occur in isolation and will almost always be accompanied by other, more obvious signs of spinal cord disease.

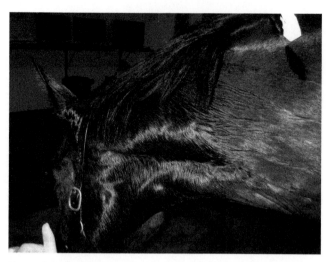

Figure 10.17 Sweating to approximately the level of C2 caused by perivascular injection of xylazine. The horse also had left-sided ptosis and miosis consistent with Horner's syndrome.

A common cause of Horner's syndrome is perivascular injection of substances in the jugular groove and the subsequent inflammatory reaction affecting the sympathetic trunk as it travels deep to the jugular vein. If Horner's syndrome is evident from a perivascular injection reaction, the larynx should be endoscoped as the recurrent laryngeal nerve runs with the vagosympathetic trunk and could result in development of laryngeal hemiplegia or roaring. Function often returns to the sympathetic trunk after perivascular injections. In more chronic cases of Horner's syndrome, horses normally adapt well and there are minimal complications.

10.6.4 Spinal cord disease

Most spinal cord disease in horses is caused by external compression. With increasing compression, more functional deficits occur, usually in the following order.
- Loss of proprioception
- Upper motor neuron weakness
- Loss of sensory perception, touch
- Loss of pain

Clinical signs include ataxia, postural deficits, paresis, hypermetria, hypometria and recumbency (tetraparesis) in severe lesions. Lower motor neuron signs of weakness and areflexia will be seen in the thoracic limb with lesions located between C6 and T2 and the pelvic limb for lesions between L4 and S3. The forelimbs are often less severely affected than the hindlimbs with cervical spinal cord and brainstem lesions.

In Australia and the UK, the majority of equine spine lesions are the result of trauma or cervical vertebral malformation-malarticulation (CVM). In the USA, equine protozoal myelitis (EPM) is also very common. Other diseases include congenital malformations (e.g. atlantooccipital/axial malformation in Arabians), infection (e.g. EHV-1), degenerative myelo(encephalo)pathies and neoplasia.

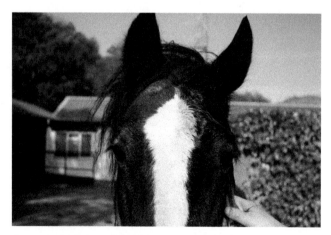

Figure 10.16 Unilateral left-sided sweating over the face and left-sided ptosis caused by Horner's syndrome.

Spinal trauma

Spinal trauma is relatively common in the horse. Of 450 horses examined for neurological disease in one study, 119 were due to trauma and of these 60 were localised to the spine (Tyler *et al.* 1993). Spinal trauma usually presents with a history of sudden onset of ataxia or recumbency, and only sometimes is the incident observed. If there is not an unstable fracture, there may be no progression and frequently improvement, although later compression of the spinal cord may occur due to callus formation. Trauma may play a role in the acute exacerbation of CVM, i.e. the horse is already neurologically abnormal, more likely to fall, and only after acute exacerbation do the owners notice the abnormalities.

The cervical spine is the region most commonly injured (Tyler *et al.* 1993; Williams *et al.* 2003). Other areas can also be injured; fracture of the mid back usually requires considerable force and frequently results in an unstable fracture, paraplegia and recumbency (dog sitting). Spinal shock and Schiff–Sherrington phenomenon should be considered in equine spinal trauma but are poorly described compared to other species (Mayhew 2009).

Management

Management usually includes analgesia, antiinflammatory therapy (non-steroidal), box rest if standing, and nursing care. Use of corticosteroids remains controversial in spinal cord injury (Tennent-Brown 2007). Surgical stabilisation or decompression has been described and can be considered in some cases. In the great majority of cases, manipulation of vertebrae is contraindicated, but successful treatment has been described in a foal with atlantooccipital and atlantoaxial dislocation (Licka 2002).

Recumbency presents particular challenges. Turning and taking care of a recumbent horse are difficult and a 24-hour-a-day concern (Figure 10.18). The rule of thumb is that serious myositis will occur following 6 h of lateral recumbency in a large animal (Cox *et al.* 1982; Nout & Reed 2005). They are also susceptible to pressure sores, urine scalding, ocular damage and other problems of recumbency seen in other species (Nout & Reed 2005).

Prognosis

Prognosis is guarded, but remarkable recoveries have been made. Prognosis is generally worse with luxations, unstable fractures, poor initial response to treatment (24–48 h) or continued recumbency.

Cervical vertebral malformation-malarticulation (CVM)

This is a common cause of cervical spinal cord compression, resulting in proprioceptive ataxia and UMN weakness. A confusing array of alternative names have been used for CVM, including cervical vertebral stenotic myelopathy (CVSM), cervical vertebral compressive myelopathy (CVCM), cervical spondylotic myelopathy and cervical vertebral instability (CVI). CVM is sometimes referred to as 'wobbler syndrome' but this term should be avoided as it is non-specific, also being used to refer to ataxia or wobbliness in the horse from any cause.

Cervical vertebral malformation-malarticulation can be divided into two types (Mayhew 2009). Type I CVM is a form of developmental orthopaedic disease (DOD), and normally occurs in younger horses (0–2 years). Various deformities of the cervical vertebrae and their articulations are included in type I CVM, and it generally affects the midcervical region. CVM foals tend to be heavier and taller during some time intervals than normal foals, but there were no significant differences between the two groups in any of the skeletal growth measurements. Bodyweight gain was faster in CVM foals from 31 to 60 days (Ruff *et al.* 1993).

Type II CVM tends to present in older horses, caused by enlargement of the articular processes secondary to osteoarthritis. C5–6 and C6–7 are most commonly affected (Levine *et al.* 2007).

Any age or breed can be affected, but risk factors that have been identified include young, males, Thoroughbreds, Quarterhorses and Warmbloods, and rapid growth. It is estimated that 1–3% of Thoroughbreds are affected (Oswald *et al.* 2010). Aetiology is multifactorial but includes congenital, familial, dietary and managemental (including exercise) factors.

Signs of spinal cord disease occur with progressive ataxia and paresis in all four limbs, most notable in the pelvic limbs (or only in pelvic limbs in chronic cases). Onset is usually gradual but there may be acute exacerbation after an injury. Neck pain is rarely seen.

Diagnosis

Veterinary diagnostic work-up typically includes lesion localisation and plain radiography. Plain radiography is often the only additional diagnostic procedure that is required to reach a diagnosis. Lesions may include stenosis of the vertebral canal (dynamic or static), abnormal articular processes, angular deformity of vertebrae on flexion (C2–5) or extension (C5–T1) of

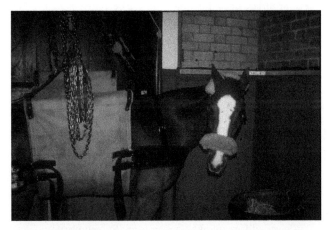

Figure 10.18 A horse with a traumatic thoracic spinal cord lesion being managed using a sling. Splinting of the pelvic limbs and bales of straw and shavings were also used in an attempt to support the mare.

the neck, enlarged vertebral physeal growth regions, overriding of the vertebral arch and next caudal vertebral body causing dynamic stenosis during flexion or extension, or proliferation of articular and periarticular soft tissues (Mayhew 2009). Plain lateral radiographs can be used to identify stenosis of the cervical vertebral canal by calculating the minimal intra- and intervertebral sagittal diameter ratios, which correct for the size of the horse and for magnification (Hahn *et al.* 2008). It is doubtful whether myelography has any advantage over sagittal diameter ratios from plain radiographs for diagnosing CVM (Mayhew & Green 2000; van Biervliet *et al.* 2004). It is, however, recommended in order to confirm the site of stenosis prior to surgical intervention (Mayhew 2009).

Management

Early detection in young foals (6 months) and dietary restriction have resulted in resolution of ataxia and successful racing careers (Donawick *et al.* 1993). Rest and systemic or intraarticular anti-inflammatory medication are used, particularly for type II CVM where there is soft tissue swelling associated with osteoarthritis of the intervertebral articulations. Once disease is advanced, prognosis for a suitable riding animal is poor. The fundamental problem is that a horse with any degree of ataxia should not be ridden.

Surgical intervertebral fusion has been performed and produced some promising results in early, mild cases of CVM (Walmsley 2005).

Cauda equina syndrome

Cauda equina syndrome (CES) describes lesions involving the sacrococcygeal spinal cord segments, cauda equina, sacral plexus and peripheral nerves to the bladder, rectum, anus, tail and perineum. CES may or may not involve lumbosacral nerve roots to the lumbosacral plexus producing gait abnormalities.

Signs

Signs are predominantly LMN of the tail, anus and perineal region presenting as various degrees of hypotonia, hyporeflexia and hypalgesia of the tail, anus and perineal region. There may be urinary bladder paresis, rectal dilation and penile prolapse.

There may also be LMN weakness and paresis of pelvic limbs tending to result in a 'dog sitting' posture or recumbency. In these cases it can be difficult to distinguish from UMN disease with urinary retention and secondary contusion of tail and anus from recumbency.

Causes

Causes of CES include:

- trauma, e.g. sacrococcygeal fracture and luxation, avulsion of the cauda equina. There may be a history of rearing and falling on the rump or backing into a wall with the tail raised
- infections, inflammatory, immune, e.g. polyneuritis equi, EHV-1

- toxicity, e.g. *Sorghum* spp. ingestion
- congenital anomalies
- neoplasia.

Equine herpes virus-1 myeloencephalopathy is an uncommon manifestation of EHV-1 infection, which more commonly causes respiratory disease and abortion. The neurological form may occur sporadically or as an outbreak. There may be a recent history of abortion or respiratory disease among in-contact horses, and pyrexia and/or swollen limbs often precede neurological signs in an individual (Henninger *et al.* 2007). Affected horses normally develop sudden-onset signs of CES including ataxia, paresis and urinary incontinence, with early stabilisation of signs. Some animals can be maintained with good nursing care including bladder catheterisation, faecal evacuation and physiotherapy during recovery. Recovery can take months to years. Prognosis is better if the animal remains standing, owing to the complications of recumbency.

Equine protozoal myelitis (EPM)

This disease predominantly occurs in North America, and is exotic to Australia and the UK as these countries lack the definitive hosts (small carnivores) required to complete the life cycle of the parasite. The two known infectious agents that cause EPM are protozoan parasites called *Sarcocystis neurona* and *Neospora hughei*, for which the horse is an aberrant host.

The disease can affect any part of the CNS (UMN, LMN), causing selective focal, multifocal or more widespread lesions. A hallmark of the parasitic disease is asymmetrical lesions, or a combination of UMN and LMN signs. Diagnosis is challenging and is by compatible clinical signs, supported by testing of serum and CSF for antibodies. Not all horses infected with these protozoa develop neurological disease, which complicates interpretation of antibody concentrations. With treatment, most horses will improve by at least one neurological grade, and with early, prolonged therapy the prognosis for a full recovery is good (Furr 2008). Depending on the neurological lesion, physiotherapy may be appropriate once the protozoa have been inactivated.

10.6.5 Neuromuscular disease

Disease of the neuromuscular unit can involve the LMN, the neuromuscular junction or the muscle, and some aspects of the clinical presentation of these can be very similar. Abnormalities in muscle contraction, including tetany and weakness, can also occur as part of an underlying metabolic problem rather than a primary neuromuscular disease. Differentiation is possible with a thorough veterinary diagnostic work-up.

Signs

- Weakness – which may be localised or diffuse.
  - Diffuse weakness can be episodic.
  - Severe diffuse weakness may result in recumbency.
- Increased tone, e.g. myotonia, tetany, spasm, synchronous diaphragmatic flutter.

- Muscle atrophy, which is particularly severe with LMN lesions.
- Abnormal gait due to:
  - decreased muscle contraction/range of movement
  - increased muscle contraction, e.g. stringhalt type gaits with stringhalt and equine motor neuron disease (EMND).
- Muscular pain.

Equine neuromuscular disorders may be grouped according to the major clinical presentations. These are localised weakness, abnormal hindlimb gait, diffuse weakness and localised or generalised muscle contraction.

Localised weakness

Peripheral neuropathies are the most common cause of localised weakness. However, localised weakness and atrophy can also occur as a result of inflammatory myositis and have been described in the neck (Barrott *et al.* 2004), back (Sponseller *et al.* 2005) and masseter muscles (Schefer *et al.* 2011). These are diagnosed by muscle biopsy. Localised weakness might also need differentiating from orthopaedic disease. For example, radial nerve paralysis and fracture of the olecranon both result in an inability to extend the elbow and can initially have a similar presentation.

Peripheral neuropathies

Peripheral neuropathies are usually traumatic in origin, although in horses they commonly occur after prolonged general anaesthesia with poor positioning and long surgical times and are associated with a type of compartment syndrome (Lindsay *et al.* 1989).

In the pelvic limb, sciatic nerve injury results in reduced flexion of the stifle and hock, and flexion of the fetlock. It can occur due to inappropriate injection of irritant drugs over the nerve, especially in foals. Femoral nerve injury results in lack of stifle extension. Obturator nerve injury may occur during parturition and results in loss of adductor function. It is particularly common in cattle associated with injury during calving.

In the thoracic limb, damage to the brachial plexus will result in loss of extension of the entire limb (Figure 10.19). Branches of the brachial plexus include the suprascapular nerve, radial nerve, axillary nerve and musculocutaneous nerve. Injury over the point of the shoulder can specifically damage the suprascapular nerve, resulting in atrophy and dysfunction of the supraspinatus and infraspinatus muscles, termed 'sweeney'. Radial nerve paralysis commonly occurs post anaesthesia or from trauma, particularly as part of brachial plexus injury. Depending on the level affected, it results in a lack of elbow, carpus and fetlock extension.

Diagnosis of peripheral nerve injuries relies on accurate localisation of clinical signs and is supported/monitored by mapping areas of reduced skin sensation or use of an electromyogram. However, skin dermatomes in the horse are difficult to detect as areas are smaller than in man and inconsistent in response (Blythe 1997b).

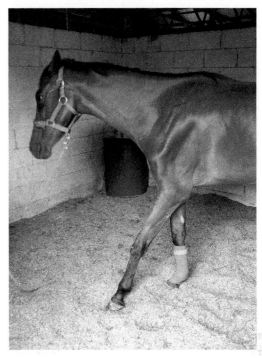

Figure 10.19 Horse with brachial plexus injury of 4 weeks' duration. Note the marked atrophy. This horse recovered fully with extensive teamwork rehabilitation by a veterinarian and physiotherapist.

Treatment

Medical treatment initially includes antiinflammatory medication. It is vital to ensure the contralateral limb is supported and monitored in horses that are non-weight bearing. Splinting may be indicated to assist in weight bearing, in radial nerve paralysis for example. Surgery may be indicated especially in chronic, adhered suprascapular nerve paralysis. Physiotherapy is indicated (see Chapter 17) to reduce the contracture and fibrosis and subsequent loss of function in denervated muscles (Figure 10.20).

There are three categories of peripheral nerve injury. Determining which is present usually depends on whether function returns within 2–4 weeks.
- *Neurapraxia* (temporary loss of function only, with no permanent structural damage). Function returns spontaneously over hours to days, usually within 3–4 weeks of injury.
- *Axonotmesis* (severance of axons, but with preservation of the myelin sheath). This is normally the worst outcome for closed injuries with no underlying fractures. The axon degenerates distally and then regenerates at approximately 1 mm/day.
- *Neurotmesis* (severance of the entire nerve fibre). This occurs only when there is open trauma or fractures with sharp fragments which can lacerate the nerve. There is denervation and regeneration of both the axon and the myelin sheath.

In both axonotmesis and neurotmesis, nerve regeneration occurs at approximately 1 mm/day. A better return to function is usually expected with axonotmesis but prognosis is guarded

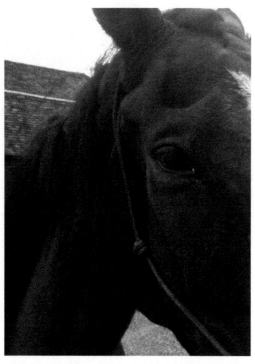

Figure 10.20 Chronic trigeminal nerve paralysis causing marked neurogenic atrophy of the muscles of mastication on the right side. This horse also had total loss of sensation to the right side of its face, consistent with loss of trigeminal nerve function.

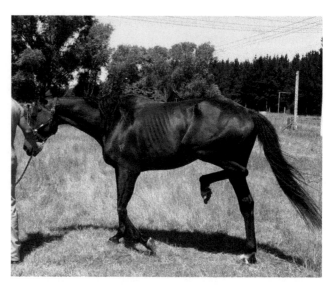

Figure 10.21 A Thoroughbred with Australian or pasture-associated stringhalt. Note the hyperflexed left pelvic limb.

with both, especially with complete loss of function. Restoration of neural pathways and maintaining muscle function and length in the affected groups are the priorities of management in peripheral nerve injury. Limiting damage to other structures and development of compensatory mechanisms are also often required. Scarring, fibrous tissue or callus formation may lead to permanent worsening of nerve injury. Physiotherapy plays an important role in the management of peripheral nerve injury.

Abnormal hindlimb gait
Shivers

Affected horses have muscle spasms that generally affect one or both pelvic limbs and the tail. The horse will generally lift the affected pelvic limbs, holding each up or shifting, while muscle fasciculation occurs. The tail is normally elevated, and muscle fasciculation may occur along the trunk.

Shivering can be incited with backing, lifting one limb and excitement, and a common history involves difficulty shoeing the hind feet. It most often occurs in tall, young male horses and in most cases signs are progressive (Draper *et al.* 2015). The cause is unknown and diagnosis is based on clinical signs and exclusion of other diseases. Treatment is based around dietary modification, but prognosis is guarded to poor.

Stringhalt

There are two forms of stringhalt – 'classic' or 'sporadic' and 'Australian' or 'pasture associated'.

Signs

Signs involve sudden, excessive flexion and adduction of one (classic) or both (Australian) pelvic limbs (Draper *et al.* 2015) (Figure 10.21). Signs are usually worse when backing and turning. Classic stringhalt frequently occurs after an injury (Crabill *et al.* 1994).

Australian stringhalt is a neurological disease due to a toxin, probably found in flatweed (*Hypocaeris radicata*) (Araujo *et al.* 2008). It frequently occurs as an outbreak, especially during hot dry weather and on poor pastures, and has been reported in several countries, but particularly in Australia and New Zealand. The lesion is a peripheral neuropathy (axonopathy) affecting branches of the sciatic and also the recurrent laryngeal nerve (Slocombe *et al.* 1992). Both forms of stringhalt may respond to surgical therapy (myotenectomy, removal of about 10 cm of the lateral digital extensor tendon).

Prognosis

Australian stringhalt often results in marked generalised atrophy and prolonged recovery but eventual improvement usually occurs (Domange *et al.* 2010). Classic stringhalt may result in permanent gait abnormalities.

Diffuse weakness

There are many causes of diffuse weakness including:
- neurological disease, e.g. equine motor neuron disease
- metabolic disease, e.g. hyperkalaemic periodic paralysis, equine polysaccharide storage myopathy
- neuromuscular toxins, e.g. botulism, ionophore toxicity.

The role of the physiotherapist in these conditions is in management of recumbency and rehabilitation during recovery (Nout & Reed 2005). Some examples of diseases are presented below.

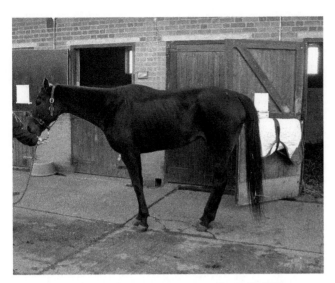

Figure 10.22 A horse with equine motor neuron disease (EMND) exhibiting diffuse muscle atrophy and generalised weakness, demonstrated by his narrow-based stance, elevated tail head and low head carriage.

Equine motor neuron disease (EMND)

This is an acquired neurodegenerative disease associated with oxidative damage to lower motor neurons (Cummings *et al.* 1990). It affects adult horses and there have been worldwide reports. Initial reports tended to occur in horses deprived of green forage, but it has also been reported to occur in pastured horses (McGorum *et al.* 2006).

Signs

These include weight loss due to muscle wasting, muscle fasciculation, particularly in the postural muscle while standing, elevated tail head and prolonged periods of recumbency. (Divers *et al.* 2006) (Figure 10.22). Appetite is normal or increased. Horses are often said to move better than they stand, and the gait will show signs of weaknesss but no ataxia.

Treatment

Treatment is usually attempted using high doses of vitamin E (5000–7000 IU/day orally) as well as dietary addition of green pasture or alfalfa (lucerne) hay versus grass hay.

Prognosis

The prognosis is guarded to poor. Cases may either continue to progress, resulting in recumbency and euthanasia, improve after 3–6 weeks (but are at risk of relapse) or stabilise but remain weak and/or emaciated and develop further gait abnormalities, e.g. stringhalt, that eventually result in euthanasia (Divers *et al.* 2001). In this third group, adjunctive physiotherapy has been used with success (McGowan, personal communication) and this is an area for further research.

Botulism

Botulism is caused by the toxin of the bacterium *Clostridium botulinum*, which interferes with the release of acetylcholine at the neuromuscular junction of both skeletal and smooth muscle. It often occurs in outbreaks, which can devastate a herd.

The disease is most commonly associated with spoiled forage (e.g. poor-quality silage) (Whitlock & McAdams 2006). Botulism can also be associated with multiplication and elaboration of toxin in an animal, especially in foals (toxicoinfectious botulism) where it multiplies in the gut, or in wounds if appropriate anaerobic conditions are present.

Clinical signs

Clinical signs are normally progressive and include dysphagia, weakness, recumbency and faecal and urinary incontinence. Horses may also present with colic. The disease in foals is often referred to as 'shaker foal' due to the pronounced muscle tremors when the foal tries to stand. The 'botulism grain test' and 'tongue strain test' can both be used to detect early cases (Whitlock & McAdams 2006).

Treatment

Treatment involves supportive care and antitoxin where available.

Prognosis

Prognosis is poor for adult horses if they are unable to stand (Johnson *et al.* 2015). Management of mild cases may be rewarding, especially if antitoxin is available. Intensively treated foals can have a very good prognosis (Wilkins & Palmer 2003). Nursing care is critical to successful treatment. Physiotherapy would be appropriate to consider during recovery of muscle function.

Postanaesthetic myoneuropathy

This occurs particularly in fit performance horses, but any large animal is at risk of developing prolonged recumbency, tetraparesis or monoparesis after general anaesthesia. Compartmental pressure elevations, ischaemia of muscle, pressure neuropathy and reperfusion injury are all thought to be involved.

Treatment includes rest with or without slinging and medical support (fluids, antiinflammatory medication, dantrolene). While recovery is often good with more localised lesions, generalised myoneuropathy has a poor prognosis. There is a role for physiotherapy and undetermined strategies, but intervention would need to be aggressive.

Hyperkalaemic periodic paralysis (HYPP)

This inherited disease affects young adult Quarterhorses of Impressive lineage (Impressive was a prolific Quarterhorse stallion in the 1970s and 1980s). A mutation of the muscle sodium channel gene causes muscle hyperexcitability, and affected horses have episodic trembling, sweating and weakness, often associated with exercise or stress. The disease is an autosomal dominant inherited trait with an identifiable genetic marker, so breeders can avoid the disease. Cases can be normally managed with long-term management changes and medication.

Tetany
Tetanus

Horses are highly susceptible to generalised tetanus caused by the toxin of the bacterium *Clostridium tetani*. Spores of this organism are found very commonly in soil and in the gastrointestinal tract. The usual route of infection is via penetrating wounds that allow bacteria to multiply in an anaerobic environment. Multiplication results in release of toxin, which is transported via motor neuron axons to the spinal cord.

Clinical signs

Clinical signs include an elevated tail head and stiff gait. The horse appears anxious with their ears back, eyelids wide open, prominent nictitating membranes, nostrils flared and head extended. Hyperaesthesia and prolapse of the nictitating membrane are particularly common early signs (Figure 10.23) (Green *et al.* 1994). Another classic sign is 'lock jaw', with dysphagia, drooling and an inability to swallow. Severely affected horses will become recumbent with relatively increased extensor tone.

Treatment

Treatment of tetanus is largely supportive: quiet, dark, low-stimulation room, hydration, good footing, deep bedding, elimination of the original infection by careful wound management, antibiotics, sedation and muscle relaxants. Reports of dose, route and efficacy of antitoxin are variable. Physiotherapy has been used successfully in the management of generalised tetanus in a foal (Mykkänen *et al.* 2011).

Mortality for tetanus in horses is high, but it is a preventable disease with vaccination highly effective and inexpensive.

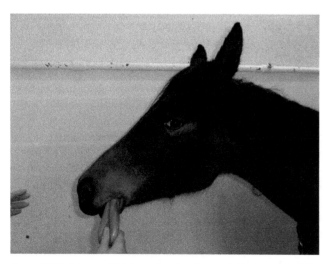

Figure 10.23 A horse with tetanus showing characteristic protrusion of the third eyelid, anxious facial expression and difficulty in opening the mouth to replace the tongue.

10.7 Equine intrinsic muscle disease

Differential diagnosis for muscle disease includes the following.
- Traumatic, e.g. delayed-onset muscular soreness (DOMS), muscle strain
- Inflammatory/infectious (bacterial, viral, protozoal, traumatic, immune mediated)
- Metabolic, e.g. polysaccharide storage myopathy, hypocalcaemia, hypokalaemia and exhaustion
- Nutritional, e.g. vitamin E deficiency
- Genetic, e.g. polysaccharide storage myopathy, and calcium regulation disorders

Equine muscle disorders are also often classified as 'exertional' (occurring during or shortly after exercise) and 'non-exertional'.

10.7.1 Laboratory diagnosis of muscle disease

Skeletal muscle cell damage ('rhabdomyolysis') will result in the release of muscle enzymes and the protein myoglobin into the blood. The main measured muscle enzymes are creatine kinase (CK) and aspartate aminotransferase (AST). CK and AST have very different kinetics, which need to be taken into consideration when diagnosing the extent and time frame of muscle damage. CK rises rapidly, peaking at 6–12 h, and if there is no ongoing muscle damage, will be back to normal rapidly, with a plasma half-life of approximately 2 h. AST takes 24–48 h to peak and has a much longer half-life, of 3–7 days. CK tends to be used for acute monitoring of muscle enzymes and AST for evaluation of changes over a longer period. While CK is specific for muscle, AST is also a liver enzyme in horses. Myoglobin is rapidly filtered by the kidney, and so can be detected in urine. In high concentrations, it makes the urine dark red/brown.

Muscle biopsy

Taking a biopsy is a simple and only mildly invasive procedure, but can yield vital information (Ledwith & McGowan 2004). The biopsy is examined for inflammatory cells, regeneration, degeneration and central nuclei. It is quite straightforward to make many diagnoses, e.g. neurogenic atrophy, myositis and polysaccharide storage myopathy, although biopsies from some horses with significant muscle disease may not reveal any information.

10.7.2 Delayed-onset muscle soreness and muscle strain injury

Delayed-onset muscle soreness (DOMS) and muscle strain injury are types of traumatic muscle damage unrelated to metabolic or other diseases and probably both common and underdiagnosed (Mack *et al.* 2014). They typically present as lameness or poor performance rather than an episode of 'tying up'. DOMS is virtually unreported in the veterinary literature but is likely to occur in animals, especially animals used for athletic activities, as it does in man (Cheung *et al.* 2003; Lewis *et al.* 2012). There have been reports of unexplained elevations of muscle enzymes in horses starting to be trained for the first time that were hypothesised to be due to DOMS (Mack *et al.* 2014). Increases in inflammatory cytokine expression have been shown in muscle and blood of horses following high-intensity exercise (Liburt *et al.* 2010). Increases in muscle enzymes have also been shown to occur without evidence of muscle disease during a training season in racehorses, correlated with cumulative training days (Mack *et al.* 2014).

Muscle strain injury occurs as a result of overstretching of muscle leading to disruption of fibres, which can subsequently lead to inflammation and healing with fibrosis. While it certainly can be a cause of lameness in horses, it can be difficult to definitively diagnose and is sometimes overlooked. It occurs particularly in those muscles that cross two or more joints, especially near the myotendinous junction (Fitch *et al.* 1997; Steiss 2002; Walmsley *et al.* 2010).

Based on the system in humans, there are four grades.

1 Tearing of a few fibres
2 Pain
3 Local spasm
4 Complete muscle rupture

Recovery is rapid with low-grade injuries, but fibrous tissue may predispose to reinjury or contracture.

Diagnosis

Muscle injury should be considered as a differential in horses presenting for lameness. Palpation may reveal pain or even a defect in the normal contour of the muscle. Ultrasonography is probably the most appropriate imaging technique for muscle injuries themselves, although if the injury occurs at the origin or insertion of a muscle, radiography is important to determine if there has been an avulsion fracture at the site. Nuclear scintigraphy may also reveal the inflammation associated with muscle injury (Walmsley *et al.* 2010).

Common sites of injury in the horse include the gluteal muscles, especially with hill work (e.g. rapid acceleration on an inclined treadmill), and lumbar muscles. Injury to the serratus ventralis, which particularly occurred in carriage horse injury from slippery roads, is no longer common but can occur.

Treatment of traumatic muscle disease

Rest, analgesia and a gradual return to work are the main principles of treatment. DOMS and low-grade muscle strain injuries may benefit from conservative physiotherapy using principles and techniques appropriate for similar injuries in humans (also see Chapter 18). High-grade muscle strain injuries may be amenable to surgical treatment, including surgical debridement, repair or tenomyectomy.

Fibrotic or ossifying myopathy

This gait abnormality involves the semitendinosus, semimembranosus or biceps femoris muscles, and most commonly affects Quarterhorses, probably as a result of repeated muscle injury. Horses present with a characteristic gait that involves a shortened cranial phase in the pelvic limb, where the hind foot is jerked caudally at the end of protraction. Sometimes a scar or mineralisation can be palpated in the body of the affected muscle. Treatment is by surgical correction, either by removal of the scar tissue or tenotomy of the tibial insertion of the semitendinosus (Gomez-Villamandos *et al.* 1995; Janicek *et al.* 2012).

10.7.3 Equine rhabdomyolysis syndrome (ERS or tying up)

Equine rhabdomyolysis syndrome is a common disorder of muscles associated with physical exertion or exercise. In horses, signs range from a stiff gait and muscle cramping to reluctance to move or recumbency. It has been referred to using a variety of synonyms including Monday morning disease, setfast, azoturia, tying up and exertional rhabdomyolysis. In the UK, it is most commonly referred to as equine rhabdomyolysis syndrome or ERS. It is common, affecting 4–7% of racing Thoroughbreds, polo, endurance and competition horses (McGowan *et al.* 2002a, b; Upjohn *et al.* 2005; Wilberger *et al.* 2015). ERS may occur sporadically or be recurrent. The recurrent form is the most problematic, and requires accurate diagnosis and management.

Two main causes for recurrent ERS have been found.

- Polysaccharide storage myopathy (PSSM). This was first described in Quarterhorses (Valberg *et al.* 1992) but has subsequently been recognised in Warmbloods, draft breeds and many other breeds of horse and pony (Stanley *et al.* 2009; Valentine & Cooper 2005). It is caused by the accumulation of abnormal polysaccharide in muscle cells and is often, but not always, associated with a glycogen synthase (GYS1) mutation.
- Recurrent exertional rhabdomyolysis (RER). Affected horses have abnormal regulation of muscle contraction owing to a defect in intracellular calcium regulation. This form is found in Thoroughbreds as a distinct disorder from EPSM (Lentz *et al.* 2002). The condition is thought to have a familial basis, but a single mutation has not been identified.

Since the underlying causes of ERS are both inherited and both are prevalent in the population, the most crucial factor in managing the condition is the avoidance of risk factors. These include change in exercise pattern (e.g. several days off and then resumption of normal work), increased carbohydrate in diet, stress, oestrus and insufficient electrolyte supplementation. These risk factors are not the same for all horses and so recommendations cannot be assumed to be beneficial for all.

Diagnosis

Diagnosis of recurrent tying up is quite straightforward and is primarily based on history, clinical signs and laboratory findings. A history of more than one episode of tying up is a good indication that the condition is recurrent, but should be combined with a thorough management history and serum muscle enzyme results. It is important to realise that a single episode may be one of many more to come and that subclinical episodes can occur.

Some horses may not show overt signs of tying up. In young horses with PSSM being backed or broken in, there may be behavioural problems such as unwillingness to go forward, bucking or rearing instead of classic tying up signs of hard contracted muscle, sweating, pain and unwillingness to walk.

Differential diagnoses include lameness, aortoiliac thrombosis, colic (many horses paw and sweat because of the pain and look as if they are having colic), atypical myopathy, laminitis and pleuritis (both of these cause the horse to be reluctant to walk, and laminitis in particular can cause such pain that all the muscles are hard and tense, mimicking a horse that has tied up).

In subclinical or chronic/recurrent cases, an exercise test to detect elevations in CK can confirm the problem. The horse is lunged at a trot or worked on the track at similar exercise intensity for 15–20 minutes. Serum CK is measured before and 4 h after exercise. Many horses with recurrent ERS will show at least a doubling of CK concentration.

Knowing the specific cause for ERS can help in determining optimal management, heritability and prognosis. A muscle biopsy is useful in differentiating PSSM as a specific cause for ERS, especially in combination with genetic testing for the GSY1 mutation. In biopsies, muscle changes are often apparent in horses with recurrent disease, even without clinical signs. Interestingly, and importantly when considering physiotherapy treatment, despite the severity of signs in episodes of tying up, fibrosis is rarely seen (as opposed to neurogenic conditions).

Treatment

The acute case/episode should be examined by a veterinary surgeon because of the risk of renal disease or complications. Immediate treatment might include analgesia (NSAIDs) and fluid and electrolyte therapy.

The mainstays of treatment of the chronic or recurrent case are threefold.

- *Diet.* The level of carbohydrate should be relative to exercise and weight and minimised by use of other energy sources, e.g. oil or fat. A high-fat diet is essential, even for horses fed 100% roughage, and helps prevent episodes of ERS (McKenzie *et al.* 2003; Ribeiro *et al.* 2004). Fat should constitute 10–20% of the caloric intake.
- *Exercise.* For prevention, it is important to allow the horse to move and not be confined. Therefore, maximise turnout (although be careful of excessively rich pasture as it may have the same effect as excessive carbohydrates). Resume exercise early; do not give prolonged periods of box rest following an episode – resume when the horse is able to walk freely without pain. Be careful of overreliance on muscle enzymes, as prolonged elevations are likely for 4 months after dietary intervention (Valentine *et al.* 2001). In some horses, restricted low-intensity exercise (excitable horses held back on a tight rein) can be more likely to induce attacks so moderate-intensity exercise on a loose rein, with minimal warm-up, can be beneficial. Ensure exercise is consistent throughout the week – ideally no days of rest.

- *Drug therapy* can be employed in Thoroughbreds on a temporary basis to get horses back into regular training. Dantrolene sodium helps reduce the severity of RER episodes when administered before exercise (McKenzie *et al.* 2004).

Prognosis

With appropriate preventive strategies, overall prognosis for ERS is good and most horses can continue an athletic career, although prognosis can be compromised in horses on restricted pasture turnout.

References

Araujo, J.A., Curcio, B., Alda, J., Medeiros, R.M., Riet-Correa, F. 2008, Stringhalt in Brazilian horses caused by Hypochaeris radicata. *Toxicon* 52(1): 190–193.

Barrott, M.J., Brooks, H.W., McGowan, C.M. 2004, Suspected immune-mediated myositis in a pony. *Equine Vet. Educ.* 16: 58–61.

Blythe, L. 1997a, Otitis media and interna and temporohyoid osteoarthropathy. *Vet. Clin. North Am. Equine Pract.* 13: 21–42.

Blythe, L. 1997b, Peripheral neuropathy. In: Robinson, N.E. (ed), *Current Therapy in Equine Medicine*, 4th edn. W.B. Saunders, Philadelphia, PA, pp. 314–319.

Butler, J., Colles, C., Dyson, S., Kold, S., Poulos, P. 2008, *Clinical Radiology of the Horse*. Wiley-Blackwell, Oxford.

Cheung, K., Hume, P., Maxwell, L. 2003, Delayed onset muscle soreness: treatment strategies and performance factors. *Sports Med.* 33: 145–164.

Cox, V.S., Mcgrath, C.J., Jorgensen, S.E. 1982, The role of pressure damage in pathogenesis of the downer cow syndrome. *Am. J. Vet. Res.* 43: 26–31.

Crabill, M.R., Honnas, C.M., Taylor, D.S., Schumacher, J., Watkins, J.P., Snyder, J.R. 1994, Stringhalt secondary to trauma to the dorsoproximal region of the metatarsus in horses: 10 cases (1986–1991). *J. Am. Vet. Med. Assoc.* 205: 867–869.

Cummings, J.F., de Lahunta, A., George, C. et al. 1990, Equine motor neuron disease: a preliminary report. *Cornell Vet.* 80: 357–379.

De Lahunta, A., Glass, E. 2009, *Veterinary Neuroanatomy and Clinical Neurology.* Elsevier Saunders, St Louis, MO.

Divers, T.J., de Lahunta, A., Hintz, H.F., Riis, R.C., Jackson, C.A., Mohammed, H.O. 2001, Equine motor neuron disease. *Equine Vet. Educ.* 13: 63–67.

Divers, T.J., Mohammed, H.O., Hintz, H.F., de Lahunta, A. 2006, Equine motor neuron disease: a review of clinical and experimental studies. *Clin Tech Equine Pract.* 5: 24–29.

Domange, C., Casteignau, A., Collignon, G., Pumarola, M., Priymenko, N. 2010, Longitudinal study of Australian stringhalt cases in France. *J. Anim. Physiol. Anim. Nutr. (Berl).* 94: 712–720.

Donawick, W.J., Mayhew, I.G., Galligan, D.T. et al. 1993, *Results of a low-protein, low-energy diet and confinement on young horses with wobbles.* Proceedings of the American Association of Equine Practice, Lexington, KY.

Draper, A.C., Trumble, T.N., Firshman, A.M., et al. 2015, Posture and movement characteristics of forward and backward walking in horses with shivering and acquired bilateral stringhalt. *Equine Vet. J.* 47(2): 175–181.

Dyce, K.M., Sack, W.O., Wensing, C.J. 2010a, The neck, back and vertebral column of the horse. In: Dyce, K.M., Sack, W.O., Wensing, C.J. (eds), *Textbook of Veterinary Anatomy*, 4th edn. Elsevier Saunders, St Louis, MO.

Dyce, K.M., Sack, W.O., Wensing, C.J. 2010b, The nervous system. In: Dyce, K.M., Sack, W.O., Wensing, C.J. (eds), *Textbook of Veterinary Anatomy*, 4th edn. Elsevier Saunders, St Louis, MO.

Fitch, R.B., Jaffe, M.H., Montgomery, R.D. 1997, Muscle injuries in dogs. *Comp. Contin. Educ. Pract. Vet.* 18: 20–36.

Furr, M. 2008, Equine protozoal myeloencephalitis. In: Furr, M., Reed, S. (eds), *Equine Neurology*. Wiley-Blackwell, Ames, IA.

Gomez-Villamandos, R., Santisteban, J., Ruiz, I., Avila, I. 1995, Tenotomy of the tibial insertion of the semitendinosus muscle of two horses with fibrotic myopathy. *Vet. Rec.* 136: 67–68.

Green, S.L., Little, C.B., Baird, J.D., Tremblay, R.R., Smith-Maxie, L.L. 1994, Tetanus in the horse: a review of 20 cases (1970 to 1990). *J. Vet. Intern. Med.* 8: 128–132.

Hahn, C.N., Handel, I., Green, S.L., Bronsvoort, M.B., Mayhew, I.G. 2008, Assessment of the utility of using intra- and intervertebral minimum sagittal diameter ratios in the diagnosis of cervical vertebral malformation in horses. *Vet. Radiol. Ultrasound.* 49: 1–6.

Henninger, R.W., Reed, S.M., Saville, W.J. *et al.* 2007. Outbreak of neurologic disease caused by equine herpesvirus-1 at a university equestrian center. *J. Vet. Intern. Med.* 21: 157–165.

Janicek, J., Lopes, M.A., Wilson, D.A. *et al.* 2012. Hindlimb kinematics before and after laser fibrotomy in horses with fibrotic myopathy. *Equine Vet. J.* 136(suppl): 126–131.

Johnson, A.L., McAdams-Gallagher, S.C., Aceto, H. 2015, Outcome of adult horses with Botulism treated at a veterinary hospital: 92 cases (1989–2013). *J. Vet. Intern. Med.* 29(1): 311–319.

Kristoffersen, M., Puchalski, S., Skog, S., Lindegaard, C. 2014, *Cervical computed tomography (CT) and CT myelography in live hoses: 16 cases.* Proceedings of the BEVA Congress, Birmingham, UK.

Ledwith, A., McGowan, C.M. 2004, Muscle biosy: a routine diagnostic procedure. *Equine Vet. Educ.* 16: 62–67.

Lentz, L.R., Valberg, S.J., Herold, L.V., Onan, G.W., Mickelson, J.R., Gallant, E.M. 2002, Myoplasmic calcium regulation in myotubes from horses with recurrent exertional rhabdomyolysis. *Am. J. Vet. Res.* 63: 1724–1731.

Levine, J.M., Adam, E., Mackay, R.J., Walker, M.A., Frederick, J.D., Cohen, N.D. 2007, Confirmed and presumptive cervical vertebral compressive myelopathy in older horses: a retrospective study (1992–2004). *J. Vet. Intern. Med.* 21: 812–819.

Lewis, P.B., Ruby, D., Bush-Joseph, C.A. 2012, Muscle soreness and delayed-onset muscle soreness. *Clin. Sports Med.* 31: 255–262.

Liburt, N.R., Adams, A.A., Betancourt, A., Horohov, D.W., McKeever, K.H. 2010, Exercise-induced increases in inflammatory cytokines in muscle and blood of horses. *Equine Vet. J.* 38(suppl): 280–288.

Licka, T. 2002, Closed reduction of an atlanto-occipital and atlantoaxial dislocation in a foal. *Vet. Rec.* 151: 356–357.

Lindsay, W.A., Robinson, G.M., Brunson, D.B., Majors, L.J. 1989, Induction of equine postanesthetic myositis after halothane-induced hypotension. *Am. J. Vet. Res.* 50: 404–410.

Mack, S.J., Kirkby, K., Malalana, F., McGowan, C.M. 2014, Elevations in serum muscle enzyme activities in racehorses due to unaccustomed exercise and training. *Vet. Rec.* 174: 145.

Mayhew, I.G. 2009, *Large Animal Neurology.* Wiley-Blackwell, Oxford.

Mayhew, I.G., Green, S.L. 2000, *Accuracy of diagnosing CVM from radiographs. Proceedings of the 39th British Equine Veterinary Association Annual Congress*, Newmarket, pp. 74–75.

Mayhew, I.G., de Lahunta, A., Whitlock, R.H., Krook, L., Tasker, J.B. 1978, Spinal cord disease in the horse. *Cornell Vet.* 68(suppl 6): 1–207.

McGorum, B.C., Mayhew, I.G., Amory, H. *et al.* 2006, Horses on pasture may be affected by equine motor neuron disease. *Equine Vet. J.* 38: 47–51.

McGowan, C.M., Fordham, T., Christley, R.M., Posner, R.E. 2002a, Incidence and risk factors for exertional rhabdomyolysis in thoroughbred racehorses in the United Kingdom. *Vet. Rec.* 151: 623–626.

McGowan, C.M., Posner, R.E., Christley, R.M. 2002b, Incidence of exertional rhabdomyolysis in polo horses in the USA and the United Kingdom in the 1999/2000 season. *Vet. Rec.* 150: 535–537.

McKenzie, E.C., Valberg, S.J., Godden, S.M. *et al.* 2003, Effect of dietary starch, fat, and bicarbonate content on exercise responses and serum creatine kinase activity in equine recurrent exertional rhabdomyolysis. *J. Vet. Intern. Med.* 17: 693–701.

McKenzie, E.C., Valberg, S.J., Godden, S.M., Finno, C.J., Murphy, M.J. 2004, Effect of oral administration of dantrolene sodium on serum creatine kinase activity after exercise in horses with recurrent exertional rhabdomyolysis. *Am. J. Vet. Res.* 65: 74–79.

Mykkänen, A.K., Hyytiainen, H.K., McGowan, C.M. 2011, Generalised tetanus in a 2-week-old foal: use of physiotherapy to aid recovery. *Aust. Vet. J.* 89: 447–451.

Nout, Y.S., Reed, S.M. 2005, Management and treatment of the recumbent horse. *Equine Vet. Educ.* 17: 324–336.

Oswald, J., Love, S., Parkin, T.D., Hughes, K.J. 2010, Prevalence of cervical vertebral stenotic myelopathy in a population of thoroughbred horses. *Vet. Rec.* 166: 82–83.

Ribeiro, W.P., Valberg, S.J., Pagan, J.D., Gustavsson, B.E. 2004, The effect of varying dietary starch and fat content on serum creatine kinase activity and substrate availability in equine polysaccharide storage myopathy. *J. Vet. Intern. Med.* 18: 887–894.

Ruff, S.J., Wood, C.H., Aaron, D.K., Lawrence, L.M. 1993, A comparison of growth rates of normal Thoroughbred foals and foals diagnosed with cervical vertebral malformation. *J. Equine Vet. Sci.* 13: 596–599.

Schefer, K.D., Hagen, R., Ringer, S.K., Schwarzwald, C.C. 2011, Laboratory, electrocardiographic, and echocardiographic detection of myocardial damage and dysfunction in an Arabian mare with nutritional masseter myodegeneration. *J. Vet. Intern. Med.* 25: 1171–1180.

Slocombe, R.F., Huntington, P.J., Friend, S.C., Jeffcott, L.B., Luff, A.R., Finkelstein, D.K. 1992, Pathological aspects of Australian Stringhalt. *Equine Vet. J.* 24: 174–183.

Sponseller, B.T., Valberg, S.J., Tennent-Brown, B.S., Foreman, J.H., Kumar, P., Timoney, J.F. 2005, Severe acute rhabdomyolysis associated with Streptococcus equi infection in four horses. *J. Am. Vet. Med. Assoc.* 227: 1753–1754, 1800–1807.

Stanley, R.L., Mccue, M.E., Valberg, S.J. *et al.* 2009, A glycogen synthase 1 mutation associated with equine polysaccharide storage myopathy and exertional rhabdomyolysis occurs in a variety of UK breeds. *Equine Vet. J.* 41: 597–601.

Steiss, J.E. 2002, Muscle disorders and rehabilitation in canine athletes. *Vet. Clin. North Am. Small Anim. Pract.* 32: 267–285.

Stubbs, N.C., Hodges, P.W., Jeffcott, L.B., Cowin, G., Hodgson D.R., McGowan C.M. 2006, Functional anatomy of the caudal thoracolumbar and lumbosacral spine in the horse. *Equine Vet. J.* 36(suppl): 393–399.

Tennent-Brown, B.S. 2007, Trauma with neurologic sequelae. *Vet. Clin. North Am. Equine Pract.* 23: 81–101.

Tyler, C.M., Davis, R.E., Begg, A.P., Hutchins, D.R., Hodgson, D.R. 1993, A survey of neurological diseases in horses. *Aust. Vet. J.* 70: 445–449.

Upjohn, M.M., Archer, R.M., Christley, R.M., McGowan, C.M. 2005, Incidence and risk factors associated with exertional rhabdomyolysis syndrome in National Hunt racehorses in Great Britain. *Vet. Rec.* 156: 763–766.

Valberg, S.J., Cardinet, G.H. 3rd, Carlson, G.P., Dimauro, S. 1992, Polysaccharide storage myopathy associated with recurrent exertional rhabdomyolysis in horses. *Neuromusc. Disord.* 2: 351–359.

Valentine, B.A., Cooper, B.J. 2005, Incidence of polysaccharide storage myopathy: necropsy study of 225 horses. *Vet. Pathol.* 42: 823–827.

Valentine, B.A., van Saun, R.J., Thompson, K.N., Hintz, H.F. 2001, Role of dietary carbohydrate and fat in horses with equine polysaccharide storage myopathy. *J. Am. Vet. Med. Assoc.* 219: 1537–1544.

Van Biervliet, J., Scrivani, P.V., Divers, T.J., Erb, H.N., de Lahunta, A., Nixon, A. 2004, Evaluation of decision criteria for detection of spinal cord compression based on cervical myelography in horses: 38 cases (1981–2001). *Equine Vet. J.* 36: 14–20.

Walmsley, E.A., Steel, C.M., Richardson, J.L., Hesse, K.L., Whitton, R.C. 2010, Muscle strain injuries of the hindlimb in eight horses: diagnostic imaging, management and outcomes. *Aust. Vet. J.* 88: 313–321.

Walmsley, J.P. 2005, Surgical treatment of cervical spinal cord compression in horses: a European experience. *Equine Vet. Educ.* 17: 39–43.

Whitlock, R.H., McAdams, S. 2006, Equine botulism. *Clin. Tech. Equine Pract.* 5: 37–42.

Wilberger, M.S., Mckenzie, E.C., Payton, M.E., Rigas, J.D., Valberg, S.J. 2015, Prevalence of exertional rhabdomyolysis in endurance horses in the Pacific Northwestern United States. *Equine Vet. J.* 47: 165–170.

Wilkins, P.A., Palmer, J.E. 2003, Botulism in foals less than 6 months of age: 30 cases (1989–2002). *J. Vet. Intern. Med.* 17: 702–707.

Williams, N.M., Allen, G., Powell, D. 2003, Equine neurologic disease. *J. Equine Vet. Sci.* 23: 431–433.

CHAPTER 11

Physiotherapy assessment for animals*

Lesley Goff

Lecturer, Equine Science, School of Agriculture & Food Sciences, The University of Queensland, Gatton, Australia; Director, Active Animal Physiotherapy, Toowoomba, Australia

Summary

Physiotherapy assessment of the animal is the first step the physiotherapist takes in delivering optimal physiotherapeutic intervention to the animal. This chapter outlines the history, physical assessment and special considerations for the animal patient assessment.

11.1 Introduction

The aim of this chapter is to provide the animal physiotherapist with guidelines for comprehensive physiotherapy assessment of the dog and horse. Emphasis lies with communication with the veterinarian, clinical reasoning, accurate history taking and physical assessment to guide the physiotherapist in selection of treatment. The chapter is designed to be used in conjunction with other chapters in this text such as orthopaedics, neurology, biomechanics and manual therapy.

In many countries, physiotherapists have been granted professional autonomy, and as such they are able to diagnose and treat human patients as primary contact practitioners. Yet most veterinary Acts, for example the Veterinary Surgeons Act 1966 in the United Kingdom, currently preclude physiotherapists from being primary contact practitioners when providing physiotherapy for animals. The UK Act clearly states that: 'only veterinary surgeons registered with the Royal College of Veterinary

---

*Adapted from the first edition chapter, which was written by Tracy Crook and Lesley Goff

Animal Physiotherapy: Assessment, Treatment and Rehabilitation of Animals, Second Edition. Edited by Catherine M. McGowan and Lesley Goff.
© 2016 John Wiley & Sons, Ltd. Published 2016 by John Wiley & Sons, Ltd.

Surgeons have the right to practise veterinary surgery'. Veterinary surgery is defined in the Act as follows.

The art and science of veterinary surgery and medicine, without prejudice to the generality of the foregoing, shall be taken to include:

a The diagnosis of diseases in, and injuries to animals, including tests performed upon them for diagnostic purposes.

b The giving of advice based on such a diagnosis.

c The medical and surgical treatment of animals.

d The performance of surgical operations on animals.

It is essential that animal/veterinary physiotherapists obtain veterinary diagnosis of the animal's condition requiring treatment from the referring veterinarian, before carrying out physiotherapy assessment and devising a physiotherapy treatment plan. Good communication between physiotherapist and veterinarians is paramount, not only to comply with legislation but to maintain high standards of professional conduct in animal physiotherapy.

Physiotherapy assessment of the animal involves the integration of skills, which include:

• knowledge of anatomy, functional anatomy and biomechanics
• the ability to observe movement and analyse movement patterns of the musculoskeletal system
• animal husbandry skills
• sound clinical reasoning based on the latest research evidence
• ability to communicate with and educate the owner/carer
• ability to communicate with veterinarians.

Historically, veterinarians' initial diagnosis of a condition, injury or disease in the animal has focused on both the anatomical location and the specific pathology involved, that is, pathoanatomical diagnosis. While a pathoanatomical diagnosis is ideal, it is not always possible to establish a pathoanatomical diagnosis prior to initialising patient management based on the identified problems. Physiotherapy treatment decisions can then be based on the patient's signs and presenting movement disorders.

Pathoanatomical diagnoses may be difficult where the conditions affecting an animal's performance are either non-specific in origin or are difficult to diagnose with traditional veterinary diagnosis. For example, there is much written about the difficulty in diagnosing conditions such as chronic sacroiliac disease and temporomandibular disorders in the horse, due to the non-specific nature of clinical signs and, in the case of the former, difficulty diagnosing with traditional veterinary diagnostic modalities (Jeffcott et al. 1985; Moll & May 2002). An example of a condition of non-specific origin in a horse, for which physiotherapy may be of benefit, is a restriction of cervical spine mobility affecting the horse's ability to flex laterally on a small circle. A mechanical, musculoskeletal condition such as this in a horse may show no obvious lameness. A work-up involving lameness assessment, joint blocks or imaging techniques readily available to veterinarians will be unlikely to reveal pathology. Imaging techniques available to most veterinarians, for example ultrasound or radiography, do not show the presence of movement dysfunction. The veterinarian may instead classify the cervical restriction as part of the 'problem list'. In the above case, a physiotherapy assessment involving movement analysis, physical examination and the employment of sound clinical reasoning should be able to ascertain the cause of the mechanical dysfunction, and lead to development of a treatment plan for restoring mechanical function.

There are many instances where combined assessment by veterinarian and physiotherapist will deliver the best outcome for the animal patient. Veterinary expertise can be utilised to discover the source of many conditions and pathologies in animals, and physiotherapy expertise can be utilised to assess any secondary or associated mechanical dysfunctions. In some cases, veterinary assessment and management will need to be instigated before physiotherapy assessment and treatment are warranted. In cases where there are contraindications or precautions to a physiotherapy assessment, or where a new development occurs within the presenting condition, the physiotherapist should discuss with the referring veterinarian.

11.2 Clinical reasoning

Clinical reasoning and medical and veterinary problem solving require the practitioner to develop the critical clinical skill of communication (Adams & Kurtz 2012). Communication with the owner/trainer/handler is paramount when dealing with the animal patient and is linked to significant outcomes of care, including accuracy, efficiency, supportiveness, adherence to treatment plans and client and veterinarian satisfaction (Adams & Kurtz 2012). Communication with the animal is addressed in Chapter 2, and is also an important part of clinical reasoning and assessment.

Clinical reasoning forms the basis for assessment and ongoing reassessment, which in turn is essential for, and concurrent with, delivery of the most effective treatment. Clinical reasoning is an essential part of each step of the animal physiotherapy assessment. It is influenced by the clinician's knowledge base, beliefs or values and skills associated with clinical practice (Refshauge & Latimer 1995). Unlike a human patient, an animal patient cannot describe to you their resting symptoms or tell you that assessment is causing an increase in their symptoms. An animal can only show signs of problems. Thus clinical reasoning is an essential skill for delivering animal physiotherapy safely.

As mentioned above, clinical reasoning begins with communication and the clinician's interpretation of clues from the patient. These initial clues help the clinician to formulate a preliminary working hypothesis. The working hypothesis should be considered throughout the rest of the subjective and physical examination, as well as during ongoing patient management (Jones 1994).

The following is a brief example of the clinical reasoning process.

A horse presents with lameness in the right hindlimb, which is apparent when trotted on a right-hand circle in deep sand. Lameness is absent on the straight line or on a hard surface. Lameness was unaffected by nerve blocking the lower limb or tibial and peroneal nerves by the referring veterinarian. The clinician forms a working hypothesis by making a note of the possible pain-producing structures (e.g. coxofemoral joint, sacroiliac joint, neuromeningeal structures, pelvic limb soft tissues). Further information is then sought through the subjective and physical examination with the working hypothesis in mind (Jones 1994). Information may include specific questioning of the owner (if not already carried out) such as previous episodes of lameness, horse's working history and performance, veterinary investigations, medications and previous trauma. This subjective information may then guide the clinician on 'where to start' with the physical examination.

The history directs the physiotherapist towards the starting point of the physical examination, which in the above case may include sacroiliac joint palpation and functional tests, including neural tension tests, to help narrow down the area or structure from which the signs are most likely to arise. It is important, however, to realise that the physical examination is not a routine series of tests (Jones 1994). Whilst it is useful to have a systematic manner in which to carry out assessment, the physical tests should be an extension of the hypothesis testing performed through the subjective examination. If the history has provided the physiotherapist with no working hypothesis, however, then it is essential to test and 'clear' all possible structures from contribution to the signs.

Hypotheses regarding precautions and contraindications (see Chapter 12) to physical examination and treatment will guide the extent to which physical examination and initial treatment can be performed without risk of aggravation of signs (Jones 1994). The physical examination is used to test the hypothesis regarding potential sources of signs and contributing factors in such a way that each structure that could be implicated is specifically examined. In summary, the clinical reasoning process guides the examination and the treatment.

A clinical reasoning form, which can be used in clinical practice, is shown in Figure 11.1, along with further notes on clinical reasoning.

11.2.1 The assessment

Although the physical examination is not a routine 'recipe' of tests, it is useful to perform the physiotherapy examination in a systematic manner, to optimise efficiency (Refshauge & Latimer 1995). Following a routine of examination also helps to ensure that crucial components of the examination are not omitted, especially where there are complications such as multiple or difficult signs reported by the animal's owner, or distractions such as behavioural issues with the animal at time of examination.

An example of a systematic approach to the assessment process is set out below but individual physiotherapists may find their own order of systematic approach to be more suitable. The order of the components of the physical assessment is interchangeable, depending on the direction in which clinical reasoning takes the clinician.

- History/subjective information from the owner
- Observation and conformation (willingness to move, postural deformities, conformation)
- Analysis of provoking activity/gait – sport and occupation specific
- Functional tests
- Active physiological movements
- Passive physiological movements
- Passive accessory movements
- Soft tissues – palpation and testing
- Nervous system – testing relative spinal cord and peripheral nerve function plus status of neuromeningeal system

11.2.2 History

Taking an effective history is fundamental to optimal physiotherapy treatment; therefore it is arguably the most important part of the whole examination (Refshauge & Latimer 1995).

Following the diagnosis given by the veterinarian, it is important to take an extensive clinical history from a physiotherapist's point of view, to document the degree of functional disability perceived by the owner/handler/trainer, onset and progression of the disorder and the past history related to the disorder. The physiotherapist can employ a variety of questioning methods, but should avoid posing leading questions. Open-ended questions provide reliable and valid information. Taking a history requires good interpersonal skills as well as a good knowledge base. The time spent with the owner obtaining information allows the physiotherapist to observe the animal's general demeanour and behaviour, and its general condition, conformation, gait and posture.

The history of the animal's presenting condition should be taken from the owner and recorded in the physiotherapy records, supplemented by notes obtained from the referring veterinarian. A typical veterinary referral should include details of the breed, age and sex of the animal, veterinary diagnosis, previous medical history, history of the present complaint, current medication and veterinary management. If the veterinary referral does not include all this information, it is important for this to be followed up by the physiotherapist with the veterinarian.

The owner should be asked when they first became aware that their animal had a problem or dysfunction, and whether or not the problem is becoming worse or better. The questioning should cover whether there are observed changes in the animal's demeanour, and if the owner feels the animal is in pain, or is depressed or anxious. In the case of lameness, it is useful to ask the owner to identify the affected limb and to report any observed gait abnormalities. The owner may be questioned regarding activities or situations that exacerbate or ease their animal's condition. It is often these observations that will affect in the owner's view whether or not the physiotherapy intervention is of benefit to their animal.

Immediately following the history (BEFORE physical examination)

1. List, in order of importance, three structures most likely to be contributing to presenting signs and symptoms. Even though there is unlikely to be ONE joint, muscle or other tissue solely responsible, you need to be identifying structures down to a high level of accuracy, so be specific (e.g. upper cervical vertebrae; left brachial plexus; right cranial ligament of the stifle; right peroneus tertius).

	Structure	Justify your reasoning (e.g. distribution of symptoms; history of specific trauma)
1.		
2.		
3.		

If you wish to include more contributing structures, please justify.

2. In consideration of breed and/or conformation of the animal, are there any precautions or contraindications, prior to going on with physical examination?
No:
Yes: a) Are you confident it is safe to proceed with FULL physical examination?
    Yes/No
    b) Are there any veterinary or physiotherapy tests, which can carried out to indicate it safe to proceed with FULL physical examination?
    Yes/No
If yes, list.
    c) Is it safe to proceed with a modified examination? Justify.

Following the physical examination, BEFORE treatment
3. Do you agree with your hypothesis of structures most likely to be contributing to presenting condition?
Yes?
No? If no, please revise list

	Structure	Justify your reasoning (e.g. specific gait pattern, specific pain response or motion restriction)
1.		
2.		
3.		

4. At this point on the assessment, are there any precautions or contraindications to treatment?
    Y/N
If yes: a) Do you feel safe to proceed with treatment? Please justify
     b) Do you feel neurological test or further veterinary investigation is warranted? Justify.
5. If your answer to the question above was No, do you feel it is appropriate to begin initial treatment today? Justify.
6. What treatment will you implement as initial treatment and why? (Include dosage)
7. What response/s do you expect from treatment and the dosage?
    a) Immediate response
    b) Response after 24 hours
8. Do you envisage an exercise programme as being appropriate for this patient? If so, at what stage will it be introduced?
9. When would you like to implement the second treatment? Justify.
10 If the response is as hypothesised, explain what is likely to be implemented as second treatment, including dosage.
11. Can you predict the outcome from the second treatment? If no, please justify.

To be completed after 2nd treatment
12. Is your outcome as expected? If no, please give reasons,

Notes regarding use of Clinical Reasoning Form
This clinical reasoning form has been prepared to assist the animal physiotherapist in the process of clinical reasoning and to help the clinician avoid examination or treatment when it is NOT warranted, or when it will be detrimental to the animal. Knowing when to cease examination of the animal or when it is not appropriate to provide a full physical examination, is even more important than knowing which examination procedures to include in your assessment. There may be dire consequences in performing a physiotherapy examination or treatment when contraindicated.
When treating animals, clinical reasoning is possibly more important a skill to possess, than when treating humans (not detract from the importance of clinical reasoning in human physiotherapy). A human patient can tell you they are feeling worse (e.g. pain, paraesthesia) during assessment or can alert you to their resting symptoms of numbness, dizziness or if they arent feeling well, but an animal can only do it to a certain degree.
It may be useful to make a copy of the form and take it with your patient records, so it can be filled in as you proceed with your examination- this may be more time-consuming initially, but worthwhile to avoid exacerbating an animals condition and to improve your animal patient outcomes.

Figure 11.1 A clinical reasoning form.

In summary, for animal physiotherapy, the structure of a history includes the following.

- Recording of the area affected/effect of dysfunction
- Current history of condition/current veterinary diagnosis
- Past history (including past treatments)
- Questions to determine contraindications and precautions to treatment
- Questions related to the animal's occupation/activity (including equipment and tack used)
- Owner/handler expectations of future occupation/activity
- For ridden horses, questions related to rider biomechanics/existing injuries

All information must be recorded in detail for legal purposes as well as liaison with the veterinarian and owner.

11.2.3 Observation

The patient should be observed statically and dynamically.

Static observation

The purpose of observing the animal is to glean information about any visible functional deficits and other abnormalities such as swellings, muscle atrophy, scarring, alignment of extremities and spine, and also the animal's conformation (see also Chapters 7, 8) and condition score. The physiotherapist may observe the animal from a lateral, cranial, caudal and sometimes dorsal aspect.

Lateral aspect

- Weight distribution between limbs
- Limb alignment (angles of long bones, hocks, stifles, carpi, placement of limbs caudocranially, hoof–pastern axis in the equine)
- Obvious swellings or scarring of limbs, body and head
- Angle of scapula, spinal curves and set of tail
- Head position
- Coverage of muscle/other soft tissue

Cranial aspect

- Mentation and head position (including head tilt)
- Limb alignment (angles at carpus, placement of limbs mediolaterally, foot/hoof alignment relative to metacarpals/proximal phalanges, hoof/claw growth)
- Trunk symmetry (including ribcage)
- Weight distribution between limbs
- Obvious swellings or scarring of limbs, body and head

Caudal aspect

- Symmetry and development of muscle/other soft tissues over pelvis and trunk
- Height of pelvic bony landmarks
- Set of tail
- Trunk symmetry (including ribcage)
- Limb alignment (hock height, angles at hock, stifles, fetlock (metacarpal/tarsal phalangeal) joints, placement of limbs mediolaterally)
- Weight distribution between limbs
- Obvious swellings or scarring of limbs, body and head

Dorsal aspect (especially applicable to canines)

- Spinal curvatures
- Trunk symmetry (including ribcage)
- Alignment of pelvic bony landmarks
- Set of tail

Ideally, relevant abnormalities or asymmetries should be measured if the physiotherapist intends to alter them (Goodsell & Refshauge 1995). Useful measurement equipment includes tape measure, goniometer and digital camera. Goniometry and algometry have been shown to be reliable and useful measurement tools (Haussler & Erb 2006; Liljebrink & Bergh 2010). Figure 11.2 shows goniometry and tape measure used to record cervical spine range of motion. Measurement and outcome measures in animal physiotherapy are explored further in Chapter 22.

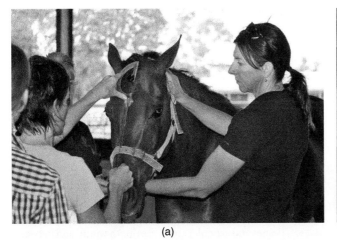
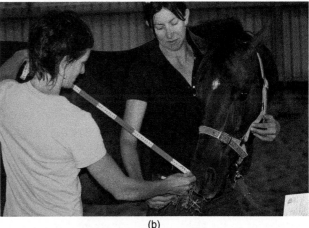

(a)   (b)

Figure 11.2 (a) Preparing to measure craniocervical rotation via goniometer placed along midline of maxilla. (b) Recording the amount of midcervical lateral flexion with a tape measure.

Dynamic observation

Dynamic observation has been included in sections of this chapter specific to the dog and the horse.

Other gait tests (analysis of provoking activity)

It may be necessary to 'challenge' the animal if gait patterns are normal and the animal displays no functional disability during gait. These can be performed at this point of the examination but will be detailed in section 11.3.

In the case of dogs, obstacle courses are a useful means by which to challenge gait; for example, stairs or steps, poles to walk, trot or run over, or performing serpentine manoeuvres. Transitions from sit to walk and vice versa are also useful tests. Many of these gait tests fall under the category of 'functional tests' and may relate to the animal's occupation. If there is no opportunity to use stairs or obstacles, the therapist can apply a challenge to the dog, for example, assess the ability of the dog to bear weight on a fore–hind diagonal. It can be thought of as assessing what the dog can achieve in stance, balance and/or proprioceptive ability. Obstacle courses may also be used to emphasise functional disabilities in the horse, including challenges such as slopes (up and down), poles and serpentine manoeuvres. As for the dog, if there are no such obstacles in the testing vicinity, then simple tests such as small circles, walking backwards and displacing the horse's pelvis laterally during walk or stance may also be used. Testing the horse's gait on different surfaces, such as hard concrete, soft, deep sand or grass, may be required to emphasise functional disabilities as well as lameness.

11.3 Physical assessment

The physical examination is aimed at confirming the hypotheses and ideas suggested by the history and observation and identifying the most appropriate treatment (Refshauge & Latimer 1995). It involves the physiotherapist carrying out active movements, passive motion tests, palpation and functional tests. As mentioned above, the latter often involve sport- or occupation-specific manoeuvres or challenges. Functional tests may also look at integrity of groups of muscles and/or neuromeningeal status. Neurological assessment, which involves testing of neural system conductivity, may be grouped under functional tests (see Chapters 9, 10).

For adequate physical assessment, it is essential to have an understanding of the anatomy, functional anatomy and biomechanics of the animal, conditions and diseases occurring in animals as well as practical skills in animal handling, and experience in the practice of physiotherapy. This knowledge enables the physiotherapist to be accurate, identifying the structures underlying the surface during observation, palpation, active and passive movements; to ascertain which anatomical structures are contributing to the global or local movement dysfunction or painful condition; and to ascertain when it is not appropriate to continue with physiotherapy treatment for the animal. The

veterinarian may have already diagnosed a disease or condition, but if at any point in the examination the physiotherapist is unsure of whether a disease or condition exists that has not been addressed, or if the condition has progressed, the veterinarian should be consulted or the animal returned for veterinary examination.

During the physiotherapy physical assessment process, continual reassessment is essential as signs may be altered by the examination process itself.

11.3.1 Active movement tests

Understanding the normal pattern and amount of movement available at a joint or body segment allows detection of abnormalities of movement (Lee 1995). In addition to overall body motion and gait, it is important to assess active movements of regions of the animal patient. The physiotherapist needs to know what movements the animal is willing to do, as, unlike humans, they cannot tell us which activities cause pain or difficulty. Active movement testing enables the physiotherapist to ascertain which movements are affected, in what way the movements are altered, the effect of pain on movement and the range of movement available (Refshauge & Latimer 1995). Importantly, baseline measures are made for reassessment so that it can be established whether the patient has improved as a result of treatment. The physiotherapist may need to set up tasks to view certain active movements as the animal patient cannot be asked to specifically move an affected body part (see Other gait tests, earlier in this chapter).

Facilitated active movements may be part of the manual examination and can be achieved using food treats or reflexes inherent in the animal. An example of an active movement readily facilitated by a treat is cervical lateral flexion range of motion. The vertebral level at which the lateral flexion occurs can be approximately guided by the physiotherapist's positioning of the food treat (Figure 11.3). Reflexes, such as the rounding reflex in the horse, can facilitate the general movement of flexion of the vertebral column (Figure 11.4).

It may be desirable to reproduce the signs in an animal to establish a baseline so that treatment effect and its dosage can be monitored. Applying further stress to the active movement may be required for the reproduction of signs. Examples of further stressing active movements are the hock, fetlock and carpal flexion tests. Further stressing a joint or applying overpressure can also 'rule out' a joint or segment as being responsible for signs, if there is no pain response or no worsening of movement pattern following the overpressure.

11.3.2 Palpation

To carry out effective palpation, it is essential that the clinician has a sound knowledge of the animal's anatomy, and has developed skills that enable differentiation between varying states of the soft tissues and articular structures, both within and between individual animals. For example, the musculature of a racing Greyhound will feel completely different from that of a more

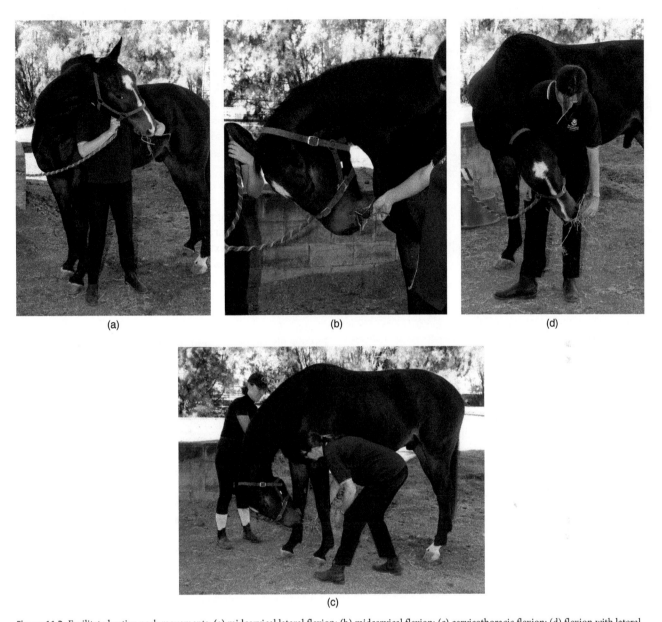

Figure 11.3 Facilitated active neck movements: (a) midcervical lateral flexion; (b) midcervical flexion; (c) cervicothoracic flexion; (d) flexion with lateral flexion.

sedentary lap dog, and the joints of the thoracolumbar region of a Thoroughbred will have a different feel from those of a Welsh Mountain Pony, from a conformational aspect as well as possibly range of motion.

General soft tissue palpation

This may be performed safely on all animal patients and gives the physiotherapist information regarding temperature, soft tissue irritability, muscle spasm/hypertonicity/hypotonicity, bony anomalies, soft tissue thickening/tightness/swelling and pain response. General palpation is also an important part of the physiotherapist's communication with the animal patient, as

a precedent to deeper palpation and further manual examination. This may be carried out before active movements if appropriate.

Specific soft tissue palpation

Muscles can be a source of pain and can be palpated for pain response as well as the parameters mentioned in the above paragraph. Muscle palpation is a subjective assessment technique based on the physiotherapist's experience in feeling the quality of soft tissue. Algometry has been found to be a more objective measure of muscle pain pressure threshold (PPT) and has been used in both human and animal research (Brown *et al.* 2000;

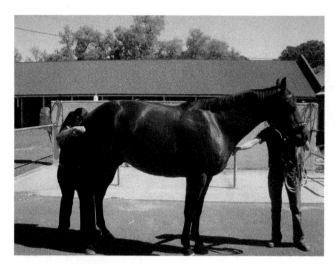

Figure 11.4 Rounding reflex.

Haussler & Erb 2006; Ohrbach & Gale 1989). In veterinary literature, PPT has been referred to as mechanical nociceptive threshold (MNT) (Haussler & Erb 2006). Algometry has been shown to be a repeatable modality for assessment (Varcoe-Cocks *et al.* 2006), and can be used in baseline assessment as well as reassessment.

Specific muscle palpation should be carried out when the working hypothesis suggests that groups or individual muscles are the primary source of signs of pain. Experience will help the physiotherapist to determine whether a pain response on deeper muscle palpation is due to reactivity of muscle groups or symptomatic pain. Often, the quadruped is tender or 'reactive' along the epaxial muscles as a secondary aspect to another injury elsewhere. It is therefore necessary to compare palpation side to side, and develop a feel for localised spasm or alteration in muscle texture, as opposed to general reactivity. Alteration in muscle texture may manifest as strong, hypertonicity (spasm), hypotonicity, 'boggy' (oedematous), woody or fibrous. Occasionally the fascia covering the muscle group is not continuous. This may represent a recent or chronic fascial or muscle disruption.

Specific soft tissue palpation can also divulge the presence of scar tissue, effusions, oedema or general soft tissue thickening. These are signs that can readily be measured for reassessment during and after treatment.

Peripheral nerves may be palpated where they are found superficially, for example the distal limb of horses. Careful palpation of the peripheral nerves may provide information regarding pain response, quality of the tissue surrounding the nerve (including protective muscle spasm or muscle atrophy) and this should be carefully compared with the contralateral side.

11.3.3 Passive movement tests

The results of the passive movement examination in terms of the direction of motion loss or instability, the nature of the resistance perceived (tissue resistance of muscle spasm) and the nature and intensity of the pain provoked direct the selection and application of manual therapy techniques. The physiotherapist is looking for reproduction of signs or pain response in the animal, and local discrepancies in movement of the body part or segment such as increased or decreased stiffness. Comparison of movements or components of the movement to the contralateral side is essential while the physiotherapist gains experience in feeling for 'normal' motion, for any given part of the animal. Passive testing may be of body regions or more localised to specific joints or soft tissues.

Passive joint tests

Passive testing of joint motion affects intraarticular and periarticular structures (joint surfaces, joint capsule, ligaments) and to an extent also affects extraarticular structures (musculature, fascia and neuromeningeal tissue) (Coppieters *et al.* 2004). Passive joint movement tests can be divided into passive physiological and passive accessory or translatory joint movements (see also Chapter 12).

Passive physiological joint testing

Passive physiological movements involve the movement patterns observed in active movements, but these are performed on the animal by the physiotherapist when the patient is passive. In the case of the horse, which for physiotherapy examination is usually conscious and standing, true passive physiological movement of certain joints is not possible. This is because of the tonicity of the postural muscles, particularly of the vertebral column. If required, the horse can be sedated by a veterinarian for physiotherapy examination, but the postural stabilising muscles remain recruited in standing. Depending on the state of relaxation of the dog patient, passive physiological joint movements can be carried out on most joints, especially if the dog is recumbent. If required, dogs can be sedated by the veterinarian for physiotherapy assessment. This enables true passive physiological assessment.

Passive physiological joint testing requires knowledge of the normal pattern and amount of movement available at a joint or body segment, to enable the physiotherapist to detect abnormalities of movement (Lee 1995). 'End-feel' of joint range of motion is an important guide as to the status of the joint. A joint may have abnormal range of motion but in addition, qualifying the nature of the end-feel may help with assessment and reassessment and establish more clearly the structures involved in the dysfunction.

Passive accessory joint testing

Passive accessory motion tests are translatory movements applied by the physiotherapist to articular structures, and may be applied to the spine and the extremities. As for passive physiological joint movements, assessment using translatory joint movements involves the judgement of any pain response of the patient and the physiotherapist's perception of the quality and range of movement that result from the translatory forces

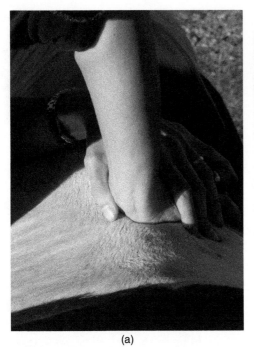
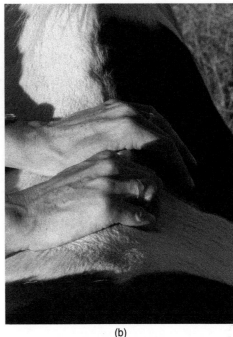

(a) (b)

Figure 11.5 (a) Dorsoventral accessory translation of thoracic vertebral level. (b) Rotational accessory translation of thoracic vertebral level.

applied to the joint. As these applied movements are passive, the same issue with postural muscles and passive physiological movement tests exists. However, translatory movements are small gliding motions, and with careful hand placement and positioning of direction of forces parallel to the 'plane' of the articular surface, information regarding the quality of motion at the joint and pain response can be gathered. It is suggested that in assessment of vertebral levels in humans, a complete examination should include application of forces in a number of angulations of directions to the sagittal plane, to investigate the effect on stiffness, pain and muscle activity surrounding the segments (Caling & Lee 2001) (Figures 11.5, 11.6).

Combined movements are another means by which to perform a more detailed passive movement assessment. Combined movements may allow a more accurate choice of manual treatment technique to be made, and may also help predict the outcome of a technique (Edwards 1994). The increase or decrease in signs produced when combining movements can help the physiotherapist to establish the direction of passive movement best suited as a treatment, as well as predicting response (Edwards 1994). For example, a combined movement in examination of extension and lateral flexion of the thoracolumbar spine may exacerbate a dysfunction at reassessment. A useful technique to relieve signs may then involve flexion and lateral flexion in the opposite direction. If the same technique had improved the dysfunction (say, improved lateral flexion at the thoracolumbar spine), then placing that segment or segments into lateral flexion and extension to apply the chosen technique may be useful.

Combined movements may be performed in the extremities or the vertebral column. In the equine vertebral column,

facilitated movement can be combined with overpressure to result in a combined movement (Figure 11.7). As the canine patient can be made recumbent, it is a little easier to obtain a 'true' passive combined movement in the spine (Figure 11.8). Peripheral joints in the horse may have combined movements applied in standing.

Combined movements may also give information about joint integrity in the periphery. An example is akin to the collateral ligament tests of the human knee, which indicate the possibility of damage of articular structures and will direct the type of management. Periarticular structures in peripheral joints in

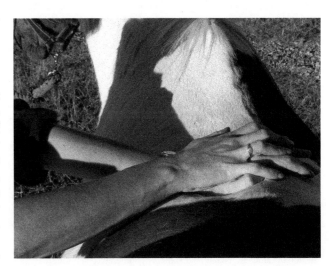

Figure 11.6 Obliquely directed translation over costotransverse joint.

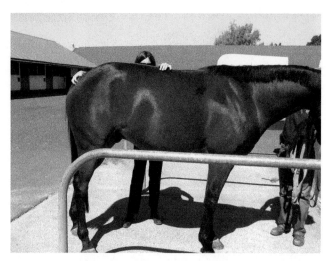

Figure 11.7 Combined movement assessment of flexion and left lateral flexion of equine thoracolumbar spine (using unilateral rounding reflex and overpressure with physiotherapist's left hand at desired level of vertebral column).

both the canine and equine can be similarly assessed using combined movements.

11.3.4 Functional tests

Muscles can be a source of pain but, as previously addressed, can also be examined as a functional unit. Manual muscle testing is carried out in human patients to ascertain the ability of the individual muscles or muscle groups to contract through range and against resistance (Herbert 1995). Muscle testing can also help to localise pain, but it has been argued that strong muscle contraction, particularly isometric, can stress other pain-sensitive structures such as joint surfaces and ligaments. As manual muscle testing is a voluntary activity for the patient to perform at

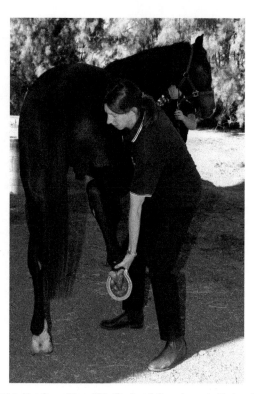

Figure 11.9 Test for unilateral hindlimb stability – horse is displaced toward the left by the physiotherapist. Note, this horse demonstrates hindlimb stability as there is no increase in lateral displacement of the pelvis over the weight-bearing hindlimb.

the request of the clinician, the value of such tests is difficult to determine in animals.

Human research has shown altered patterns of muscle recruitment with functional activities such as balancing on one leg (Hungerford *et al.* 2003) and straight leg raising (O'Sullivan *et al.* 2002). In the animal patient, we can test patterns of functional muscle recruitment. An example is the ability of a horse or dog to unilaterally stabilise on one hind leg: the clinician lifts the contralateral hind leg and displaces the animal towards the standing leg, which allows measurement of the integrity of the muscle groups of the hindlimb and pelvis on the weight-bearing limb (Figure 11.9).

Neural provocation tests

Other manual tests to be grouped into functional tests include testing of the status of the neuromeningeal structures, specifically the ulnar, median and radial nerve of the forelimb, femoral and sciatic nerves in the hindlimb and the meninges of the spinal cord. As is the case in humans, neural provocation tests can be used in animals to assess the effects upon the neural tissue of the structures adjacent to the nervous system (the mechanical interface), and neurobiomechanics, that is sliding of nerve alongside the interface and elongation (Butler 2000). Neurodynamics are also affected by intraneural and extraneural oedema and circulation (Coppieters *et al.* 2004). Results from neural

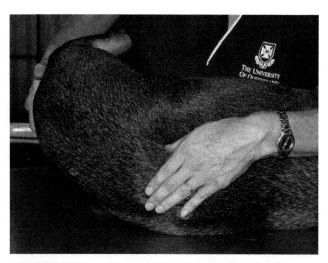

Figure 11.8 Combined movement assessment of flexion and left lateral flexion of canine thoracolumbar spine. Physiotherapist's left thumb is palpating approximation of spinous processes in a relatively flexed position.

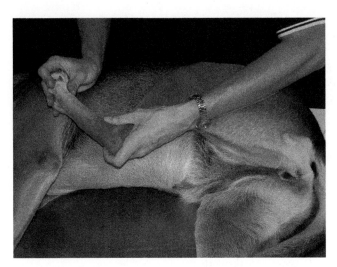

Figure 11.10 Neural provocation test of canine sciatic nerve. *Source:* Babbage *et al.* 2007. Reproduced with permission from Elsevier.

provocation testing may be sensitised by adding or removing a 'central' component such as cervicothoracic or thoracolumbar flexion (equivalent to the slump test in human physiotherapy) (Coppieters & Butler 2001). A pain response may be reproduced during tension testing, and increased stiffness in neural tissue may limit movement (Boland 1995). Animal patients cannot report reproduction of symptoms, so the physiotherapist must be sensitive to increase in perceived tension of the neuromeningeal structures, and compare side to side. Neural provocations tests are used not only to establish the contribution of the structure to symptoms, but for reassessment and treatment (Figure 11.10).

Neurological examination

Neurological examination is an important part of the functional assessment and is carried out when there are signs suggesting that neural conductivity is abnormal. Neurological tests may be used to monitor the progress of the patient (see Chapters 9, 10). When providing physiotherapy assessment or treatment, it is important to know where the neurological system may be compromised and to what degree. This will ensure the physiotherapy assessment does not further compromise the neural conductivity in the relevant part of the nervous system and the appropriate technique is eventually chosen for treatment. In all manual assessment, particularly when the vertebral column is involved, it is vital to perform a neurological examination focusing on the spinal cord to determine if there are neurologically based contraindications to manual therapy. Much of the neurological assessment will have been performed during the examination of the animal's gait (see Chapters 7, 8) and it is pertinent to always include specific neurological provocation tests in your gait assessment. Examples are, in the horse, small circles, walking up and down hills and backing (see Chapter 10) and in the dog, the hindlimb placing reflex (see Chapter 9). Scuffing of the

toenails or areas of wear on the dorsum of the pad or hoof can alert the examiner to the likelihood of reduced proprioception and this should be investigated further.

11.4 Special considerations in canine physiotherapy assessment

11.4.1 History

During the history taking, the physiotherapist may gain clues or red flags (contraindications or precautions for examination) as to breed-typical diseases, just from observing the breed and conformation of the dog. For example, some toy breeds are predisposed to patella subluxation; young, large breed dogs are predisposed to ununited anconeal process, osteochondritis dissecans and panosteitis; and old, large breed dogs are predisposed to chronic hip dysplasia. It is important, however, not to make assumptions regarding the dog's condition based only on the breed or conformation.

Recording the age of the patient is essential. Immature animals may have skeletal developmental growth disorders, and aged dogs may have degenerative conditions that require modification of examination techniques. Information should be gathered from the owner concerning the animal's home environment, diet, exercise levels and occupation (companion animal or working dog).

The following are suggested questions that may be useful.
- Does the dog live inside or out?
  If the dog lives inside, ask the following questions.
- Has there been a change in the home which coincides with the onset of their symptoms, for example have wood floors, tiled floors or vinyl floors recently been fitted?
- Do they live with other animals, cats, dogs, etc.?
- Is there a boisterous puppy or child in the house that they regularly play with?
- Where is their bed, and what type of bedding is used? For example, is it a hard or soft surface? Could it possibly be in a draft? Are they confined to a cage?
- Do they regularly climb the stairs or are there steps in or out of the house?
- Do they jump in or out of the car, on and off the owner's bed/settee, etc.?
  If the dog lives outside, ask the following questions.
- Are they chained?
- What type of shelter do they have?
- Has there been a change to the garden layout or surfaces?
- Plus any of the questions already listed for indoor dogs.

It is useful to ask the owner to describe in detail the animal's daily routine from the time it wakes in the morning to the time it goes to sleep. This will gather information of the amount and type of exercise that the dog has.

The following questions may be of benefit when discussing the patient's exercise levels.
- Is it a working dog or companion animal?

If it is a working dog, specific information related to the discipline undertaken should be gathered. If it is a companion animal, ask the following general questions.

- What is the frequency of exercise – once, twice daily, weekly, etc.?
- How long is the typical exercise session in terms of minutes?
- Is the dog leash-walked or allowed free exercise, or a combination of both?
- Does the dog play with other dogs when out?
- What type of lead/harness does it wear?
- Does it play with toys, e.g. chase balls/frisbees/squirrels/ rabbits?

In addition, the owner should be asked if exercise seems to exacerbate or lessen signs. For example, the animal may initially appear stiff on an affected limb and may subsequently warm up and move more freely after exercise. Conversely, some animals may appear more uncomfortable after exercise. Discomfort/lameness may become more apparent several hours later or the next morning.

11.4.2 Canine static observation

It is useful to consider individual breed differences when conducting a visual examination. Each breed will have its own stance and posture; for example, chondrodystrophic breeds such as Bull Dogs and Bassett Hounds will stand completely differently from breeds such as the German Shepherd and Labrador Retriever. Any deviation from the breed standard should be recorded, together with information relating to the patient's general condition in terms of weight and muscling. Obesity is known to exacerbate chronic lameness in dogs and condition scoring can be a useful objective measure during treatment (see Chapter 3).

Observation of the position of the head and neck and trunk will often give clues as to the amount of weight that an animal is putting through its limbs. Observation has been covered in section 11.2.3 of this chapter.

11.4.3 Canine dynamic observation and gait assessment

The dog should be observed both statically and when moving, to determine information about its static and dynamic conformation and posture. Its willingness to move in general, coupled with the fluidity of motion when changing postures, should be noted. For example, is the animal able to get from lying to sitting, sitting to standing with ease and vice versa? Is it symmetrical in its movement patterns, and equally weight bearing on each limb? Does it appear to be in pain? Does it vocalise? When changing position, does it do so in a consistent pattern?

If possible, it is preferable to observe the dog ambulating on a number of different surfaces at different gait speeds. This should be done in a controlled environment, without evident distractions for the patient. Ideally, the dog should be observed on and off the lead. If it is only possible to see the animal moving on the lead, the owner should be asked to walk on either side of the animal with a slack lead to allow the dog to move freely without interference. The dog should be observed from different angles.

11.4.4 Canine palpation

Before beginning palpation of a dog, it is important to carry out a risk assessment. Part of this will have been done by observing the dog during the subjective assessment, and observation of static and dynamic postures. The physiotherapist needs to be aware that one of the dog's defence mechanisms is biting, especially if it is in pain (see Chapter 2). A restraint such as a muzzle is a useful piece of equipment to carry when providing physiotherapy for dogs. The owner may need to acclimatise the animal to wearing a muzzle in advance of the physiotherapy sessions.

Many dogs become tense when standing on an examination table, making it difficult to assess muscle tone accurately. A 'vet bed' can provide a useful alternative.

Pain response as a result of palpation is often dependent on the pain tolerance of the animal concerned. Some breeds are known to be more stoic than others.

Every clinician will develop his or her own examination sequence when palpating a dog. Some prefer to start with the head and work caudally; others will start at the toes and work dorsally. All parts of the dog should be palpated sequentially, even if the presenting problem is an obvious injury such as a 'knocked-up/sprung toe' in a competitive animal. All animals learn compensatory movement patterns, very often resulting in secondary musculoskeletal problems.

11.5 Assessment and palpation of canine extremities

11.5.1 General palpation of the limbs

The dog's limbs may be palpated with the patient in the standing or recumbent position, or both. The advantage of having the dog in lateral recumbency is that they can be more readily restrained by the physiotherapist or handler, allowing a more thorough examination of the limb in question. Palpation of animals in standing allows a comparison of left and right limbs, by palpating both sides simultaneously. Both limbs should be similarly positioned.

It is preferable to start proximally and work distally following the lie of the coat, initially applying gentle pressure with the flat of the hand to allow the patient to become acclimatised to contact by the physiotherapist. Differences in muscle definition, atrophy/hypertrophy, soft tissue swelling, bony anomalies and temperature and pain responses between the left and right side should be noted. Differences noted may be examined in more detail when the animal is later placed in lateral recumbency.

11.5.2 Palpation of the canine limbs

The joints of the thoracic and pelvic limbs should be assessed, including palpation of:

- bony landmarks
- ranges of motion
- joint stability.

A detailed assessment of each muscle is beyond the scope of this chapter. However, it is expected that the examining physiotherapist will have an excellent grasp of the regional muscle anatomy, so that they are able to evaluate systematically each muscle in turn, noting clinical signs of atrophy, hypertrophy, spasm, haematomas, tears, adhesions and discomfort. Specific muscle and tendon pathologies related to individual joints will be highlighted. When assessing joint range of motion, the affected and the contralateral joint should be simultaneously tested, comparing the quality and resistance of the joint movement, crepitus and end-feel. Ranges of motion vary between breeds and have been published for the Labrador Retriever (Crook *et al.* 2007; Jaegger *et al.* 2002) and Greyhound (Nicholson *et al.* 2007). If joint instability is suspected following physiotherapy examination, the referring veterinarian should be consulted so that any underlying pathologies can be further evaluated. Orthopaedic assessment of the thoracic and pelvic limbs is detailed in Chapter 8.

11.5.3 Palpation of the canine vertebral column

Assessment of the head, vertebral column and pelvis often requires detailed neurological evaluation. For further details refer to Chapter 9.

Head and cervical spine

The position of the head on the neck should be observed from above, the front and either side. Any obvious neurological signs such as head tilt, nystagmus and paralysis/paresis of the facial muscles should be investigated fully before commencing further examination. The general demeanour of the animal should be noted, together with its responsiveness to verbal stimulation.

Palpable bony landmarks of the head

- Occipital protuberance
- Nuchal line
- Mastoid process
- Temporomandibular joint

Palpable bony landmarks of the cervical spine

- Wings of the atlas
- Vertebral bodies of C2–6
- Vertebral body of C7? This depends on the size of the dog but is generally difficult to palpate.

Active range of motion

The dog should be encouraged to go through the full active range of neck motion. This can be done in the form of a baited stretch where the dog reaches for a treat. For the caudal cervical spine, the dog is asked to flex fully to the middle of the chest, extend, side-flex and rotate throughout the whole cervical spine to either side. The cranial cervical spine motion can be differentiated from the caudal cervical spine by gently stabilising dorsally over C2 region and guiding the nose in a forward and upward motion to simulate upper cervical extension. The nose can be guided closer toward the cranial chest to gain the upper cervical 'nodding' motion. Upper cervical rotation can be guided with a food treat, in a motion simulating the nose rotating around the longitudinal axis of the dens of C2.

Passive range of motion

With the animal in the sitting or standing position, one hand is used to stabilise the shoulder girdle, while the other hand gently guides the head through available range, noting any resistance from the animal, the quality of the movement and end-feel. Care should be taken not to exceed the range of motion achieved by the dog actively, or past the dog's comfortable range. Again, with careful hand placement, upper cervical motion can be differentiated from the caudal cervical motion. (Refer to contraindications to cervical manual techniques for dogs in Table 12.2.)

Ranges of motion in the cranial cervical spine (O–C1–C2)

- Flexion (O–C1): nose to upper chest
- Extension (O–C1): nose moved in a forward direction first then up toward ceiling
- Rotation (C1–2): nose 'pivots' around the estimated longitudinal axis of the dens of C2

Ranges of motion in the caudal cervical spine (C2–7)

- Flexion: nose to lower chest
- Extension: nose to ceiling (90°) to remainder of vertebral column
- Sideflexion/rotation: nose to lateral chest wall

The greatest amount of flexion and extension (nodding movement) occurs at the atlantooccipital joint. Rotation is greatest at the atlantoaxial joint, with smaller amounts of flexion, extension, sideflexion and rotation occurring throughout the rest of the cervical spine. It should be noted that coupled motion occurs throughout the spine owing to the orientation of the facet joints; hence, lateral flexion is accompanied by rotation (Johnson *et al.* 2011) (see also Chapter 4).

Assessing for pain/restricted motion

If the dog is unwilling to go through full active/passive range of motion, this may be because of pain or restriction of soft tissues or articular structures. Palpation of the muscles, soft tissues and joints may give further clues as to the source of the limitation. Pain response or altered motion arising from vertebral segments can be determined by palpating ventrolaterally, dorsolaterally and via a lateral translatory glide (Figure 11.11). The plane of the articular facets should guide the direction of passive movement assessment (see Chapter 4). The accuracy of palpation of vertebral levels is dependent on the size of the dog.

Thoracic spine

The dog should be observed for degree of thoracic lordosis or kyphosis from the front, above and either side, plus symmetry of the ribcage noted.

Palpable bony landmarks of the thoracic spine

- Spinous processes T1–13 inclusive
- Anticlinal vertebrae T10–11

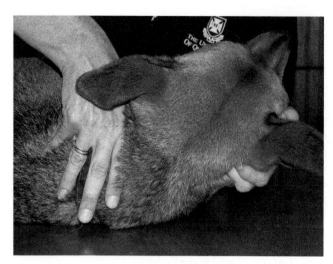

Figure 11.11 Lateral accessory translation of C3–4.

- Ribs 1–13
- Sternum

Ranges of motion of the thoracic spine

Specific ranges of intervertebral motion have not been documented for the thoracic spine in the dog. Research by Takeuchi *et al.* (1999) revealed increases in neutral zone in the thoracic spine joints of the dog following partial discectomy, which further increased after resection of the rib head at one level studied. It is thought that orientation of the articular facets, intervertebral discs and rib articulations guide the direction and amount of available motion (see Chapter 4).

Active assessment of thoracic spine

The dog may be observed in various positions and activities which move the thoracic spine, such as scratching or stretching. Lateral flexion-baited stretches can be utilised, similar to those for the cervical spine, but encouraging the dog's nose to approximate the flank. Lateral flexion can be combined with extension and flexion of the thoracic spine by directing the treat appropriately.

Passive assessment of motion of the entire thoracic spine

With the animal in the standing position, perform the following.
- Dorsal flexion: the flat of one hand is placed under the dog's chest on the sternum and applies pressure in a dorsal direction, encouraging the dog to round its back.
- Ventral flexion: the flat of one hand is placed on the thorax of the dog at about the level of T6–10 and applies pressure in a ventral direction, encouraging the animal to arch its back.
- Sideflexion/rotation: the flat of one hand applies dorsolateral pressure to the side of the chest wall, while the other hand stabilises at the shoulder/hip region.

Assessing individual joint mobility in the thoracic spine and ribcage

The spinous processes in the dog are readily palpable, so it is possible to determine joint mobility at each segmental level. As for the cervical spine, accuracy of individual vertebral level palpation is dependent upon the size of the dog.

Thoracic dorsoventral mobility

This can be assessed by applying digital dorsoventral pressure either side of the spinous process, and repeating at each level.

Thoracic rotation

This can be tested by applying unilateral dorsoventral pressure either side of the spinous process. In both cases, the quantity and quality of the movement and the end-feel should be noted, together with any indication of discomfort from the animal.

Mobility of the ribcage

With the dog in the standing position, it is possible to determine mobility of the ribcage, by laying the flat of each hand laterally on either side of the chest wall at approximately the same level, comparing left and right sides. Rib excursion may be felt during respiration.

Mobility of the costovertebral and costosternal joints

This can be achieved by applying digital pressure in a ventral direction over the costovertebral joints and by applying a dorsal pressure over the costosternal joints. Range and quality of motion are noted, and compared side to side.

Lumbar spine
Palpable bony landmarks
- Spinous processes L1–7
- Lumbosacral junction
- Wings of the ilia

Ranges of motion of the lumbar spine

The facet joints of the canine lumbar spine display mostly sagittal alignment, with interlocking of the caudal and cranial articular processes; therefore flexion–extension tends to be the main movement available at this part of the vertebral column. Preliminary data from *in vitro* study suggest that flexion–extension is variable throughout the lumbar spine, increasing from 5–10° at L4–5, to 40° at L7–S1. The greatest amount of lateral bend occurs at L4–5, and very little axial rotation was observed at all lumbar segments. Flexion–extension is coupled with slight axial rotation, which increases cranial to caudal. During lateral flexion and axial rotation, the coupling of motion is greatest in the lumbosacral segment, followed by L4–5 (Benninger *et al.* 2004).

At the lumbosacral junction, the caudal articular facets face mediodorsally and cranial facets face lateroventrally – they are more angled to the transverse plane than the more cranial lumbar joints. Flexion–extension is significant at this articulation (Benninger *et al.* 2006). Dogs who have undergone partial discectomy and dorsal laminectomy at the lumbosacral junction have significant spinal instability, so care should be taken when palpating dogs with such a surgical history (Early *et al.* 2013).

Passive assessment of movement of the entire lumbar spine

With the animal in the standing position, perform the following.

- Dorsal flexion: the flat of one hand is placed under the dog's belly and applies pressure in a dorsal direction, encouraging the animal to round its back.
- Ventral flexion: the flat of one hand is placed on the dorsal lumbar spine of the animal at the level of L1–6 and applies pressure in a ventral direction, encouraging the animal to arch its back.
- Sideflexion/rotation: the flat of one hand applies dorsolateral pressure to the side of the lumbar spine, while the other hand stabilises at the thoracic/hip region.

Assessing individual joint mobility in the lumbar spine

The spinous processes in the dog are readily palpable so it is possible to determine joint mobility at each segmental level.

Lumbar dorsoventral mobility

This can be assessed for extension of a given vertebral motion segment by applying dorsoventral pressure either side of the spinous process, and repeating at each level for comparison of range of motion, end-feel and pain response. The relative 'opening' or fanning out between spinous processes, as an indication of flexion at a given motion segment, can be localised between vertebral segments by careful palpation with one hand and application of ventral 'lift' via the abdomen with the other hand.

Assessment of dorsoventral mobility can also be carried out via passive physiological movement tests in lateral recumbency. This is described in detail for thoracic segments in Chapter 12, and can be applied to any vertebral level.

Lumbar lateroflexion/rotation

This can be tested by applying unilateral dorsoventral pressure either side of the spinous process, in a direction obliquely angled toward the midline. This is mostly applicable for more caudal levels. Comparison between levels and from side to side should be performed. See Chapter 12 for passive physiological movement test in lateral recumbency as described for thoracic vertebral levels.

Pelvis and sacroiliac joints
Palpable bony landmarks

- Iliac crest
- Tuber sacrale
- Sacrum
- Cranial dorsal iliac spine
- Cranial ventral iliac spine
- Greater ischiatic notch
- Lesser ischiatic notch
- Greater trochanter
- Caudal vertebrae

Note any differences in the relative positions of the bony landmarks on the left and right sides.

Ranges of motion of the pelvis and sacroiliac joints

The main movements available at the sacroiliac joint are flexion–extension with a total of range of 7° thought to be available (Gregory *et al.* 1986).

Assessing passive mobility of the sacroiliac joints

Palpation of the ilial wing and the sacral body simultaneously (with flat of hand or two fingers) allows relative motion between the ilium and the sacrum to be assessed during protraction/retraction of the hindlimb. This may be done in lateral recumbency or in standing (Figure 11.12). A dorsal glide of the ilium on the sacrum can be applied via the hindlimb and any relative dorsoventral motion between ilium and sacrum assessed. Gapping and approximation of the sacroiliac joint can be assessed via the described palpation of ilium and sacrum, with adduction and abduction of the hindlimb.

11.6 Special considerations in equine physiotherapy assessment

As for dogs, there are certain breeds of horse which tend to carry certain conditions. Examples are atlantoaxial/occipital malformation in Arabians, cervical vertebral malformation (CVM or 'wobbler') in Thoroughbreds and Warmbloods, and developmental (congenital) peripheral joint disease in Warmbloods and also miniature breeds. It is important, however, to take a full, unbiased history without 'labelling' the horse into a category.

Special questions pertaining to the equine patient include:

- horse's occupation or use – current and past, including current level of training
- tack – type, fit, recent changes
- nutrition
- shoeing/trimming
- rider musculoskeletal dysfunction existing concurrently.

11.6.1 Equine static observation

General static observation of the quadruped has been covered in section 11.2.3. Specifically for horses, it is important to observe the following.

Trunk

- Areas of white hair under girth or saddle region (may indicate poor tack fit).

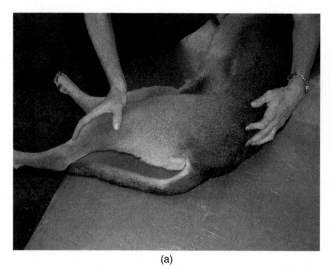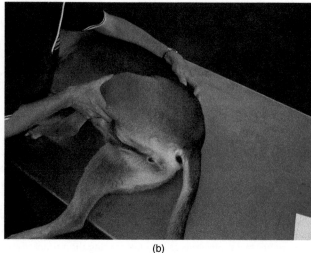

(a)   (b)

Figure 11.12 (a) Palpation of cranial rotation of ilium relative to sacrum via hindlimb retraction. (b) Palpation of caudal rotation of ilium relative to sacrum via hindlimb protraction. Fingers palpate the sacral spine and ilium.

- The curves of the cervical, thoracolumbar and lumbosacral spine in relation to the horse's age, breed and conformation.

Extremities
- Specific detail to hoof wear, hoof axes and shoes.
- Observe closely for scars, swelling and asymmetries of limb alignment.

Head
- Asymmetries of facial features
- Mentation, ear position

11.6.2 Equine dynamic observation and gait assessment

Observation of gait will ascertain the degree of lameness of the animal, if present. Lameness scoring will not be dealt with in detail here; rather, the observation of gait from a physiotherapy movement analysis point of view is discussed.

At the walk

In the absence of obvious lameness, the walk may bring out subtle movement dysfunction that faster gaits may mask. This is because in the walk cycle, there are stages where a limb must be able to stabilise unilaterally at a given point. Kinematic data reveal greater ranges of motion for the thoracolumbar spinal segments at the walk compared with the trot (Roethlisberger *et al.* 2006), giving another reason for the subtle dysfunction of gait being more apparent to the observer at the walk. The horse may be led in hand or observed on the lunge. For the slower gaits of walk and trot, it may be useful to assess both in a straight line and on the circle.

From the lateral aspect (straight line or circle)
- Timing of limb contact with the ground (audible as well as visual)
- Placement of hindlimb with respect to forelimb (degree of 'overreach')
- Placement of hoof (flat/toes first/toes up)
- Head carriage/head 'bob'
- Maintenance of spinal curves
- Tail carriage
- Recruitment of abdominal musculature
- General mobility of trunk, pelvic and neck fascia

From the caudal aspect (straight line)
- Timing of limb contact with the ground (audible as well as visual)
- Tracking of hindlimbs compared with forelimbs
- Specifically for hindlimb – plaiting/winging/mediolateral placement
- Mediolateral placement of hind hoof with ground
- Tail carriage
- Symmetry of rise of gluteal musculature
- Symmetry of lateral swing of pelvis
- Symmetry of lateral swing of ribcage/abdomen

From the cranial aspect (straight line)
- Head carriage/head 'bob'
- Tracking of forelimbs compared with hindlimbs
- Specifically for forelimb – winging/mediolateral placement
- Mediolateral placement of fore hoof with ground
- Symmetry of shoulder motion
- Symmetry of swing of ribcage/abdomen

At the trot

Concussive limb lameness may be more apparent at the trot than the walk, owing to increased loading forces. In the absence of lameness, the following are some useful points regarding gait analysis at the trot.

From the lateral aspect

- Head carriage/'bob'
- Symmetry of the diagonal limbs striking the ground
- Tail carriage
- Maintenance of spinal curves
- Recruitment of abdominal musculature
- General mobility of trunk, pelvic and neck fascia
- (On the circle) ability of inside hind leg to 'drive' on the circle – often it will adduct if there is difficulty stabilising
- Degree of overreach

From the caudal aspect

- Timing of limb contact with the ground (audio as well as visual)
- Tracking of hindlimbs compared with forelimbs
- Specifically for hindlimb – plaiting/winging
- Tail carriage
- Symmetry of rise of gluteal musculature
- Symmetry of lateral swing of pelvis
- Symmetry of lateral swing of ribcage/abdomen

From the cranial aspect

- Head carriage/head 'bob'
- Tracking of forelimbs compared with hindlimb
- Specifically for forelimb – winging/mediolateral placement
- Symmetry of shoulder motion
- Symmetry of swing of ribcage/abdomen

At the canter

Important in assessment of gait is the transition from trot to canter and back to trot again. The physiotherapist looks for ease of transition, coordination of limbs and ability of the horse to engage the hind (pelvic) limbs, which involves some lumbosacral flexion as well as recruitment of pelvic and abdominal stabilising musculature (Faber *et al.* 2001). It is important to assess the recruitment of hindlimb musculature with each direction of the canter on the lunge. Canter assessment is usually performed on the lunge owing to the speed of gait.

11.7 Equine palpation

11.7.1 Head, neck and temporomandibular joint

The physiotherapy history should follow on from the veterinary history and examination, in which a *full dental examination* should have been undertaken, along with any other diagnostic tests described above.

Special questions regarding temporomandibular joint (TMJ) dysfunction include asking the owner about the following clinical signs (Moll & May 2002):

- head shaking
- quidding
- apparent masticatory problems

as well as:

- bitting problems.

The above list is not exhaustive, and there may be more subtle clinical signs, which are associated with TMJ dysfunction, such as minor deviations of the poll during work or inability of the horse to accept the bit on one rein.

Observation

- Symmetry of the visible muscles of mastication, primarily the masseter and temporalis muscles at rest
- Symmetry of facial bones, especially mandible
- Position of upper cervical spine regarding extension and flexion, plus symmetry of occipital and upper cervical muscles
- Mastication during eating
- Mentation

Palpation

Careful palpation of the horse's TMJ and comparison with the other side can detect joint effusion. The TMJ is located by following a horizontal projection from the lateral aspect of the eye directly caudal (Moll & May 2002). The distance between the condyle of the mandible and the mastoid process can be palpated and compared side to side, as can the distance between the mastoid process and the atlas. Gentle movement of the mandible in a lateral direction can be used to confirm the location of the mandibular condyle, as the joint line is palpated.

Muscles of mastication should be palpated bilaterally for symmetry of bulk, quality of the muscle belly and pain response. The masseter, temporalis, medial pterygoid (jaw closure) and anterior belly of digastric (jaw opening) are the most easily palpable muscles. The anterior belly of digastric and medial pterygoid muscle are palpated on the medial aspect of the mandible. The strap-like digastric belly can be distinguished medially and rostrally from the medial pterygoid. The occipitomandibular part of the caudal belly of digastric, which assists in raising the tongue and hyoid bone, can be palpated just caudal to the mandible. Other muscles assisting jaw opening are geniohyoid, inferior genioglossus, sternohyoid and omohyoid (Baker 2002). The latter two muscles can be palpated just caudal to the hyoid bone and run caudally to the scapula, crossing the larynx (Sisson 1975).

Algometry has been used in assessment of pain in the muscles of mastication in human TMJ dysfunction (Farella *et al.* 2000; Michelotti *et al.* 2004), and has been shown to be useful in assessment of pain response in horses (Varcoe-Cocks *et al.* 2006). Algometry therefore may be an objective measure of TMJ dysfunction where there is muscular adaptation or spasm.

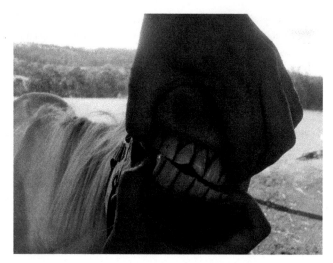

Figure 11.13 Lateral excursion test to examine dental/temporomandibular joint movement.

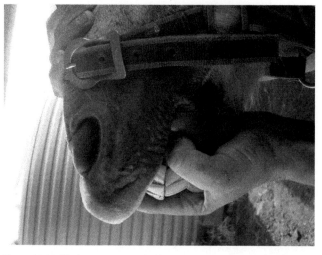

Figure 11.14 Flexion test to examine jaw movement relative to head position.

Motion tests
Lateral mandibular glide
Symmetry of lateral glide of the mandible may give an indication of altered mediolateral excursion. The mandible can be moved laterally in relation to the stabilised maxilla, where the examiner should see an initial lateral displacement of the mandible, followed by an oblique glide of the mandible relative to the maxilla which 'gaps' the upper and lower incisor rows (Figure 11.13).

Flexion test
This tests the rostral movement of the mandible relative to the maxilla. The front incisors are palpated by the examiner's index finger while the head is flexed on the upper cervical spine. There should be a relative rostral movement of the lower incisors compared with the upper incisors, indicating a slight rostral movement of the mandible. If the head is moved into a relative upper cervical extension, then the lower incisors should be felt to glide caudally on the upper incisors (Figure 11.14).

11.7.2 Equine cervical spine
Palpation
The muscles of the occiput, temporal and hyoid region should be palpated for symmetry, tone, thickening, tenderness and spasm. This can be done bilaterally, taking care of your position if in front of the horse when palpating the occipital region, as the horse can throw its head up if there is a pain response. The larger muscles of the cervical spine should also be palpated with the same parameters in mind.

Each vertebral body can be palpated from C1 to C6. When palpating horses with a lot of soft tissue coverage, it is often useful to count the spaces between the vertebral bodies to enable identification of each vertebral level.

Active movements
Observation of the horse during gait, on small circles and ridden, during grazing/feeding will give an overall impression of cervical range of active motion.

Baited active movements for cranial cervical spine
- Extension: guide horse's muzzle forward and up (with a treat), so effecting upper cervical extension.
- Flexion: guide horse's muzzle towards upper chest to effect a nodding movement (at the poll).

For caudal cervical spine
- Flexion: for lower cervical/upper thoracic flexion, guide horse's muzzle down between fetlocks (or observe horse grazing – check for even weight distribution between forelimbs); also guide horse's muzzle towards sternum to check midcervical flexion.
- Lateral flexion: guide muzzle around along horse's lateral trunk towards the flank and compare range side to side.
- Lateral flexion/flexion: guide muzzle around towards the carpal region and compare range side to side (see Figure 11.3).

Passive physiological movements
Many of these manoeuvres are passive-assisted movements (not true passive physiological movement tests) as the horse is not truly relaxed in the standing position.

Cranial cervical spine
- Extension: guide muzzle as described above (with or without treat); stabilise with one hand over C1 and apply 'lifting' overpressure from underneath the muzzle. Assess end-feel and any asymmetrical deviation (laterally or rotatory) of the occiput on C1.

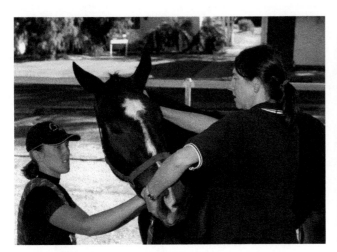

Figure 11.15 Passive physiological assessment of equine atlantoaxial (C1–2) joint.

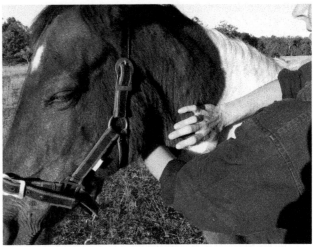

Figure 11.16 Oblique dorsoventral translation at C3–4. Near hand is applying translation to C4 vertebral body while far hand is stabilising C3 contralaterally.

- Flexion: guide muzzle towards the upper chest; stabilise with one hand over C1 and apply gentle overpressure to the front of the muzzle or maxilla. Assess end-feel and any deviation of occiput on C1.
- Rotation: stabilise with one hand over C2 and guide horse's muzzle toward you on an axis that is approximately through the longitudinal axis of the dens. Apply overpressure via the muzzle, rotating it towards you. Compare range of motion and end-feel side to side (Figure 11.15).

Caudal cervical spine
- Flexion: passive neck flexion is difficult to assess as it requires the horse to initiate the action.
- Extension: as above.
- Lateral flexion: motion at each cervical level between C3 and C6 can be assessed by palpating the 'opening' of the cervical vertebrae when an assistant laterally flexes the horse's neck away from the assessor.
- *Or*: stabilise with one hand over the vertebral body to effectively 'block' motion from the chosen level caudal, and gently guide the horse's muzzle toward you, in a lateral flexion direction. Apply gentle overpressure; assess range of motion and end-feel and compare side to side.

Passive accessory palpation
Lateral glide technique to caudal cervical spine
This technique is described in detail in Chapter 12, and involves assessing the relative lateral glide of the more cranial level on the more caudal level. Range of motion and end-feel are compared side to side.

Oblique dorsoventral translation
This technique assesses the combined ventral and lateral glide of a vertebral level relative to the segment above and below. Translation is applied in an oblique dorsoventral direction on the body

of the vertebra, while stabilising the level cranial to that from the contralateral side (Figure 11.16).

Oblique ventrodorsal translation
Translation is applied in an oblique ventrodorsal direction on the body of the vertebra, while stabilising the level caudal to that from the contralateral side.

11.7.3 Thoracic and thoracolumbar spine
Palpation
The musculature of the trunk, including the epaxial muscles, abdominal muscles and wither region, should be palpated for symmetry, tone, thickening, swelling, tenderness and spasm. The spinous processes of T4–18 should be identified and the corresponding rib angles. Often it is helpful to identify the last thoracic vertebra via the 18th rib and palpate cranially. The sternum and manubrium and costal cartilages should be palpated ventrally.

The lumbar spinous process should be identified from L1 to L6 – often it is easier to count back cranially from the lumbosacral junction. The transverse processes can be palpated, depending on the depth of soft tissue coverage. Note that some horses may only have five lumbar vertebrae and/or transitional thoracolumbar and sacral vertebrae (see Chapter 4) (Stubbs *et al.* 2006).

Active movements
Active movements are assisted with either baited stretching or using reflexes inherent in the horse.
- Lateral flexion: observation of the relative contribution of the cranial thoracic spine to a baited lateral flexion test of the cervical spine, or making the horse perform a tight circle; can be compared side to side. The lateral flexion reflex can be initiated by stimulating the contralateral gluteal region of the horse

with a firm object such as fingernail, pen cap or blunt hoof pick. The horse will tend to shift the pelvis away from the irritant, and as there is minimal lateral flexion in the lumbar vertebral column, much of the movement occurs at the thoracic spine (this is often combined with some flexion of the thoracolumbar region).

- Flexion: a ventrodorsal 'lift' reflex can be performed via the manubrium/sternum or more caudally at the level of the girth. A firm pressure with fingernails, pen cap or blunt hoof pick applied to the midline of the above-mentioned regions can cause the horse to 'lift' the cranial thoracic region. The motion at the thoracic spinous processes is observed.
- Extension: dorsoventral extension or 'hollowing' of the thoracic spine can be induced by stimulating as mentioned above along the epaxial muscles. This can be performed bilaterally for extension or unilaterally for a combined extension/lateral flexion movement. Differences side to side can be noted.

Passive physiological movements

As for the cervical spine, these manoeuvres are passive-assisted movements (not true passive physiological movement tests) as the horse is not truly relaxed in the standing position.

- Lateral flexion: use of the lateral flexion reflex can be localised to a given level of the thoracic spine by stabilising with one hand over the lateral aspect of the spinous process, and causing the horse to flex laterally. The amount of intervertebral lateral flexion can be compared between levels and then side to side. Depending on the size of horse and examiner, the horse's pelvis may also be pulled towards the examiner to create a lateral flexion movement as an alternative to using the reflex (Figure 11.17). Motion can also be assessed between ribs and rib angles with this technique.
- Flexion: using reflexes described above, the horse can be encouraged to perform a ventrodorsal 'lift'. The physiotherapist can palpate the relative 'opening' movements between the spinous processes and compare between levels.

Passive accessory palpation

- Extension: a dorsoventral translation can be applied in a direction perpendicular to the spinous process, to effect an extension movement between vertebral segments (or groups of vertebral levels). Care should be taken to be aware of the angles of the individual spinous processes, as cranial thoracic processes tend to override the body of the next caudal vertebra. T1–15 spinous processes are angled dorsocaudally, change at the anticlinal vertebra T16 to an upright position, and are angled dorsocranially from T16 to T17.
- Lateral flexion/rotation: a relative latero-rotatory translation of one vertebra relative to the next can be applied in a variety of ways, and it is to be noted that lateral flexion is coupled with rotation in the thoracic spine (see Chapter 5 for definition).

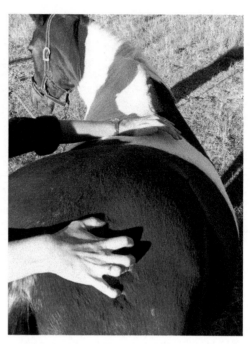

Figure 11.17 Use of reflex to induce left lateral flexion at thoracolumbar spine. Physiotherapist localises the lateral flexion at desired level with hand.

- Digital pressure may be used to 'pull' a spinous process towards you from the contralateral side, effecting a lateral flexion at that level combined with an ipsilateral rotation. Comparison between levels and side to side, regarding range and quality of motion, should be performed.
- Translation of the vertebral body via the spinous process from the ipsilateral side may achieve a relative movement between adjacent vertebrae – it is useful to provide a 'counter' stabilisation at the spinous process cranial or caudal.
- Rotation/lateral flexion: an obliquely, medially and ventrally directed glide applied over the costotransverse joint (between transverse process and tubercle on rib) may effect a relative rotation and lateral translation between vertebral levels in the thoracic spine. The quality of movement and end-feel should be compared between levels and side to side.

11.7.4 Lumbopelvic and sacroiliac/hip region
Palpation

The gluteal musculature in particular (note middle gluteal; extends as far cranial as the lumbar spine) should be palpated for symmetry, tone, thickening, swelling, tenderness and spasm, along with biceps femoris, hamstring group, tail head muscles, adductor and medial and lateral thigh muscles. The lumbosacral junction, tuber coxae, tuber sacrale, ischial tuberosity, sacral spinous processes, caudal vertebrae, pelvic symphysis and greater trochanter should be identified – in particular, symmetry of the tubera coxae and sacrale, sacral spines and pelvic symphysis. The dorsal sacroiliac ligament is palpable running from tuber sacrale to abaxial surface of sacral spine.

The sacrotuberous ligament is palpable medial and cranially to the ischial tuberosity.

Active movements

Active movements of the lumbopelvic and sacroiliac region can be observed during straight line gait (look for symmetry at walk and trot), tight circles, canter transitions, rein-back, walking up and down hills, and unilateral hindlimb stance. Rounding reflex via the gluteal musculature can indicate ability to rotate the pelvis caudally and extension reflex can indicate ability to rotate the pelvis cranially.

Passive movements

The tail can be extended and moved laterally to ascertain tail head muscle tone, as well as comparison of motion side to side, as far cranial as the sacrum (one hand moves the tail while the other palpates over the relevant vertebral level).

The hindlimb can be moved into protraction to assess relative caudal rotation of the pelvis on that side, and retraction to assess relative cranial rotation (Figure 11.18). It is difficult to differentiate between coxofemoral joint and pelvic motion when using the hindlimb to cause physiological movement, so these joints could be considered a functional unit. The limb can be adducted and abducted to assess relative motion of the hip in these ranges. Compare range and quality of motion side to side.

Passive physiological and passive accessory movements

- Ilium on sacrum: cranial, caudal and oblique rotations can be applied to the ilium around the sacrum as well as dorsoventral translations via the tuber coxae and tuber sacrale. The latter may be angulated laterally to follow the plane of the ilial wing. Compare range and quality of motion, and end-feel side to side (Figure 11.19).
- Sacrum on ilium: the sacrum can be translated laterally by stabilising the ipsilateral tuber sacrale and gripping the sacral spines and gliding towards the operator. Compare range and quality of motion, and end-feel side to side (Figure 11.20).
- A dorsoventral translation can be applied to the sacrum, centrally, and a relative longitudinal distraction translation can be applied by 'cupping' the most anterior sacral spinous process and gliding the sacrum caudally.

11.7.5 Scapulothoracic articulation
Palpation

The borders and surfaces of the scapula, including the supraglenoid tubercle, the dorsal scapular cartilage as well as the superficial muscles such as deltoid, supraspinatus, infraspinatus, triceps group, serratus ventralis, subclavius and trapezius, should be palpated and compared side to side. The muscles on the ventral thorax, that is the pectoral groups (ascending, transverse and descending), sternocephalicus and brachiocephalicus should also be palpated.

Active movements

The movement of the scapula on the thorax can be observed during varieties of gait, including changes of direction that involve adduction and abduction of the forelimb.

Passive movements

Gliding or translatory movements of the scapula can be performed in craniocaudal, dorsoventral and abduction directions.

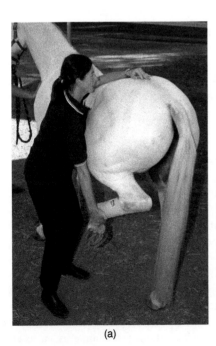
(a)

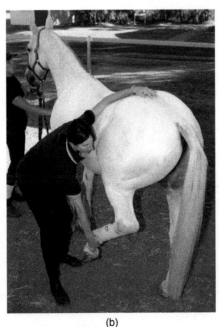
(b)

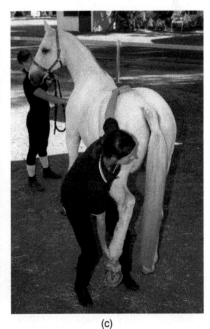
(c)

Figure 11.18 Palpating relative iliosacral motion at tuber sacrale and sacrum via movement of hindlimb. (a) Neutral; (b) in protraction; (c) in retraction.

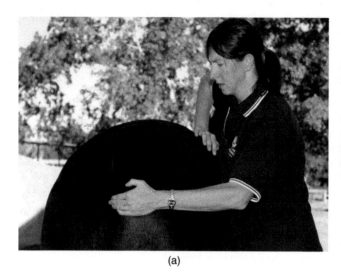
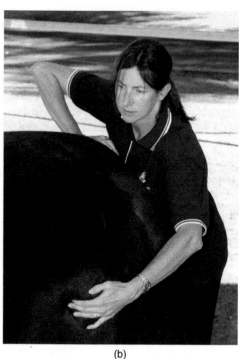

(a)   (b)

Figure 11.19 Assessing movement of ilium on sacrum: (a) cranial rotation; (b) oblique rotation.

The forelimb is elevated and flexed at the carpus, elbow and shoulder and the physiotherapist faces the scapula, holding the flexed forelimb and supporting underneath the elbow. The scapula is then translated as described above, in its plane against

Figure 11.20 Lateral translation of sacrum relative to the ilia – physiotherapist's right hand stabilises against right tuber sacrale and left hand glides sacrum laterally towards the right.

the thorax. Range and quality of movement are noted and compared side to side.

Relative flexion/extension excursion of the scapula can also be observed and/or palpated with full retraction and protraction of the forelimb. Relative abduction and adduction of the forelimb can provide an observable assessment for abduction/adduction excursion of the scapula.

11.7.6 Glenohumeral joint
Palpation

The greater and lesser tubercles of the humerus are readily palpated, and the joint line can be identified with the shoulder in flexion, applying a slight cranial force along the axis of the humerus. The biceps tendon, from supraglenoid tubercle via the intertubercular groove, can be palpated.

Active movements

Active movements of flexion and extension can be observed during various gaits.

Passive movements
Passive physiological movements

The humerus lies at right angles to the scapula and may be further flexed, with the rest of the forelimb also flexed for ease of handling. The physiotherapist faces the trunk of the horse and applies flexion to the shoulder via the distal humerus. The integrity of the muscular support of the joint can be assessed by applying medial and lateral rotations to the humerus, via its distal end, and comparing end-feel and range of motion side to side.

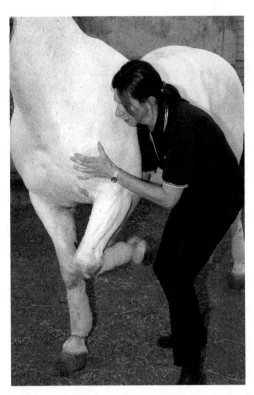

Figure 11.21 Assessing cranial translation of the humerus at glenohumeral joint – left hand is palpating the joint line, while cranial translation of humerus is applied along the humeral longitudinal axis via the physiotherapist's forearm.

Extension of the glenohumeral joint is most easily assessed when combined with a caudal translation of the scapulothoracic articulation (see earlier in this chapter).

Passive accessory movements
The forelimb is flexed for ease of handling with the physiotherapist facing slightly cranially, palpating the glenohumeral joint line. Cranial and caudal translation of the humerus can be performed to assess joint range of motion (Figure 11.21). Medial and lateral rotations can be applied via the humerus (as above) and assessed via palpation of the joint line.

11.7.7 Elbow joint
Palpation
Medial and lateral epicondyles of the humerus, olecranon, lacertus fibrosus (crossing the flexor aspect of the elbow), brachialis and triceps may be palpated and compared side to side. Musculature distal to the elbow (muscles of the forearm) includes the extensor and flexor groups.

Active movements
Active movements of the elbow may be observed during various gaits.

Passive movements
Passive physiological movements
The elbow may be flexed passively and extended via the radius/ulna (with the carpus in flexion for ease of handling), using counter-pressure on the distal humerus. Medial and lateral movements may be applied to the joint at various angles of flexion and extension to test joint integrity. For all passive physiological movements, joint end-feel, quality and range of motion are compared side to side.

Passive accessory movements
With the elbow in a neutral flexed/extended position, a longitudinal force can be applied along the radius/ulna, and the relative translation palpated via the heel of the hand at the olecranon (humerus is stabilised distally). Medial and lateral translation can be applied, and joint end-feel, quality and range of motion are compared side to side.

11.7.8 Carpal joint
Palpation (including metacarpal region)
In extension (standing), the styloid processes of distal radius, extensor tendons and accessory carpal bone are readily palpable. In flexion, the radiocarpal joint space (which has greatest mobility) and midcarpal joint space can be palpated on the extensor aspect, for relative range of motion and the presence of any joint distension. The joint line of the carpometacarpal joint may also be palpated on the extensor aspect. The palmar carpal ligament can be palpated on the flexor aspect and, just distally, the accessory (check) ligament of the deep digital flexor tendon. Distal to these structures, the superficial and deep digital flexor tendons should be distinguishable from each other. The third metacarpal should be palpated for irregularities, as should the second and fourth metacarpals (medial and lateral splint bones).

Active movements
Active movements of the carpal joint may be observed during various gaits.

Passive movements
Passive physiological movements
The carpus as a whole may be fully flexed, and mediolateral movements and medial and lateral rotations applied to the fully flexed position, via the metacarpal, to test joint integrity and range of motion. The carpus is in extension in standing, but overpressure may be applied with the forelimb in protraction, and via application of force over the flexor surface of the carpus (the physiotherapist may differentiate the articular rows) (Figure 11.22). Joint end-feel, quality and range of motion are compared side to side.

Passive accessory movements
In flexion, cranial translation of the proximal carpal row on the radius may be performed. The physiotherapist faces cranially and supports the metacarpal and applies translation with thumb

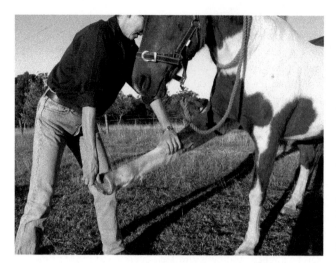

Figure 11.22 Assessment of carpal extension via overpressure.

or web of hand. The translation may be biased towards the radial carpal bone or ulna/intermediate carpals, and the amount of flexion of the carpal joint required to access the proximal carpals varies between horses. Joint end-feel, quality and range of motion are compared side to side.

The amount of appreciable motion at the middle carpal joint and carpometacarpal joint make accessory translation a difficult task. As extension is the close-packed position of the carpal joint, translation of the carpals in a caudal direction is also a difficult task.

11.7.9 Metacarpophalangeal joint (fetlock)
Palpation

The distal third metacarpal, proximal sesamoids and proximal phalanx (PI) should be palpated for irregularities and compared side to side. Proximally and palmolaterally, the interosseous ligament may be identified. The palmar ligament, collateral and straight sesamoidean ligament may be palpated at the palmar aspect. Distension of the joint capsule ('wind puffs') may be palpated between the interosseous ligament and the sesamoid bones.

Active movements

Active movements of the metacarpophalangeal joint may be observed during various gaits.

Passive movements
Passive physiological movements

The joint is extended in standing and thus may be further flexed in non-weight bearing, and overpressure applied to assess the end-feel, quality and range of motion, and compared side to side. Even though the shape of the joint restricts the motion to flexion-extension, medial and lateral rotation may be applied to the joint in various flexed positions to assess its integrity. Joint end-feel, quality and range of motion are compared side to side.

Passive accessory movements

A relative cranial translation of the proximal phalanx may be performed upon the metacarpal. The physiotherapist may face cranially or caudally and, stabilising the distal metacarpal, apply the cranially directed translation close to the joint line of the proximal phalanx. Joint end-feel, quality and range of motion are compared side to side.

11.7.10 Proximal interphalangeal joint (PIP) – PI/PII (pastern joint)
Palpation

Palpation of the bony surface of PI and PII and along the coronet band for irregularities can be performed and compared side to side. Axial and abaxial ligaments may be palpated along the palmar aspect of PI.

Active movements

Active movements at the PIP joint may be more difficult to observe than more proximal joints when observing gait, but should be compared from side to side.

Passive movements
Passive physiological movements

Passive flexion and extension can be assessed by stabilising PI and flexing or extending PII. Overpressure may be applied in the flexion-extension direction, and also medial and lateral rotation, and abduction/adduction applied at various angles of flexion-extension. Joint end-feel, quality and range of motion are compared side to side.

Passive accessory movements

Cranial translation of PII relative to PI is achieved by stabilising PI and gliding PII in a cranial direction, holding close to the joint line (Figure 11.23). Accessory rotations may be delivered using the same stabilisation and handholds. Joint end-feel, quality and range of motion are compared side to side.

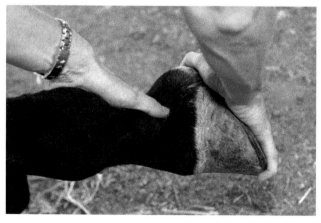

Figure 11.23 Accessory translation of distal phalanx (PIII) on middle phalanx (PII). Left hand stabilising proximal phalanx (with joint in neutral) as right hand applies translation.

11.7.11 Distal interphalangeal joint (DIP) – PII/PIII (coffin joint)
Palpation

The distal phalanx (PIII) is contained within and conforms to the interior of the hoof, so it is not readily palpable. The hoof should be observed and palpated for irregularities and compared side to side (see Chapter 7).

Active movements

Active movements are difficult to ascertain by observation but are thought to mirror those of the PIP joint.

Passive movements

Careful stabilisation of the middle phalanx (PII) can allow a relative translation of the distal phalanx via the hoof. A relative cranial glide of PIII on PII may be achieved, and medial and lateral rotation accessory glides can be assessed and compared, as for other joints, side to side.

11.7.12 Coxofemoral joint (hip)
Palpation

The greater (cranial and caudal parts) trochanter and the third trochanter, plus the musculature covering the region (gluteal muscles, tensor fascia latae, biceps femoris, semitendinosus, semimembranosus, adductors, pectineus, gracilis, sartorius, quadriceps femoris), should be palpated and compared side to side.

Active movements

The active movements of the hip joint as part of the lumbopelvic-hip complex should be observed during gaits (including movements which cause abduction/adduction of the hindlimb). (See also section 11.7.4 on the lumbopelvic and sacroiliac/hip region.)

Passive movements
Passive physiological movements

The hindlimb can be moved into protraction to assess relative caudal rotation of the hip/pelvis on that side, and retraction to assess relative cranial rotation. It is difficult to differentiate between coxofemoral joint and pelvic motion when using the hindlimb to cause physiological movement, so these joints could be considered as a functional unit. The limb can be adducted and abducted to assess relative motion of the hip in these ranges. Palpation of the greater trochanter or third trochanter during these hindlimb movements may give an indication of relative coxofemoral movement as opposed to that of the ilium/hemipelvis. Compare range and quality of motion side to side.

Passive accessory movements

Due to the depth of the coxofemoral joint, passive accessory glides are difficult to deliver. (See passive accessories delivered via the ilium; section 11.7.4.)

11.7.13 Stifle (tibiofemoral and patellofemoral joints)
Palpation

The patella and the three patellar ligaments should be palpated – often these ligaments are more accessible to palpation when the stifle is in flexion. Medial and lateral femoral condyles may be palpated as well as insertions of musculature of the anterior, medial and lateral thigh.

Active movements

The active movements of the stifle as a whole should be observed during gaits, with particular attention to the presence of any patellar locking.

Passive movements
Passive physiological movements

The tibiofemoral joint may be flexed, as well as extended (both these movements are coupled with the hock due to the reciprocal apparatus – see Chapter 5), and medial and lateral rotation applied to the joint via the tibia to assess the integrity of the joint. Quality of movement, end-feel and range of motion should be compared side to side.

The patellofemoral joint may be palpated as the tibiofemoral joint is flexed and extended to ascertain its pattern of passive glide in the femoral trochlea. It also may be palpated as the horse walks, to ascertain the quality of the movement. Mild locking can sometimes be identified in this way.

The proximal tibiofibular joint has little movement (there is no distal tibiofibular joint in the horse).

Passive accessory movements

The patella may be translated in the trochlea of the femur in a craniocaudal direction and a mediolateral direction.

11.7.14 Tarsal joint (hock)
Palpation

The muscles covering the tibia (craniolateral group and caudal group) should be palpated, as well as the medial and lateral malleoli, the calcaneal tuber and calcaneal tendon (gastrocnemius). Proximal metatarsal, fourth (lateral) and third (medial) tarsal bones may also be palpated. Superficial and deep digital flexor tendons may be palpated on the flexor aspect from an area proximal to the calcaneal tuber. On the medial (extensor) aspect of the hock, the cunean tendon (medial branch of tibialis cranialis) is palpable.

Active movements

Hock action is readily observed during a variety of gaits.

Passive movements
Passive physiological movements

The hock as a whole may be fully flexed and compared side to side. Most of the motion occurs at the tarsocrural joint. Extension of the hock is coupled with stifle movements (see reciprocal apparatus in Chapter 5) and if full extension is independently available at the hock, then partial or full rupture of the peroneus tertius should be considered.

Passive accessory movements

It is difficult to apply translatory joint movements to the hock because the hock movement is coupled with stifle movement, and the 'stack' of tarsal bones and the tarsometatarsal joint allow little appreciable movement. Small amounts of mediolateral translation may be applied to the calcaneal tuber, which may reflect accessory lateral movement of the calcaneus.

11.7.15 Metatarsophalangeal joint and interphalangeal joints

See similar in forelimb: sections 11.7.9, 11.7.10 and 11.7.11.

11.8 Conclusion

This chapter has provided a summary of the key components of physiotherapy assessment for animals. The importance of an accurate history and the use of clinical reasoning, careful and logical motion analysis, and palpation skills have been emphasised in guiding selection of treatment. Physical examination of the main joints and soft tissues of the dog and horse vertebral column and extremities has also been outlined. Please refer to orthopaedic (Chapters 7, 8), neurological (Chapters 9, 10), manual therapy (Chapter 12) and other chapters in this book to provide information necessary for a comprehensive assessment of the animal patient.

References

Adams, C., Kurtz, S. 2012, Coaching and feedback: enhancing communication teaching and learning in veterinary practice settings. *J. Vet. Med. Educ.* 39(3): 217–228.

Babbage, C., Coppieters, M., McGowan, C. 2007, Strain and excursion of the sciatic nerve in the dog: biomechanical considerations in the development of a clinical test for increased neural mechanosensitivity. *Vet. J.* 174(2): 330–336.

Baker, G. 2002, Equine temporomandibular joint (TMJ): morphology, function and clinical disease. *AAEP Proc.* 48: 442–447.

Benninger, M.I., Seiler, G.S., Robinson, L.E. *et al.* 2004, Three-dimensional motion patter of the caudal lumber and lumbosacral portions of the vertebral column of dogs. *Am. J. Vet. Res.* 65(5): 544–551.

Benninger, M., Seiler, G., Robinson, L. *et al.* 2006, Effects of anatomic conformation on the three-dimensional motion of the caudal lumbar and lumbosacral portions of the vertebral column of dogs. *Am. J. Vet. Res.* 67(1): 43–50.

Boland, R. 1995, Tension tests. In: Refshauge, K., Gass, L. (eds), *Musculoskeletal Physiotherapy – Clinical Science and Practice*. Butterworth Heinemann, Oxford.

Brown, F., Robinson, M., Riley, J. *et al.* 2000, Better palpation of pain: reliability and validity of a new pressure pain protocol in TMD. *Cranio* 18: 58–65.

Butler, D. 2000, *The Sensitive Nervous System. Noigroup Publications*, Adelaide, Australia.

Caling, B., Lee, M. 2001, Effect of direction of applied mobilisation force on the posteroanterior response in the lumbar spine. *J. Manip. Physiol. Ther.* 24(2): 71–78.

Coppieters, M., Butler, D. 2001, In defense of neural mobilisation. *J. Orthop. Sports Phys. Ther.* 31(9): 520–521.

Coppieters, M., Bartholomeeusen, K., Stappaerts, K. 2004, Incorporating nerve-gliding techniques in the conservative treatment of cubital tunnel syndrome. *J. Manip. Physiol. Ther.* 27(9): 560–568.

Crook, T.C., McGowan, C.M., Pead, M. 2007, The effect of passive stretching on canine osteoarthritic joints. *Vet. Rec.* 160(16): 545–547.

Early, P., Mente, P.,Dillard, S. *et al.* 2013, In vitro biomechanical comparison of the flexion/extension mobility of the canine lumbosacral junction before and after dorsal laminectomy and partial discectomy. *Vet. J.* 196(3): 533–535.

Edwards, B. 1994, Examination of high cervical spine using combined movements. In: Boyling, J.D., Palastanga, N. (eds), *Grieve's Modern Manual Therapy, The Vertebral Column*, 2nd edn. Churchill Livingstone, Edinburgh.

Faber, M., Johnston, C., Schamhardt, H. *et al.* 2001, Three-dimensional kinematics of the equine spine during canter. *Equine Vet. J.* 33(suppl): 145–149.

Farella, M., Michelotti, A., Steenks, M. *et al.* 2000, The diagnostic value of pressure algometry in myofascial pain of the jaw muscles. *J. Oral Rehabil.* 27: 9–14.

Goodsell, M., Refshauge, K. 1995, The physical examination. In: Refshauge, K., Gass, L. (eds), *Musculoskeletal Physiotherapy – Clinical Science and Practice*. Butterworth Heinemann, Oxford, pp. 115–119.

Gregory, C., Cullen, J., Pool, R. *et al.* 1986, The canine sacroiliac joint – preliminary study of anatomy, histopathology and biomechanics. *Spine* 11(10): 1044–1048.

Haussler, K., Erb, H. 2006, Mechanical nociceptive threshold in the axial skeleton of horses. *Equine Vet. J.* 38(1): 70–75.

Herbert, R. 1995, Adaptations of muscle and connective tissue. In: Refshauge, K., Gass, L. (eds), *Musculoskeletal Physiotherapy – Clinical Science and Practice*. Butterworth Heinemann, Oxford, pp. 27–32.

Hungerford, B., Gilleard, W., Hodges, P. 2003, Evidence of altered lumbopelvic muscle recruitment in the presence of sacroiliac joint pain. *Spine* 28(14): 1593–1600.

Jaegger, G., Marcellin-Little, D.J., Levine, D. 2002, Reliability of goniometry in Labrador Retrievers. *Am. J. Vet. Res.* 63(7): 979–986.

Jeffcott, L., Dalin, G., Ekman, S. *et al.* 1985, Sacroiliac lesions as a cause of chronic poor performance in competitive horses. *Equine Vet. J.* 17(2): 111–118.

Johnson, J., da Costa, R., Bhattacharya, S. *et al.* 2011, Kinematic motion patterns of the cranial and caudal canine cervical spine. *Vet. Surg.* 40(6): 720–727.

Jones, M. 1994, Clinical reasoning process in manipulative therapy. In: Boyling, J.D., Palastanga, N. (eds), *Grieve's Modern Manual Therapy, The Vertebral Column*, 2nd edn. Churchill Livingstone, Edinburgh.

Lee, M. 1995, Biomechanics of joint movements. In: Refshauge, K., Gass, L. (eds), *Musculoskeletal Physiotherapy – Clinical Science and Practice*. Butterworth Heinemann, Oxford.

Liljebrink, Y., Bergh, A. 2010, Goniometry: is it a reliable tool to monitor passive joint range of motion in horses? *Equine Vet J.* 42(suppl): S676–682.

Michelotti, A., Steenks, M., Farella, M. *et al.* 2004, The additional value of a home physical therapy regimen versus patient-only education for the treatment of myofascial pain of the jaw muscles: short-term results of a randomised clinical trial. *J. Orofac. Pain* 18(2): 114–125.

Moll, H., May, K. 2002, A review of conditions of the equine temporomandibular joint. *AAEP Proc.* 48: 240–243.

Nicholson, H.L., Osmotherly, P.G., Smith, B.A. *et al.* 2007, Determinants of passive hip range of movement in adult Greyhounds. *Aust. Vet. J.* 85(6): 217–221.

Ohrbach, R., Gale, E. 1989, Pressure pain thresholds in normal muscles: reliability, measurement effects and topographic differences. *Pain* 37: 257–263.

O'Sullivan, P., Beales, D., Beetham, J. *et al.* 2002, Altered motor control strategies in subjects with sacroiliac joint pain during active straightleg-raise test. *Spine* 27(1): E1–E8.

Refshauge, K., Latimer, J. 1995, The history (Chapter 5) and The physical examination (Chapter 6). In: Refshauge, K. Gass, L. (eds) *Musculoskeletal Physiotherapy – Clinical Science and Practice*. Butterworth Heinemann, Oxford, pp. 95 and 111–115.

Roethlisberger, K., Wennerstrandt, J., Lagerquist, U. *et al.* 2006, Effect of local analgesia on movement of the equine back. *Equine Vet. J.* 38(1): 65–69.

Sisson, S. 1975, Peripheral nervous system. In: Getty, R. (ed.), *Sisson and Grossman's The Anatomy of the Domestic Animals*, 5th edn. WB Saunders, Philadelphia, PA, p. 508.

Stubbs, N., Hodges, P., Jeffcoat, L. *et al.* 2006, Functional anatomy of the caudal thoracolumbar and lumbosacral spine in the horse. *Equine Vet. J.* 36(suppl): S393–399.

Takeuchi, T., Abumi, K., Shono, Y. *et al.* 1999, Biomechanical role of the intervertebral disc and costovertebral joint in the stability of the thoracic spine. A canine model study. *Spine* 24(14): 1414–1420.

Varcoe-Cocks, K., Sagar, K., Jeffcott, L., *et al.* 2006, Pressure algometry to quantify muscle pain in racehorses with suspected sacroiliac dysfunction. *Equine Vet. J.* 38(6): 558–562.

CHAPTER 12

Manual therapy*

Lesley Goff

Lecturer, Equine Science, School of Agriculture & Food Sciences, The University of Queensland, Gatton, Australia; Director, Active Animal Physiotherapy, Toowoomba, Australia

Summary

Manual therapy is an important aspect of physiotherapy for both the assessment and treatment of animals. In this chapter, the concepts of manual therapy for animals are introduced, along with some explanations for the efficacy of and mechanisms behind the effectiveness of manual therapy techniques. Examples of some manual therapy techniques are provided.

12.1 Introduction

Manual therapy (or manipulative therapy) refers to the practice, within musculoskeletal physiotherapy, of therapist-applied passive or assisted active movement techniques for the management of pain and impairments in the articular, neural and muscle systems. Its use is based on a detailed assessment of the presenting pathophysiological features in the neuro-musculoskeletal system underlying the pain and loss of normal function, for the purposes of diagnosis and management.

Manual therapy is a vital component of the multimodal management approach to musculoskeletal disorders within the field of musculoskeletal physiotherapy. Manual therapy complements other management strategies inclusive of therapeutic exercise, electrophysical agents, functional retraining, education and self-management procedures. The passive movement techniques of manual therapy are used as both assessment and management techniques.

The theory and practice of manual therapy are well established in the management of human musculoskeletal disorders. This chapter will review the practice of manual therapy and how it may be applied to animals. While there can be some direct transfer of principles and practices from the human to the animal, there are obviously issues unique to the animal patient. For example, there are anatomical, kinesiological and functional differences, and animals cannot be instructed to relax, unlike human patients. As a consequence of these factors, the animal physiotherapist is required to modify techniques. This chapter offers some suggestions on the manner in which techniques may be modified as well as providing some insight into the rationale and application of manual therapy. It will offer some examples of treatment for selected extremity and vertebral column articular regions in the dog and the horse.

---

*Adapted from the first edition chapter, which was written by Lesley Goff and Gwendolen Jull

Animal Physiotherapy: Assessment, Treatment and Rehabilitation of Animals, Second Edition. Edited by Catherine M. McGowan and Lesley Goff.
© 2016 John Wiley & Sons, Ltd. Published 2016 by John Wiley & Sons, Ltd.

12.2 Technical aspects of manual therapy

Passive mobilisation is often discussed in terms of effects on intraarticular and periarticular structures (joint surfaces, joint capsule, ligaments). The movements also affect extraarticular structures (muscles, fascia and neuromeningeal tissue). In the application of manual therapy or passive movement, treatment techniques can be applied at different amplitudes, velocities and positions within a joint's range of movement (Maitland *et al.* 2006).

Manual therapy encompasses two predominant technique types.

- Joint manipulation
- Passive joint mobilisation

Joint manipulation is differentiated from joint mobilisation by the speed of application of a single movement (high-velocity thrust). Passive joint mobilisation includes any manual therapy directed at joint or soft tissue structure that does not involve a high–velocity thrust (Hurwitz *et al.* 1996). Passive joint mobilisation involves the rhythmical application of movement, which is performed at a comfortable speed (approximately 2–3 oscillations per second). Passive mobilisation, as its name implies, is traditionally performed as a passive technique, but evolution of the practice has seen the introduction of components of active mobilisation in combination with the therapist-applied passive technique (Mulligan 1995).

The movements performed passively include the joint's physiological movements as well as its accessory (or translatory) movements. Passive physiological movements refer to the rotations that occur around the joint's three axes and are performed by the physiotherapist, usually without the patient's active assistance. Passive accessory movements are the translations which automatically accompany the rotations but, in contrast to the physiological movements, cannot be performed voluntarily by the patient. In a typical joint, translation of a joint surface upon another tends to involve a combination of rolling and sliding (MacConnail 1964). This is partly due to the concavo-convex nature of most joint surfaces (Lee 1995). The direction of translation is related to the plane of the joint and the direction of motion that the physiotherapist wishes to effect. Passive physiological and passive accessory movements may be applied to both the spine and extremity joints in both humans and animals.

Either of the movement types can be performed in assessment or treatment. The physiological or accessory movements can be performed singularly or in combination (Edwards 1994), or the passive mobilisation may be combined with the patient performing directed active movement, termed *mobilisation with movement* (Mulligan 1995). In mobilisation with movement (MWM), the translatory movement of a painful or restricted joint is performed passively by the therapist and the painful or restricted physiological movement is performed simultaneously. The physiological movement may be accomplished actively by the patient or in an assisted active or passive manner (Mulligan 1995). In the case of the animal, the physiological movement is accomplished by instigating an active assisted, passive movement, or reflex movement (Figure 12.1). MWM can be applied to both spinal and extremity joints. When applied to spinal joints, this manual technique is termed the *sustained natural apophyseal glide* (SNAG). Mulligan (1995) points out that the technique applied to the joints in the spine is generally in the direction of the physiological movement that is restricted, and in the extremity joints, the sustained translation is often applied in a related but often different direction from the physiological movement.

12.2.1 Proposed physiological effects of manual therapy

There is a growing bank of research regarding beneficial effects of manual therapy with studies carried out using animal and human models. Randomised control trials in humans have

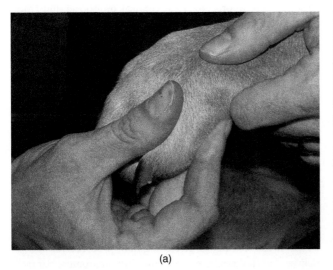
(a)

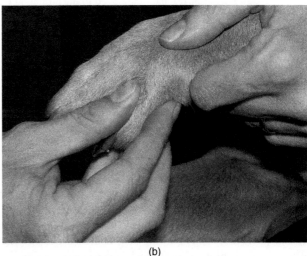
(b)

Figure 12.1 (a) Flexion of canine metacarpophalangeal joint. (b) MWM (flexion/external rotation) of canine metacarpophalangeal joint.

provided evidence of the effectiveness of manual therapy for relief of pain and increase in function (Boline *et al.* 1995; Childs *et al.* 2004; Jull *et al.* 2002; Nilsson *et al.* 1997). Research in more recent times has also attempted to explain these beneficial effects on a physiological basis.

Many theories have been proposed to explain the mechanism of manual or manipulative therapy. Theories on the effect have ranged from biomechanical, for example, movement of the nucleus pulposus in a discal disorder (Haldeman 1978), to effects on the muscle system such as a reduction in paraspinal muscle hypertonicity (Herzog *et al.* 1999). The biomechanical effects were thought to correspond with an alteration in electromyographical activity and/or a temporary increase in degree of joint displacement due to a hysteretic effect (Herzog *et al.* 1999).

There are biomechanical effects of movement-based manual therapy; however, the evidence is not secure for a predominant biomechanical basis to explain the effect of manipulative therapy when used as a single modality. For example, Hearn & Rivett (2002) investigated the reported biomechanical effects of a cervical mobilisation technique – the sustained natural apophyseal glide. The technique was proposed to cause a repositioning of the articular facet as well as affecting the whole functional spinal unit (Mulligan 1995). Hearn & Rivett (2002) found no empirical evidence to support such a biomechanical effect. Likewise, in a single case study with a similar technique applied to a subluxed carpometacarpal joint of the thumb, Hsieh and colleagues (2002), using MRI imaging, were not able to measure any improvement in the positional fault, despite the patient achieving pain relief. Immediate gains in range of movement from a manipulation in an acute neck pain model were lost within 48 hours of treatment (Nansel *et al.* 1990), which highlights the need and supports the evidence (Gross *et al.* 1996) for a multimodal approach inclusive of exercise to assist in maintaining range of movement gains. In a randomised controlled trial, immediate reduction in quadriceps stretch reflex following passive and dynamic oscillations applied to the human knee lasted less than 1 minute (Newham & Lederman 1997). Thus, although biomechanical features are inherent in a movement-based treatment technique, they do not seem to explain, in large part, the beneficial effects of manual and manipulative therapy techniques at this stage of research.

In more recent times there has been a shift toward investigations of neurophysiological mechanisms to explain the pain-relieving effects of manipulative therapy. Neurophysiological studies have investigated models of pain relief resulting from the afferent input and stimulation provided by the locally induced movement. It was thought that such afferent input may stimulate neural inhibitory systems at various levels in the spinal cord (Christian *et al.* 1988; Terrett & Vernon 1984; Wyke 1985), as well as in higher centres in the central nervous system (Wright 1995). A growing body of evidence is showing that one mechanism of pain modulation could be through activation of descending inhibitory pathways via the lateral periaqueductal grey area of the midbrain, suggesting that manipulative therapy produces a non-opioid-mediated hypoalgesia (Vicenzino *et al.* 1994, 1998, 2001; Wright 1995; Wright *et al.* 1994). Recent evidence indicates that spinal manual therapy produces a treatment-specific initial hypoalgesic and sympathoexcitatory effect beyond that of a placebo or control condition (Sterling *et al.* 2001; Vicenzino *et al.* 1998, 2007). A concurrent motor response, a decrease in superficial neck flexor activity, was also noted in the study by Sterling *et al.* (2001) of manual therapy to the C5–6 segment, which would further support the proposal of activation of the periaqueductal grey region. Furthermore, in a series of studies of a manual therapy technique applied to the elbow for lateral epicondylalgia, Paungmali and colleagues (Paungmali *et al.* 2003a,b, 2004) again confirmed the concurrent hypoalgesic and sympathoexcitation effects of manual therapy, and that the initial effect was not antagonised by naloxone, in concordance with a non-opioid mechanism of action. Changes in local and remote skin blood flow (Zegarra-Parodi *et al.* 2015) and local pressure-pain thresholds (Voogt *et al.* 2015) occur immediately following the application of manual therapy.

Manual therapy has also been shown to produce mechanical, not thermal hypoalgesia (Vicenzino *et al.* 1998). This implicates an endogenous noradrenergic over a serotonergic mechanism – that is, a non-opioid form of analgesia. In animal studies, following the injection of inflammatory mediators around the L5 dorsal root ganglion (DRG) in rats, Song *et al.* (2006) demonstrated that spinal manipulation reduced inflammation and hyperexcitibility of the DRG neurons, which was accompanied by a reduction of thermal and mechanical hyperalgesia. Similarly, peripheral joint mobilisation in rats produced an antihyperalgesic effect in conjunction with a normalisation of glia activation in the dorsal horn of the spinal cord (Martins *et al.* 2011).

Manipulative therapy is likely to exert its effects via multiple mechanisms. For example, Heikkila and colleagues (2002) showed some improvement in cervical proprioception (measured as joint position error) following manipulative therapy to the cervical spine. Further research is required to fully understand all mechanisms of effect of manipulative therapy techniques on the sensory, muscular, articular and postural control systems.

12.2.2 The broader scope of manual therapy

The use of manual therapy is not restricted to articular structures. The muscle and neural systems can also contribute to restriction of movement, pain and functional loss. The prevention and treatment of adaptations of muscle and connective tissue that impede the performance of motor tasks is a core part of manual therapy (Herbert 1995). Manual therapy can be utilised to effect muscle length changes via stretching, various massage or soft tissue techniques. Stretching may be sustained, static or delivered via hold–relax or 'proprioceptive neuromuscular facilitation' (PNF) techniques. PNF techniques involve lengthening of target muscles and contraction of opposing muscle groups (Chalmers 2004). This involves a voluntary contraction at command of the therapist; thus sustained or static stretching of muscles and soft tissue, as a technique, may be more applicable to animals than PNF techniques. A recent review of the literature suggests that the effects of mobilisation of muscle via sustained or static stretch, that is, a lengthening of the muscle, are achievable because of the viscoelastic properties of muscle (Chalmers 2004). This may also partly explain the efficacy of other soft tissue manual techniques such as trigger point therapy and myofascial release, both of which involve applying sustained pressure to the muscle and connective tissue. Recent research indicates that compression for myofascial triggers points is effective for acute low back pain (Takamoto *et al.* 2015). Myofascial trigger points have also been described in dogs (Frank 1999; Janssens 1991), horses (Macgregor & Graf von Schweinitz 2006), rabbit and rat muscles (Hong & Simons 1998).

The other soft tissue system that is viscoelastic and must slide and extend in response to the body's movement is the neural system. The neural system is innervated and of itself can cause pain if its movement is impeded or the neural structures are irritated by movement (Butler 2000; Elvey 1994, 1997). The involvement of neural structures is elicited clinically in humans through the use of neural tissue provocation tests (Butler 2000; Elvey 1994, 1997), which involve a combination of limb movements that stress neuromeningeal structures to a greater extent than non-neural structures (Boland 1995). Although little evidence exists as to the physiological effects of neural mobilisation, Butler (2000) has hypothesised that these include dispersion of intraneural oedema, lengthening of neural tissue, improved intraneural blood supply and improved axonal transport. A recent study in rats with a severe peripheral nerve injury showed that passive neurodynamic exercises (sliding and gliding of the nerve in relation to its interface via limb movements) are capable of reducing nociceptive behaviour in combination with a normalisation of the satellite glial cell response in the DRGs and astrocyte response in the spinal cord (Santos *et al.* 2012).

In human physiotherapy, neural tissue provocation tests are performed with standardised procedures, which are based on the pathways that the peripheral nerves take through the body, from emergence of the nerves from the intervertebral canals into the formation of the plexuses. Standardisation of neural tissue provocation tests in animal physiotherapy has been explored in the canine sciatic nerve (Babbage *et al.* 2007). The sequence proposed for the straight leg raising (SLR) test in dogs is hip flexion, stifle extension, hock flexion and extension of the digits. The cumulative increase in strain in the sciatic nerve recorded in this study is comparable to measurements in humans (Figure 12.2).Until further research on neural tissue provocation tests in animals is carried out, knowledge of anatomy of the neural plexuses of the thoracic and pelvic limbs in the quadruped will guide the physiotherapist in the application of neural tissue provocation tests in animals.

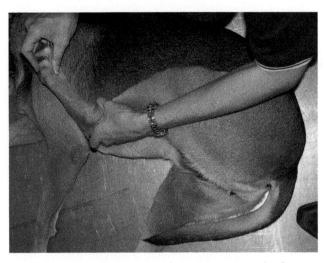

Figure 12.2 Neural provocation tests of canine sciatic nerve – hip flexion, stifle extension, hock flexion and digit extension. *Source:* Babbage *et al.* 2007. Reproduced with permission from Elsevier.

Mobilisation of neuromeningeal structures invariably imparts movement to the physiological mechanical interface, which is the tissue of the nervous system that can move independently from the system (Butler 2000). The interface may include muscle and fascia, ligaments and joints. Pathological interfaces may include scar tissue, osteophytes, ligamentous swelling or oedema (Butler 2000). In contrast, accessory and physiological joint mobilisations and manipulations are commonly performed in patients with neuropathies (Schmid *et al.* 2013). These techniques may facilitate the descending pain inhibitory system (Bialosky *et al.* 2009; Vicenzino *et al.* 2007).

12.3 Manual therapy in practice

12.3.1 Assessment

Assessment of the movement impairment in the articular, muscle and neural systems as well as the reactions to the movement test, in terms of pain response, tissue resistance and muscle guarding, is fundamental to guiding the application of manual therapy techniques. Specific tests are used to examine each system.

With respect to the articular system, both active movements and functional performance are assessed in the first instance. This is followed by a passive examination of the joint's movements. Both passive physiological and accessory movements of the joint are examined in all directions. Physiotherapists using passive physiological movements in the vertebral column of animals need to be aware that different spinal levels demonstrate varying ranges of motion. Range of movement varies between species and is related to biomechanics of the spinal column (see Chapter 4). For example, there is minimal intervertebral lateral flexion available in the equine lumbar spine, owing to the size of the transverse processes and the presence of extra articulations between the transverse processes (Denoix 1999). In the limbs, there is variation in range of motion and resting positions of the peripheral joints, which is breed or species specific. For example, the resting weight-bearing position of the wrist (carpus) is more extended in dogs such as Collies compared with dogs with more upright carpi such as Boxers.

In the tests of physiological and accessory movements, the physiotherapist assesses:

- the range, quality and end-feel of movement that result from the gentle manual forces applied to the joint during the test
- the pain response of the patient to the test.

A thorough knowledge of the normal patterns and ranges of movement available at a joint or body segment provides the basis for decisions on abnormalities of movement (Lee 1995). The results of the passive movement examination in terms of the direction of motion loss or instability, the nature of the resistance perceived (tissue resistance of muscle spasm) and the nature and intensity of the pain provoked direct the selection and application of manual therapy techniques. Passive movements can also be examined with simultaneous performance of an active movement. Assessment for the potential efficacy of an MWM as a treatment involves the reduction of pain or improvement in the range of a joint motion, when the passive translation is applied as the physiological movement is undertaken.

12.3.2 Reliability

It is important that assessment techniques are reliable. Interrater reliability refers to the ability of raters to assign scores in a consistent fashion and is determined when two or more raters judge a given event at the same point in time (Domholdt 2000). Studies of intertherapist reliability of spinal joints have indicated that judgements of joint stiffness or motion by experienced manual therapists have poor to moderate interrater reliability (Hoving et al. 2005; Maher & Adams 1994; Smedmark et al. 2000). A more recent study showed that inter- and intrarater reliability of therapists observing cervical movement control dysfunction tests was good (Segarra et al. 2015). Schneider et al. (2013) showed that experienced physiotherapists using standardised clinical tests (including assessment of cervical spine ROM using measurement devices, and palpation of articular structures for stiffness and for pain response) were moderately to substantially reliable, when assessing cervical spine pain. Judgements that include a pain response (pain provocation tests) have generally shown good to excellent reliability (Hoving et al. 2005; Jull et al. 1988, 1997; Maher & Adams 1994; Potter & Rothstein 1985). The studies on interrater reliability and pain response involve human subjects verbalising the presence of pain during a manual assessment technique. Animals give various signals as pain responses, which include vocalisation, but this is not always the case. This poses a challenge for physiotherapists in animal physiotherapy. It is suggested that animal physiotherapists need to become very sensitive with their manual palpatory skills, as they cannot rely on the pain response alone in assessment and treatment. There is some evidence that it is the complexity of biological tissue that

is responsible for the poor reliability in joint stiffness and movement judgement. Physiotherapists have been shown to be accurate and reliable when testing stiffness and very small ranges of motion on non-biological models (Goff et al. 2004; Latimer et al. 1998).

12.3.3 Selection of manual therapy technique

The selection of technique evolves via clinical reasoning processes that require careful consideration of hypotheses such as sources of symptoms, precautions, prognosis and further contributing factors (Butler et al. 1994). Information to form the hypotheses is derived from questioning, handling skills and previous clinical reasoning experiences that must include due attention to what is known about the presenting pathoanatomy, pathophysiology and psychological traits of the animal. Thus, it goes without saying that a sound knowledge of the anatomy, physiology, conditions and diseases which can affect the animal, as well as animal behaviour, is crucial in such reasoning processes. Close liaison with veterinary professionals is important for knowledge of disease processes and when further examination by a veterinary surgeon is indicated.

There are no recipe approaches for the selection and application of manual therapy interventions in animal or human treatment. Neither is there one correct treatment approach for a given patient's presentation or condition. There are several manual therapy approaches within physiotherapy and randomised clinical trials in humans have shown that they have similar efficacy (Hoving et al. 2002; Jull et al. 2002; Rosenfeld et al. 2000). The skill of the physiotherapist is to select the most appropriate manual therapy intervention for the particular patient, based on the clinical examination of that patient's pain and movement impairments.

Selection of a specific passive mobilisation technique is based on several factors (Maitland et al. 2006). These are inclusive of the specific direction of movement impairment, the limiting features to that movement (pain, tissue resistance or muscle guarding) and the response to the manual tests that have been applied. The technique selected usually relates to the physiological direction (or its associated translatory movement) with the most restriction. In addition, the pain response to that movement will guide how gently or firmly the technique can be applied. The selection and application of the initial passive mobilisation technique are further guided by assessment of the responsiveness to the technique in the examination (Maitland et al. 2006). During the reassessment phase of the examination, if an animal's condition is improved following a passive mobilisation technique, then it is likely that implementing such a technique in treatment will be beneficial. Similarly, if the animal's condition is improved following deep muscle palpation or testing of extensibility in a certain muscle or group of muscles, then it is possible that techniques designed to lengthen or relax those tissues may be of benefit. Neural tissue provocation tests, as discussed, are an important component of the physical examination. If the animal's active movements, pain responses or other signs such as

Table 12.1 Contraindications to manual therapy

Contraindication	Species	Breed/signalment	Action
Severe splinting spasm often seen at a spinal segment	Canine Equine	Spinal fracture, any breed Chondrodysplastic dog breeds for thoracolumbar lesions	Diagnostic imaging or neurological testing by veterinarian. Avoid manual testing of affected segment
Ataxia ± upper motor neuron signs – usually indicates spinal cord disease	Canine Equine	Cervical vertebral malformation in Doberman, Weimeraner, Great Dane (canine), Thoroughbred, Warmblood (equine). Atlantoaxialocciptal deformity in Arabian horses	No treatment should be initiated without accurate diagnosis – further veterinary and diagnostic imaging investigation
Severe progressive pain or non-weight bearing in any limb that does not seem to follow a mechanical pattern on manual testing	Canine	Osteosarcoma of the long bone, particularly in canine breeds such as Rottweiler. Sites of predilection include proximal humerus and distal femur, but can be anywhere	Further veterinary and diagnostic imaging investigation
Non-weight bearing in horses – infection and fracture are main two causes	Equine	Any	Precaution – diagnostic imaging. If hot, swollen peripheral joint, may be infective arthropathy – a veterinary emergency

joint signs are improved after such tests, then selection of gentle neural tissue mobilisation techniques may be warranted at some stage in the management.

12.3.4 Safety

Safety in initial selection and application of manual therapy techniques is a prime consideration for the welfare of the animal. Contraindications to the use of manual therapy techniques are presented in Table 12.1 and precautions are presented in Table 12.2. Precautions and contraindications to manual therapy assessment and treatment are related to certain syndromes or diseases in animals, which can be breed or species specific. This list is not exhaustive. During the assessment, these should be considered as possible breed- and signalment-related red flags. It is the physiotherapist's responsibility to assess each case and to request more information or refer back to a veterinarian for further tests if there are concerns.

As well as the safety of the animal, the safety of the physiotherapist is also paramount. Physiotherapists must be able to apply techniques without the risk of being kicked, bitten or crushed. Injuries from large animals such as horses can be life threatening. Handling animals, large and small, has occupational risks for physiotherapists and other animal handlers. Physiotherapists must always be aware of optimal positioning for themselves. Manual therapy techniques can be physically demanding and

require postures and positions that are potentially causative of injuries.

12.3.5 Treatment dosage

Ongoing reassessment as the treatment is progressing is of fundamental importance. Reassessment is the key to delivering the optimal dosage of treatment. It provides guidance as to the effectiveness of the particular technique chosen and, importantly, provides the direction for the progression of technique as the animal improves. If any improvement within or between treatments does not continue, this indicates that the selection of the particular technique needs to be reappraised and another technique chosen. Continual assessment for responsiveness is integral to the practice of manual therapy. A lack of responsiveness to a technique or an aggravation of the condition can also be a useful guide as to what may help to ease symptoms. Past experience and expected responsiveness of an intervention can also guide the physiotherapist in judging whether the animal has a condition that will or will not respond to manual therapy.

Ideally, the animal should receive as many treatments as are required to effect the change desired by the owner, within the limits of the presenting condition, the animal's age and activity/skill requirements, and the length of time the condition has been present. Improvement in function should be measured and

Table 12.2 Precautions to manual therapy techniques

Precaution	Species	Breed/signalment	Action
Brachycephalic dogs – may have underlying cervical vertebral malformation	Canine	Basset Hounds, Pugs, Pekinese	Active movements only for cervical spine followed by very careful palpation
Lethargy, vomiting, unexpected deterioration of hindlimb weakness	Canine	Any	Any medical problem which may arise needs to be referred back to veterinarians – these could indicate metabolic, toxic or organ disease unrelated to the initial complaint

recorded between sessions. If functional improvement does not occur, then the physiotherapist should reappraise the treatment approach. Other factors such as possible reinjury, compliance with home programmes by the owner, activity levels and other interventions may need to be considered.

It must be stressed that manual therapy is one component of the multimodal management programme provided to the animal. Within the multimodal programme, specific exercises to facilitate the muscle system and functional muscle lengthening exercises, as required, are conducted with the animal. Such procedures capitalise on the improved mechanical function of the animal following a manual therapy intervention and facilitate movement patterns and muscle groups, which may have been inhibited by pain or altered movement (see Chapter 14). A home programme is designed to be carried out by the owner and this is an essential component of overall management.

12.3.6 Considerations in manual physiotherapy for animals

There are both similarities and differences between providing physiotherapy for animals and physiotherapy for humans. From a manual physiotherapy perspective, the concepts of manual assessment and treatment are similar when dealing with human and animal patients, but there are some practical differences. For example, when noting a pain response, the physiotherapist should be very aware of the body language of the animal. Animals, particularly dogs, may vocalise when experiencing pain from palpation or movement, but often the response is to move away from the application, and sometimes to bite, kick or cause deliberate or unintentional harm to the physiotherapist or handler (see Chapter 2). This points to the need for the palpation or movement to be applied with care. With such care, subtle changes can be detected in the segment that the physiotherapist is examining. Such changes may include tissues retracting or moving away from palpation or pressure, a mild spasm reaction or change in surrounding musculature or soft tissue. It is essential for a manual physiotherapist treating animals to develop their palpatory and tissue perception skills to be able to detect subtle changes and response of tissues, especially as a pain response is not always indicative of movement dysfunction.

12.4 Dogs

Dogs, like humans, can be examined in functional positions as well as recumbent positions. The advantage of recumbency is that joints and soft tissue may be palpated or moved through a range of motion in a relaxed state. Being able to perform passive accessory movements as part of manual assessment gives the physiotherapist information regarding movement occurring at the joint's surface, in relation to the movements that take place during physiological movements. The degree of relaxation available when undertaking manual assessment for a dog depends on the arousal or distress levels of the dog and its willingness to be in a recumbent position. Unlike in a human patient, the therapist cannot request a dog to relax in a prone position on a treatment couch, although practice and calm, skilful handling may induce relative relaxation in a dog. Owner cooperation is paramount here. The canine physiotherapist may instruct the owner in appropriate mannerisms and handling to maximise the cooperation of the canine patient. Assistance from a veterinarian regarding sedation or anaesthesia may occasionally be required to complete a full manual examination on a dog that is very anxious.

It is good practice to conduct all relevant tests in one position to maximise comfort of the dog before moving on to the next position. For example, an efficient approach might be to first observe gait and active movements, then carry out manual testing procedures which may be done in standing, such as preliminary neurological tests and certain passive physiological tests. The assessment can then be conducted in recumbency for relevant tests, such as reflex testing, passive accessory spinal or peripheral movements and neural tissue testing. Manual testing must be tailored to that with which the dog will comply. Most manual tests can be modified for position or an alternative test can be devised to minimise distress to the dog. Use of a checklist or consistent examination routine will minimise the chance of omitting parts of the examination.

Breed variation is another consideration when performing a manual musculoskeletal examination of a dog. There are vast differences in size and conformation within the canine species, and the physiotherapist's examination may need to be tailored accordingly. An example is palpation of thoracic spine segments. Palpation of individual spinous processes will not be as specific in a small dog such as a Miniature Fox Terrier compared with a middle-sized or large dog. A skilled manual physiotherapist should be able to modify the examination to account for this, without missing vital information. The canine physiotherapist should be familiar with the conformational differences that exist between dog breeds, as well as related differences in gait.

It is not possible in this section to describe all manual therapy techniques that may be used in the management of dogs, but the following examples illustrate a range of techniques and, importantly, suggest modifications for animals.

12.4.1 Extremity joints

As for human extremity joints, the joints of dog forelimbs and hindlimbs can be moved through their passive physiological and accessory ranges of motion for purposes of both assessment and treatment. Principles of manual handling for both passive physiological and accessory techniques ordain that the proximal segment is usually stabilised and the distal segment moved. The physiotherapist's hands support the limb and joint as close to the joint line as possible, without blocking movement at the joint. In relation to the accessory (translatory) movements, the physio-therapist needs to be aware of the plane of the articular surfaces and the direction of glide of the moving segment. The planes of the articular surfaces are listed in Table 4.1.

Practical descriptions of manual therapy techniques for assessment and treatment of the stifle joint are presented as an example of the process of adaptation for dogs. These concepts can be applied to any peripheral joint in the dog, where the functional anatomy and biomechanics of the joint are understood. These techniques may be applied to the dog in any position, but a position of lateral recumbency is ideal to allow manual handling of joints and relative relaxation of the dog.

Techniques for the canine stifle joint
Passive physiological movements of tibiofemoral and patellofemoral joint complex

The physiotherapist stabilises the femur with one hand while the other hand grasps the proximal tibia. The stifle may be flexed or extended to the end of the available physiological range, or the movement is ceased at a certain point in response to pain. In assessment, the end-feel and pain response are noted and compared with the other side. The joint may be further stressed if more information is required by flexing or extending the joint in differing ranges of hindlimb protraction or retraction. This may be done with the dog recumbent or standing.

Ligamentous integrity of tibiofemoral joint

Ligament tests should be performed in lateral recumbency to ensure the dog is as relaxed as possible. The therapist tests ligamentous integrity by applying medial and lateral stresses (testing joint capsule and collateral ligaments) with the stifle in neutral and then various positions of flexion and extension. The cranial cruciate ligament test involves a cranially directed draw of the tibia upon the femur, with the stifle flexed approximately 120°. The physiotherapist faces cranially, grasping the distal femur, with the thumb stabilising over the lateral femoral condyle and index finger palpating close to the joint line cranially. The other hand grasps the proximal tibia, with the thumb stabilising via the lateral condyle of the tibia and index finger palpating close to the joint line at the tibial tuberosity. The hand stabilising the tibia performs a cranial translation of the tibia upon the femur. Index fingers palpate the distance travelled cranially by the tibial tuberosity relative to the distal femur (joint line), and the physiotherapist notes the quality of end-feel (Figure 12.3). The test should be compared with the other stifle. Sedation may be required to attain a true passive cranial drawer test (for further details, see Chapter 8).

Passive accessory (translation) movements

- Patellofemoral joint: the patella is grasped between the index finger and thumb, and may be translated medially and laterally or dorsoventrally in the trochlea of the distal femur. A comparison of the relative amount of lateral and medial excursion should be made, and the directions of glide compared overall

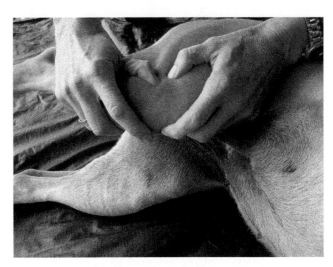

Figure 12.3 Cranial drawer test of canine stifle.

with the contralateral joint. Patella translations or glides may be performed in various tibiofemoral joint angles.

- Tibiofemoral joint: the therapist grips the distal femur and the proximal tibia with both hands close to the joint line. The primary accessory movement glide or translation of the tibia on the femur in relation to physiological flexion–extension will be in a cranial and caudal direction. This can be performed in various angles of flexion–extension. Other accessory movements or glides that are assessed at the tibiofemoral joint include mediolateral glides, internal and external rotation of the tibia on the femur and distraction–compression of tibia on the femur. Again, a judgement is made regarding quality of the translatory movements and/or pain response and responses compared with the contralateral side. Crepitus or meniscal clicks may be felt if there is degenerative change or meniscal pathology. To further assess the medial and lateral compartment of the tibiofemoral joint and the associated menisci, a test similar to McMurray's test in the human can be applied. The tibia can be medially or laterally rotated relative to the femur, whilst passively extending or flexing the stifle.

Treatment

Treatment decisions regarding the direction of treatment movement and dosage are based on the assessment findings of range, tissue resistance and pain response. For example, if there has been primarily a pain response to passive testing, this directs that treatment by either passive physiological or accessory movements should be delivered within a pain-free range. In the tibiofemoral joint, this may be gentle passive flexion or extension mobilisation, a mid-range translatory glide in a neutral position of the stifle or the stifle position is found that allows a more pain-free delivery of either the passive physiological or accessory movement. This could involve positioning into directions other than the main physiological movement; for example, flexion of the joint in slight internal rotation of the tibia or reducing neuromeningeal tension by slightly ipsilaterally laterally flexing the thoracolumbar spine.

If passive testing has revealed that stiffness or restriction is the main problem, then the technique chosen may be to end of range. Techniques to improve flexion or extension include end-range passive physiological movements into flexion or extension, applied in a rhythmical oscillation at a comfortable speed, or using a passive accessory mobilisation, stabilising the femur and translating the tibia upon it in a craniocaudal direction towards end of range, with the stifle in a physiologically flexed or extended position.

An MWM may involve holding the tibia or patella in a position that allows greater flexion or extension to be achieved (rotation, deviation, compression or distraction for tibia and mediolateral or dorsoventral glide for patella) and then applying the passive physiological or accessory movement.

The treatment can be progressed in several ways: the stifle can be held in greater ranges of the movement direction to be achieved; the mobilisation can be performed more towards end range or at end range; neuromeningeal tension may be superimposed on the joint; or number and/or vigour of mobilisation repetitions increased.

12.4.2 Canine vertebral joints

Passive physiological and translatory movements of the vertebral joints are likewise used in both assessment and treatment. The orientation of the facet (zygapophyseal) joints directs the movements that can occur at each level of the vertebral column, so it is important for the physiotherapist to be aware of their anatomical orientation. Intervertebral discs will also affect motion available at a given vertebral level (see Chapter 4). The example presented here will be passive movement assessment of the canine midthoracic spine. With an understanding of anatomy, these principles can be applied throughout the vertebral column. Passive movements to any area of the vertebral column can be applied to the dog in sitting, standing or recumbency (lateral recumbency or supine).

Assessment of joints of the midthoracic spine (T7–8)

The facet joints of T1–9 tend to be orientated in a transverse plane, with the cranial articular processes facing dorsally and the caudal processes facing ventrally. The main movement available from T1–9 is lateral flexion, which tends to be coupled with contralateral rotation (see Chapter 4). The ribs attach to the vertebral bodies of two thoracic vertebrae and the intervening disc to form the costovertebral joints (e.g. the second rib attaches to T1 cranially and T2 caudally). These joints have a small role in limiting motion in the thoracic spine. The costotransverse joints attach to the transverse process and the rib level corresponds to the vertebral level. Thus passive physiological and accessory movement examination of, for example, the T7–8 motion segment involves the facet joints, intervertebral joints and costotransverse joint of T7 and T8 plus the costovertebral joints of ribs 6, 7, 8 and 9. During palpation, it should also be noted that

the spinous processes of this section of thoracic spine overlap the body of the next most caudal vertebra.

Examination of passive physiological movements

- T7–8 (R) lateral flexion with dog standing: the physiotherapist is positioned standing over the dog and faces the dog's head. Depending on the size of the dog, the T8 level is stabilised with the right hand over the side of the vertebral body or with the thumb on the spinous process. The dog's trunk from T7 cranially is guided into right lateral flexion with the left hand down to the T8 segment. The right hand palpates for closing of the vertebral body and ribs on the right side and the therapist notes range of motion, quality of motion and end-feel of the movement. Alternatively, the physiotherapist may face the tail of the dog and, stabilising T7 with the left hand, move the trunk caudal to this level into right lateral flexion.
- Examination of T7–8 (R) lateral flexion in left lateral recumbency: the physiotherapist faces the dog's ventral trunk. The T8 spinous process is stabilised with the left hand and the dog's upper trunk is lifted into right lateral flexion. The stabilising hand palpates either opening or closing movement between T7 and T8 just lateral to the spinous process. Alternatively, the spinous process of T7 is stabilised with the right hand and the dog's lower trunk is lifted into right lateral flexion. Palpate with the right hand as described above (Figure 12.4).

Examination of T7–8 segmental flexion and extension

The relative flexion–extension mobility of the T7–8 motion segment can be assessed by palpating the interspinous space of T7–8 with the dog in lateral recumbency or standing. In standing, the spine and ribcage are moved into relatively flexed and extended positions via the sternum and the ribcage. The relative opening or fanning out of the spinous processes, or rib angles (flexion), or the relative closing of the spinous processes and ribs is palpated. In lateral recumbency, the spinous process of T7 or T8 is palpated while either the caudal or cranial trunk of the dog is moved into flexion and extension. Again, the relative opening and closing are palpated between T7 and T8 as for standing position. Passive physiological movements are compared with levels cranial and caudal to T7–8.

Accessory movement for right lateral flexion of T7–8 in standing or left lateral recumbency

The physiotherapist stabilises the spinous process/laminar region of T7 with the left thumb and uses the right thumb to apply a lateral glide on the right side of T8 towards the left (Figure 12.5a). The amount and quality of motion and end-feel are assessed. The glide may also be performed at the costotransverse joint and the accuracy of application depends on the size of the dog's vertebra. The lateral translations are compared with cranial and caudal levels and compared with motion in left lateral flexion.

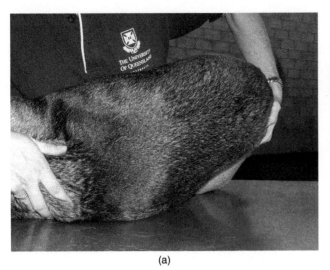
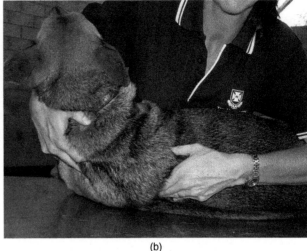

(a)   (b)

Figure 12.4 (a) Passive physiological right lateral flexion of T7–8, stabilising T7 and moving T8. (b) Stabilising T8 and moving T7.

12.5 Horses

As a general rule, equine manual physiotherapy techniques will be carried out with the horse in standing. Horses are rarely assessed in recumbency, as this mostly requires the horse to be anaesthetised. Horses may be sedated by veterinarians for manual examination but even when sedated, the horse can remain in the standing position. As the postural muscles of the horse are active when standing, true passive accessory movement testing is not possible for some joints, such as those of the thoracolumbar region. Palpation of some soft tissues in a relaxed state may not be possible. Modified passive physiological joint movements can be carried out in standing.

Horses requiring physiotherapy are generally accustomed to being handled by owners, farriers and veterinarians, so are quite receptive to manual physiotherapy examination. Great care must always be taken with regard to safety of the physiotherapist at all times. Even under sedation, horses may deliver accurate kicks. Owner cooperation regarding handling of the equine patient is paramount to the safety of the physiotherapist.

12.5.1 Extremity joints
Passive physiological movements may easily be performed on equine limb joints. The approach to accessory/translatory joint movements of the equine limb joints, however, differs slightly from that of the canine, as some of the joints, especially the carpus and hock, are stable and the small flat bones, which comprise part of those joints, are difficult to palpate. The coxofemoral joint is also difficult to approach in a translatory manner owing to its coverage by large musculature. The example of the equine

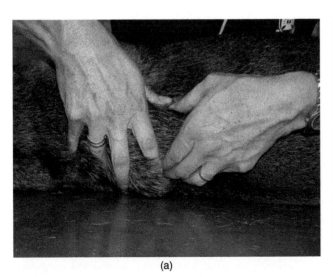
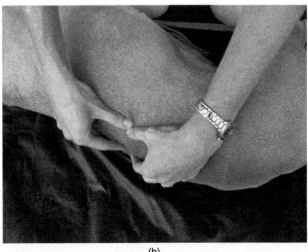

(a)   (b)

Figure 12.5 (a) Right lateral flexion passive accessory translation of T7–8 (left thumb is applying translation to T8 spinous process relative to T7). (b) Hand position for passive accessory translation in caudal thoracic vertebral column.

fetlock (metacarpophalangeal joint) will be used, but principles can be applied to all peripheral joints. As equine limbs can be heavy and dangerous if the horse strikes or kicks, the physiotherapist must be careful with positioning at all times.

Techniques for the metacarpophalangeal (fetlock) joint
Passive physiological movements of equine fetlock joint – flexion and extension

For the technique to be performed in a safe manner, the physiotherapist faces the caudal end of the horse and picks up the hoof. For the assessment of flexion, the toe or front of the hoof is grasped and the fetlock is fully flexed. Any pain response, range, quality and end-feel of the movement are assessed. When flexed, the fetlock has accessory lateral and rotatory movements (see Chapter 5). To further stress the joint, medial and lateral stresses are added to the flexed fetlock. The stress can be applied at various angles of flexion and the amount of medial versus lateral motion is noted and compared. The same process is conducted for medial and lateral rotatory accessory movement. All movements should be compared with the contralateral fetlock.

The fetlock takes up an extended position when the horse is weight bearing, but extension can be further stressed in the following way. The forelimb is picked up and brought into a protracted position. The fetlock is extended further via the toe of the hoof. Overpressure may be applied to the dorsal surface of the fetlock, and the therapist assesses the very slight accessory motion in extension (Figure 12.6). The movement should be compared to the contralateral fetlock.

Assessment of craniocaudal translation of the metacarpophalangeal (fetlock) joint

The physiotherapist picks up the hoof in a safe manner, holding the fetlock in a semi-flexed position (non-close-packed position). The metacarpal is stabilised and the proximal phalanx is grasped close to the joint line. A dorsal glide of the phalanx is directed upon the metacarpal (Figure 12.7). The range

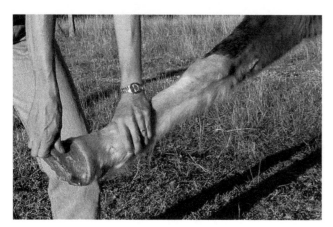

Figure 12.6 Extension with overpressure for equine metacarpophalangeal (fetlock) joint.

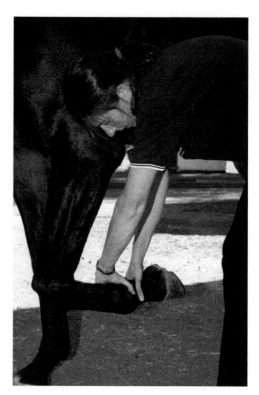

Figure 12.7 Craniocaudal accessory translation of the equine metacarpophalangeal (fetlock) joint – left hand stabilising distal metacarpal, right hand directing glide of proximal phalanx.

of motion, quality of motion and the end-feel of the joint are assessed. The glide can be repeated in various degrees of flexion and also in relative extension. Medial and lateral rotations may be applied to the fetlock joint via the proximal phalanx. All translations should be compared with the contralateral side.

12.5.2 Equine vertebral joints

As for dogs, joints of the equine vertebral column may be taken through passive physiological and translatory movements in both assessment and treatment. Again, the orientation of the facet (zygapophyseal) joints directs the movements that can occur at each level of the vertebral column; the intervertebral discs will also affect motion available at a given vertebral level. The illustrative example will be the passive movement assessment of the midcervical spine. Passive movements are applied to the horse in standing.

Techniques for midcervical spine (C4–5)
Passive physiological movements, lateral flexion C4–5

Note this is a modified passive physiological movement, as the horse's cervical spine is not relaxed in standing. To examine the movement of lateral flexion at the C4–5 segment, the C5 level is stabilised with one hand. The horse's head and neck are guided by the therapist into lateral flexion by directly pulling the head around, or using an active stimulus such as a carrot. The range

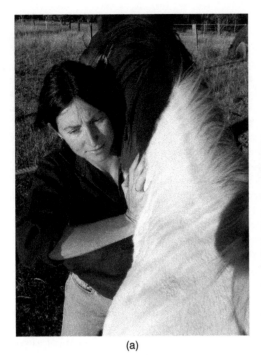
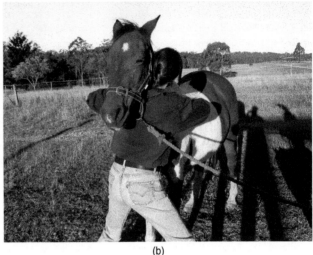

(a)   (b)

Figure 12.8 Accessory lateral flexion glide of equine cervical vertebral. (a) Right hand directs glide to C4 towards the right. (b) Forearms are positioned perpendicular to vertebral body level.

of lateral flexion and the end-feel are assessed via the stabilising hand and the motion is compared with lateral flexion in the opposite direction. Lateral flexion can be tested in various positions of cervicothoracic flexion and extension.

Accessory lateral glide of C3–4

The physiotherapist stands facing the horse's rump and places one hand on either side of the vertebral body. The forearms are positioned perpendicular to the horse's neck to enable a lateral glide to be delivered through the body of the vertebra. To test for left lateral flexion of C3–4, stabilise either side of C3 and glide the vertebral body towards the right (Figure 12.8). The same can be repeated for level C4. The quantity and quality of the movement are assessed and the perceived motion is compared between levels.

12.6 Conclusion

Manual therapy is an essential part of the multimodal approach to assessment and treatment of musculoskeletal disorders in animal physiotherapy. The basic requirements for the application of effective manual therapy are knowledge of the functional anatomy of the musculoskeletal and neuromeningeal systems, and how these systems are affected by pathology and movement dysfunction. Good palpation skills enhance the effectiveness of the manual therapist in both assessment of disorders and delivery of treatment techniques. Manual therapy may be the sole

form of treatment chosen for a given condition, but is usually delivered in conjunction with other therapeutic modalities such as electrotherapy and functional exercise programmes.

References

Babbage, C., Coppieters, M., McGowan, C. 2007, Strain and excursion of the sciatic nerve in the dog: Biomechanical considerations in the development of a clinical test for increased neural mechanosensitivity. *Vet J.* 174(2): 330–336.

Bialosky J., Bishop M., Price, D. *et al.* 2009, The mechanisms of manual therapy in the treatment of musculoskeletal pain: a comprehensive model. *Man. Ther.* 14(5): 531–538.

Boland, R. 1995, Tension tests. In: Refshauge, K., Gass, L. (eds), *Musculoskeletal Physiotherapy – Clinical Science and Practice*. Butterworth Heinemann, Oxford.

Boline, P.D., Kassak, K., Bronfort, G. *et al.* 1995, Spinal manipulation vs. amitriptyline for the treatment of chronic tension-type headaches: a randomised clinical trial. *J. Manipulative Physiol. Ther.* 18: 148–154.

Butler, D. 2000, *The Sensitive Nervous System*. Noigroup Publications, Adelaide. Australia.

Butler, D., Shacklock, M., Slater, H. 1994, Treatment of altered nervous system. In: Boyling, J.D., Palastanga, N. (eds), *Grieve's Modern Manual Therapy, The Vertebral Column*, 2nd edn. Churchill Livingstone, Edinburgh.

Chalmers, G. 2004, Re-examination of the possible role of golgi tendon organ and muscle spindle reflexes in proprioceptive neuromuscular facilitation muscle stretching. *Sports Biomech.* 3(1): 159–183.

Childs, J., Piva, S., Erhard, R. 2004, Immediate improvement in side-to-side weight bearing and iliac crest symmetry after manipulation in patients with low back pain. *J. Manipulative Physiol. Ther.* 27(5): 306–313.

Christian, G.F., Stanton, G.J.,Sissons, D. *et al.* 1988, Immunoreactive ACTH, beta-endorphins and cortisol levels in plasma following spinal manipulative therapy. *Spine* 13: 1411–1417.

Denoix, J-M. 1999, Spinal biomechanics and functional anatomy. *Vet. Clin. North Am. Equine Pract.* 15(1): 27–60.

Domholdt, E. 2000, *Physical Therapy Research, Principles and Applications*, 2nd edn. WB Saunders, Philadelphia, PA.

Edwards, B. 1994, Examination of high cervical spine using combined movements. In: Boyling, J.D., Palastanga, N. (eds), *Grieve's Modern Manual Therapy, The Vertebral Column*, 2nd edn. Churchill Livingstone, Edinburgh.

Elvey, R.L. 1994, The investigation of arm pain. Signs of adverse responses to physical examination of the brachial plexus and related neural tissues. In: Boyling, J.D., Palastanga, N. (eds), *Grieve's Modern Manual Therapy of the Vertebral Column*. Churchill Livingstone, Edinburgh, pp. 577–585.

Elvey, R. 1997, Physical evaluation of the peripheral nervous system in disorders of pain and dysfunction. *J. Hand Ther.* 10: 122–129.

Frank, E.M. 1999, Myofascial trigger point diagnostic criteria in the dog. *J. Musc. Pain* 7(1-2): 231–237.

Goff, L., Gilleard, W., Adams, R. 2004, Physiotherapist reliability in assessment of the stork test. Proceedings of the Australian Physiotherapy Association 8th International Physiotherapy Congress, Adelaide.

Gross, A., Goldsmith, C., Hoving, J. *et al.* 2007, Conservative management of mechanical neck disorders. A systematic review. *J. Rheumatol.* 34(5): 1083–1102.

Haldeman, S. 1978, The clinical basis for discussion of mechanisms of manipulative therapy. In: Korr, I. (ed.), *The Neurobiologic Mechanisms in Manipulative Therapy*. Plenum Press, New York, pp. 53–57.

Hearn, A., Rivett, D. 2002, Cervical SNAGS: a biomechanical analysis. *Man. Ther.* 7(2): 71–79.

Heikkila, H., Johansson, M., Wenngren, B. 2000, Effect of acupuncture, cervical manipulation and NSAID therapy on dizziness and impaired head repositioning of suspected cervical origin: a pilot study. *Man. Ther.* 5(3): 151–157.

Herbert, R. 1995, Adaptations of muscle and connective tissue. In: Refshauge, K., Gass, L. (eds), *Musculoskeletal Physiotherapy – Clinical Science and Practice*. Butterworth Heinemann, Oxford.

Herzog, W., Scheele, D., Conway, P. 1999, Electromyographic responses of back and limb muscles associated with spinal manipulative therapy. *Spine* 24(2): 146–153.

Hong, C., Simons, D. 1998, Pathophysiological and electrophysiological mechanisms of myofascial trigger points. *Arch. Med. Phys. Rehab.* 79: 863–872.

Hoving, J.L., Koes, B.W., de Vet, H. *et al.* 2002, Manual therapy, physical therapy or continued care by a general practitioner for patients with neck pain. *Ann. Intern. Med.* 136(10): 713–722.

Hoving, J., Pool, J., van Mameren, H. *et al.* 2005, Reproducibility of cervical range of motion in patients with neck pain. *BMC Musculoskelet. Disord.* 6: 59.

Hsieh, C., Vicenzino, B., Yang, C. *et al.* 2002, Mulligans mobilization with movement for the thumb: a single case report using magnetic resonance imaging to evaluate the positional fault hypothesis. *Man. Ther.* 7(1): 44–49.

Hurwitz E., Aker, P., Adams, A. *et al.* 1996, Manipulation and mobilisation of the cervical spine. A systematic review of the literature. *Spine* 21(15): 1746–1759.

Janssens, L.A. 1991, Trigger points in 48 dogs with myofascial pain syndromes. *Vet. Surg*, 20(4): 274–278.

Jull, G., Bogduk, N., Marsland, A. 1988, The accuracy of manual diagnosis for cervical zygapophyseal joint pain syndromes. *Med. J. Aust.* 148(5): 233–236.

Jull, G., Zito, G., Trott, P. *et al.* 1997, Inter-examiner reliability to detect painful upper cervical joint dysfunction. *Aust. J. Physiother.* 43(2): 125–129.

Jull, G., Trott, P., Potter, H. *et al.* 2002, A randomised controlled trial of exercise and manipulative therapy for cervicogenic headache. *Spine* 27(17): 1835–1843.

Latimer, J., Adams, R., Lee, M. 1998, Training with feedback improves judgements of non-biological linear elastic stiffness. *Man. Ther.* 3(2): 85–89.

Lee, M. 1995, Biomechanics of joint movements. In: Refshauge, K., Gass, L. (eds), *Musculoskeletal Physiotherapy – Clinical Science and Practice*. Butterworth Heinemann, Oxford.

MacConnail, M. 1964, Joint movements. *Physiotherapy* 50: 359–367.

Macgregor, J., Graf von Schweinitz, D. 2006, Needle electromyographic activity of myofascial trigger points and control sites in equine cleidobrachialis muscle – an observational study. *Acupunct. Med.* 24(2): 61–70.

Maher, C., Adams, R. 1994, Reliability of pain and stiffness assessments in clinical manual lumbar spine examination. *Phys. Ther.* 74(9): 801–811.

Maitland, G.D., Hengeveld, E., Banks, K. 2006, *Maitland's Vertebral Manipulation*, 7th edn. Butterworth, London.

Martins, D., Mazzardo-Martins, L., Gadotti, V. *et al.* 2011, Ankle joint mobilization reduces axonotmesis-induced neuropathic pain and glial activation in the spinal cord and enhances nerve regeneration in rats. *Pain.* 152: 2653–2661.

Mulligan, B. 1995, *Manual Therapy, NAGS, SNAGS, MWMs etc.*, 3rd edn. Plane View Services, New Zealand.

Nansel, D., Peneff, A., Cremata, E., Carlson, J. 1990, Time course considerations for the effects of unilateral lower cervical adjustments with respect to the amelioration of cervical lateral-flexion passive end-range asymmetry. *J. Manipulative Physiol. Ther.* 13: 297–304.

Newham, D., Lederman, E. 1997, Effect of manual therapy techniques on the stretch reflex in normal human quadriceps. *Disabil. Rehabil.* 19(8): 326–331.

Nilsson, N., Christensen H.W., Hartvigsen, J. 1997, The effect of spinal manipulation in the treatment of cervicogenic headache. *J. Manipulative Physiol. Ther.* 20(5): 326–330.

Paungmali, A., O'Leary, S., Souvlis, T., Vicenzino, B. 2003a, Hypoalgesic and sympathoexcitatory effects of mobilization with movement for lateral epicondylalgia. *Phys. Ther.* 83(4): 374–383.

Paungmali, A., Vicenzino, B., Smith, M. 2003b, Hypoalgesia induced by elbow manipulation in lateral epicondylalgia does not exhibit tolerance. *J. Pain* 4(8): 448–544.

Paungmali, A., O'Leary, S., Souvlis, T., Vicenzino, B. 2004, Naloxone fails to antagonize initial hypoalgesic effect of a manual therapy treatment for lateral epicondylalgia. *J. Manipulative Physiol. Ther.* 27(3): 180–185.

Potter, N., Rothstein, J. 1985, Intertester reliability for selected clinical tests of the sacroiliac joint. *Phys. Ther.* 65(11): 1671–1675.

Rosenfeld, M., Gunnarsson, R., Borenstein, P. 2000, Early intervention in whiplash associated disorders: a comparison of two treatment protocols. *Spine* 25(14): 1782–1787.

Santos F, Silva J., Giardini, A. *et al.* 2012, Neural mobilization reverses behavioral and cellular changes that characterize neuropathic pain in rats. *Mol Pain* 8: 57.

Schmid, A., Nee, R., Coppieters, M., 2013, Reappraising entrapment neuropathies – mechanisms, diagnosis and management. *Man. Ther.* 18: 449–457.

Schneider G., Jull G, Thomas, K. *et al.* 2013, Intrarater and interrater reliability of select clinical tests in patients referred for diagnostic facet joint blocks in the cervical spine. *Arch. Phys. Med. Rehabil.* 94(8):1628–1634.

Segarra, V., Dueñas, L., Torres, R. *et al.* 2015, Inter-and intra-tester reliability of a battery of cervical movement control dysfunction tests. *Man. Ther.* 20(4): 570–579.

Smedmark, V., Wallin, M., Ardvisson, I. 2000, Inter-examiner reliability in assessing passive intervertebral motion of the cervical spine. *Man. Ther.* 5(2): 97–101.

Song, X., Gan, Q., Cao, J. *et al.* 2006, Spinal manipulation reduces pain and hyperalgesia after lumbar intervertebral foramen inflammation in the rat. *J. Manipulative Physiol. Ther.* 29: 5–13.

Sterling, M., Jull, G., Wright, A. 2001, Cervical mobilisation: concurrent effects on pain sympathetic nervous system activity and motor activity. *Man. Ther.* 6(2): 72–81.

Takamoto, K., Bito, I., Urakawa, S. *et al.* 2015, Effects of compression at myofascial trigger points in patients with acute low back pain: a randomized controlled trial. *Eur. J. Pain.* Mar 24. Doi: 10.1002/ejp 694

Terrett, A.C., Vernon, H. 1984, Manipulation and pain tolerance. A controlled study of the effect of spinal manipulation on paraspinal cutaneous pain tolerance levels. *Am. J. Phys. Med.* 63(5): 217–225.

Vicenzino, B., Collins, D., Wright, W. 1994, Sudomotor changes induced by neural mobilisation techniques in asymptomatic subjects. *J. Man. Manip. Ther.* 2: 66–74.

Vicenzino, B., Collins, D., Benson, H., Wright, A. 1998, An investigation of the interrelationship between manipulative therapy-induced hypoalgesia and sympathoexcitation. *J. Manipulative Physiol. Ther.* 21: 448–453.

Vicenzino, B., Paungmali, A., Buratowski, S., Wright, A. 2001, Specific manipulative therapy treatment for chronic lateral epicondylalgia produces uniquely characteristic hypoalgesia. *Man. Ther.* 6(4): 205–212.

Vicenzino, B., Paungmali, A., Teys, P. 2007 Mulligan's mobilization-with-movement, positional faults and pain relief: current concepts from a critical review of literature. *Man. Ther.* 12: 98–108.

Voogt, L., Devries, J., Meeus, M. *et al.* 2015, Analgesic effects of manual therapy in patients with musculoskeletal pain: a systematic review. *Man. Ther.* 20: 250–256.

Wright, A. 1995, Hypoalgesia post-manipulative therapy: a review of the potential neurophysiological mechanisms. *Man. Ther.* 1: 11–16.

Wright, A., Thurnwald, P., O'Callaghan, J. *et al.* 1994, Hyperalgesia in tennis elbow patients. *J. Musculoskel. Pain* 2: 83–97.

Wyke, B.D. 1985, *Articular Neurology and Manipulative Therapy.* Churchill Livingstone, Edinburgh.

Zegarra-Parodi, R., Park, P., Heath, D. *et al.* 2015, Assessment of skin blood flow following spinal manual therapy: a systematic review. *Man. Ther.* 20: 228–249.

CHAPTER 13

Electrophysical agents in animal physiotherapy

Tim Watson[1] and Katie Lawrence[2]

[1] University of Hertfordshire, Hatfield, UK

[2] Justo Development Ltd, Oxford, UK

Summary

The electrophysical agents (EPAs) offer a range of therapy tools that have an evidenced role to play in veterinary physiotherapy practice. It is rarely the case that their use in isolation offers the optimal outcome but in combination with other interventions, their inclusion in the treatment package can add significant benefit. It is critical to select the most efficacious tool for the required task (whether related to tissue healing, pain management or muscle function) and this chapter explores the key issues for the most commonly available EPA modalities, together with their mode of action, key research evidence and practice issues.

13.1 Introduction

Whilst electrotherapy (now more correctly called the electrophysical agents (EPAs)) has been employed as a component of practice in physiotherapy for many decades, there has been a progressive shift in emphasis with the development of new intervention options and the continued refinement of those which are long established. There is an increased emphasis on evidence-based practice, by which the practitioner is encouraged to employ the best available evidence in any particular circumstance. Whilst there is a very substantial evidence base to support the use of EPAs as a component of the treatment package, there remains a lack of case-by-case specific evidence covering every eventuality with a randomised controlled trial (RCT) or systematic review (the same is true in human-based therapy). This notwithstanding, it is the aim of this chapter to briefly identify those EPA interventions which have sufficient evidence to justify their inclusion and to further elaborate their value as a therapeutic tool. This is presented under several key topic areas (tissue repair, muscle function and pain management) rather than as a detailed account working through each available modality. No attempt is made to provide a recipe-based chart which negates the need for thorough assessment and sound clinical decision making. The principles presented herein can be applied across a wide variety of clinical encounters.

Extensive literature (textbook and research-based publications) can be employed should higher levels of detail be required. This chapter provides an overview rather than detail – this is a deliberate strategy rather than a means to avoid problematic material. Supporting references are provided at the end of the chapter from where the interested reader can pursue the detail. The modalities included in the chapter certainly do not represent the full range of EPAs currently available, but they do represent those which are most commonly employed in animal-based therapy.

Animal Physiotherapy: Assessment, Treatment and Rehabilitation of Animals, Second Edition. Edited by Catherine M. McGowan and Lesley Goff.

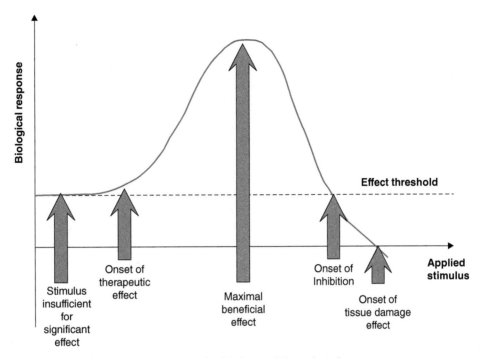

Figure 13.1 Graphical representation of the dose–response curve related to the use of electrophysical agents.

13.2 General principles of electrophysical agent decision making and application

Whilst this has been covered extensively in all major texts (e.g. Belanger 2014; Robertson *et al.* 2006; Watson 2008a) and in several discussion papers (e.g. Sutton & Watson 2011; Watson 2010), the key issues will be briefly summarised before heading into the main sections.

It is strongly argued that the introduction of any energy type into the tissues (e.g. electrical, mechanical, electromagnetic) will instigate a physiological response in the tissue provided that sufficient energy has been employed to surpass the response threshold. The physiological response can be used to provide a therapeutic effect, whether this relates to tissue repair, muscle function or pain management. The dose (a complex matter, but one that takes into account energy, energy density, frequency, intensity, pulsing parameters and treatment time, for example) is a critical aspect of this delivery. The current evidence supports the contention that there are doses which are more and doses which are less effective (as there would be with exercise, manual therapy, drug therapy or any other intervention). Underdosing is not dangerous, nor does it put the tissue at risk, but it is ineffective in that too little energy is delivered to reach the optimal therapeutic outcome. Overdosing can put the tissues at risk – too much energy is delivered or the energy is delivered at high density. The evidence from published research enables the physiotherapist to establish effective doses for the intervention being employed. It is generally possible to identify optimal dose parameters across a wide range of applications. The

dose–response relationship has been presented by numerous researchers and practitioners in the EPA field and is summarised in Figure 13.1. Clearly, the aim of EPA-based therapy is to employ the treatment dose which reaches the peak of the biological response curve and a more detailed consideration of the dose–response issue is reviewed in Watson (2010).

Decision making in practice starts with the problem presented rather than with the machine. The physiotherapist makes an informed decision regarding the aim or intention of the treatment (e.g. to stimulate tissue repair or to increase muscle strength) based on a detailed and thorough assessment (see Chapter 11). From this, it is possible to identify the key physiological events that need to be stimulated, promoted or in some way enhanced. Once the intended physiological outcomes are known, using the best available evidence, it is possible to make a modality choice (e.g. ultrasound, laser, shockwave, muscle stimulation – neuromuscular electrical stimulation (NMES)). This is a critical decision in that if the most effective modality is selected, a positive therapy outcome is a reasonable option. If a less effective modality is used, the result of the treatment cannot be optimal. Having selected the preferential modality, it is important to apply this energy at the dose which the evidence supports as being the most effective (Figure 13.2). Figure 13.2 illustrates the decision-making model used with EPAs. Whilst the theoretical model runs left to right, the clinical decision-making model runs right to left. Details of dosing are not generally included in this chapter, nor are recipes employed for muscle tear or tendon injury. It is not possible to detail all the dose options for a modality (e.g. therapeutic ultrasound) covering

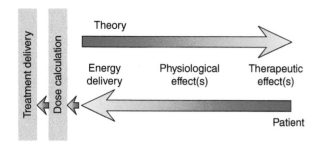

Figure 13.2 Basic model proposed for electr physical agents in practice. *Source:* Watson and Young 2008. Reproduced with permission from Elsevier.

acute tendon presentations in a small animal (a small dog, for example) right through to a long-standing (chronic) tendinopathy in a much larger animal (e.g. a racehorse).

As with all physiotherapy treatment modalities, it is crucial to assess the response to therapy both during therapy and afterwards, with reassessment of the patient at each treatment, and to ensure the expected response has occurred or outcome achieved (see also Chapters 11 and 22). If the expected response does not occur, it is essential to reevaluate the treatment plan or refer back to the veterinary surgeon. It is also important for the physiotherapist to remember that electrotherapeutic agents are rarely used in isolation in physiotherapy. They are combined with other treatment approaches, including manual therapy and exercises, to achieve optimum outcome.

The division of the remainder of this chapter into three main sections reflects the current range of clinical practice areas in animal physiotherapy: the management of damaged/healing/repair tissue; the management of muscle function issues, most commonly muscle strengthening; and pain management issues.

13.3 Modalities to influence healing and tissue repair

Several of the commonly available modalities are evidenced as being able to influence the process of tissue repair in a positive way. These include ultrasound, laser and pulsed shortwave, though the latter has been less commonly employed in animal practice, mainly due to the relatively cumbersome nature of the equipment. In addition, two newer modalities – microcurrent-based therapy and shockwave therapy – have more recently gained ground and join this group with supportive evidence. Whilst each is capable of stimulating repair in damaged tissue, they are not equal in their effect, and thus not universal in their applicability. Each is briefly considered in turn together with the prime evidence to underpin their application in this arena. None of these are used primarily as pain relief interventions, though by virtue of their capacity to positively influence repair in damaged tissue, pain relief can reasonably be expected as a secondary outcome. In the following sections, both ultrasound and laser therapies will be given greater consideration based on the strength of

their evidence and their higher usage in the animal physiotherapy environment.

13.3.1 Therapeutic ultrasound

Therapeutic ultrasound is one of the mainstay modalities in practice, with a substantive evidence base and a long track record. Ultrasound energy is mechanical in nature, thus it is clearly one of the electrophysical agents whilst not actually constituting an electrotherapy modality.

Technically, a sound wave vibrating at a frequency greater than 20 kHz (20,000 vibrations a second) is classified as ultrasound. Whilst horses (audible range up to 33.5 kHz) and dogs (audible range typically up to 45 kHz) clearly have the capacity to hear sound at higher ranges than humans, the frequencies employed in therapy ultrasound are most commonly in the MHz range (millions of cycles a second), and hence are significantly beyond the known hearing frequency of any animal likely to be encountered in practice (even a bat has an upper limit of some 100 kHz).

The delivery of mechanical energy at frequencies in the MHz range will generate heat in the tissue if applied at sufficient power, though in recent years, the use of ultrasound as a thermal intervention has diminished, given that the strongest evidence is in favour of its use at low levels (often cited as being nonthermal). At lower levels, especially when used in a pulsed mode, the dominant effect of ultrasound is to stimulate cell activity (cellular upregulation) and it is this mechanism which is primarily responsible for its capacity to stimulate tissue repair (Nussbaum 1997). The frequencies most often employed are at 1 and 3 MHz, with the 1 MHz being used to reach the deeper tissues (down to 5 or 6 cm) and the 3 MHz for the more superficial lesions (down to a depth of some 2 cm). The absorption of ultrasound energy is optimal in the dense collagen-based tissues (tendon, ligament, fascia, joint capsule and established scar tissue), and it is in these tissues that it is at its most effective.

In the inflammatory phase, ultrasound does not have, as previously proposed, an antiinflammatory effect, but rather stimulates the cells which are responsible for driving the inflammatory events through the release of numerous growth factors, cytokines and other chemical messengers (reviewed in Watson 2008d; Watson & Young 2008). The result is not a more intense set of inflammatory events, but rather a normal set of inflammation events which take place with enhanced efficiency. Tissue exposed to ultrasound at therapeutic levels will progress through the inflammatory events with greater efficiency (in less time) and hence provide a clinical advantage. Whilst used in practice on many different tissues, given the preferential absorption of the ultrasound energy in the dense collagen-based tissues, it is in these locations where maximal effect will be achieved.

In the proliferative (early repair) phase, the effect of ultrasound is to stimulate fibroblasts and myofibroblasts, both of which make a significant contribution to the generation of the newly forming scar tissue. Additionally, ultrasound has been shown to enhance the angiogenic (neovascular) response which provides essential support to the cells producing the new scar tissue (collagen). The result is not a greater scar by virtue of volume but, as with the inflammatory phase, an increased efficacy of the normal sequence of events.

In remodelling, ultrasound serves to stimulate collagen fibre orientation which in turn provides enhanced functional capacity, quality and maturity of the developing scar tissue. The oft claimed but incorrect concept that ultrasound at this later stage removes excess scar tissue can be dismissed. Ultrasound cannot remove scar tissue – it can, however, stimulate and promote remodelling events, resulting in a higher quality scar with enhanced functional capacity.

At all stages, the current evidence identifies that the mechanism common to all these events and processes relates to the enhanced release of mediators, growth factors and cytokines (reviewed in Watson 2008d; Watson & Young 2008).

A subtle variation of the classic therapeutic ultrasound is to employ the same energy but at significantly lower intensity (effectively lower density), and this is a particularly strongly evidenced application in fracture management – both acute fractures and those demonstrating delayed and non-union. The specific dose known to be effective in these cases is at 1.5 MHz, 0.03 W/cm^2 (30 mW/cm^2), pulsed at 1000 Hz and delivered daily for 20 minutes with a stationary applicator. It is not currently possible to replicate this dose with a standard therapy machine, though future developments and machine refinements make this a highly likely option. The application of ultrasound at this low level is most commonly referred to as low-intensity pulsed ultrasound (LIPUS) and has a substantive base of clinical efficacy, increasing the rate at which fresh fractures transit to union and stimulating a repair response in those with slowed or stalled healing. The mechanisms of effect are reviewed in Padilla *et al.* (2014). This type of ultrasound is currently being evaluated across a range of different soft tissue presentations (e.g. muscle; Montalti *et al.* 2013), but the fracture-based treatments are currently the most strongly evidenced. The main indications for both traditional and low-intensity ultrasound in animal practice are shown in Table 13.1 and Figures 13.3 and 13.4.

13.3.2 Low-level/low-intensity laser therapy

Laser is an acronym for 'light amplification by stimulated emission of radiation'; it is a form of electromagnetic radiation in the visible and near visible part of the spectrum. Numerous other terms are employed in the therapy environment, the two most recent being low-level laser therapy (LLLT) and low-intensity laser therapy (LILT). In principle, the laser light is applied at a low intensity/energy level, and the aim of delivering in this fashion is to have a biostimulative effect rather than the destructive effect which is achieved at higher levels, such as employed in surgical and ablative procedures. Useful material can be found in Tuner & Hode (2004), which includes sections reviewing laser use in animal-based therapies, and Prindeze *et al.* (2012), who evaluate and review the current literature relating to mechanism

Table 13.1 Main indications for both traditional and low-intensity ultrasound in animal practice

Traditional ultrasound	Low-intensity pulsed ultrasound (LIPUS)
Ligament damage (from overuse/overstretch through to grade IV tears)	Fresh fracture
Tendon damage, post tendon (surgical) repair, tendon presentations including tendinitis and tendinopathy	Fracture with delayed union
Joint capsule damage/irritation, including post dislocation and as a consequence of degenerative joint changes	Fracture with non-union
Improving the quality and functional capacity of developing scar tissue in any musculoskeletal/soft tissue	Stress fractures
	Avulsion fractures

of action, whilst Millis & Levine (2014a) include animal-specific material related to laser therapy.

Lasers used in therapy are of low power (typically 500 mW or less) and may include both true laser sources and superluminous diodes or light-emitting diodes (LEDs). They emit light in a range from the red end of the visible spectrum to the first part of the infra-red range (typically 600–1000 nm). They are most commonly used either as a single probe (i.e. one light source in a pen-type applicator) or a cluster probe which will incorporate numerous sources (typically around 20, but can be 60 or more), which provides a straightforward method to treat larger areas

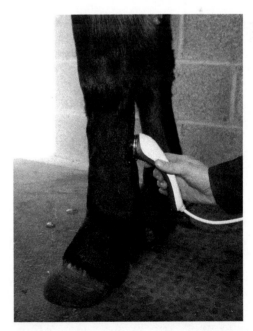

Figure 13.3 Ultrasound therapy treatment of the superficial digital flexor tendon to stimulate collagen fibre orientation and therefore the functional capacity of scar tissue during remodelling. The area can be shaved and extra gel/70% alcohol in water used to improve contact if necessary.

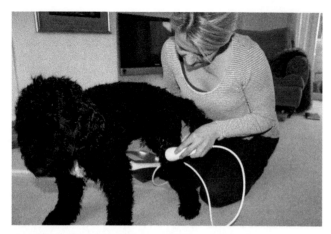

Figure 13.4 Application of ultrasound therapy using a gel contact technique. For smaller limb segments, immersion of the limb segment and the ultrasound treatment applicator in a bowl of water can help to eliminate contact issues.

(Figure 13.5. Figure 13.6). Most devices offer both continuous and pulsed output modes, though it is difficult to identify convincing evidence that the mode is critical to treatment outcome.

Laser light is absorbed in the tissues, primarily by the chromophores (within the mitochondria), resulting in increased levels of cellular reactions, and thus, in a similar way to ultrasound, the delivered energy results in cellular upregulation, a variety of secondary reactions, which lead to modulation of cellular functions, and typically the stimulation of tissue repair mechanisms. Laser irradiation has been shown to enhance the production of

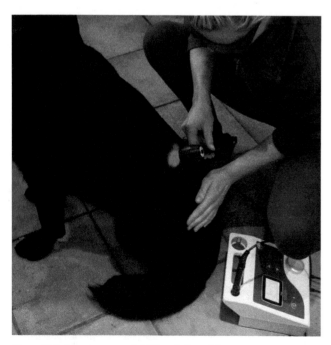

Figure 13.5 Laser treatment (*visible red cluster*) for acute trigger point stimulation. Protective goggles should be worn by the physiotherapist and handler and the animal's eyes should be protected.

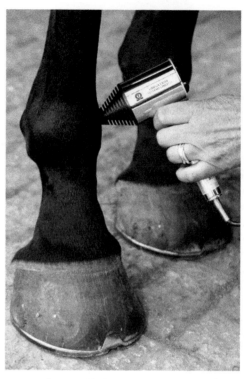

Figure 13.6 Laser therapy applied to treat a periarticular inflammatory lesion. *Source:* Reproduced with permission from Omega Laser Systems Ltd.

adenosine triphosphate (ATP) within cells, and thus mediate or modulate a variety of other events, including release of growth factors and cytokine reactions; the ultimate effect of these events is acceleration of delayed tissue healing. This is the primary effect of laser therapy; hence the terms 'photobiostimulation' or 'photobiomodulation' are employed as generic descriptors of physiological and cellular effects. Useful summaries can be found in Baxter (2008), Bjordal (2012) and in all standard texts such as Michlovitz *et al.* (2012).

Laser light itself will not penetrate the tissues for any significant distance. It is cited that 15 mm is probably the realistic limit to effective penetration, though it is also pointed out that it is the absorption of the energy that is critical to bring about the therapy effects rather than how far the light reaches into the tissue. The main indications for laser-based applications in animal practice are shown in Table 13.2.

13.3.3 Pulsed shortwave

Whilst pulsed shortwave has not been widely employed in animal-based therapies historically, the recent advent of smaller, battery-powered, portable devices makes this a potential area for expansion. Pulsed shortwave most commonly employs radiofrequency (RF) electromagnetic energy (usually delivered at 27.12 MHz) as a means to facilitate tissue repair. It is at its most effective in the tissues which absorb this type of energy, primarily the ionic tissues of low impedance – such as muscle, nerve and tissues where there is a high water content following

Table 13.2 Main indications for laser therapy in animal practice

Indication	Remarks
Wounds: employed as a means to stimulate wound healing in both fresh and delayed wound environments	Traumatic and surgical wounds. Ulcers, pressure lesions and similar slow-to-heal lesions
	Burns, abrasions
Acute injuries/trauma	Muscle lesions/tears/overuse (also ligament, tendon lesions)Haematoma, tenosynovitis, bursitis
Subacute and chronic soft tissue lesions	Repetitive strain and overuse injuries, surpraspinatus lesions, flexor carpi ulnaris strain/carpal hyperextension injury
Degenerative joint lesions	Periarticular involvement in degenerative arthritis, quiescent inflammatory arthropathies
Trigger points	Both acute (irritable) and chronic (established) trigger points can be effectively treated

injury, such as areas of oedema, joint effusion and haematoma. Its effects when used at low dose in the more acute stages are similar to those of ultrasound (though in a different target tissue). In the more chronic lesions, it is typically delivered at higher doses, with heat generating in these tissues becoming a more dominant intended outcome. Millis & Levine (2014b) review shortwave/pulsed shortwave along with other magnetic and pulsed magnetic applications in animal-based therapy.

The small portable units deliver insufficient power to generate any significant tissue heating and are therefore more useful in the acute injury phase. Their energy is delivered at low power, but over prolonged periods of time (hours – commonly overnight) rather than clinic sessions lasting for minutes (typically 10–20 min).

At the present time, there is supportive research evidence (e.g. Al Mandeel & Watson 2008; Rawe & Vlahovic 2012) for both intervention methods, though no direct comparison of the two, so it is not yet possible to categorically identify whether the low power delivery over several hours is more or less effective than the higher power applications (usually clinic based) lasting tens of minutes. The main indications for pulsed shortwave-based therapies in animal practice are shown in Table 13.3.

13.3.4 Shockwave therapy

This is a relatively new modality as a therapy tool. It is a lower powered version of lithotripsy which was developed as a means to conservatively manage renal stones. A shockwave is

essentially a pressure disturbance that propagates rapidly through a medium. Whilst there are several different types of shockwave generator, the most commonly employed in therapy are the radial devices (hence it is sometimes called radial shockwave therapy). The energy wave generated by such devices is delivered to the tissue by means of a 'gun' type device, using a gel medium which serves to increase the efficacy of the energy transfer. There are numerous clinical reviews (Wang 2012) and some papers which summarise the essentials of shockwave generation and associated issues (Wilbert 2002). Focused shockwave therapy can be destructive in nature, and is not routinely employed in therapy at the present time though both are usefully considered in a recent review (Speed 2014).

The energy wave consists of a high-powered but short duration pressure wave which, as it travels through the tissue, will, at any interface, result in reflection, refraction or onward transmission as would be the case with any other energy (ultrasound, light, electromagnetic radiation). The absorption of the delivered energy is not equal between tissues, and the dense soft tissues appear to be the strongest absorbers of the energy and thus, the tissues which respond preferentially to this modality (Ogden *et al.* 2001).

Treatment typically consists of 1–2000 shocks delivered in a session at 1–3 bar (for most machines this falls into the low-energy shockwave band of up to 0.08 mJ/mm^2 though may include the lower end of the medium energy range (up to 0.28 mJ/mm^2). The shocks are delivered at 5–20 Hz (shocks per second), though there is no evidence that identifies a particular rate as being more effective. A 2000 shock treatment delivered at 10 Hz would take a little over 3 min to deliver, and whilst it cannot be considered to be soothing, it is at worst uncomfortable rather than painful. Treatment is evidenced as being effective when delivered 1 × weekly, typically for 3–5 sessions (reviewed in Wang 2012). When used in focused mode (as opposed to the radial application described in this section), it can be a painful intervention, and some animals require sedation which clearly adds to both the cost and the complexity of the treatment, which is normally carried out by a veterinary surgeon.

The effect of this type of treatment is provocative in nature. It instigates an acute reaction in the tissues, taking the tissue from a chronic, unresponsive, recalcitrant state to a more responsive, acute lesion. Having instigated this acute reaction in the tissues,

Table 13.3 Main indications for pulsed shortwave therapy in animal practice

Clinic-based pulsed shortwave	Low-power pulsed shortwave
Acute injury in tissues such as muscle and nerve (with relatively high water content)	Post acute injury/trauma/surgery
Treatment of oedema in soft tissue and effusion in synovial joints	Bruising of muscle
Treatment of tissue haematoma following injury/trauma/surgery	Superficial haematoma
Used for more chronic conditions of similar lesions. Employed at higher power with overt tissue heating	Local swelling post injury/surgery

Table 13.4 Main indications for shockwave therapy in animal practice

Established	Emerging
Chronic tendinopathy	Chronic open wounds
Chronic presentations in fascia, e.g. plantar fasciitis	Chronic lesions of cartilage, muscle and ligament
Local analgesia	Poorly or non-responding fractures
	Chronic (unresponsive) bursitis

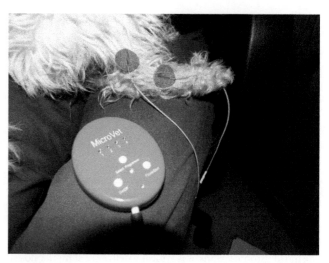

Figure 13.7 Microcurrent therapy (applied with small electrodes due to limb size) to the tarsal area following acute injury.

treatment for an acute lesion can be pursued in the normal way. The role of the shockwave is to take the tissue from its more chronic to a more acute state.

In terms of the research evidence to date, the strongest evidence is in favour of using it in the management of chronic tendon-type lesions – most especially, the chronic tendinopathies. There is an emerging evidence base to support the potential value of this treatment across a range of other clinical conditions, including analgesia, open wound management, bone healing issues (delayed and non-union), chronic soft tissue problems other than in tendons (e.g. cartilage, ligament, muscle) and a widening range of other musculoskeletal presentations. A useful review of the use of shockwave-based therapy in animal practice together with emerging applications is found in Durant & Millis (2014). The main indications for radial shockwave therapy in animal practice are shown in Table 13.4.

13.3.5 Microcurrent-based therapy

Using very small electric currents is not a new therapy, though it is often presented as such. Unlike TENS, NMES, interferential and similar modes of electrical stimulation, microcurrent therapies employ subsensory-level stimulation (by definition, less than 1 mA) as a means to stimulate repair in damaged tissue. It is long established as a means to facilitate repair in bone lesions and skin wounds (reviewed in Poltawski & Watson 2009), but has more recently been employed in a range of soft tissue conditions with good effect.

The devices are small (no larger than a TENS device), battery powered (thus portable) and relatively inexpensive. They are best evidenced when used for hours a day rather than for short clinic treatment sessions. The current is delivered via disposable, skin surface electrodes, and in the veterinary therapy arena, this is normally carried out by the owner as a home-based intervention. There are several animal therapy-specific devices available on the market, but they are not fundamentally different from those employed in human-based treatments (Figure 13.7 and Figure 13.8).

The principle on which the treatment is based has been extensively documented in the literature, but is summarised thus. All tissues, not just nerve and muscle, exhibit small, internally generated bioelectric potentials which are essential to the normal physiology and response to injury. These are commonly referred to as the 'tissue batteries' which is a generic, but nonetheless useful term. On injury, these local bioelectric potentials shift in both polarity and magnitude. It is evidenced that this local adjustment

in bioelectric activity is responsible, at least in part, for driving the repair sequence.

After injury, in some tissues, these currents appear to be insufficient to instigate or maintain the repair sequence (the so-called 'flat battery'). The fundamental purpose of the microcurrent therapy is to stimulate (or support) these endogenous potentials using an externally applied current – in some way, mimicking the missing internal current. The background evidence, core

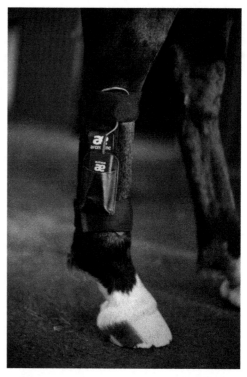

Figure 13.8 Microcurrent therapy applied for a soft tissue injury in the region of the cannon bone. *Source:* Reproduced with permission from Peter Bulman, Expo Life.

Table 13.5 Main indications for microcurrent-based therapy in animal practice

Indication	Remarks
Wound healing	Both acute and chronic (slow and/or unresponsive) wounds
Musculoskeletal injury	Facilitated repair in muscle, ligament and tendon lesions
Bone injury	Stimulated repair, especially in fractures demonstrating delayed or non-union
Postoperative recovery	Facilitated recovery following orthopaedic surgical procedures

literature and evidence base are reviewed in numerous papers including Watson (2008b) and Kloth (2005).

These currents are widely employed in veterinary-based therapy, most commonly for tissues which are slow to heal or which have reached a plateau in their healing response. They have additionally been used with good effect in acute lesions, including postsurgical cases, as a means to support tissue repair right from the start.

Whilst they are advocated as a means to provide pain relief, with supportive research evidence, their inclusion in this chapter is on the basis of their capacity to stimulate/facilitate repair of damaged tissue. The main indications for microcurrent-based therapy in animal practice are shown in Table 13.5.

13.3.6 Tissue repair summary

The modalities briefly outlined in this section are all evidenced as being capable of positively influencing repair in tissue which has suffered overt injury, has been subjected to repeated minor trauma (overuse) or tissue in a postsurgical situation. None are universally applicable, and the selection of the most appropriate modality is essential for optimal outcome.

13.4 Modalities to influence muscle function

The preferred term for electrical stimulation applied to effect contractions of muscle is neuromuscular electrical stimulation or NMES. There are many alternatives proposed such as MES (muscular electrical stimulation) and FES (functional electrical stimulation). The latter is used to describe therapy using units that aim to mimic the stimulation patterns of intact nerves and has limited current uptake in animal-based therapy. Many of the available devices are named with some variation of the NMES acronym, though the principles of their application and effect are the same. The aim of this section is to briefly summarise how NMES might be usefully employed as a means to influence muscle function, most commonly muscle strength, in an animal therapy environment.

It is noteworthy that the waveforms used in TENS (next section) and NMES (this section) are essentially the same and the

units that generate these currents can both be small, portable and battery powered, though both stimulation modes are routinely available from mains-powered, clinic machines. The key differences are that motor nerve stimulation (NMES) devices employ different frequencies – those which are optimal in achieving motor-level rather than sensory-level outcomes – and that the pulse duration delivered from a typical NMES unit is longer (usually in the range 300–600 μsec) than those from a TENS device.

There is a move towards using NMES units in a similar way to TENS, the physiotherapist teaching the owner or other responsible person how to operate the device and where to place the electrodes and explaining the stimulation protocol (e.g. 30 min once daily or whatever is appropriate). Whilst this can clearly be delivered by the physiotherapist, once the stimulation parameters and protocol have been identified through a clinical reasoning process, effective therapy can be delivered by a responsible owner. It is more effective for the owner to deliver this on a daily basis than for the physiotherapist to be only able to deliver once or twice weekly. The application of NMES-type electrical stimulation in animals is usefully reviewed in Levine & Bockstahler (2014) and Schils (2009), and the integration of stimulation with exercise programmes in Paulekas & Haussler (2009) and Berté et al. (2012).

Electrical stimulation has been used for strengthening of normal muscle, but the evidence for electrical stimulation over voluntary exercise is limited. The best evidence strongly suggests that the use of electrical stimulation in conjunction with an active exercise/activity programme is most likely to result in optimal outcome. Electrical stimulation has also been used for muscle stimulation in neurological damage, promoting both motor recovery and strength, and additionally for the reduction of muscle spasticity. In animal therapy, the primary use is the treatment of muscle atrophy (recovery from and prevention of), which may be associated with an imbalance of muscle groups, to underpin reeducation of muscle function, and muscle strengthening. As in humans, muscle strengthening in muscle atrophy resulting from neurological lesions has also been successfully achieved with electrical stimulation. The use of NMES as a means to strengthen muscles and promote muscle recovery in the postoperative environment (Johnson et al. 1997; Millis et al. 1997) is a logical and supported application so long as sufficient awareness of the potential impact of the stimulation on the surgical site is maintained.

The most straightforward application method is to use electrodes of a similar size which are placed at either end of a muscle belly (or muscle group) (Figure 13.9). This method obviates the necessity to locate the motor point, which is a valid consideration if the treatment is being delivered by an owner who is simply following instruction rather than having a detailed knowledge of anatomy and motor point location. If using this technique, electrodes should be large enough to ideally cover a substantial proportion of the muscle (without touching one another); the standard-sized electrodes which come with most units are

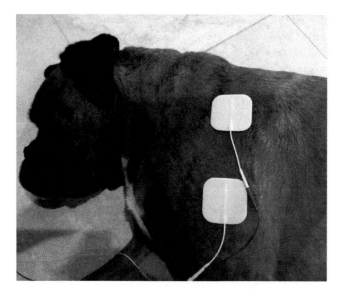

Figure 13.9 NMES used for neuromuscular reeducation of the shoulder flexor, elbow extensor muscle group.

likely to be too small for some larger animals. Clipping of the area may be required in patients with longer coats and additional gel can be used to improve conduction of the current and electrode adhesion. The skeletal structures should be in a functional position during stimulation for optimal outcome.

Regular treatment (at least every other day) is preferable, though results are likely to be stronger with daily stimulation so long as adequate rest periods are employed. It should be stressed that overstimulation (as might be delivered by overenthusiastic owners several times a day) can be detrimental, in the same way that overuse of voluntary exercise has detrimental effects. The fundamental difference with NMES is that the muscle is being forced to undergo a contraction, whereas in the voluntary exercise scenario, fatigue will be encountered at an earlier stage.

Most stimulators have a ramp option which enables the stimulation to build up rather than coming on at full power from a zero start. Ramping is both more comfortable and a closer mimic of the physiological position and therefore should be employed if the option is available. There is no definitive evidence with regard to ramp times but typically, the ramp up (at the start of the contraction) would be longer than the ramp down (at the conclusion of a contraction). Two seconds ramp up and 1 second ramp down has been shown to be acceptable and effective.

Treatment times during the early recovery phase should be shorter, with 10–15 min on alternate days being adequate. In later rehabilitation, longer daily sessions (up to 60 min) can be entirely appropriate. For strengthening effects, stimulation should be initiated with the device set to deliver at 30–35 Hz.

The intensity should be adjusted to suit the outcome. In animals with very poor motor activity or atrophy of musculature, it may be useful for the physiotherapist to palpate the muscle being stimulated so that the threshold of activation via NMES is established. The intensity, length of time of application and frequency

of application can then be judged as the animal responds. Treatment should be started with stimulation of 8–15 contractions per session, with sessions provided 3–5 times per week. Treatment should be continued for at least 4–6 weeks of training in order for significant effects to be achieved. As identified previously, using NMES alone as a means to enhance muscle strength is unlikely to produce optimal results. Employing it in conjunction with an exercise programme (or activity schedule of some form) is likely to be most beneficial.

13.5 Modalities to influence pain

The use of various electrophysical agents to assist in pain management is a common intervention in human-based therapies, predominantly employing electrical stimulation strategies. This approach can be effective in the animal therapy world, though there are some additional issues which need to be managed as, in classic delivery modes, patient feedback with regard to the sensation levels is key to determining the stimulation intensity. This approach cannot be simply transferred to pain management work with animals.

In addition to symptomatic pain management using electrical stimulation, modalities which are capable of influencing tissue repair after injury, insult or trauma will clearly have an effect on pain, though this is most commonly considered to be a secondary effect rather than primary. For example, following a ligament tear, ultrasound will have a positive effect by facilitating tissue repair. As a result, the modulation of the inflammatory and repair sequences will result in diminished chemically mediated irritation of the local nerve endings, and thus there will be a diminution in pain. Ultrasound and other modalities in the tissue repair group are therefore not employed primarily for their pain relief effects, though this will be a beneficial or bonus effect which is supported by the research-based evidence.

This section will focus on the capacity to have a direct effect on pain perception using electrical stimulation modalities, and thus providing symptomatic pain relief. More detailed explanations can be found in the standard texts (Veenman & Watson 2005) and an animal-specific consideration is published in Levine & Bockstahler (2014).

13.5.1 Transcutaneous electrical nerve stimulation (TENS)

This is an evidenced and widely used modality in human pain management, somewhat less so in the animal therapy arena. In principle, a small, battery-powered, inexpensive stimulator is used to deliver low-level (sensory, submotor) stimulation to the peripheral nerves with the primary intent of either increasing activity in the CNS opioid system or encouraging closure of the pain gate at spinal cord level. The effectiveness of TENS varies with the clinical pain being treated, but research would suggest that when used well, it provides significantly greater pain relief than a placebo intervention. There is an extensive research base for TENS in both the clinical and laboratory settings (Johnson 2014; Sluka *et al.* 2013).

In therapy practice, the majority of practitioners consider TENS as a treatment option in circumstances when a patient is experiencing chronic pain. This is not a problem as there is evidence to support this mode of application (e.g. Johnson 2014; Sluka *et al.* 2013; Vance *et al.* 2014). There is, however, a significant and growing body of evidence that supports the use of TENS as a valid and effective intervention in acute pain conditions (e.g. Silva *et al.* 2012; Simpson *et al.* 2014).

The current intensity (strength) will typically be in the range of 0–80 mA, though some machines may provide outputs up to 100 mA. Although this is a small current, it is sufficient because the primary target for the therapy is the sensory nerves, and so long as sufficient current is passed through the tissues to depolarise these nerves, the modality can be effective. The actual milliamperage delivered is based (see below) on the animal response to the stimulation rather than on a specific (numeric) level.

The machine will deliver discrete pulses of electrical energy, and the rate of delivery of these pulses (the pulse rate or frequency) will normally be variable from about 1 or 2 pulses per second (pps) up to 200 or 250 pps (sometimes the term hertz or Hz is used here). To be clinically effective, it is suggested that the TENS machine should cover a range from about 2 to 150 pps (Hz).

In addition to the stimulation rate, the duration (or width) of each pulse may be varied from about 40 to 250 microseconds (μsec). Recent evidence would suggest that this is possibly a less important control than the intensity or the frequency and the most effective setting in the practice environment is probably around 200–250 μsec.

The reason that such short-duration pulses can be used to achieve these effects is that the targets are the sensory nerves which tend to have relatively low thresholds (i.e. they are quite easy to excite) and that they will respond to a rapid change of electrical state. There is generally no need to apply a prolonged pulse in order to force a sensory nerve to depolarise, therefore stimulation for less than a millisecond is sufficient. In addition, most modern machines will offer a burst mode in which the pulses will be allowed out in bursts or 'trains', usually at a rate of 2–3 bursts per second.

Most machines offer a dual-channel output, i.e. two pairs of electrodes can be used simultaneously. In some circumstances, this can be a distinct advantage, though it is interesting that most physiotherapists tend to use just a single channel application. Widespread and diffuse pain presentations can be usefully treated with a four-electrode (two-channel) system, as can a combined treatment for local and referred pain.

The type of stimulation delivered by the TENS unit aims to excite (stimulate) the sensory nerves and by so doing, activate specific natural pain relief mechanisms. For convenience, if one considers that there are two primary pain relief mechanisms that can be activated – the pain gate mechanism and the endogenous

opioid system – the variation in stimulation parameters used to activate these two systems will be briefly considered.

Pain relief by means of the pain gate mechanism involves activation (excitation) of the A beta sensory fibres and by doing so, reduces the transmission of the noxious stimulus from the c fibres, through the spinal cord and hence on to the higher centres. The A beta fibres respond preferentially to stimulation at a relatively high rate (in the range of 80–130 Hz or pps).

Alternatively, stimulation of the A delta fibres, which respond preferentially to a much lower rate of stimulation (in the order of 2–5 Hz, though some authors consider a wider range of 2–10 Hz), will activate the opioid mechanisms and provide pain relief by causing the release of an endogenous opiate (encephalin) in the spinal cord which will reduce the activation of the noxious sensory pathways.

There is an option to stimulate both nerve types at the same time by employing the stimulation in burst mode. In this instance, the higher frequency stimulation output (typically at about 100 Hz) is interrupted (or burst) at the rate of about 2–3 bursts per second. When the machine is on, it will deliver pulses at the 100 Hz rate, thereby activating the A beta fibres and the pain gate mechanism, but by virtue of the rate of the burst, each burst will produce excitation in the A delta fibres, therefore stimulating the opioid mechanisms. This type of TENS stimulation can result in a variable amount of muscle twitching, and whilst it is effective, may be less well tolerated than the straightforward higher frequency (pain gate) or lower frequency (opioid) options.

This theory would support the translation of the two basic modes of TENS to animal therapy. The lower frequency option is most often used in chronic pain cases and higher frequency for the more acute pain presentations. Furthermore, the evidence from humans would suggest that stimulation for periods less than 30 min is unlikely to be effective in either mode.

With the higher frequency stimulation, the significant pain relief is achieved during the stimulation period, in that its carry-over effect is limited. The low-frequency stimulation does have a longer carry-over, and thus is most commonly employed with periods of stimulation (typically 30 min to 1 h) at intervals of 2–3 h.

The issue of stimulation intensity is the main difference between human and animal-based methods of intervention. In the human case, the stimulation is increased until a definite sensation (paraesthesia) is felt. Recent research supports the concept that strong but not uncomfortable is likely to be the most effective stimulation intensity. The stimulator intensity will need to be increased at intervals (varies from around 10 to 20 min) to maintain its effect, based on the fact that sensory nerves will accommodate to a stimulus of constant magnitude. In animal-based therapy, the same machine, same electrode system and same stimulation parameters are effective, but clearly this sensory feedback is less easy to manage. The practitioner may palpate over the area of the electrode whilst the stimulation is being carefully increased. This allows the practitioner to detect either the onset of the stimulation, which can be felt through the back of the electrode, or a slight motor response. If a motor response is detected then the stimulation intensity is reduced to submotor threshold, as the former level is a higher intensity of stimulation than is required when using TENS

Whilst this may appear to be a very subjective way of determining the treatment dose, it is both effective and manageable by the practitioner.

In terms of electrode placement, whilst there are a lot of options, the most straightforward option is to place them either side of the tissue giving rise to the pain. It does not matter whether they are orientated proximal-distal or medial-lateral (or any other combination), as long as they effectively lie either side of the problem area. The most obvious alternative to the local electrode placement is to apply the TENS electrodes directly over the relevant peripheral nerve that supplies the affected area, proximal to the pain site (i.e. between the pain source and the spinal cord), or over the relevant spinal nerve roots. In the latter case, the electrodes are placed lateral to the spine (paravertebral) for optimal effect.

The electrodes most commonly used in current practice are pregelled and self-adhesive. They are designed to be used repeatedly on a single person and are available in numerous sizes, most commonly 5 × 5 cm or about 10 × 5c m which will cater for most common circumstances. Extra-large (20 × 20 cm or more) or particularly small (1 cm diameter circular) electrodes can be obtained from manufacturers and distributors where circumstances dictate (for example, when treating a horse or larger animal). In some animal therapy circumstances, it might be necessary to employ additional gel and/or to use adhesive tape to ensure that the electrodes stay where they are placed. Some physiotherapists prefer to shave the fur/coat, which is perfectly acceptable with the owner's consent. This is more to do with adhesion of the electrode than it is to do with increased transmissivity of the current. Additional gel, rubbed into the coat prior to the application of the standard pregelled electrodes, achieves the same effect. Some physiotherapists simply wet the coat at the electrode location and this, too, appears to be effective.

Clearly, a more comprehensive analysis of this intervention is beyond the space available in this brief overview. Further (animal-specific) information can be found in Levine & Bockstahler (2014) and an excellent recent consideration of TENS applications in a wider context can be found in Johnson (2014).

13.5.2 Interferential therapy

Interferential therapy (IFT) is probably the second most common type of electrical stimulation employed in the context of pain management. It has a less strong evidence base than TENS, though sufficient to justify its inclusion as a means of achieving significant pain relief in practice.

The essential difference between interferential therapy and TENS relates to the means of generating stimulus rather than the physiological responses achieved. In TENS, discrete pulses

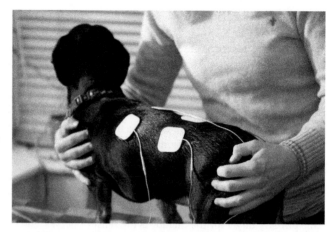

Figure 13.10 Interferential therapy as a treatment for established back pain in a small dog.

are generated and delivered through the electrodes to the tissue. With interferential therapy, two sinusoidal electrical currents are simultaneously delivered, such that a pattern of interference is generated in the deeper tissues. The sinusoidal current is delivered at several thousand hertz, and therefore cannot directly generate nerve action potentials. The interference achieved between the two currents is at a low frequency, and the nerve action potentials are instigated by the interference rather than the sinusoidal carrier *per se*. As with the TENS section above, there is a lot more detail which could be described, but the interested reader is referred to the standard core texts and publications for more detailed explanation (Robertson *et al.* 2006; Watson 2008a).

The useful alternative to using the classic four-electrode interferential system (four electrodes, two separate currents) is to employ a premodulated sinusoidal wave; the effects – physiological and clinical – are the same, though the interference is generated within the system unit rather than in the tissues (Ozcan *et al.* 2004). The clinical advantage is clearly that only two electrodes need to be located on the animal (Figure 13.10).

The main significant difference between using interferential currents and TENS pulses is that whilst IFT is less effective in terms of the magnitude of the pain relief response, it is less irritating by virtue of the sinusoidal wave being passed through the skin rather than discrete pulses. For animals that do not appear to tolerate the TENS stimulation well, IFT is a useful alternative. The amount of pain relief achieved might be at a lower level, but it is still worthy of consideration.

When selecting stimulation parameters with IFT for pain management, the same stimulation frequencies have been shown to be effective (between 80 and 130 Hz for the pain gate – acute pain – and 2–5 Hz for the opioid system – chronic pain). The electrode systems on modern machines also employ the pregelled units, electrode placement follows the same principles, and the additional gel or wetting of the coat is also effective in the same way.

The one other difference between an interferential unit and a typical TENS machine is that the interferential offers an automatic sweep option such that you do not need to select a specific stimulation frequency – a range can be identified (e.g. set to 80–130 Hz or 2–5 Hz).

Historically, interferential units were large, mains-powered machines, and whilst these remain useful in the clinic setting, the recent increased availability of small battery-powered units has meant that owners can use them in the home environment following appropriate instruction, in much the same way as TENS which has been used as a home-based therapy for several decades.

13.6 Conclusion

In summary, a range of electrophysical agents have the capacity to make a positive difference to treatment outcomes. They are least likely to be effective when employed in isolation but as an integrated component of the treatment package, they have significant added value.

Some of the modalities are best evidenced as a means to facilitate tissue repair after injury, surgery or overuse/training. Others (NMES) have the capacity to influence muscle function, whilst a variation of the electrical stimulation (TENS, interferential) can result in clinically useful pain relief.

These are not magical in their capacity to influence therapy outcome. Biophysical principles and the rules of good clinical practice remain; for example, the need for thorough physiotherapy assessment, reassessment and determination of outcome measures are all essential. Electrotherapies can, however, be of value when employed in an optimal fashion. These include the importance of the selection of appropriate treatment parameters (including treatment intensity, time and site of application) for the desired effects or clinical benefits. Frequently, physiotherapists are unclear on the relevance of treatment parameters, and thus fail to achieve the desired or anticipated benefits of electrotherapy treatment. Beyond this, the effectiveness of the therapy is dependent upon the quality of the machine and regular testing and servicing, especially in situations where the machine can be subjected to high levels of wear and tear.

Given the potential risks associated with some treatments, care should be taken with anxious or temperamental animals, where application of electrophysical agents may not be appropriate. General contraindications to treatment with electrophysical agents include application over the eyes, the pregnant uterus or the gonads. In addition, caution should be exercised in all such applications, as animals are unable to provide the therapist with the requisite feedback, such as feelings of discomfort or heating.

Both treatment protocols and the available modalities are likely to change as research and technical developments ensue. The key issues identified in this review summarise the position at the current time, which is expected to change with emerging evidence and the development of technology.

References

Al Mandeel, M., Watson, T. 2008, Pulsed and continuous shortwave therapy. In: Watson, T. (ed.), *Electrotherapy: Evidence Based Practice*. Churchill Livingstone/Elsevier, Edinburgh, pp. 137–160.

Baxter, D. 2008, Low intensity laser therapy. In: Watson, T. (ed.), *Electrotherapy: Evidence Based Practice*. Churchill Livingstone/Elsevier, Edinburgh, pp. 161–178.

Belanger, A.Y. 2014, *Therapeutic Electrophysical Agents: Evidence Behind Practice*. Lippincott Williams & Wilkins, Philadelphia, PA.

Berté, L., Mazzanti, A., Salbego, F.Z. *et al.* 2012, Immediate physical therapy in dogs with rupture of the cranial cruciate ligament submitted to extracapsular surgical stabilization. *Arq. Bras. Med. Vet. Zootec.* 64: 01–08.

Bjordal, J.M. 2012, Low level laser therapy (LLLT) and World Association for Laser Therapy (WALT) dosage recommendations. *Photomed. Laser Surg.* 30(2): 61–62.

Durant, A., Millis, D. 2014, Applications of extracorporeal shockwave in small animal rehabilitation. In: Millis, D., Levine, D. (eds), *Canine Rehabilitation and Physical Therapy*, 2nd edn. Elsevier/Saunders, Cambridge, pp. 381–392.

Johnson, J.M., Johnson, A.L., Pijanowski, G.J. *et al.* 1997, Rehabilitation of dogs with surgically treated cranial cruciate ligament-deficient stifles by use of electrical stimulation of muscles. *Am. J. Vet. Res.* 58(12): 1473–1478.

Johnson, M.I. 2014, *Transcutaneous Electrical Nerve Stimulation (TENS): research to support clinical practice*. Oxford University Press, Oxford.

Kloth, L.C. 2005, Electrical stimulation for wound healing: a review of evidence from in vitro studies, animal experiments, and clinical trials. *Int. J. Low. Extrem. Wounds* 4(1): 23–44.

Levine, D., Bockstahler, B. 2014, Electrical stimulation. In: Millis, D., Levine, D. (eds), *Canine Rehabilitation and Physical Therapy*, 2nd edn. Elsevier/Saunders, Cambridge, pp. 342–358.

Michlovitz, S.L., Bellew, J.W., Nolan, T.P. 2012, *Modalities for Therapeutic Intervention*, 5th edn. F.A. Davis, Philadelphia, PA.

Millis, D., Levine, D. 2014a, *Canine Rehabilitation and Physical Therapy*, 2nd edn. Elsevier/Saunders, Cambridge.

Millis, D., Levine, D. 2014b, Other modalities in veterinary rehabilitation. In: Millis, D., Levine, D. (eds), *Canine Rehabilitation and Physical Therapy*, 2nd edn. Elsevier/Saunders, Cambridge, pp. 393–400.

Millis, D., Levine, D., Brumlow, M., Weigel, J. 1997, A preliminary study of early physical therapy following surgery for cranial cruciate ligament rupture in dogs. *Vet. Surg.* 26(2): 434.

Montalti, C.S., Souza, N.V., Rodrigues, N.C., Fernandes, K.R., Toma, R.L., Renno, A.C. 2013, Effects of low-intensity pulsed ultrasound on injured skeletal muscle. *Braz. J. Phys. Ther.* 17(4): 343–350.

Nussbaum, E. 1997, Ultrasound: to heat or not to heat – that is the question. *Phys. Ther. Rev.* 2(2): 59–72.

Ogden, J., Toth-Kischkat, A., Schultheiss, R. 2001, Principles of shock wave therapy. *Clin. Orthop. Relat. Res.* 387: 8–17.

Ozcan, J., Ward, A.R., Robertson, V.J. 2004, A comparison of true and premodulated interferential currents. *Arch. Phys. Med. Rehabil.* 85(3): 409–415.

Padilla, F., Puts, R.L., Vico, L., Raum, K. 2014, Stimulation of bone repair with ultrasound: a review of the possible mechanic effects. *Ultrasonics* 54(5): 1125–1145.

Paulekas, R., Haussler, K.K. 2009, Principles and practice of therapeutic exercise for horses. *J. Equine Vet. Sci.* 29(12): 870–893.

Poltawski, L., Watson, T. 2009, Bioelectricity and microcurrent therapy for tissue healing – a narrative review. *Phys. Ther. Rev.* 14(2): 104–114.

Prindeze, N.J., Moffatt, L.T., Shupp, J.W. 2012, Mechanisms of action for light therapy: a review of molecular interactions. *Exp. Biol. Med. (Maywood)* 237(11): 1241–1248.

Rawe, I.M., Vlahovic, T.C. 2012, The use of a portable, wearable form of pulsed radio frequency electromagnetic energy device for the healing of recalcitrant ulcers: a case report. *Int. Wound J.* 9(3): 253–258.

Robertson, V.J., Ward, A., Low, J., Reed, A. 2006, *Electrotherapy Explained: Principles and Practice.* Elsevier, Oxford.

Schils, S.J. 2009, Review of electrotherapy devices for use in veterinary medicine. Annual Convention of the American Association of Equine Practitioners (AAEP) Proceedings, Las Vegas, NA, pp. 68–73.

Silva, M.B., de Melo, P.R., de Oliveira, N.M., Crema, E., Fernandes, L.F. 2012, Analgesic effect of transcutaneous electrical nerve stimulation after laparoscopic cholecystectomy. *Am. J. Phys. Med. Rehabil.* 91(8): 652–657.

Simpson, P.M., Fouche, P.F., Thomas, R.E., Bendall, J.C. 2014, Transcutaneous electrical nerve stimulation for relieving acute pain in the prehospital setting: a systematic review and meta-analysis of randomized-controlled trials. *Eur. J. Emerg. Med.* 21(1): 10–17.

Sluka, K.A., Bjordal, J.M., Marchand, S., Rakel, B.A. 2013, What makes transcutaneous electrical nerve stimulation work? Making sense of the mixed results in the clinical literature. *Phys. Ther.* 93(10): 1397–1402.

Speed, C. 2014, A systematic review of shockwave therapies in soft tissue conditions: focusing on the evidence. *Br. J. Sports Med.* 48(21): 1538–1542.

Sutton, A., Watson, T. 2011, Electrophysical agents in physiotherapy. In: Ross, M.W., Dyson, S.J. (eds), *Diagnosis and Management of Lameness in the Horse.* Elsevier Saunders, St Louis, MO.

Tuner, J., Hode, L. 2004, *The Laser Therapy Handbook.* Prima Books, Grangesberg, Sweden.

Vance, C.G., Dailey, D. L., Rakel, B.A., Sluka, K.A. 2014, Using TENS for pain control: the state of the evidence. *Pain Manag.* 4(3): 197–209.

Veenman, P., Watson, T. 2005, A physiotherapy perspective on pain management. *UK Vet.* 10(8): 87–91.

Wang, C.-J. 2012, Extracorporeal shockwave therapy in musculoskeletal disorders. *J. Orthop. Surg. Res.* 7(1): 11.

Watson, T. (ed.) 2008a, *Electrotherapy: Evidence Based Practice.* Churchill Livingstone/Elsevier, Edinburgh.

Watson, T. 2008b, Electrical properties of tissues. In: Watson, T. (ed.), *Electrotherapy: Evidence Based Practice.* Churchill Livingstone/Elsevier, Edinburgh, pp. 37–52.

Watson, T. 2008c, Introduction: Current concepts and clinical decision making in electrotherapy. In: Watson, T. (ed.), *Electrotherapy: Evidence Based Practice.* Churchill Livingstone/Elsevier, Edinburgh, pp. 3–10.

Watson, T. 2008d, Ultrasound in contemporary physiotherapy practice. *Ultrasonics* 48(4): 321–329.

Watson, T. 2010, Narrative review: key concepts with electrophysical agents. *Phys. Ther. Rev.* 15(4): 351–359.

Watson, T., Young, S. 2008, Therapeutic ultrasound. In: Watson, T. (ed.), *Electrotherapy: Evidence Based Practice.* Churchill Livingstone/Elsevier, Edinburgh.

Wilbert, D.M. 2002, A comparative review of extracorporeal shock wave generation. *BJU Int.* 90: 507–511.

CHAPTER 14

Aquatic therapy

Michelle Monk

Dogs in Motion Canine Rehabilitation, Moorabbin, Australia

Summary

Aquatic therapy is an important component of the physiotherapy management of animal patients. This chapter explores the physical properties of water that contribute to the benefits patients receive when therapy is provided in water, along with some recommendations for types of aquatic therapy for common conditions.

14.1 Introduction

Aquatic therapy has become an increasingly valuable component of the rehabilitation of many animal patients. Many facilities around the world now have purpose-built animal swimming pools and underwater treadmill systems installed. For the animal patient, exercising in water allows unloading of painful joints, as well as earlier weight bearing on otherwise very weak or painful limbs (Steiss 2003). Therapy in the water can assist with increases in range of motion and fitness, while other land-based exercise is limited or contraindicated (Jackson *et al.* 2002).

Hydrotherapy allows for earlier intervention, with patients being able to begin moving within days of injury or surgery with little or no risk of reinjury (Konilan 1999).

While therapy in the water often forms an important component of the rehabilitation programme, it should not be the sole source of therapy. A complete rehabilitation programme that includes aquatic therapy, manual therapy and land-based exercises will provide the best outcome for the patient.

14.2 Physical properties of water

Movement and exercise performed in water are very different from those performed on land. We are unable to simply transfer land exercises over to similar practice in water. To do so would be to ignore the opportunities available to us through exercising in water and the physiological effects of immersion on the body.

Animal Physiotherapy: Assessment, Treatment and Rehabilitation of Animals, Second Edition. Edited by Catherine M. McGowan and Lesley Goff.
© 2016 John Wiley & Sons, Ltd. Published 2016 by John Wiley & Sons, Ltd.

There are several properties of water we must understand, in order to develop efficient hydrotherapy programmes for animals.

- Density
- Specific gravity
- Buoyancy
- Hydrostatic pressure
- Viscosity
- Surface tension
- Refraction

14.2.1 Density

The density of a substance is the relationship between its mass and volume, measured in kg/m^3. Density = mass/volume, kg/m^3. Water is most dense at 4°C, expanding at both higher and lower temperatures. Density increases with dissolved substances; hence seawater is denser than pure water. The *relative density* of a substance compares its density using water as a standard.

Densities of various substances are defined by a number value called *specific gravity*. The specific gravity of pure water is 1.0. Relative density and specific gravity of an object will depend on the composition of the object and will determine whether an object will float or sink. If the ratio of an object's specific gravity to that of water is greater than 1.0, the object will tend to sink; if the ratio is less than 1.0, the object will float. The upper and lower limits of body density in the human community are typically 0.939 g/mL in the very obese and 1.10 g/mL in the leanest individuals (Edlich *et al.* 1987). The relative density of the substance also determines how much of it will sit outside the water. If the specific gravity of a cork is 0.2, only 20% of it will sit under the water. A human with air in the lungs, with a specific gravity of 0.95–0.97, will have 95–97% of their body under the water.

Implications for animal patients (Figure 14.1)

- Lean animals and heavily muscled animals have a tendency to sink, and may need to use a buoyancy vest to reduce effort.
- Lean or heavily muscled animals will have to work harder to keep their heads above water when swimming; they may become tired more quickly so there is a need to monitor all sessions for each patient individually.
- Animals with a greater amount of body fat will float more easily.
- Animals with osteoporosis will have reduced specific gravity and will float.
- Adding flippers or weights will increase specific gravity and cause the animal to sink, so increased effort will be required to keep the head above water.

14.2.2 Buoyancy

When a body is immersed in water, it is subject to the forces of gravity and buoyancy. The principle of buoyancy was discovered by Archimedes, whose principle states that 'when a body is wholly or partially immersed in a fluid at rest, the body experiences an upthrust, equal to the weight of the water it has displaced' (Edlich *et al.* 1987). Buoyancy is the force experienced as an upthrust, which acts in the opposite direction to the force of gravity. The body immersed in the water appears to lose weight, and the weight loss is equal to the weight of water displaced.

So the body at rest in water is subject to two opposing forces.

- Gravity – acting through the centre of gravity (COG)
- Buoyancy – acting through the centre of buoyancy, which is the centre of gravity of the volume of the displaced liquid (Edlich *et al.* 1987)

In women, the percentage weight bearing when immersed to the level of C7 is 6–9%, when immersed to the xiphoid process is 25–31% and when immersed to the anterior superior iliac spine, 40–51% (Harrison & Bulstrode 1987).

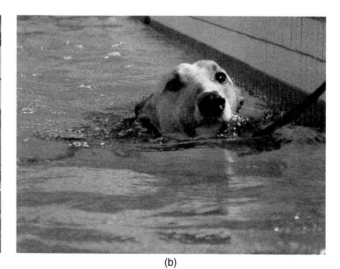

(a)　　　　　　　　　　　(b)

Figure 14.1 (a, b) Comparison of dogs swimming with different buoyancies.

In dogs, a similar study comparing weight bearing in standing as a percentage of bodyweight borne on land demonstrated that when dogs were immersed to the level of the greater trochanter, weight bearing was 38%, at the lateral femoral condyle weight bearing was 85% and at the lateral malleolus 91% (Tragauer & Levine 2002). Further studies need to be performed in various breeds and sizes of dog to confirm these values. Additionally, there are no studies available that investigate the percentage of weight bearing that occurs while the patient is ambulating on the underwater treadmill.

If the centres of gravity and buoyancy are in the same vertical line, the body is kept in *equilibrium*. If the centres of gravity and buoyancy are not in a vertical line, the resultant effect of the two forces will cause a turning force called a *moment* about a pivot point. The body will continue rotating until it finds a point of equilibrium. The *moment of force* = the force of buoyancy × distance between the centre line of buoyancy and a vertical line through the axis of rotation/pivot point. Buoyancy will have a greater effect on a long lever than on a short lever. We can also use the force of buoyancy to assist movement in weak or injured limbs, and provide support and reduced loading to painful or healing structures.

Implications for animal patients

- Left hindlimb amputee swimming: COG moves towards right, will rotate up on right side to reach equilibrium.
- A right hindlimb held up in flexion: moves COG to left, will rotate down on the affected side to reach equilibrium – a dog may struggle to overcome this.
- Spinal-injured patients or those with asymmetrical tone may not be able to control trunk rotation that occurs during swimming – may use buoyancy vest in early stages, but then progress to the dog having to strengthen trunk against moment of force.
- Care with position of flotation devices as they will alter buoyancy and, if asymmetrical, can cause the dog to tip over.
- If a limb is very painful, increased depth of immersion will provide less weight bearing and increase comfort.

14.2.3 Hydrostatic pressure

Pascal's law states that fluid pressure is exerted on all surfaces of an immersed body, while at rest, and at any given depth. Hydrostatic pressure is the sum pressure exerted on all surfaces of a body immersed in water, for any given depth. Pressure is directly proportional to the depth of the part immersed and the density of the water (Edlich *et al.* 1987). Pressure increases with increased depth and increased density of the fluid.

Implications for animal patients

- The principles of hydrostatic pressure tell us that peripheral pooling of blood can be reduced in extremities deep in the water, assisting reduction of oedema and promotion of healing.

- Hydrostatic pressure will affect lung volumes so care needs to be taken with patients with respiratory distress or compromise.

14.2.4 Viscosity

The resistance to movement through water is caused by the friction between water molecules. Water acts as a resistance to movement, as the molecules tend to adhere to the surface of the body moving through it. Viscosity *decreases* as water temperature *increases*. This means weaker and smaller muscles move more easily in warmer water.

Reynolds' theorem

Reynolds demonstrates that there are three types of flow.
- *Laminar flow*: streamlines of molecules in even and regular patterns. The rate of movement at any fixed point is constant.
- *Transitional flow*: as velocity increases, molecules make small movements sideways.
- *Turbulent flow*: velocity increases further; fluid moves irregularly, giving rises to 'eddies'.

Turbulence is the term describing the 'eddies' that follow in the wake of an object moving through fluid. The degree of turbulence will depend on the speed of movement and the shape of the object. Increased speed produces increased turbulence. The more unstreamlined, the more turbulence will be produced. When there is turbulence, there is *drag*. Drag is also increased when the velocity of the limb movement is increased.

Skin friction drag

Water molecules are attracted to a submerged body. This accounts for 56% of the drag experienced by a moving object. Movement in the water is 799 times slower than in air. This is due to the weight of the water, plus the skin friction drag.

Implications for animal patients

- Animals with poor swimming technique, limbs thrashing out of the water, or those that are poorly balanced, cause increased turbulence and increased drag, or resistance to movement – increased difficulty and effort.
- We also use turbulence to provide resistance for strengthening such as the reciprocal movement of limbs in the water, or swimming against a swim-jet, or adding floats or aqua-fins.
- Drag is reduced when a limb moves in the same direction as the turbulent flow, and can be used to assist movement, e.g. hip extension may be aided by swimming against swim-jets or walking on the underwater treadmill.
- Other smaller animals in the water may be affected by turbulence created by larger animals.
- Animals with poor balance on land may be able to stand in water, with less chance of falling as they can correct themselves before falling over. We often see patients with spinal injury able to walk in the underwater treadmill before they can on land.

14.2.5 Surface tension

Surface tension is the force exerted between the surface molecules of the fluid. Water molecules have a greater tendency to adhere together at the surface. Resistance to movement is slightly greater at the surface as there is more cohesion of the molecules here. That's why an insect can land on the surface of the water, or dog hair can float on the top.

Implications for animal patients

- Weak animals may be able to move a limb under the surface of the water, but have difficulty lifting the limb out of the water.
- More effort is required for swimmers thrashing limbs out of the water.

14.2.6 Refraction

Bending of light occurs as it passes from a denser medium to a less dense medium, or vice versa, e.g. air to water. This means that objects can appear shallower than they are, or steps can appear deeper. It also makes viewing limb movement through the top of the water more difficult.

Implications for animal patients

- Limb movements look different from below the water rather than through the top. Observing gait pattern through the surface of the water in the underwater treadmill is much more difficult than through a side glass panel due to refraction
- Animals can be initially nervous walking on the underwater treadmill due to difficulty seeing the walking surface
- Animals may misjudge steps.

14.3 Physiological responses to exercising in water

Exercising in the water causes different physiological responses from exercising on land. A number of studies have compared energy expenditure of exercising in water with the same activity on land (Evans 1978; Gleim & Nicholas 1989).

14.3.1 Energy expenditure

Energy expenditure in the water is the same, or less, compared with the same exercise performed on land, depending on the activity, the water depth, the temperature of the water and the speed at which the activity is carried out. Energy expenditure in the water is different for the same movement pattern performed on land owing to the buoyancy of the water, which reduces the bodyweight, so less force is required to lift the body against gravity (Cureton 1997). Also the viscosity of water increases the energy required to overcome the resistance to movement through water (Cureton 1997). The resistance encountered is directly related to the bodyweight, size, shape, position and speed of movement (Cureton 1997). In addition, exercising in cool water may require more energy to be expended in an attempt to maintain core body temperature, because of the greater conductivity of heat to water (Cureton 1997).

Walking in water

Walking in water has become a common form of hydrotherapy for rehabilitation for humans and animals, and is thought to be particularly beneficial for injuries of the limbs (Cureton 1997). Evans (1978) found that only half to one-third of the speed was needed to walk or jog across a pool in waist-deep water at 31°C, to achieve the same energy expenditure as walking or jogging on a dry treadmill (1.6–3.5 miles/h in water; 3.4–8.3 miles/h on treadmill). Evans found that the resistance to movement through the water had a greater effect on energy expenditure than the reduction in bodyweight caused by the force of buoyancy.

Gleim & Nicholas (1989) investigated the effect of water depth on energy expenditure while walking at different speeds on a land treadmill and an underwater treadmill. They found that there were complex opposing effects of buoyancy and water resistance on energy expenditure in water. They found that the rate of oxygen uptake (VO_2) was increased during water walking in ankle- (25–55%), knee- (26–67%), thigh- (34–72%) and waist-deep (14–67%) water at speeds of 2–4.5 miles/h. At these speeds, VO_2 increased in a curvilinear fashion with speed for both dry and water treadmill walking. At speeds above 5 miles/h, VO_2 during jogging in ankle-, knee- and thigh-deep water was higher than jogging on the dry treadmill, but by a lesser amount than at lower speeds. In waist-deep water at speeds above 5 miles/h, there was no difference in the VO_2 compared with jogging on the dry treadmill. It appears that at this depth, the effect of buoyancy offset the effect of water resistance so that energy expended in the water and on the dry treadmill was the same.

Swimming

Swimming tends to be the other common form of hydrotherapy used in the rehabilitation of animals, and there have been several studies looking at energy expenditure during swimming in humans. There are dramatic differences in energy expenditure, depending on the swimming stroke used and the skill of the swimmer, making it difficult to predict the energy cost of swimming (Cureton 1997). In general, the energy cost of swimming a given distance is about four times the cost of running the same distance.

Implications for animal patients

- Recipe dosages for swimming animal patients should be avoided. Each patient needs to be closely monitored and have an individual programme prescribed based on swimming style, experience in the pool and current pathology.

Water temperature

Energy expenditure during exercise in water may be increased when exercising in cold water owing to the additional effect of shivering (Cureton 1997). The size of the effect is a function of the fatness of the participant, the exercise intensity and duration and the water temperature. At rest in the water, shivering tends to occur in humans when the water temperature is below 28–34°C (Craig & Dvorak 1970), depending on the degree of body fitness and duration of immersion. Even with light to moderately heavy submaximal exercise, energy expenditure is increased when water temperature is below 26°C (Craig & Dvorak 1970).

14.3.2 Maximal oxygen uptake

Maximal oxygen uptake is generally lower in water compared with similar exercise on land (Cureton 1997). Maximal heart rate and blood lactate are also lower during maximal water running, suggesting that the work rate achieved at exhaustion is less in the water than on the land (Cureton 1997).

These findings are important as they suggest that we cannot base exercise prescriptions in water on maximal heart rates or oxygen uptakes measured on land. Reduced maximal heart rate accounts for much of the reduced maximal oxygen uptake observed (Cureton 1997).

14.3.3 Circulation

During upright, head-out-of-water immersion in humans, there is a shift of blood volume from the lower limbs and the abdomen to the thorax. This shift of blood increases central venous pressure, left ventricular end-diastolic volume, stroke volume and cardiac output, and decreases systemic vascular resistance at rest and during submaximal exercise.

While the body is at rest, or exercising at lower intensities, the heart rate remains mostly unchanged during immersion. At higher intensities of submaximal and at maximal exercise intensities, heart rate is decreased compared with exercise on land.

It is commonly, but not always, observed that heart rate is lower during exercise in the water compared with exercise at the same maximal oxygen uptake on the land. This is dependent on exercise intensity and water temperature. During moderately light head-out-of-water exercise in water 31–33°C, heart rate does not differ from when exercise is performed on land at the same VO_2. During strenuous exercise, the heart rate is usually, but not always, lower by approximately 10 beats/min (Craig & Dvorak 1970; Evans 1978).

These studies demonstrate that the relationship of VO_2 to heart rate during exercise in water compared with that on land is variable and depends on several factors including exercise intensity, exercise mode and water temperature. Therefore, we must be very careful in using heart rate to prescribe or monitor exercise intensity in the water, or using a maximal heart rate derived from a land-based test, to determine expected exercise intensity in the water.

14.3.4 Thermoregulation

In humans, the regulation of body temperature in water is very different than it is in air because the primary means of dissipation of heat during exercise on land, evaporation of sweat, is not possible. The loss or gain of heat is also much greater in water through convection and conduction (Cureton 1997). Heat conductance is about 25 times greater in water than air, so when water temperature is above or below skin temperature, heat gain or loss, respectively, is greater in water than in air (Cureton 1997). In the water, there is a much narrower range of water temperatures through which core temperature is not affected by exercise compared with the land.

During exercise in the air, environmental temperatures of between 5°C and 35°C do not affect the rise in central body temperature caused by increased exercise intensity (Cureton 1997). During exercise in water, the temperature needed to prevent a rise in core temperature during prolonged exercise varies from 34°C to 17°C, depending on the intensity of the exercise performed and the degree of body fat of the person (Craig & Dvorak 1970).

Exercising in warm water over 33°C can cause a feeling of fatigue and exhaustion, owing to elevated core temperature. Exercising in cold water below 25°C causes thermal stress and brings about metabolic and cardiovascular adjustments geared towards maintaining core body temperature, because the heat flow from the body is substantial. Exercising in water at 18°C can cause the muscles to fatigue, and an inability to contract the muscles fully. For most humans, the optimal water temperature for exercising is around 28–30°C, where little heat would be stored and performance would not be impaired (Edlich *et al.* 1987). Most pools for human hydrotherapy are kept at 'thermo-neutral' temperature, 32–34°C, as we are not 'swimming'.

The optimal water temperature for small animal hydrotherapy is unknown, but will vary somewhat, depending on the size of the animal, how fast it can swim or walk, how fit or old it is, how fat it is, the duration of the exercise session, the depth of the water and any preexisting respiratory or cardiac conditions.

It is expected that lower temperatures will be required for dogs that are swimming or generating considerable body heat, or if the dog will spend extended periods in the water. Pools for swimming should be kept at subthermal temperatures: 25–27°C. However, a small puppy will quickly chill if left standing in cooler water and may need temperatures up to 32°C.

When using the underwater treadmill to exercise patients after neurological or orthopaedic surgery, exercise intensity will mostly be low. Hence, water temperature should be in the therapeutic range of 27–32°C, depending on the needs of the individual patient, speed of exercise and depth of immersion.

Rectal temperatures may need to be taken if there is concern for hyperthermia.

Implications for animal patients

- Exercising in colder water may cause an increased work of swimming and increase oxygen uptake due to shivering, as well as difficulty contracting muscles.
- Thinner animals will feel the effects more in colder water.
- If the water is cold, sessions should be shorter (e.g. in the sea in winter).

- Similarly, water should not be too warm for swimming (suggest no more than 30°C), due to the thermal load on the body, the risk of fatigue and exhaustion.
- Monitoring of animal patients is imperative – and strict home exercise instructions should be given regarding water temperature, depth of immersion and duration of exercise (difficult to control for intensity).

There are several important differences between the physiological responses to exercise on land and in water, but as long as the therapist is aware of these differences, the benefits of exercising in an environment with reduced weight-bearing stresses on the limbs and the increased resistance offered by the water make it an ideal environment for rehabilitating many injuries.

Just with any rehabilitation programme, animals who are rehabilitating from injury or surgery and have been prescribed swimming or walking in the water as a 'home therapy programme' must be fully assessed by a trained animal aquatic therapist. This therapy should then be trialled under the guidance and supervision of the therapist to ensure it is appropriate and a specific dosage can be prescribed, prior to completing subsequent sessions away from the clinic.

14.4 Evidence for effectiveness of hydrotherapy

In humans, the benefits of exercising in water have long been recognised and more recently, evidence has been provided to confirm that hydrotherapy is beneficial for pain, function, self-efficacy, joint mobility, strength and balance (Davis & Harrison 1988; Geytenbeek 2002; Hall et al. 1990; Kelly et al. 2000; Konilan 1999; Langridge & Phillips 1988).

Aquatic therapy is used widely in humans by therapists and patients for the management of osteoarthritis and rheumatoid arthritis. Aquatic therapy has been shown to reduce pain and improve function in patients with hip osteoarthritis, and increase strength and range of motion in joints affected by osteoarthritis. Reduction in pain, improved range of joint motion and reduced difficulty in the performance of functional tasks for those affected by rheumatoid arthritis have also been demonstrated as a result of hydrotherapy programmes. Patients with rheumatoid arthritis also experienced an improved emotional and psychological state, along with improved joint range of motion and reduced pain, following a hydrotherapy programme (Hall et al. 1990). Hydrotherapy has also been shown to improve function in subjects with back pain.

Aquatic therapy is also commonly used by physiotherapists for postoperative therapy. Following shoulder surgery, movement of the shoulder in the water requires much less muscle activation than on land, meaning that rehabilitation can begin earlier, with less stress on the injured structures (Kelly et al. 2000). An investigation of the effects of exercise in water and on land, following intraarticular anterior cruciate ligament reconstruction, showed that exercising in the water was more effective in reducing joint effusion and hastened return to function, and that hydrotherapy was as effective for increasing knee range of motion and quadriceps muscle strength.

While aquatic therapy appears to be widely used for the rehabilitation of animals, currently there are few studies investigating the benefits of this form of exercise, or the parameters to use when prescribing exercise. Unlike human hydrotherapy, much of the hydrotherapy performed on animals consists of swimming or walking through the water. Fewer one-to-one therapist–patient treatments are performed, largely due to the danger of performing such activities, particularly in horses, or the inability of the patient to relax in the water. More one-to-one treatments may be performed in dogs, and with acclimatisation, the animals can become quite relaxed in the water and allow limbs or body parts to be moved for them.

Swimming is often used as part of the rehabilitation programme for the canine patient following surgery for cranial cruciate ligament deficiency. A programme of physiotherapy exercise and swimming, commenced at 3 weeks after surgery, was shown to improve limb function over cage confinement, with no difference evident between the affected and unaffected limbs measured with a force-plate at 6 months after surgery (Marsolais et al. 2002).

Range of motion of the stifle was compared in a group of dogs swimming versus those exercising on a land treadmill following cranial cruciate ligament stabilisation surgery. More stifle flexion was achieved while swimming than while exercising on the treadmill, so swimming was recommended if increasing stifle flexion is the goal (Marsolais et al. 2003).

There have been several investigations of the physiological responses of horses to swimming (Hobo et al. 1998) but as with humans, it is very difficult to standardise the intensity and velocity of the movement of the horse in the pool, therefore measurements are often inaccurate.

Underwater treadmill therapy has become very popular for the rehabilitation of both canine and equine injuries. Joint kinematics of dogs studied while walking on an underwater treadmill showed that joint flexion is greatest when the water is filled higher than the joint of interest, but that full joint extension is also achieved with underwater treadmill walking, which is not the case in swimming (Jackson et al. 2002).

More recently, the effects of an early intensive underwater treadmill, physiotherapy exercise and home-walking programme was compared with a typical home-walking programme, for their effects on limb function following tibial plateau-levelling osteotomy surgery in dogs with cranial cruciate ligament deficiency (Monk et al. 2006). Dogs in the underwater treadmill physiotherapy group increased thigh circumference, and stifle flexion and extension range of motion, so no difference was evident between the affected and non-affected limbs at 6 weeks after surgery, while the home-walking group continued to lose muscle mass and their stifle joints became stiffer.

14.5 Benefits of hydrotherapy for animals

Based on the evidence we have for human and animal hydrotherapy, the suggested benefits of hydrotherapy or exercising in water for animals include the following.

- Reduces loading on painful or healing structures – exercise can be commenced earlier with less muscle activation required and less load on limbs.
- Provides additional support to limbs, reducing likelihood of injury to muscles, tendons and ligaments.
- Allows exercise to continue while land-based exercise is restricted or contraindicated.
- Eases performance of difficult activities and movements through the force of buoyancy.
- Water provides more resistance/drag than air: great for strengthening.
- Prevents atrophy.
- Increases in muscle mass and strength.
- Increases cardiovascular fitness and endurance.
- Increases joint range of motion, reduces stiffnes.
- Increases soft tissue extensibility.
- Reduces muscle spasm and hyertonicity.
- Increases tone in hypotonic body parts.
- Allows gradual progression and return towards more normal function.
- Assists in management of oedema through hydrostatic pressure.
- Provides relaxation.
- Reduces pain in joints with degenerative joint disease.
- Increases circulation and assists in promotion of healing.

14.6 Assessment of the small animal patient for hydrotherapy

Although this subject will not be covered in detail, it is expected that all patients attending for hydrotherapy will be assessed and cleared by their veterinarian before commencing hydrotherapy.

As with all human physiotherapy patients, a thorough assessment, including documentation of findings, needs to be performed. The physiotherapist needs to consider which patients will be suitable for hydrotherapy. Apart from their current medical or physical conditions, factors to consider include temperament, previous history of swimming, including good and bad experiences. On the whole, most patients are suitable for hydrotherapy in some form.

All horses, dogs and cats can swim. How well they do it and with how much anxiety will depend on prior experience, and experience of the handler now attempting to swim them.

Most animals will become acclimatised in a few visits, and it is worth trying to persevere with even the most anxious patients. Use of buoyancy vests and equipment to lead the animal, extra staff members to assist and a short session help to reduce anxiety and enable acclimatisation.

14.6.1 Subjective questioning

In addition to your standard subjective questioning of the owner or handler, further questions specific to hydrotherapy, which will help you determine the type of hydrotherapy that will be suitable and where to start, include the following.

- Date of last vaccination and worming?
- Previous level of exercise/fitness?
- Has the animal swum previously and where? In a pool/beach/dam – be aware that those that swim well at the beach may not swim well in your pool. Also, those that are fearful of water often are more relaxed in an underwater treadmill where feet can still touch the bottom.
- Did they actually initiate the swimming or did you place them in the water?
- Do they like the bath? The hose?
- Any incontinence?
- Any ear problems?
- When did they last eat?
- Did the vet advise you how much hydrotherapy to do?

14.6.2 Objective assessment

Along with your standard objective assessment, if you are planning to take a patient into the water, things to check before include the following.

- Skin condition – any dryness, redness, flaking (not contraindicated, just be aware).
- Ear problems – check inside.
- Make sure the dog has toileted.
- Any open wounds, torn nails, etc.
- Heart rate and respiratory rate assessment at rest.

14.6.3 Contraindications to hydrotherapy for animals

Hydrotherapy is not recommended for animals with any of the following conditions.

- Open, infected or draining wounds
- Unhealed surgical incisions without a waterproof cover
- Active gastrointestinal disease (vomiting and/or diarrhoea)
- Elevated body temperature, infection
- Systemic compromise such as severe cardiac, liver, kidney disease, hypotension or hypertension
- Respiratory compromise or distress
- Advanced debility
- Uncontrolled epilepsy
- Kennel cough in dogs (contagious)

14.6.4 Precautions

Animals with any of the following conditions may still be suitable for hydrotherapy, depending on the equipment and facilities available. No animal should *ever* be left unattended while participating in hydrotherapy in any form.

- Faecal incontinence – use nappies or evacuate bowel beforehand in dogs
- Urinary incontinence if urinary tract infection

- Laryngeal paralysis (no swimming, but underwater treadmill if closely monitored and head remains out of the water)
- Wounds that have been given the 'OK' by the veterinarian – get written permission
- Older patients
- Mild systemic compromise – monitor
- Extremely obese patients
- External fixators
- Skin problems
- Ear problems
- Epilepsy

14.6.5 Treatment plan

After assessment, a treatment programme and plan should be written and discussed with the owner, including expected time frames for improvement. Goals of treatment need to be devised and discussed with the owner. The owner may simply want the dog to return to getting up the back steps independently or walking to the local shops for the paper, or they may wish to return them to high-level agility or hunting and retrieving.

Objective measures need to be used to determine the effectiveness of treatment.

- Lameness score/gait analysis with video; there are many applications that are inexpensive and easily available now for analysing gait video
- Range of motion of affected limb
- Muscle mass/limb circumference
- Functional measures: able to sit squarely/use stairs/get into the car
- Force-plate or pressure – mat gait assessment if available

14.6.6 Reassessment and progression of treatment

Regular reassessment of the whole dog should be performed to determine if the patient is progressing as expected with the current treatment, and the programme modified accordingly. Frequency of reassessment is dependent on the type of pathology and severity of the condition, with more severely affected dogs requiring more frequent reassessment to ensure they remain on track with rehabilitation.

Each time the patient attends for a hydrotherapy session, the owner should be questioned about response to the previous session. This will help guide the therapist on the dosage of hydrotherapy for that day.

14.7 Types of hydrotherapy for animals

Following your assessment, you will have to determine the most suitable form of hydrotherapy, and the expected dosage for that day (or for home exercise).

This will be determined not only by your assessment findings, but by the size of the animal, their pathology, severity of their problem, experience of hydrotherapy, general response to

handling and new situations, the equipment you or the owners have available, assistants on hand to help you, equipment available to help you, and the goals of treatment.

Small animals
- Sink
- Bathtub
- Whirlpool
- Swim-spa
- Children's wading pool
- Beach
- Dam
- Lake
- River
- Above-ground or in-ground human swimming pools – swimming and therapist-assisted hydrotherapy
- Purpose-built dog pools – swimming and hydrotherapy (Figure 14.2)
- Underwater treadmills (Figure 14.3)

Large animals
- Swimming in purpose-built pools (Figure 14.4)
- Beach
- Dam
- River
- Water walker/underwater treadmill (Figure 14.5)

14.7.1 Equipment

There are several different pieces of equipment that can be useful when working in an aquatic environment. These may be used to

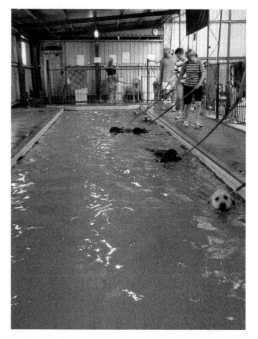

Figure 14.2 Dog pool.

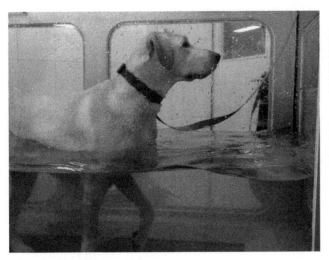

Figure 14.3 Underwater treadmill.

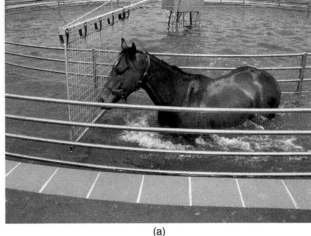

(a)

either reduce or increase effort of the animal or body part in the water.

- *Floats*: may be used to assist joint flexion when placed below the joint of interest, or increase the work required to overcome the buoyancy. They may help to increase weight bearing in an affected limb if placed on the contralateral limb while walking in the underwater treadmill. Floats may also be used under the abdomen to help keep the hindlimbs up while swimming, or prevent a dog from sitting in the underwater treadmill.
- *Pool noodles:* can be used to keep dogs away from the sides of the underwater treadmill and keep their feet on the treadmill belt. They can also be used under the abdomen to help keep dogs afloat.
- *Theraband*: can be used to provide assistance or resistance to movement: looping around both hindlimbs will increase the work of walking while in the treadmill. Be sure it can be easily released if the animal becomes distressed.

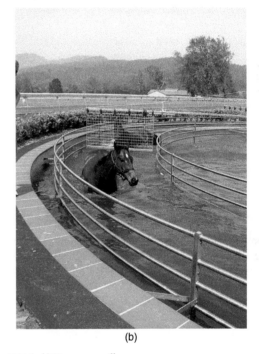

(b)

Figure 14.5 (a, b) Horse aquawalker.

- *Weighted straps around limbs*: can increase the work of swimming or walking to increase strength.
- *Buoyancy vests*: good for initial swimmers, those with poor trunk control and anxious dogs. Can reduce the work of swimming on the heart and lungs, meaning dogs can exercise their limbs for longer before tiring (Figure 14.6).
- *Harnesses*: to assist front, rear or the entire dog; sometimes a buoyancy vest gives too much support and we want the animal to work a little harder. Harnesses can be helpful to provide support and assistance to particular body areas, for example holding the rear end higher in the water for a dog with spinal injuries, but still making it use its trunk muscles to control body rotation.

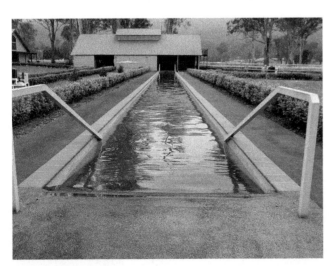

Figure 14.4 Horse pool.

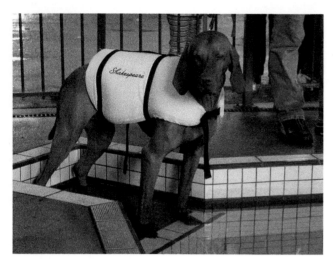

Figure 14.6 Buoyancy vest.

- *Hoists*: useful for assisting large animals and those quite disabled in and out of the pool or treadmill.
- *Aquatoys*: great for motivation to encourage swimming.
- *Steps*: can be used to provide alternating terrain to negotiate while walking through the water.
- *Ramps/inclines/declines*: to assist entry/exit as well as increasing work of hindlimbs if walking uphill, or forelimbs if walking down hill
- *Swim snoods:* to keep water out of the ears if dogs have an ear complaint.

14.7.2 Hydrotherapy for specific conditions – small animals

There are many conditions that will benefit from hydrotherapy in some form, including joint surgeries, fracture repairs, non-use of a limb, spinal injuries or surgeries and many degenerative conditions such as arthritis. Where possible, hydrotherapy should not be the only form of therapy the animal receives, and each patient should be assessed by a physiotherapist before commencing a hydrotherapy programme. The following information disregards the land-based therapy and is intended as a general guideline only. It is by no means a recipe for treatment, and each patient case must be assessed individually and an individual programme devised which considers the patient's condition, other health conditions, fitness, previous experiences, fear of water, etc. Programmes should be revised regularly and progressed as needed.

Stifle surgery

Hydrotherapy has an important place in the rehabilitation of all dogs recovering from the various forms of stifle surgery such as those for cranial cruciate ligament deficiency or patella luxation. Hydrotherapy would generally be commenced 10 days to 2 weeks after surgery, when the wound has healed. When deciding on a type of hydrotherapy, it is important to determine your

goals of treatment, and not simply choose hydrotherapy for all patients with this condition.

In the early stages post surgery (weeks 2–6), we are aiming to increase weight bearing, increase strength and gently work on range of motion. In the later stages of rehabilitation (weeks 7–16), while strength and range of motion still need to be addressed, we are working towards more muscle endurance and increased load on the limb.

The underwater treadmill is particularly beneficial in the early stages of recovery as it is much more controlled and precise. Recommendation for frequency of underwater treadmill sessions is dependent on degree of muscle atrophy, but typically 2–3 times per week is ideal for the first month (weeks 2–6 post surgery). Water level should be as deep as is possible without the patient trying to swim, for maximal unloading of the surgical limb. After this, frequency will be determined by reassessment findings and how the patient is progressing. The author typically recommends underwater treadmill for 6–8 weeks post surgery in most patients (weeks 2–8 or 10 post surgery). If the patient has not been able to attend as frequently as this, then the programme may need to be extended until muscle mass of the affected limb is normal or near normal, and lameness has resolved. As the patient improves, intensity and duration of exercise can increase and water depth can be reduced, to provide greater challenge.

Swimming can be beneficial for increasing stifle joint range of motion but it is more of an endurance exercise so strength gains are slower in comparison to underwater treadmill. There is also much less control over intensity of limb motion and speed of swimming in comparison to underwater treadmill therapy. It can be very vigorous for some patients who are not seasoned swimmers and can actually aggravate their pain and inflammation. It is, however, a great form of exercise in postacute stages of stifle surgery rehabilitation, when pain and inflammation have settled down. At this stage, around 6 weeks post surgery, endurance can start to be worked upon and the pool still provides protection for the surgery site which won't yet have full strength. Land-based rehabilitation exercises should still be performed at this stage.

Swimming is also a great alternative form of long-term exercise for dogs that have had stifle joint surgery, so they can exercise safely without loading.

Fracture repair

Hydrotherapy is often extremely beneficial after fracture repair to allow exercising of the injured part, thus increasing joint range of motion and preventing atrophy, contractures and non-use of limbs, and then building muscle strength but in a controlled fashion, without compromising repair. The physiotherapist should check with the referring veterinarian as to how much weight they are happy for the animal to take on the limb and the stability of the repair. In general, hydrotherapy would start when the wound has healed and any casts or bandages have been removed. Sometimes hydrotherapy will be performed when a dog attends for a bandage change, then the limb is dried and the bandage reapplied. This is very useful for preventing excessive joint stiffness and muscle wastage. Depending on the area fractured and type of fixation used, some animals may be more suitable for underwater treadmill initially as it is more controlled than swimming. If water quality is kept at human standards, and the referring veterinarian is happy, dogs with external fixators may be suitable to commence hydrotherapy also, as long as the limb is dried and kept clean afterwards.

Once radiographs demonstrate bone healing, weights and floats may be added to increase resistance.

Femoral head and neck excisional arthroplasty

Aquatic therapy forms an important component of the rehabilitation of the femoral head and neck excisional arthroplasty patient. These patients can be reluctant to use the limb, and progress slowly with land-based exercises while scar tissue forms to fill the pseudo hip joint. Supplementing land-based therapy with walking on the underwater treadmill can help weight bearing in the surgical limb and assist with more normal muscle activation. The treadmill belt can also assist with increasing the protraction phase of stance during the gait cycle. Swimming can have varied outcomes with these patients. Some patients will swim with the hindlimbs tucked up as their regular swimming action, resulting in no benefit to progression or improvement of limb use on land. Others may swim very vigorously if they are nervous, which can make the operation site painful afterwards. If swimming is chosen as a form of aquatic therapy, the patient must be monitored very closely and progressed gradually as they improve.

Non-use of a limb

Non-use of a limb can occur after any limb injury or surgery, but is typically worse in dogs with complex injuries, multiple surgeries, those that have been immobilised for lengthy periods and anxious dogs. Complications of prolonged non-use of a limb include joint contractures, muscle shortening, muscle wasting, altered mechanics of other body parts, anxiety, muscle pain and hypersensitivity. It is important for the referring veterinarian to assess and treat the dog for any condition that may continue to promote non-use, such as pain or implant irritation.

Hydrotherapy can be very beneficial to encourage gentle limb use, stretching and strengthening of the limb, often with swift carry-over to the land. The warmth of the water can relax the muscles holding up the limb and allow the limb to begin to be used. The buoyancy of the water reduces the load on the limb and often makes walking in the underwater treadmill possible. Even if the dog is still reluctant to use the limb outside the pool or treadmill, the water provides an avenue to start to stretch and strengthen in the interim. Assisting the dog's limb to move either in the pool or treadmill can also be very beneficial to start limb movement in those somewhat more reluctant. Standing in the water and performing weight shifting or non-affected limb lifting exercises can also be very beneficial for reeducating normal movement and facilitating weight bearing.

Spinal injury or surgery

Dogs with paralysis and paresis and one or multiple limbs affected benefit greatly from hydrotherapy. Hydrotherapy can commence once the spine is stable. Patients are exercised in the underwater treadmill from day 2 after surgery, where they are assisted to move their limbs gently, with buoyancy supporting them, keeping the wound out of the water. Limbs that are very weak can be assisted to swim and walk, often resulting in a faster return to walking on the land. Dogs that are too weak to walk on the land will often swim or walk on the underwater treadmill first, then using the hydrotherapy to gain strength and control, can transfer over to independent walking on land. The use of a buoyancy vest is beneficial to assist in trunk control, and can be removed as the dog strengthens, to help development of trunk muscles. Even if limb movement is not initially seen in the water, perseverance is worthwhile, as the weightless environment means small muscle contractions are often possible here initially, compared with attempting to move against gravity out of the water. Where possible, daily hydrotherapy is recommended for these patients until they can walk independently on land. This group of patients often benefits from ongoing weekly hydrotherapy where available, particularly if they have any deficits remaining after rehabilitation is complete.

Whether in the swimming pool or in the underwater treadmill, facilitating correct limb sequencing and motion in patients with reduced or absent proprioception helps to facilitate return of neuromuscular control through neural plasticity. Tail stimulation – squeezing the tail intermittently – in patients with hindlimb paresis or paralysis can cause reflexive limb movement through stimulation of the central pattern generators in the spine. This can be done intermittently throughout an aquatic therapy session.

Arthritis

Hydrotherapy is very beneficial in this group of patients for allowing strengthening without loading, increasing and maintaining joint range of motion, maintaining cardiovascular fitness and assisting with weight loss, when exercise on land may be difficult. This group of patients benefits from ongoing hydrotherapy, where available, once or twice a week. A variety of devices can be used to make the work of swimming or walking in the water more or less difficult, depending on how the dog is affected and in which joints. Dogs may need assistance in and out of the water, but often cope well once the buoyancy of the water supports them, and can exercise in the water with minimal assistance.

14.7.3 Exercise prescription and monitoring
Warm-up, exercise component and cool-down

As with all exercise programmes, each hydrotherapy session should have a warm-up, exercise component and cool-down. This may simply be that exercise commences slowly, increases in intensity and then slows down before ceasing. Alternatively, the warm-up and cool-down may be done outside the pool. In the case of exercising for particular conditions, massage, stretching or other land-based exercises may also make up part of the warm-up and cool-down, or be done during the rests breaks between bouts of exercise.

Intensity of treatment

Intensity is also a consideration for each animal's hydrotherapy programme. Intensity of exercise in the underwater treadmill is easily controlled through depth of water and speed of walking. Swimming intensity cannot be so easily controlled, but control over the number of laps swum before a rest, rest time, and use of a buoyancy vest are all ways to control exercise intensity while swimming. In general, as animals improve, the intensity of exercise is increased so they can adapt and strengthen.

Duration of treatment

Treatment time will be affected by several factors, including the dog's prior experience of being in water, anxiety, age, weight, preexisting conditions, e.g. heart problems, recent limb surgery, previous fitness level.

In general, the more debilitated the animal is, the shorter the treatment time will need to be. The initial session may consist of swimming three or four half-laps in the pool, with several minutes rest in between, or walking for three sets of 1 minute at a time on the underwater treadmill, with rests in between.

Monitoring

Monitoring of heart rate can help determine the length of exercise and rest sessions. Alternatively, watching for breathing rate and signs of distress can be helpful to avoid exhaustion.

Normal resting heart rates for dogs range between 50 bpm and 160 bpm, depending on size and fitness. Some puppies and toy breeds may have heart rates up to 180 bpm at rest.

At this stage, there are no documented 'target heart rates' for dogs. It has been suggested that the desirable difference between pre- and postexercise heart rates is 20–50 bpm (Lamoreaux 2002). Until further studies are performed to determine appropriate heart rates for exercising dogs in water, it is better to do a small amount of hydrotherapy initially and increase slowly each session as the animal allows.

Normal respiratory rate is 16–20 breaths/min, with larger, fitter dogs having a rate as low as 10 breaths/min, and overweight or unfit dogs may be at 30 breaths/min. There are no values for exercising respiratory rates at present.

Further studies are required to determine the best way to monitor and when to monitor.

Frequency of treatment

As in human physiotherapy, we generally attain faster return to function with more intensive rehabilitation. The same occurs with rehabilitation and hydrotherapy in small animals.

For *orthopaedic* cases, the recommendation is two or three times per week for the first 4–6 weeks. After this time, depending on how the patient is progressing, they may reduce down to one or two per week until the 12-week mark. This will not be possible for many owners and once a week or fortnight has to suffice. Hydrotherapy will still benefit these patients but the rehabilitation process will take longer.

For *neurological* cases, daily hydrotherapy is recommended, especially in the first 2–3 weeks, to make use of neural plasticity.

Progression of treatment

Treatment needs to be progressed in order to overload the body slightly, and cause it to adapt and strengthen. Following each session, ask the owner to monitor their animal at home over the next 24 h and record anything that indicates we may have done too much.

Questions to ask on the next visit.

- How was the animal after the session? (Lameness same/worse/better; may have been tired, developed muscle soreness, been a little stiff)
- If the animal was more lame, how long did it last? (Few hours or until the next morning is OK, 24 h+ and we have done too much)
- How has the animal been since then? (May have been same, continued to improve, got worse)
- Did you increase any other exercises? (May have increased walk or other home exercises – decide if this contributed to lack or progression or deterioration if occurred)
- Did you give the dog any NSAIDs or ice/heat/massage, etc. if worse?
- How is the dog today and what exercise have you done before coming here today?

The answers to these questions will help you decide how to progress the patient's exercises for that day's session, as well as advising on what home exercise to do afterwards.

References

Craig, A.B., Dvorak, M. 1970, Thermal regulation during immersion. *J. Appl. Physiol.* 21: 1577–1585.

Cureton, K.J. 1997, Physiologic responses to water exercise. In: Routi, R.G., Morris, D.M. (eds), *Aquatic Rehabilitation*. Lippincott, Philadelphia, PA, pp. 39–56.

Davis, B.C., Harrison, R.A. 1988, *Hydrotherapy in Practice*. Churchill Livingstone, Melbourne, pp. 158–159.

Edlich, F.R., Towler, M.A., Goitz, R.J., *et al.* 1987, Bioengineering principles of hydrotherapy. *J. Burn Care Rehab.* 8(6): 580–584.

Evans, B.W. 1978, Metabolic and circulatory responses to walking and jogging in water. *Res. Q.* 49: 442–449.

Geytenbeek, J. 2002, Evidence for effective hydrotherapy. *Physiotherapy* 88(9): 514–529.

Gleim, W.G., Nicholas. J.A. 1989, Metabolic costs and heart rate responses to treadmill walking in water at different depths and temperatures. *Am. J. Sports Med.* 17(2): 248–252.

Hall, J., Bisson, D., O'Hare, P. 1990, The physiology of immersion. *Physiotherapy* 79(9): 517–521.

Harrison, R.A., Bulstrode, S. 1987, Percentage weight-bearing during partial immersion in a hydrotherapy pool. *Physiotherapy Pract.* 3: 60–63.

Hobo, S., Yoshida, K., Yoshihara, T. 1998, Characteristics of respiratory function during swimming exercise in Thoroughbreds. *J. Vet. Med. Sci.* 60(6): 687–689.

Jackson, A.M., Millis, D.L., Stevens, M., Barnett, S. 2002, Joint kinematics during underwater treadmill activity. Second International Symposium: on Rehabilitation and Physical Therapy in Veterinary Medicine. Knoxville, TN.

Kelly, B.T., Roskin, L.A., Kirkendall, D.T., *et al.* 2000, Shoulder muscle activation during aquatic and dry-land exercises in non-impaired subjects. *J. Orthop. Sports Phys. Ther.* 30(4): 204–210.

Konilan, C. 1999, Aquatic therapy: making a wave in the treatment of low back injuries. *Orthop. Nurs.* 18(1): 11–20.

Lamoreaux, A. 2002, Integrating hydrotherapy and physical therapy in canine rehabilitation. Westcoast Seminar, USA.

Langridge, J.C., Phillips, D. 1988, Group hydrotherapy exercises for chronic back-pain sufferers – introduction and monitoring. *Physiotherapy* 74(6): 269–273.

Marsolais, G.S., Dvorak, G., Conzemius, M.G. 2002, Effects of post-operative rehabilitation on limb function after cranial cruciate ligament repair in dogs. *J. Am. Vet. Med. Assoc.* 220: 1325–1330.

Marsolais, G.S., McLean S., Derrick, T. *et al.* 2003, Kinematic analysis of the hind limb during swimming and walking in healthy dogs and dogs with surgically corrected cranial cruciate ligament rupture. *J. Am. Vet. Med. Assoc.* 222(6): 739–743.

Monk, M.L., Preston, C.A., McGowan, C.M. 2006, Effects of early intensive post-operative physiotherapy on limb function after tibial plateau leveling osteotomy in dogs with deficiency of the cranial cruciate ligament. *Am. J. Vet. Res.* 67(3): 529–536.

Steiss, J.E. 2003, Canine rehabilitation. In: Braund, K.G. (ed.), *Clinical Neurology in Small Animals – Localization, Diagnosis and Treatment.* IVIS, New York.

Tragauer, V.L., Levine, D. 2002, Percentage of normal weight bearing during partial immersion at various depths in dogs. Second International Symposium on Rehabilitation and Physical Therapy in Veterinary Medicine, Knoxville, TN.

CHAPTER 15

Acupuncture and trigger points*

Brooke Marsh

Holistic Animal Physiotherapy, Maroochy River, Australia

Summary

Oriental medicine is a highly complex system of diagnosis and treatment that was developed over 4000 years ago. Acupuncture may be considered as one of the principal elements used in Oriental medicine for the treatment of many conditions, including those treated predominantly by physiotherapists such as musculoskeletal pain and disability.

Essentially, acupuncture stimulates the body's own remarkable pain-relieving and healing mechanisms. It has long been used as part of veterinary practice, with good results being reported for disorders of the musculoskeletal, cardiovascular, respiratory and gastrointestinal systems.

This chapter will outline the use of acupuncture, potential mechanisms for its effect, and evidence of the clinical efficacy of acupuncture in the management of human and animal musculoskeletal pain conditions. The nature of trigger points in musculoskeletal pain and the role of physiotherapy, including dry needling, will also be discussed.

15.1 Introduction

Traditional Chinese Medicine (TCM) is a highly complex system that is both precise and flexible. It treats the mind-body-spirit as a single entity in harmony with nature and the environment. The Chinese view the body (human/animal) as an intricate and interdependent system in which all aspects of internal life and external environment are intimately intertwined. When the body-mind-spirit is in a state of harmony and balance with external influences, health is achieved.

Traditional Chinese Medicine initially developed in an era before the introduction of modern medicine as a preventative form of treatment. Approximately 4000 years ago, practitioners used TCM to maintain the health of livestock, a valuable resource in China. The foundations of classical acupuncture texts were transmitted to Japan from China 1200 years ago, hence for the purpose of this text I will refer to the concepts of Oriental medicine rather than specifically TCM. The first written record of acupuncture is found in the over 2200-year-old *Huang-de-nei-jing* (*Yellow Emperor's Classic of Internal Medicine*), one of the oldest medical textbooks in the world (Xie & Preast 2007).

As Kuwahara (2003) explains, 'Nowadays there are various schools of thought that govern the practice of acupuncture. Some treatments are based on modern (i.e. Western) medical concepts, some on traditional Chinese medical (i.e. TCM) ideas, and some on the classical theories'. Oriental medicine involved a complex system of diagnosis and treatment based on a number of principles formulated before therapists had any detailed knowledge of neurophysiology, or indeed physiology.

Acupuncture may be considered as one of the principal elements used in Oriental medicine for the treatment of many conditions, including those treated predominantly by physiotherapists such as musculoskeletal pain and disability. TCM or Oriental medicine is not a synonym for acupuncture as it can use many techniques including herbs, dietary advice,

---

*Adapted from the first edition chapter, which was written by Tina Souvlis

Animal Physiotherapy: Assessment, Treatment and Rehabilitation of Animals, Second Edition. Edited by Catherine M. McGowan and Lesley Goff.

meditation, exercise and massage. Acupuncture can be defined as 'the insertion of a solid needle into the body with the purpose of therapy, disease prevention or maintenance of health' (Acupuncture Regulatory Working Group 2003). Although it is primarily thought of in Oriental medicine to be a method of balancing energy flow throughout the body, research has demonstrated that it can elicit a strong multisystem physiological response. Essentially, acupuncture stimulates the body's own remarkable pain-relieving and healing mechanisms. It has long been used as part of veterinary practice, with good results being reported for disorders of the musculoskeletal, cardiovascular, respiratory and gastrointestinal systems (Lindley 2010).

Modern practice often uses a modified or 'Western' approach to acupuncture, which is based on modern physiology and anatomy instead of the ancient 'point' system. However, in order to integrate this treatment approach into a broader medical frame, knowledge of the traditional practice, the evidence base and the clinical implications of the treatment is necessary. Acupuncture can look – and feel – very different depending upon the training, approach and, sometimes, philosophy of whoever is delivering the treatment. The technique of needle insertion, for example, varies greatly amongst practitioners. Shallow insertion was adopted in Japanese acupuncture to match their sensitive bodies, compared to Chinese acupuncture techniques.

This chapter will outline:

- the use of acupuncture
- potential mechanisms for its effect
- evidence for the clinical efficacy of acupuncture in humans and animals in the management of musculoskeletal pain conditions.

The nature of trigger points in musculoskeletal pain and the role of physiotherapy, including dry needling, will be discussed.

15.2 Traditional acupuncture

Underpinning Oriental medicine and the use of acupuncture is the concept of Qi (pronounced *chi*). The life force energy infused in everything is Qi energy. It sustains movement and change and is thought to be what animates living beings. It can protect against harmful influences and flows with blood in the blood vessels and in special channels or meridians.

The concept of Yin and Yang is fundamental to the practice of Oriental medicine and acupuncture. Yin/Yang is the representation of opposite but complementary qualities that are interdependent and exist in a constant state of balance. The original meanings of Yin and Yang were 'the shady side of a hill' and 'the sunny side of a hill' respectively. These constructs apply to the universe – not just to the body. In the biological sense, Yin is considered female and Yang is male. They are opposites but not mutually exclusive, meaning that Yin always contains some Yang and vice versa. They cover a wide array of options;

for example, Yin may refer to cold, rest, passive, inward movement whereas Yang refers to heat, movement, vitality and outward movement. Yin and Yang interact with each other and can transform from one to the other. Hence a concept of constant flow and movement is represented. The health state depends on a balance between Yin and Yang, with disease states occurring when either one or the other is dominant. When Yin and Yang energies become unbalanced, Kyo (depletion/deficiency) and Jitsu (excess) occur. Treatment will therefore be focused on tonifying or filling up the Kyo points or sedating the Jitsu points. The subtle palpation skill will enable the practitioner to assess and treat appropriately. The meridians or channels in which the energy of Yin and Yang flows are thought to carry Qi to the organs and all parts of the body.

The meridians are thought to run within the body and come to the surface only at specific points. These are considered to be the acupuncture points. However, there are a few points that do not lie on channels (so called extra-meridian points). There are 12 main channels that carry acupuncture points and two extraordinary vessels (Figure 15.1, Figure 15.2). The paired channels are related to and named for the organs through which they run such as liver, gallbladder, lung, etc. Although they have the same names, the Western and TCM concept of organs are only loosely related. There are thought to be six primarily Yin channels linked to solid organs such as the liver and six Yang channels linked to hollow organs such as the stomach. The two main extra vessels are reservoirs of Qi which are used to treat certain forms of imbalance. The Governing Vessel (Yang), and the Conception Vessel (Yin) run down the centre of the body, rather than bilaterally.

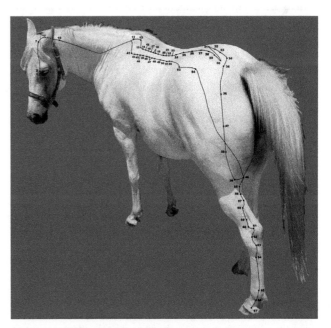

Figure 15.1 The Bladder meridian in the horse, which is commonly used in clinical practice. *Source:* Xie and Preast 2003. Reproduced with permission from John Wiley & Sons.

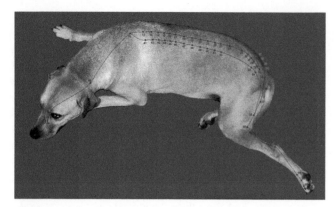

Figure 15.2 The Bladder meridian in the dog, which is commonly used in clinical practice. *Source:* Xie and Preast 2003. Reproduced with permission from John Wiley & Sons.

Meridian theory is based on the belief that when there is a blockage or some form of interruption along the meridian pathway where the Qi does not flow smoothly, it will cause an imbalance or disharmony. Meridian therapy therefore is a traditional medical system that sees all diseases as a condition of deficiency or excess of Qi or blood in the meridians, and then uses the techniques of acupuncture to tonify or disperse that deficiency or excess in order to bring about healing (Kuwahara 2003).

Acupuncture points are a mechanism for perturbing the flow of energy and restoring balance (Vickers & Zollman 1999). Modern scientific investigation has shown that the classic acupuncture points are situated at places where there are particular physical features, for example around joints, in the depressions between muscles or where nerves run superficially. There are about 360 acupuncture points located throughout the body which have various effects on pain relief and organ systems. The electrical resistance can be measured using electrical equipment on the skin at these points and has been demonstrated to be lower than elsewhere on the body's surface, but with high electrical conductivity (Brown *et al.* 1974; Reichmanis *et al.* 1975; Urano & Ogasawara 1978). Historical studies reveal that acupuncture points are located in areas where there are free nerve endings, arterioles, lymphatic vessels and aggregations of mast cells (Pan *et al.* 1986). There are a variety of ways to stimulate acupuncture points to create an effect: dry needle, electroacupuncture, aquapuncture, acupressure, laser acupuncture, moxibustion, haemoacupuncture, pneumoacupuncture and gold implantation.

15.3 Acupuncture analgesia

Although acupuncture can be used in the management of many conditions, including nausea, asthma, drug addiction and dental pain (Birch *et al.* 2004), the focus of this chapter is on the use and possible mechanisms of acupuncture in musculoskeletal pain conditions.

The analgesic effect of acupuncture is thought to be related to activation of descending pain inhibitory pathways. These pathways can be activated by a number of stimuli, including stress, pain and activity.

The perception of pain and analgesia involves a number of levels within the nervous system from periphery to cortex and, broadly speaking, two systems subserve this cognition (Kanjhan 1995). The *ascending system* relays information regarding peripheral nociception via the spinal cord to higher centres (Cross 1994). The *descending inhibitory system* also involves activation of the central nervous system at many levels, including cortex, thalamus and brainstem, and determines the response to this peripheral input by modulating the functional state of the nociceptive system at spinal cord level and at higher centres within the neuraxis (Cross 1994; Kanjhan 1995). Activation of peripheral nociceptors does not necessarily result in the perception of pain, and as such, this perception reflects the balance of ascending input and descending controls.

It has been demonstrated that descending inhibition of pain is produced by a number of mechanisms that can be categorised as either opioid or non-opioid (Watkins *et al.* 1992).

Acupuncture analgesia can occur following needling with and without associated electrical stimulation. The insertion of fine, sterile needles into specific points creates physiological responses, which are due to the stimulation of both central and peripheral nervous systems. This leads to a release of endogenous substances such as beta-endorphins, dynorphins, encephalins, serotonin, epinephrine, gamma-aminobutyric acid (GABA), cortisol and various hormones. The earliest scientific studies done on acupuncture focused on its analgesic effects (Zink & van Dyke 2013). Mayer & Price (1976) showed that naloxone (opioid antagonist) blocked the effects of acupuncture and decreased the pain threshold in acupuncture subjects. Therefore it was concluded that endogenous opioids played a role in the mechanism of action of acupuncture analgesia.

There are thought to be segmental and heterosegmental effects. In segmental acupuncture, it is thought that acupuncture stimulates the A delta fibres which are fast myelinated fibres activated by a range of noxious mechanical and thermal stimuli. These fibres signal actual or potential tissue damage, and cause the body or area damaged to withdraw from the threatening/damaging stimulus. This is a postsynaptic effect (distinct from the 'pain gate' mechanism which is presynaptic). The fast pain fibre input takes priority over the slow fibre input (chronic pain) in the dorsal horn of the spinal cord where pain is modulated (Lindley 2010). Encephalinergic interneurons are stimulated by fast pain fibres, which in turn inhibit onward transmission of C fibre (slow pain) signals, thus blocking conscious perception of pain. Therefore, the neurophysiological approach to acupuncture places needles as close to the source of pain (or dysfunction) as possible, as the presynaptic effect is most potent at the segment stimulated.

Although acupuncture needles may not cause any pain or sensation on insertion, the patient will often describe a sense of soreness or heaviness ('de Qi'), meaning 'the arrival of Qi', which the practitioner may use as evidence that the acupuncture point has been located. Afferent input from these fibres can inhibit pain through activation of the descending pain inhibitory system (DPIS) (Vickers & Zollman 1999). Once the acupuncture stimulus has passed the dorsal horn of the spinal cord, it continues via the crossed spinothalamic tracts to the brain and affects areas that include the limbic system, periaqueductal grey (PAG) and nucleus raphe magnus. This is known as the heterosegmental effect and triggers the release of beta-endorphins, serotonin and noradrenaline, amongst other neurotransmitters. The effects are both humoral and via DPIS, thus the pain-relieving effects are potent at the segment stimulated and also throughout the body. Blood concentration of serotonin precursor free tryptophan is increased with acupuncture (Costa *et al.* 1982). Acupuncture releases beta-endorphins, which in turn induce release of serotonin. This increase in serotonin has been found in the CNS after acupuncture stimulation (Zink & van Dyke 2013).

Sympathetic nervous system responses, which accompany analgesia, have also been demonstrated. Takeshige *et al.* (1992) demonstrated that an initial excitatory response is followed by subsequent sympathoinhibition within a time frame of 20–45 minutes. Acupuncture needles are commonly left *in situ* for between 10 and 40 min (Vickers & Zollman 1999) as it may take this length of time for SNS inhibitory effects to take place

Essentially, in a 'Western' approach to acupuncture, the points are selected based on neurophysiological principles and examination of the patient.

15.4 Clinical effectiveness of acupuncture

Acupuncture is a relatively safe procedure with limited reporting of serious events (Birch *et al.* 2004). However, although it is widely used clinically, there has been limited support for the effectiveness of acupuncture for the management of chronic pain (Ezzo *et al.* 2000).

In research, issues with blinding and difficulty with the development of an adequate placebo technique have led to many studies investigating the efficacy of acupuncture being poorly controlled (Sjolund 2005). However, the advent of the placebo needle (Streitberger & Kleinhenz 1998) has begun to impact positively on the quality of research in the area and recent studies have started to show efficacy for acupuncture and acupressure in a number of conditions.

The effect of acupuncture and acupressure on low back pain (LBP) has been investigated in humans. In a large study investigating the long-term benefits (over 24 months) of acupuncture compared with standard medical (GP) care for chronic LBP, 81% of patients stated that acupuncture had helped their back pain compared with 52% who had standard GP care (Thomas *et al.* 2005). Hsieh *et al.* (2006) demonstrated that acupressure had a statistically superior effect to physical therapy in reducing low

back pain, both after the course of treatment and at 6-month follow-up.

15.5 Use of acupuncture in animals

Acupuncture has become a more widely recognised treatment option in animals over the last few decades and the International Veterinary Acupuncture Society was founded in 1974 (www.ivas.org) (Chan *et al.* 2001). The more recent rapid development of veterinary acupuncture has been driven by owners following media focus on its efficacy (Chan *et al.* 2001; Scott 2001).

Acupuncture has been used for a variety of conditions including bovine reproductive disorders, canine paralysis and lameness and equine back pain (Chan *et al.* 2001). Conditions treated by physiotherapy that may also be amenable to acupuncture can include vertebral disorders, degenerative disc disease, joint disease and pain (Figure 15.3). The particular acupuncture points used are transposed from human points as TCM texts only provide points for large animals and birds (Chan *et al.* 2001; Yu & Lin 2000).

Needle lengths ranging from 10 to 50 mm should suit all purposes in small animals and needles 10–100 mm should suit all purposes in large animals. Generally, the duration of treatment is most commonly 10–30 min. Gold beads can be embedded into points for lifetime treatment of hip dysplasia or epilepsy in dogs (Xie & Preast 2007). Depending on the nature and severity of the condition, the frequency of treatment will be adjusted. In most cases, clinical results can be achieved after 2–5 acupuncture sessions (Xie & Preast 2007). For more acute or severe conditions such as laminitis in the horse, acupuncture can be used once every 12–48 h until the pain is under control. Points that are most commonly used in veterinary medicine are along the neck, back, hips and shoulders and are most easily accepted by animal patients (Table 15.1) (Xie & Preast 2007).

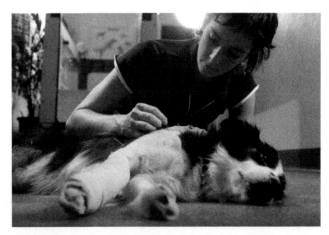

Figure 15.3 A Border Collie receiving acupuncture for treatment following carpus surgery.

Table 15.1 Commonly used acupuncture points for specific conditions

Clinical condition	Acupuncture point selection
General pain	Liv-3, GB-34, Bl-60, SI-9
Hip pain	Bl-54, GB-29, GB-30, *Jian-jiao*, Bl-40, Bl-23, Liv-3
Stifle pain	St-36, GB-33, GB-34, Sp-9, Sp-10, Bl-40, Liv-3
Hock pain	Bl-60, Kid-3, St-41, Kid-6, Liv-3
Shoulder pain	LI-15, TH-14, SI-9, Lu-1
Elbow pain	LI-10, LI-11, Lu-5, Ht-3, Pc-3
Carpal pain	Ht-7, Lu-7, Lu-9, TH-4, PC-7
Intervertebral disc disease (IVDD)	Local, cranial, and caudal BL points to site of IVDD, Kid-1, *Lui-feng*
Wobbler's syndrome	*Jing-jia-ji*, LI-4, SI-16, SI-3
Degenerative myelopathy	St-36, LI-10, Bl-23, *Bai-hui*, Bl-54, Bl-40, Kid-1, *Lui-feng*
Vestibular disease	GB-20, GB-21, GV-20, TH-21, SI-19, GB-2, *An-shen*
Urinary incontinence	Bl-39, Kid-3, Kid-6, Sp-6, CV-1
Faecal incontinence	GV-1, Bl-25, St-36, St-37, LI-10
Appetite stimulation	Bl-20, Bl-21, *Shan-gen*, *Jian-wei*

Source: Adapted from Xie & Preast 2007 and Zink & Van Dyke 2013.

Acupuncture has been used in sports medicine practice, typically 2–5 days before competition to enhance endurance and physical performance, and help to regulate heart rate and blood pressure (Ehrlich & Haber 1992). Points used for performance enhancement include ST 36, LI-10, CV-4, CV-6, Bl-24, Bl-26, LI-4 and Liv-3. It can also be used 2–4 h post performance (once the athlete has cooled down) to alleviate pain or stress on the musculoskeletal system.

As part of a rehabilitation programme post intervertebral disc disease (IVDD), acupuncture can be used alongside physiotherapy techniques to promote nerve regeneration (La *et al.* 2005) and can be used 1–5 days per week, depending on the grade of disc disease. Improvements in deep pain perception, mobility and function, proprioception and postoperative pain reduction have been attributed to electroacupuncture in dogs and cats following paralysis from IVDD (Choi & Hill 2009; Laim *et al.* 2009). Additionally, in a study on 80 paralysed dogs, the combination of electroacupuncture and acupuncture with conventional medicine was found to be more effective than conventional medicine alone in recovering ambulation, relieving back pain and decreasing relapse (Han *et al.* 2010). Electroacupuncture was found to be effective for treatment of chronic thoracolumbar pain in horses and the analgesic effect induced by this can last at least 2 weeks (Xie *et al.* 2005). Different acupuncture methods have been used to treat equine back pain, including injection acupuncture, electroacupuncture, moxa and laser acupuncture (Chan *et al.* 2001).

Acupuncture also has a calming/sedating effect for dogs, which can be used for postsurgical patients confined to a cage (Kim 2006). Points could include GV-17, GV-20, GV-21, *An-shen* and Ht-7. Additionally, postoperative analgesic requirements have been found to be reduced when electroacupuncture is applied to control pain in dogs (Cassu *et al.* 2012; Gakiya *et al.* 2011; Groppetti *et al.* 2011).

Precautions and contraindications for the use of acupuncture in animals are much the same as in humans. Points around the eyes, along the lateral thorax and abdomen should be used with caution and oblique angle used to avoid entering the pleural or abdominal cavities. Electroacupuncture is contraindicated in patients with a history of seizures, epilepsy, cardiac arrhythmias and those with a pacemaker. It should be used with caution in patients with neoplasia and congestive heart failure (Altman 1994). It should never be used in or around a tumour, into open wounds or scar tissue, or directly into skin that has severe dermatitis. In pregnancy, the following points are contraindicated: LI-4, SP-6, Bl-23/24/25/26/27/28/52, Bl-40, Bl-60, Bl-67, St-36, CV-2, CV-3, CV-4, CV-5, CV-6 and *Yan-chi* (Xie & Preast 2007). After racing/training, make sure that the animals are rested and relaxed for about an hour before conducting acupuncture procedures.

Although early studies were predominantly of low methodological quality, more recent research has begun to elucidate the mechanisms and the efficacy of acupuncture compared with both placebo treatment and more traditional therapies. A study investigating the efficacy of acupuncture on induced arthritis in the stifle joint of dogs has demonstrated a superior effect of acupuncture over non-treatment. Skin temperature was measured using infra-red thermography and following treatment for 3 weeks (1 session/week), there was a return to normal of skin temperature only in the acupuncture group (Um *et al.* 2005).

Veterinary acupuncture is becoming established to treat a variety of conditions including musculoskeletal pain and dysfunction and further well-controlled studies are required to provide an evidence base for its effectiveness.

15.6 Trigger points

Areas of increased sensitivity within a muscle are commonly referred to as 'trigger points'. It must be noted that although Travell & Simons (1993) have described trigger points to be pathognomic of myofascial pain syndrome (MPS), local muscle pathology may be only one of the mechanisms by which this hypersensitivity occurs. Tenderness or mechanosensitivity in muscle may be related to changes in muscle activity and sensitivity as a result of joint pathology, visceral pathology and nervous system pathology (Giamberardino *et al.* 1999; Johansen *et al.* 1999). It may occur due to both peripheral mechanisms of sensitisation (Graven-Nielsen & Mense 2001) and represent areas of secondary hyperalgesia related to central sensitisation mechanisms (Graven-Nielsen & Arendt-Nielsen 2002). In this chapter, the mechanisms and management underpinning so-called 'trigger point' development and their management will be discussed.

Trigger points can be described as local tender spots located in a band of skeletal muscle that produce pain on compression which is felt as pain locally, and which can also evoke pain in a referred pattern (Travell & Simons 1993). The aetiology and pathophysiology of trigger points remain speculative but clinically, trigger points are thought to produce pain, restrict movement, cause muscle weakness (Alvarez & Rockwell 2002) and alter the muscle activation patterns in both local and distal muscle groups (Lucas *et al.* 2004). Autonomic signs such as hyperaemia, vasomotor and temperature changes and symptoms including dizziness and paraesthesia may be evident in patients with trigger points (Fricton *et al.* 1985; Jay 1995).

15.6.1 Diagnosis of trigger points

In addition to local and referred pain, which reproduces symptoms, a local twitch response and presence of a taut pain on palpation are considered to be characteristic of a trigger point (Borg-Stein & Simons 2002; Borg-Stein & Stein 1996). Although trigger points have been long recognised as a pathological entity clinically, these diagnostic criteria are not universally accepted (Borg-Stein & Simons 2002) and there is equivocal support in the literature that these symptoms are reproducible between examiners. Some authors contend that there is limited agreement (Hsieh *et al.* 2000; Lew *et al.* 1997; Nice *et al.* 1992; Wolfe *et al.* 1992) whereas others have shown statistically significant reliability for location and identification of trigger points (Gerwin *et al.* 1997; Sciotti *et al.* 2001). Use of specific diagnostic criteria by specifically trained and experienced investigators for research studies could assist in reducing this discrepancy.

15.6.2 Possible mechanisms

Pathophysiology of either the motor endplate or the muscle spindle has been proposed as a potential cause of the trigger point. Measuring electromyography (EMG) activity with a needle electrode, Hubbard & Berghoff (1993) hypothesised that this activity originated in the muscle spindle. They suggested that the tenderness at the trigger point site was due to increased pressure within the spindle. However, no studies have been able to measure intrafusal muscle fibre activity (Hong & Simons 1998) and therefore allow a comparison with the activity described by Hubbard & Berghoff (1993).

It has been suggested that there are physiological characteristics that are shared by the twitch response and the stretch reflex. Rivner (2001) demonstrated bursts of activity from insertion of a needle electrode into rabbit trigger points, which showed similar profiles for amount and duration of activity and behaviours to those occurring in the stretch response resulting from muscle spindle activity.

In contrast, some researchers postulate that the activity observed by Hubbard & Berghoff (1993) is more likely to be recording of endplate noise (Simons *et al.* 2002). In their review on myofascial pain, Borg-Stein & Simons (2002) suggested that endplate noise is related to a 'pathological increase in release of acetylcholine (ACh) by the nerve terminal of an abnormal

motor endplate under resting conditions'. This assertion is supported by evidence demonstrating endplate noise significantly more frequently in trigger points than in areas outside trigger points (Couppe *et al.* 2001; Simons *et al.* 2002).

As mentioned earlier, tenderness in muscle is thought to include elements of peripheral and central sensitisation of the nervous system. The pathophysiology of the trigger point has been described as a complex interplay between peripheral and central mechanisms (Borg-Stein & Simons 2002) whereby affected endplates are thought to release excessive acetylcholine, causing sustained depolarisation of the muscle fibre and thereby producing a sustained shortening of sarcomeres. As a consequence, an increase in local energy consumption and decrease in local circulation occur, resulting in localised ischaemia and hypoxia. The release of inflammatory mediators, such as prostaglandin, bradykinin, serotonin and histamine, stimulated by the local ischaemia, is thought to sensitise afferent nerve fibres, accounting for the hyperalgesia or tenderness in the muscle (Borg-Stein & Simons 2002). A study has demonstrated that change in the muscle microcirculation is thought to play a role in the pain and development of tender points associated with trapezius overactivation. Sustained sarcomere shortening may produce contraction within the muscle and explain the presence of the palpable taut band (Borg-Stein & Simons 2002).

In order to effect the most appropriate treatment, more research is required to clarify the pathophysiology of MPS trigger points. It may be that there is not a single pathophysiology, but instead that both muscle spindles and endplates are implicated in the pathogenesis of trigger points. Peripheral and central nervous system mechanisms play a role in the development, maintenance and spread of trigger points and therefore these mechanisms should be considered when considering the effects of treatment.

15.6.3 Treatment

In order to best guide management, the physical examination of the patient should consider posture, biomechanics and joint function in order to establish the presence of underlying mechanisms for the development of local or referred pain of MPS trigger points (Borg-Stein & Simons 2002). The presence of focal tenderness and reproduction of the patient's complaints as well as taut bands within the muscle should be elicited. Treatment should then include specific interventions to modify or prevent factors that may have predisposed to the development of trigger points.

There is limited evidence for the use of pharmacological treatments in the management of MPS trigger points. Medical management of patients with pain may include the use of non-steroidal antiinflammatory drugs, antidepressants and anticonvulsants although there is no evidence for their use in MPS; however, their prescription may be based on research for these medications in fibromyalgia (Borg-Stein & Simons 2002). There is some evidence, however, for the use of botulinum toxin as it has the potential to disrupt the abnormal endplate dysfunction by blockade of the release of ACh (Borg-Stein & Simons 2002). It may also have a central mechanism at the spinal cord and brainstem (Borg-Stein & Simons 2002; Gobel et al. 2001).

Common physiotherapy interventions for trigger points include massage, stretching and exercise. Electrophysical agents such as TENS, ultrasound and laser have also been used. Whilst anecdotally these treatments can be effective, there is limited evidence of their usefulness. Well-designed placebo-controlled trials are necessary to provide therapists with support for these interventions.

Wet and dry needling have proved useful in the management of MPS trigger points to augment non-invasive stretching and exercise. Injection of steroids, local anaesthetics and, as discussed above, botulinum toxin has been used to inactivate the points. The lack of inflammatory mechanisms does not support the use of steroids, but use of anaesthetic may reduce the amount of postneedle soreness (Borg-Stein & Simons 2002).

Dry needling refers to the use of acupuncture needles to stimulate muscle or inactivate trigger points without the injection of substances such as local anaesthetics or corticosteroids. There is no evidence to support the use of wet needling over and above the effects of dry needling (Cummings & White 2001). Dry needling has shown benefits in treating musculoskeletal pain (Edwards & Knowles 2003). In previous uncontrolled clinical studies, needling of the trigger point has been reported to be effective in reducing pain (Gunn et al. 1980; Hong 1994) and is arguably the most efficient way of treating trigger points (Cummings & White 2001).

The mechanisms supporting the use of dry needling include those which were previously mentioned for acupuncture. For example, the use of superficial dry needling as advocated by Baldry et al. (2001) may activate the DPIS through stimulation of the A delta fibres. However, additional specific local effects may be produced by deeper stimulation (e.g. intramuscular stimulation) (Gunn 2003), which produces a twitch response. Alterations in peripheral circulation including an increase in muscle blood flow for tibialis anterior and in the overlying skin were demonstrated in asymptomatic and fibromyalgia patients (Sandberg et al. 2005). These authors showed that deep needling was superior to subcutaneous needling in healthy and trapezius myalgia subjects for increasing muscle blood flow. However, superficial needles produced more increase in blood flow than deep needles in fibromyalgia patients (Sandberg et al. 2005). Acupuncture can also be applied to trigger points and the location of trigger points is often coincident with traditional acupuncture points (Borg-Stein & Simons 2002). Although the needles used in the two interventions are the same, the application method differs, with acupuncture needles often left in situ for 20 min or longer whereas techniques for muscle stimulation will be introduced and removed from the muscle quickly. Electrical stimulation can be used and added to both interventions. Therefore, the type of needling used may be relevant to the patient and the mechanism of their complaint.

15.6.4 Trigger points in animals

In animals, trigger points may be associated with pain and lameness. They may also be associated with autonomic disturbance (Schoen 2001). Factors such as arthritis, trauma, stress, postoperative status and infection may predispose to the development of trigger points in animals (Schoen 2001). They are diagnosed by palpation, which produces vocalisation in the animal and may highlight the presence of the taut band. They can also cause a reduction in range of motion (Schoen 2001) and, as in humans, they may be colocalised with acupuncture points (Janssens 1992). Trigger points have been described in the triceps, infraspinatus, quadriceps, pectineus, iliocostalis lumborum, peroneus longus and gluteus medius muscles (Janssens 1991) in dogs and in the cleidobrachialis muscle in the horse (Macgregor & Schweinitz 2006).

Treatment approaches are similar to those used in humans and include stretching, massage, TENS and laser (Schoen 2001), as well as wet and dry needling. These approaches to management have very limited research support. In a study in which lame dogs were treated with needling or injection with local anaesthetic into trigger points, 60% of the animals (n = 48) showed complete recovery (Janssens 1991). These animals had previously been unsuccessfully treated with medication and acupuncture. Further research in this area would clearly be useful to guide management. It should be noted that vigorous needling would only be tolerated by a very few animal patients.

In conclusion, acupuncture has its basis in Oriental medicine and has been used for thousands of years for the management of many conditions, including those regularly managed by physiotherapists. The evidence for the mechanism of pain relief suggests that activation of the DPIS is important in mediating the effects of acupuncture. Although the location of trigger points and acupuncture points may coincide, the potential mechanisms for the development of trigger points suggest changes at either the muscle spindle or the motor endplate, including abnormal release of ACh at the motor point. Further investigation is necessary to determine conclusively the underlying pathophysiology of the trigger point and the relationship between the acupuncture and trigger point should be established so that management can be optimal. In addition, the direct effect of dry needling as an isolated treatment should be established to guide physiotherapists in the most appropriate ways to manage trigger points and musculoskeletal pain.

References

Acupuncture Regulatory Working Group 2003, *Statutory Regulation of the Acupuncture Profession, the Report of the Acupuncture Regulatory Working Group*. Prince of Wales' Foundation for Integrated Health, London, p.12.

Altman, S. 1994, Techniques and instrumentation. In: Schoen, A.M. (ed), *Veterinary Acupuncture: Ancient Art to Modern Medicine*. Mosby, St Louis, MO, pp. 86–97.

Alvarez, D.J., Rockwell, P.G., 2002, Trigger points: diagnosis and management. *Am. Fam. Physician* 65(4):653–660.

Baldry, P.E., Yunus, M.B., Inanici, F. 2001, *Myofascial Pain and Fibromyalgia Syndromes: a clinical guide to diagnosis and management.* Churchill Livingstone, Edinburgh.

Birch, S., Hesselink, J.K., Jonkman, F. *et al.* 2004, Clinical research on acupuncture: Part 1. What have the reviews of the efficacy and safety of acupuncture told us so far? *J. Altern. Comp. Med.* 10: 468–480.

Borg-Stein, J., Simons, D.G. 2002, Myofascial pain. *Arch. Phys. Med. Rehab.* 83(suppl 1): S40–S48.

Borg-Stein, J., Stein, J. 1996, Trigger points and tender points: one and the same? Does injection treatment help? *Rheum. Dis. Clin. North Am.* 22: 305–322.

Brown, M.L., Ulett, GA., Stern, J.A. 1974, Acupuncture loci: techniques for location. *Am. J. Chin. Med.* 2: 67–74.

Cassu, R.N., Silva, D.A., Genari, F. *et al.* 2012, Electroanalgesia for the postoperative control pain in dogs. *Acta. Cir. Bras.* 27(1): 43–48.

Chan, W.W., Chen, K-Y., Liu, H. *et al.* 2001, Acupuncture for general veterinary practice. *J. Vet. Med. Sci.* 63: 1057–1063.

Choi, K.H., Hill, S.A. 2009, Acupuncture treatment for feline multifocal intervertebral disc disease. *J. Feline Med. Surg.* 11: 706–710.

Costa, C., Ceccherelli, F., Ambrosio, F. *et al.* 1982, The influence of acupuncture on blood serum levels of tryptophan in healthy volunteers subjected to ketamine anaesthesia. *Acupunct. Electrother. Res.* 7: 123–132.

Couppe, C., Midttun, A., Hilden, J. *et al.* 2001, Spontaneous needle electromyographic activity in myofascial trigger points in the infraspinatus muscle: a blinded assessment. *J. Musculoskelet. Pain* 9: 7–16.

Cross, S.A. 1994, Pathophysiology of pain. *Mayo Clin. Proc.* 69: 375–383.

Cummings, T.M., White, A.R. 2001, Needling therapies in the management of myofascial trigger points: a systematic review. *Arch. Phys. Med. Rehabil.* 82: 986–992.

Edwards, J., Knowles, N. 2003, Superficial dry needling and active stretching in the treatment of myofascial pain: a randomised controlled trial. *Acupuncture Med.* 21: 80–86.

Erlich, D., Haber, P. 1992, Influence of acupuncture on physical perhformace capacity and haemodynamic parameters. *Int. J. Sports Med.* 13: 486–491.

Ezzo, J., Berman, B., Hadhazy, V. *et al.* 2000, Is acupuncture effective for the treatment of chronic pain? *Pain* 86: 217–225.

Fricton, J.R., Kroening, R., Haley, D., Siegert, R. 1985, Myofascial syndrome of the head and neck: a review of clinical characteristics of 164 patients. *Oral Surg. Oral Med. Oral Pathol.* 60: 615–623.

Gakiya, H.H., Gomes, S., Gomes, J. *et al.* 2011, Electroacupuncture versus morphine for the postoperative control pain in dogs. *Acta. Cir. Bras.* 26(5): 346–351.

Gerwin, R.D., Shannon, S., Hong, C.Z. *et al.* 1997, Interrater reliability in myofascial trigger point examination. *Pain* 69: 65–73.

Giamberardino, M-A., Affaitati, G., Iezzi, S. *et al.* 1999, Referred muscle pain and hyperalgesia from viscera. *J. Musculoskelet. Pain* 7: 61–69.

Gobel, H., Heinze, A., Henize-Kuhne, K. *et al.* 2001, Botulinum A for the treatment of headache disorders and pericranial pain syndromes. *Nervenarzt* 72: 264–271.

Graven-Nielsen, T., Arendt-Nielsen, L. 2002, Peripheral and central sensitisation in musculoskeletal pain disorders: an experimental approach. *Curr. Rheumatol. Rep.* 4: 312–321.

Graven-Nielsen, T., Mense, S. 2001, The peripheral apparatus of muscle pain: evidence from animal and human studies. *Clin. J. Pain* 17: 2–10.

Groppetti, D., Pecile, A.M., Sacerdote, P. *et al.* 2011, Effectiveness of electroacupuncture analgesia compared with opiod administration in a dog model: a pilot study. *Br. J. Anaesth.* 107(4): 612–618.

Gunn, C.C. 2003, *The Gunn Approach to the Treatment of Chronic Pain: intramuscular stimulation for myofascial pain of radiculopathic origin,* 2nd edn. Churchill Livingstone, New York.

Gunn, C.C., Milbrandt, W.E., Little, A.S. *et al.* 1980, Dry needling of muscle motor points for chronic low-back pain. *Spine* 5: 279–291.

Han, H.J., Yoon, H.Y., Kim, J.Y. *et al.* 2010, Clinical effect of additional electroacupuncture on thoracolumbar intervertebral dis herniation in 80 paraplegic dogs. *Am. J. Clin. Med.* 38(6):1015–1025.

Hong, C., Simons, D.G. 1998, Pathophysiologic and electrophysiological mechanisms of myofascial trigger points. *Arch. Phys. Med. Rehabil.* 79: 863–872.

Hong, C.Z. 1994, Lidocaine injection versus dry needling to myofascial trigger point. *Am. J. Phys. Med. Rehabil.* 73: 256–263.

Hsieh, C.Y., Hong, C.Z., Adams, A.H. *et al.* 2000, Interexaminer reliability of the palpation of trigger points in the trunk and lower limb muscles. *Arch. Phys. Med. Rehabil.* 81: 258–264.

Hsieh, L.L-C., Kuo, C.H., Lee, L.H. *et al.* 2006, Treatment of low back pain by acupressure and physical therapy: randomised controlled trial. *BMJ* 332(7543): 696–700.

Hubbard, D.R., Berghoff, G.M. 1993, Myofascial trigger points show spontaneous needle EMG activity. *Spine* 18: 1803–1807.

Janssens, L.A. 1991, Trigger points in 48 dogs with myofascial pain syndromes. *Vet. Surg.* 20: 274–278.

Janssens, L.A. 1992, Trigger point therapy. *Prob. Vet. Med.* 4: 117–124.

Jay, G.W. 1995, Sympathetic aspects of mysofascial pain. *Pain Digest* 5: 192–194.

Johansen, M.K., Graven-Nielsen, T., Olesen, A.S., Arendt-Nielsen, L. 1999, Generalised muscular hyperalgesia in chronic whiplash syndrome. *Pain* 83: 229–234.

Kanjhan, R. 1995, Opioids and pain. *Clin. Exp. Pharmacol. Physiol.* 22: 397–403.

Kim, M.S. 2006. Evaluation of sedation on electroencephalographic spectral edge frequency in 95 dogs sedated by acupuncture at GV 20 or Yingtang and sedative combination. *Acupunct. Electrother. Res.* 31: 201–212.

Kuwahara, K. 2003, *Traditional Japanese Acupuncture – fundamentals of meridian theory I.* Complementary Medicine Press, Taos, New Mexico.

La, J.L., Jalali, S., Shami, S.A. 2005, Morphological strudies on crushed sciatic nerve of rabbits with electroacupuncture or diclofenac sodium treatment. *Am. J. Chin. Med.* 33: 663–669.

Laim A., Jaggy A., Forterre F. *et al.* 2009, Effects of adjunct electroacupuncture on severity of postoperative pain in dogs undergoing hemilaminectomy because of acute thoracolumbar intervertebral disk disease. *J. Am. Vet. Med. Assoc.* 234(9): 1141–1146.

Lew, P.C., Lewis, J., Strory, I. 1997, Inter-therapist reliability in locating latent myofascial trigger points using palpation. *Man. Ther.* 2: 87–90.

Lindley, S. 2010, Acupuncture in palliative and rehabilitative medicine. In: Lindley, S., Watson, P. (eds), *BSAVA Manual of Canine and Feline Rehabilitation, Supportive and Palliative Care.* BSAVA, England, pp. 123–130.

Lucas, K.R., Polus, B.I., Rich, P.S. 2004, Latent myofascial trigger points: their effects on muscle activation and movement efficiency. *J. Bodyw. Mov. Ther.* 8: 160–166.

Macgregor, J., Schweinitz, D. 2006, Needle electromyographic activity of myofascial trigger points and control sites in equine cleidobrachialis muscle – an observational study. *Acupunct. Med.* 24(2): 61–70.

Mayer, D.J., Price, D.D. 1976, Central nervous system mechanisms of analgesia. *Pain* 2: 379–404.

Nice, D.A., Riddle, D.L., Lamb, R.L. *et al.* 1992, Intertester reliability of judgments of the presence of trigger points in patients with low back pain. *Arch. Phys. Rehabil.* 73: 893–898.

Pan, X.P., Zhao, A., Zhang, X. 1986, *Research on Acupuncture, Moxibustion and Acupuncture Anesthesia*. Springer-Verlag, New York.

Reichmanis, M., Marino, A.A., Becker, R.O. 1975, Electrical correlates of acupuncture points. *IEEE Trans. Biomed. Eng.* 22: 533–535.

Rivner, M.H. 2001, The neurophysiology of myofascial pain syndrome. *Curr. Pain Headache Rep.* 5: 432–440.

Sandberg, M., Larsson, B., Lindberg L.G. *et al.* 2005, Different patterns of blood flow response in the trapezius muscle following needle stimulation (acupuncture) between healthy subjects and patients with fibromyalgia and work-related trapezius myalgia. *Eur. J. Pain* 9: 497–510.

Schoen, A. 2001, Trigger point therapy and manual medicine for canine lameness. Proceedings of the World Small Animal Veterinary Association Congress, Vancouver, Canada.

Sciotti, V.M., Mittak, V.C., DiMarco, L. *et al.* 2001, Clinical precision of myofascial trigger point location in the trapezius muscle. *Pain* 93: 259–266.

Scott, S. 2001, Developments in veterinary acupuncture. *Acupunct. Med.* 19: 27–31.

Simons, D.G., Hong, C-Z., Simons, L.S. 2002, Endplate potentials are common to midfibre myofascial trigger points. *Am. J. Phys. Med. Rehabil.* 81: 212–222.

Sjolund, B.H. 2005, Acupuncture or acupuncture? *Pain* 114: 311–312.

Streitberger, K., Kleinhenz, J. 1998, Introducing a placebo needle into acupuncture research. *Lancet* 352: 364–365.

Takeshige, C., Sato, T., Mera, T. *et al.* 1992, Descending pain inhibitory system involved in acupuncture analgesia. *Brain Res. Bull.* 29: 617–634.

Thomas, K.J., MacPhersonm, H., Ratcliffem, J. *et al.* 2005, Longer term clinical and economic benefits of offering acupuncture care to patients with chronic low back pain. *Health Technol. Assess.* 9: 1–109.

Travell, J., Simons, D. 1993, *Myofascial Pain and Dysfunction: trigger point manual*. Williams and Wilkins, Baltimore, MD.

Um, S., Kim, M., Lim, J., *et al.* 2005, Thermographic evaluation for the efficacy of acupuncture on induced chronic arthritis in the dog. *J. Vet. Med. Sci.* 67: 1283–1284.

Urano, L., Ogasawara, S. 1978, A fundamental study on acupuncture points phenomena of dog body. *Kitasato Arch. Exp. Med.* 51: 95–109.

Vickers, A., Zollman, C. 1999, ABC of complimentary medicine: acupuncture. *BMJ*, 319: 973–976.

Watkins, L.R., Wiertelak, E.P., Grisel, J.E. *et al.* 1992, Parallel activation of multiple spinal opiate systems appears to mediate 'non-opiate' stress-induced analgesias. *Brain Res.* 594: 99–108.

Wolfe, F., Simons, D.G., Fricton, J. *et al.* 1992, The fibromyalgia and myofascial pain syndromes. A preliminary study of tender points and trigger points in persons with fibromyalgia, myofascial pain and no disease. *J. Rheumatol.* 19: 944–951.

Xie, H., Preast, V. 2007, *Xie's Veterinary Acupunture*. Wiley-Blackwell, Ames, IA.

Xie, H., Colahan, P., Ott, E.A. 2005, Evaluation of electroacupuncture treatment of horses with signs of chronic thoracolumbar pain. *J. Am. Vet. Med. Assoc.* 227(2): 281–286.

Yu, C., Lin, J.H. (eds), 2000, *Modern Complete Works of Traditional Chinese Veterinary Medicine* (in Chinese). Kangshi Books Inc, Kangshi, China.

Zink, M.C., van Dyke, J.B. 2013, *Canine Sports Medicine and Rehabilitation*. Wiley-Blackwell, Oxford, UK.

CHAPTER 16

Small animal treatment and rehabilitation for cardiorespiratory conditions

Helen Nicholson
Spring Forward Family Centre, Penrith, Australia

Summary

Literature is emerging on the effectiveness of physiotherapy to help dogs with orthopaedic, neurological and sporting injuries, but the use of respiratory physiotherapy techniques in veterinary intensive care has been largely overlooked, despite the practice of physiotherapy in human intensive care units being provided to most patients and supported by Level 1 evidence.

This chapter therefore describes how physiotherapy can augment the veterinary care of dogs in intensive care, including discussion of the tolerance and effects of CPAP and manual chest physiotherapy in two common canine populations – aspiration pneumonia and brachycephalic airways disease.

16.1 Introduction

Literature is emerging on the effectiveness of physiotherapy to help dogs with orthopaedic, neurological and sporting injuries (Canapp 2007a,b; Gandini *et al.* 2003; Kathmann *et al.* 2001, 2006; Marcellin-Little *et al.* 2007; Mlacnik *et al.* 2006; Monk

et al. 2006; Shumway 2007) but the use of respiratory physiotherapy techniques in veterinary intensive care has been largely overlooked, despite the practice of physiotherapy in human intensive care units being provided to most patients and supported by Level 1 evidence.

In this chapter, I will therefore discuss how physiotherapy can augment the veterinary care of dogs in intensive care, including discussion of the tolerance and effects of CPAP and manual chest physiotherapy in two common canine populations.

16.2 Involuntary canine recumbency

There are several conditions that can lead to respiratory compromise in the canine intensive care setting, with brachycephalic dogs particularly at risk due to their shortened skulls.

16.2.1 Collapse

Dogs may collapse from any number of conditions, including tick poisoning, intervertebral disc disease, metaldehyde ingestion, hypovolaemic shock resulting from internal haemorrhage

Animal Physiotherapy: Assessment, Treatment and Rehabilitation of Animals, Second Edition. Edited by Catherine M. McGowan and Lesley Goff.
© 2016 John Wiley & Sons, Ltd. Published 2016 by John Wiley & Sons, Ltd.

and cardiac failure. As pathophysiology and treatment vary from case to case, collapse itself will be dealt with as relevant to this literature review because of the opportunity it presents to use physiotherapy to assist with sequelae of recumbency in addition to the respiratory signs. As with all other aspects of physiotherapy, collapsed dogs should be considered as a whole, not just a set of respiratory signs.

Pressure sores occur due to ischaemia and are a risk for all recumbent dogs regardless of primary pathology (Nout & Reed 2005). Regular turning and adequate pressure-dispersing bedding are obvious measures that can be taken to reduce the risk of developing pressure sores in recumbent patients (Nout & Reed 2005). Additionally, bandages or foam may be fashioned into 'donuts' to relieve pressure around a bony prominence. The bony prominence is centred in the hole of the donut, which is ideally deep enough to prevent the bone from coming into contact with the bed, and the foam or bandage section of the donut disperses pressure over as wide a surface area as possible. Whilst a systematic review was found on the use of support surfaces for the prevention of pressure ulcers (Cullum et al. 2004), the use of donuts was not discussed, so therapists are limited to anecdotal evidence of their effect.

Limb oedema is also a potential issue for all recumbent dogs and can occur in intensive care patients for reasons including static positioning in a dependent position; for example, when the patient is lying on the left side for an extended period, the left limbs may swell. Oedema may be relieved and/or prevented in intensive care patients via the use of physiotherapy techniques such as massage (Hollis 1987) and limb passive range of motion exercises, which create a passive muscle pump to help return oedematous fluid to the heart.

16.2.2 Intervertebral disc disease

Intervertebral disc disease (IVDD) was first reported in the veterinary literature in 1824 and was classified by Hansen in 1952 (Bray & Burbidge 1998a,b; Hansen 1952). Hansen's classifications were:

- type I herniation: suffered by chondrodystrophoid breeds at any age, these herniations were large and explosive, causing spinal cord trauma and vertebral sinus haemorrhage
- type II herniation: suffered more commonly by older non-chondrodystrophoid dogs, these herniations were smaller and typically had a more regular, even symmetrical profile (Hansen 1952).

Intervertebral disc disease is most prevalent at the most mobile region of the vertebral column in horses, humans and dogs (Bray & Burbidge 1998a,b) and can lead to spinal cord compression, spinal cord contusion, nerve root entrapment, meningeal irritation, paraspinal hyperaesthesia, ataxia, paresis, urinary and/or faecal incontinence, proprioceptive deficits and even Schiff-Sherrington posture and spinal shock (Levine et al. 2007; Platt & Olby 2004).

Medical management is typically considered only for those dogs who are ambulant and have an acute history of neurological signs, although cost may also preclude surgery and mean that non-ambulant dogs or those with chronic neurological signs undergo medical treatment (Levine et al. 2007; Platt & Olby 2004).

16.2.3 Motor vehicle trauma

Dogs admitted after being hit by a motor vehicle may be recumbent due to any one of a multitude of problems, or combination of problems. Such problems may include severe orthopaedic or neurological injury, blood loss, respiratory disease or shock. Specific injuries may include fractures, peripheral nerve lesions and central upper or lower motor neuron lesions. Orthopaedic disease is the most common cause of recumbency following motor vehicle trauma and physiotherapy has great potential to assist with patient management.

Physiotherapy for orthopaedic signs may include direct treatment of the problem, for example, the non-surgical management of some fractures including application of casts and thermoplastic splinting. Physiotherapy might also include range of motion exercises for uninvolved joints in the same or other limbs, balance exercises to help prevent further injury whilst trying to ambulate with a cast and/or gait rehabilitation, and prevention or treatment of secondary complications including arthritis, muscle atrophy and joint range of motion.

The following range of motion problems may occur during recumbency in patients with preexisting arthritis. Clinical signs of arthritis are ameliorated by activity (Smidt et al. 2005) and treatment during periods of recumbency aims to maintain range of motion at the joint via prescription of active, active-assisted or passive limb exercises. This is achieved by employing techniques to relieve or minimise pain such as passive accessory or physiological joint mobilisations and massage, and by retaining or improving strength of muscles that support the joints via various active and active-assisted exercises.

With regard to the management of pain, physiotherapy has many adjunctive treatments to offer the veterinary team. In addition to manual techniques such as joint mobilisations and massage, several electrotherapy modalities, such as transcutaneous electrical nerve stimulation (TENS), may be used. TENS works by stimulating A beta fibres which have an inhibitory effect on A delta (fast pain) and C (slow pain) fibres (Low & Reed 1994). It is important to note, however, that TENS is contraindicated over skin with sensory deficits or open wounds (Low & Reed 1994) and as it is not possible to perform on dogs the same preapplication safety tests required for human treatment, not all forms of electrotherapy will be safe for dogs.

16.2.4 *Ixodes holocyclus* poisoning

Admissions with recumbency due to tick (*Ixodes holocyclus*) poisoning are common along the Eastern seaboard of Australia (with seasonal variation) and typically involve respiratory distress, paralysis or a combination of both. The respiratory signs of *Ixodes holocyclus* poisoning include initial tachypnoea; long-term progressive decrease in respiratory rate; dyspnoea; wheeze; stridor; progressive inability to reposition self to ensure optimum ventilation, prevent aspiration and allow optimum appendicular muscle health; vomiting; regurgitation; aspiration pneumonia; pulmonary oedema due to pulmonary hypertension; respiratory muscle paresis to paralysis; excessive secretions (as opposed to pulmonary oedema) requiring clearance; hypoxia; hypercapnia; and type II (i.e. hypercapnia with hypoxia) respiratory failure. A rapidly ascending flaccid paralysis may occur and has been scored as follows (Campbell & Atwell 2002).

1 Can walk – able to stand from a recumbent position and ambulate.
2 Can't walk (partially recumbent) – requires assistance to reach a standing position but can then maintain the stance position.
3 Can't stand (sternal recumbent) – unable to maintain the stance position.
4 Can't right (quadriplegic/diffuse weakness) – the animal is laterally recumbent and is unable to maintain sternal recumbency.

The respiratory score classifications used are (Campbell & Atwell 2002) as follows.

A Normal character and rate of under 30 breaths per minute.
B Normal character but increased rate of 30 or more breaths per minute.
C Altered character of breathing (restrictive or obstructive) with sighing or grunting (the rate is undefined).
D Severe dyspnoea and cyanosis accompanied by a progressive reduction in respiratory rate.

Tick poisoning occurs when holocyclotoxin, a protein neurotoxin secreted by the salivary glands of the feeding adult female tick, produces signs of paralysis (Stone *et al.* 1983). Another toxin secreted by *Ixodes holocyclus* is lethal but non-paralysing (Stone *et al.* 1983). The full number and effects of toxins secreted by the *Ixodes holocyclus* tick are still being determined.

Veterinary treatment of the respiratory signs of tick poisoning includes oxygen therapy (Baker 2004) and intermittent positive pressure ventilation (Ilkiw 1980). Advice for dogs in lateral recumbency includes turning every 4–6 h to avoid hypostatic pneumonia occurring (Ilkiw 1980) although some clinicians recommend minimal handling to prevent stress (Atwell 2005, personal communication). Postural drainage has also been suggested (Ilkiw 1980).

Physiotherapy has the potential to benefit not only the acute signs of tick poisoning, but also factors that may delay recovery, such as prolonged paralysis or chronic aspiration. Some of the main ways in which physiotherapy can assist in cases of prolonged paralysis were discussed earlier in the section on collapse, i.e. in managing the risk of pressure sores and orthostatic oedema. Prolonged paralysis with the associated inability of the animal to reposition itself to allow optimum appendicular muscle health may also lead to muscular atrophy, contracture and loss of strength.

16.2.5 Metaldehyde ingestion

Metaldehyde, a molluscicide, is a tetramer of acetaldehyde, and is a common ingredient in snail and slug baits (Dolder 2003; Provet.co.uk 2008; Yas-Natan *et al.* 2007). The LD_{50} (median lethal dose) in dogs has been reported to range between 60 and 1000 mg/kg (Dolder 2003; Provet.co.uk 2008; Yas-Natan *et al.* 2007), with signs of toxicity often evident within 20 minutes to 3 hours of ingestion (Provet.co.uk 2008; Yas-Natan *et al.* 2007).

Clinical signs include anxiety, tachycardia, nystagmus, mydriasis, hyperpnoea, panting, hypersalivation, ataxia, vomiting, diarrhoea, tremors, hyperaesthesia, continuous seizures, loss of consciousness, aggressive behaviour, loss of sphincter control, metabolic acidosis, rigidity, opisthotonos and severe hyperthermia (Dolder 2003; Provet.co.uk 2008; Yas-Natan *et al.* 2007). Death may occur from respiratory failure or organ failure due to cellular necrosis caused by hyperthermia resulting from muscle tremors (Dolder 2003).

Current veterinary treatment of metaldehyde poisoning in dogs includes preventing metaldehyde absorption (e.g. via emesis, gastric lavage or activated charcoal), controlling clinical signs (e.g. via anticonvulsants or gas anaesthesia), monitoring and correcting acidosis (e.g. via sodium bicarbonate administration) and dehydration (e.g. via lactated Ringer's solution), and providing supportive care (e.g. via oxygen supplementation for dyspnoea), although an antidote does not exist (Dolder 2003). Reported survival rates with appropriate veterinary care have been as high as 83% (Yas-Natan *et al.* 2007).

16.2.6 Respiratory distress

Respiratory distress can be caused by a wide variety of conditions, including some discussed at length in this review (e.g. BAOS, tick poisoning and metaldehyde ingestion). Left-sided cardiac failure can also lead to respiratory distress. Respiratory distress is often listed as a problem rather than a primary diagnosis upon admission to canine intensive care, and signs may include hypoxia and dyspnoea. In many cases, the primary cause of the respiratory distress is not determined prior to euthanasia or death.

One sign commonly associated with respiratory distress is dyspnoea. Wheeze or stridor are also commonly associated with respiratory distress, but no respiratory physiotherapy techniques were identified in the literature that aim solely to reduce wheeze or stridor. Instead, many techniques aim to improve these by removing secretions or alleviating bronchoconstriction. Many such techniques require medical cointerventions, such as the application of nebulised bronchodilators whilst performing postural drainage, percussion and vibrations.

There is a group of techniques that aims to normalise any respiratory pattern – these techniques are called neurophysiological facilitation (NPF) and use selective afferent input (i.e. tactile and proprioceptive stimuli) to produce reflex responses in the ventilatory apparatus (Pryor *et al.* 2002). In humans, the techniques include intercostal stretch; vertebral pressure to the upper thoracic spine; vertebral pressure to the lower thoracic spine; anterior stretch lift of the posterior basal area; moderate manual pressure; perioral pressure; and abdominal co-contraction (Pryor *et al.* 2002). Further, Japanese physiotherapists have expanded upon NPF (which originated in Canada) to develop breathing assist techniques (BATs), with interesting results (Nakano *et al.* 2003). Advantages of the techniques in humans include improved inspiratory expansion of the ribs; increased tone in the abdominal muscles; changes in breath sounds on auscultation; improved mechanical chest wall stability; a normalised breathing pattern and rate; and reduced need for suctioning (Pryor *et al.* 2002). Both NPF and BATs use tactile and proprioceptive manual stimuli to the patient's thorax and/or face to improve ventilation.

16.2.7 Brachycephalic airway obstructive syndrome

Brachycephalic dogs are designated so due to the foreshortened shape of their heads. Breeds can be identified as brachycephalic if the ratio of their skulls, as measured on the illustrated dog in the breed standard (Council 1998), from nasion to prosthion and inion to prosthion, is less than 0.378. This definition is in keeping with the average measurements of brachycephalic, mesaticephalic and dolichocephalic skull types published elsewhere (Evans 1993). Brachycephalic breeds include Bichon Frise, Boxer, Cavalier King Charles Spaniel, Chihuahua, Chow, Maltese, Papillon, Pekingese, Pomeranian, Pug, Shih Tzu and West Highland White Terrier.

The most common condition related to brachycephalic dogs in the literature was brachycephalic airway obstructive syndrome (Wykes 1991), also described as brachycephalic airway obstruction syndrome (Lorinson *et al.* 1997), brachycephalic airway syndrome (Aron & Crowe 1985; Hendricks 1992; Monnet 2003) and brachycephalic syndrome (Hobson 1995). As the pathophysiology of the condition involves obstruction of the airway, it will henceforth be referred to in this chapter as brachycephalic airway obstructive syndrome or BAOS.

Laryngeal collapse occurs when the supporting function of the cuneiform and corniculate processes of the arytenoid cartilages is lost and arises in the most advanced of cases, progressing further with time until the arytenoid cartilages ultimately collapse (Monnet 2003).

Recommended surgical treatments for BAOS include vertical, horizontal or lateral wedge resection techniques for stenotic nares; resection techniques for elongated soft palate; surgery with temporary tracheostomy to treat everted laryngeal saccules (Bray & Burbidge 1998a,b); and partial arytenochordectomy for dogs with laryngeal collapse in whom resection of the nares or soft palate does not result in sufficient clinical improvement (Hobson 1995; Monnet 2003). An alternative end-stage treatment for dogs with severe laryngeal collapse is permanent tracheostomy (Hobson 1995; Monnet 2003). Temporary tracheostomy may also be required to enhance safety during the recovery from surgery (Lorinson *et al.* 1997).

Non-invasive ventilation is a common treatment modality for respiratory conditions in human intensive care (Table 16.1, Table 16.2). The term refers to methods that enhance alveolar ventilation without the use of an endotracheal airway (Hill 1993) and includes continuous positive airway pressure (CPAP) and bilevel positive airway pressure (BiPAP). CPAP is continuously applied throughout inspiration and expiration and can be administered via a lightweight desktop machine and mask using room air with or without supplemental oxygen. DiPAP differs from CPAP in that it involves two levels of pressure, typically a higher level during inspiration and a lower level during expiration.

16.3 Description of the short-term effects of recumbency in dogs

Recumbency is commonly associated with many serious diseases in dogs, but is frequently overlooked as the primary condition is treated. However, poor responsiveness to therapy and/or prolonged recovery may be related to the sequelae of recumbency, although this has received little attention in the veterinary literature. Recumbency can also have serious implications for human patients, with documented effects on various body systems, including the circulatory, integumentary, skeletal, arthrological and respiratory systems (Allen *et al.* 1999; Martin-Du Pan *et al.* 2004).

The effects of recumbency are multifactorial and require a methodical and thorough approach to investigate. A common approach is a survey tool in which many factors are assessed and scored. For example, some survey tools were identified that aimed to assess pain or quality of life in dogs (Hielm-Bjorkman *et al.* 2003; Holton *et al.* 2001; Hudson *et al.* 2004; McMillan 2003; Morton *et al.* 2005; Wiseman-Orr *et al.* 2006; Wojciechowska *et al.* 2005), but there is no such assessment tool for recumbent dogs reported in the veterinary literature. A study was therefore undertaken to describe the short-term effects of recumbency on clinically unwell dogs admitted to veterinary hospitals in Sydney, with a long-term view to developing a baseline for investigation of the long-term effects of recumbency on dogs and comparison studies of outcome measures of dogs that do and do not receive physiotherapy whilst recumbent (Nicholson 2008). Specifically, the aims were to describe the signalment of a sample of clinically recumbent dogs, to complete repeatability trials on a number of novel measurements, and to observe the natural history of clinical recumbency in a short-term timeframe to determine whether spontaneous improvement or deterioration occurs in a number of key body systems. It was hypothesised that if a deterioration or no natural improvement was observed in the timeframe measured, that there would be justification to proceed with a trial of physiotherapy within the same clinical timeframe as measured in this study, in order to determine if physiotherapy can help speed the recovery of recumbent dogs and prevent any observed complications occurring within this timeframe.

Table 16.1 Beneficial effects of NIV demonstrated in human clinical studies

Condition	Short-term benefits from human research	Long-term effects from human research	Highest level of evidence cited

Pulmonary oedema	• Decreased need for intubation:
	  • Bersten *et al.* 1991 – *trial*;
	  • Lin *et al.* 1995 – *trial*;
	  • Pang *et al.* 1998 – *review*;
	  • Collins *et al.* 2006 – *review*
	• Increased functional residual capacity: Mehta *et al.* 1997 – *trial*
	• Increased cardiac output (via decreased left ventricular preload and afterload):
	  • Mehta *et al.* 1997 – *trial*
	• Decreased atelectasis: Mehta *et al.* 1997 – *trial*
	• Decreased work of breathing (by improving pulmonary compliance): Mehta *et al.* 1997 – *trial*
	• Improved respiratory rate: Bersten *et al.* 1991 – *trial*
	• Reduced $PaCO_2$: Bersten *et al.* 1991 – *trial*
	• Improved PaO_2: Rasanen *et al.* 1985 – *trial*;
	  • Lin *et al.* 1995 – *trial*
	• Decreased right-to-left intrapulmonary shunt: Lin *et al.* 1995 – *trial*;
	  • Mehta *et al.* 1997 – *trial*
		• Decreased in-hospital mortality rate: Pang *et al.* 1998 – *review*; Collins *et al.* 2006 – *review*	Level 1

Pneumonia	• Improved PaO_2:
	  • Miller & Semple 1991 – *trial*
	• Reduced dyspnoea:
	  • Miller & Semple 1991 – *trial*
	• Decreased respiratory rate:
	  • Miller & Semple 1991 – *trial*
	• Reduced energy expenditure:
	  • Xu *et al.* 2003 – *trial*
		• Reduced mortality:
		  • Boots *et al.* 2005 – *trial*
			Level 2

Chronic obstructive pulmonary disease (COPD)	• Reduced hypercapnia: Brochard *et al.* 1990 – *trial*;
	  • Ambrosino *et al.* 1992 – *trial*
	• Improved PaO_2:
	  • Brochard *et al.* 1990 – *trial*
	• Lower intubation rate:
	  • Brochard *et al.* 1990 – *trial*;
	  • Brochard *et al.* 1995 – *trial*
		• Shorter stay in intensive care:
		  • Brochard *et al.* 1990 – *trial*
		• Lower frequency of complications: Brochard *et al.* 1995 – *trial*
		• Shorter overall hospital stay:
		  • Brochard *et al.* 1995 – *trial*
		• Lower in-hospital mortality rate:
		  • Brochard *et al.* 1995 – *trial*
		• In non-hospitalised patients with COPD receiving nocturnal NIV:
		  • improved daytime PaO_2
		  • improved daytime $PaCO_2$
		  • improved sleep time
		  • improved sleep efficiency
		  • better quality of life
		• Claman et al. 1996 – review
			Level 1

Sleep apnoea	• Reduced apnoea and hypopnoea index: Giles *et al.* 2006 – review
	• Improved sleep efficiency: Giles *et al.* 2006 – review
	• Improved minimum oxygen saturation: Giles *et al.* 2006 – review
	• Splinting airways open: Mathru *et al.* 1996 – *trial*;
	  • Gaon *et al.* 1999 – *trial*;
	  • McNicholas & Ryan 2006 – *review*
		• Improved daytime hypercapnia: Claman *et al.* 1996 – *review*
		• Improved ventilation control: Claman *et al.* 1996 – *review*
		• Improved left ventricular ejection fraction: Naughton *et al.* 1995 – *trial*
		• Reduced apnoeas and hypopnoeas: Naughton *et al.* 1995 – *trial*
		• Improved quality of life:
		  • Giles *et al.* 2006 – *review*
			Level 1

Table 16.1 (*Continued*)

Condition	Short-term benefits from human research	Long-term effects from human research	Highest level of evidence cited
Postoperatively e.g. abdominal surgery	• Lower rate of atelectasis: Stock *et al.* 1985 – *trial*; • Ricksten *et al.* 1986 – *trial* • Lower alveolar-arteriolar oxygen difference: Ricksten *et al.* 1986 – *trial* • Higher forced vital capacity (FVC): Ricksten *et al.* 1986 – *trial* • More rapid improvement in functional residual capacity (FRC): Stock *et al.* 1985 – *trial*	• Lower postoperative pulmonary complications: Denehy *et al.* 2001 – *trial*	Level 1

Acute respiratory failure	• Decreased work of breathing (as measured by total pulmonary power): Katz & Marks 1985 – *trial*
	• Decreased mean alveolar-to-arterial oxygen partial pressure difference: Katz & Marks 1985 – *trial*
	• Improved oxygen and carbon dioxide exchange: Katz & Marks 1985 – *trial*
	• Higher mean effective lung compliance: Katz & Marks 1985 – *trial*
	• Increased tidal volume:
	  • Katz & Marks 1985 – *trial*
	• Longer inspiration time:
	  • Katz & Marks 1985 – *trial*
	• Decreased respiratory rate:
	  • Katz & Marks 1985 – *trial*;
	  • Kramer *et al.* 1995 – *trial*
		• Same amount of nursing time required as traditional therapy:
		  • Kramer *et al.* 1995 – *trial*
		• Reduced rate of endotracheal intubation: Wysocki & Antonelli 2001 – *review*
		• Lower mortality rate:
		  • Wysocki & Antonelli 2001 – *review*
			Level 1

Cystic fibrosis	• Maintenance of inspiratory muscle strength: Holland *et al.* 2003 – *trial* • Improved expiratory muscle strength: Holland *et al.* 2003 – *trial* • Improved SpO_2: Holland *et al.* 2003 – *trial* • Reduced dyspnoea: Holland *et al.* 2003 – *trial*		Level 2

Weaning from mechanical ventilation	• Reduced incidence of weaning failure: Halliday 2004 – *review*
	• Reduced incidence of apnoea:
	  • Davis & Henderson-Smart 2003 – *review*
	• Reduced respiratory acidosis:
	  • Davis & Henderson-Smart 2003 – *review*
	• Lower requirements for additional oxygen: Davis & Henderson-Smart 2003 – *review*
		• Reduced chronic lung disease at 28 days post extubation: Halliday 2004 – *review*	Level 1

Overall, the study found that the average timeframe during hospitalisation that dogs are medically stable but have a static level of recumbency is between day 3 and day 5 of admission (Nicholson 2008). It is therefore possible that a trial of physiotherapy between days 3 and 5 of hospitalisation in medically stable recumbent dogs such as these may speed recovery. However, it may be possible that this timeframe is not sufficient to assess the efficacy of any physiotherapy interventions employed and future studies may need to be designed with follow-up assessments at timepoints further along the recovery period to compare the recovery of dogs who did and did not receive the physiotherapy intervention.

16.4 Tolerance and effects of the administration of continuous positive airway pressure during recovery from general anaesthetic in dogs with brachycephalic airway obstructive syndrome

As described in section 16.2, CPAP is a form of non-invasive ventilation (NIV) that has Level 1 evidence demonstrating benefits in humans with upper airway obstructive disease. Many studies have also been performed on experimental dogs for the purposes of gaining further evidence for the human use of NIV (Caldini *et al.* 1975; Cassidy *et al.* 1978; Fewell *et al.* 1980;

Table 16.2 Conditions in dogs that may benefit from the application of non-invasive ventilation

Canine condition	Problem	Proposed mechanisms of action, from human evidence (references provided in Table 16.1)
Ixodes holocyclus poisoning (Beveridge 1991; Campbell & Atwell 2001, 2002, 2003; Fearnley 2002; Fitzgerald 1998; Ilkiw 1979, 1980; Ilkiw & Turner 1987a,b, 1988; Ilkiw *et al.* 1987, 1988; Stone 1988; Stone *et al.* 1983)	Respiratory muscle paresis	• Decreased work of breathing • Maintenance of inspiratory muscle strength • Reduced energy expenditure • Splinting airways open
	Type II (hypoxia with hypercapnia) respiratory failure	• Improved hypoxia • Reduced hypercapnia • Decreased work of breathing • Improved lung compliance • Improved respiratory rate
	Dyspnoea	• Reduced dyspnoea
	Tachypnoea	• Decreased respiratory rate
	Difficulty weaning from mechanical ventilation	• Decreased work of breathing • Reduced incidence of apnoea • Reduced respiratory acidosis • Reduced energy expenditure
	Pulmonary oedema	• Decreased ventricular preload and afterload • Increased functional residual capacity • Decreased work of breathing • Improved pulmonary compliance • Decreased right-to-left intrapulmonary shunt
	Aspiration pneumonia	• Improved hypoxia • Reduced dyspnoea • Reduced respiratory rate • Reduced energy expenditure
Brachycephalic airways syndrome (Wykes 1991; Hendricks 1992; Hobson 1995; Lorinson *et al.* 1997; Monnet 2003)	Decreased airways patency due to anatomical abnormalities	• Continuous positive pressure to splint airways open
	Pulmonary oedema	• Decreased ventricular preload and afterload • Increased functional residual capacity • Decreased work of breathing • Improved pulmonary compliance • Decreased right-to-left intrapulmonary shunt
	Decreased PaO_2	• Improved hypoxia
	Respiratory distress	• Reduced dyspnoea • Decreased respiratory rate • Improved hypoxia • Decreased work of breathing • Reduced energy expenditure
	Aspiration pneumonia	• Improved hypoxia • Reduced dyspnoea • Reduced respiratory rate • Decreased energy expenditure
	Continued airway obstruction	• Improved PaO_2 • Improved $PaCO_2$
Postoperatively, depending on the type of surgery performed	Shallow respirations from pain inhibition	• Decreased respiratory rate • Decreased work of breathing • Splinting airways open • Reduced energy expenditure
	Atelectasis	• Reduced atelectasis
	Lower FRC	• Improved FRC
	Lower FVC	• Improved FVC

FRC, functional residual capacity; FVC, forced vital capacity.

Frazier *et al.* 2000, 2001; Hubmayr *et al.* 1987; Johnston *et al.* 1989; Pare *et al.* 1983; Perel *et al.* 1983; Road & Leevers 1990; Scott *et al.* 1978; Shade *et al.* 1994). Results of these studies include decreased respiratory rate, increased tidal volume (Scott *et al.* 1978) and decreased inspiratory work (Shade *et al.* 1994) from the application of CPAP in experimental dogs. It seems logical that the beneficial effects of CPAP could also be used to assist dogs with upper respiratory tract obstruction, but no reports of its use in clinical canine patients were found in the literature.

It can be hypothesised that postoperative CPAP would have an effect on the following parameters of dogs with BAOS recovering from a general anaesthetic:

- respiratory rate
- heart rate
- heart rhythm
- level of supplemental oxygen required
- quality of respiration
- demeanour
- partial pressure of oxygen as measured in the arterial blood
- partial pressure of carbon dioxide as measured in the arterial blood
- mucous membrane colour
- blood pressure
- oxygen saturation
- time to recovery as defined as having regained consciousness and the ability to maintain the airway without assistance.

A pilot study into this intervention found that the mean time to recovery was 14.17 ± 10.70 min in the treatment group and 35.00 ± 14.49 min in the control group, which represented a significantly slower recovery in the control group ($T = -2.83$, $P = 0.20$) (Nicholson 2008). Further, there were several significant differences between the treatment and control groups in the case of both visual analogue scale (VAS) of demeanour ($P = 0.0001$) and VAS of quality of respiration ($P = 0.006$).

Several attempts were made in the design phase of the pilot study to provide CPAP via a hood delivery system to healthy dogs; in Figure 16.1, the CPAP feed is evident next to the dog's right eye, with an Elizabethan collar used to try to prevent the

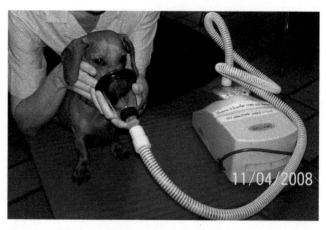

Figure 16.2 Please note that CPAP machines improve respiratory parameters with the application of room air, but that seriously unwell dogs can have supplementary oxygen supplied in addition to CPAP.

dog from feeling claustrophobic or disliking the air flow rushing at its face. Unfortunately, although attempts were made to secure the collar with vetrap to try to prevent too much leakage, pressure sphygmomanometry revealed that the desired level of pressure could not be achieved – too much air escaped between the hairs in the dog's fur.

To counter this, delivery via a facemask, when tolerated by the dog, is effective in preventing excessive pressure leak (Figure 16.2). The CPAP machine in Figure 16.2 is a common desktop machine used to treat humans with sleep apnoea in their own homes. When purchasing a CPAP machine, please check the ease with which the level of CPAP can be adjusted, as the protocol in the pilot study was to titrate the CPAP for effect, i.e. start at the lowest possible pressure and increase gradually while monitoring clinical parameters such as SpO_2 and respiratory rate. Our experience is that clinical parameters will improve for a certain time as breathing becomes easier with pressure support, but once pressure is too high, clinical parameters deteriorate as the dog works harder to breathe out against the increased pressure. Pressure can then be decreased again to a level at which clinical parameters were most satisfactorily maintained.

When the CPAP is appropriately tolerated and titrated for effect, a visual analogue scale, such as the examples in Figures 16.3 and 16.4, can be used to compare the demeanour of dogs or the quality of their respiration with and without CPAP to assist with their veterinary management.

The Nicholson (2008) study was the first report of CPAP in canine patients with upper airway disease and demonstrated that the use of CPAP postoperatively can improve time to recovery, without resulting in additional distress and is well tolerated in brachycephalic dogs recovering from general anaesthetics. It is therefore hoped that it will now be possible to expand research into the use of CPAP in other scenarios that have been shown to be effective in humans, such as weaning from mechanical ventilation, or as an adjunct to other forms of treatment for spontaneously breathing dogs with pulmonary oedema.

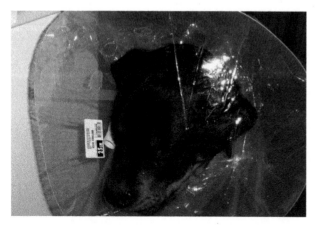

Figure 16.1 CPAP feed delivered via hood using an Elizabethan collar.

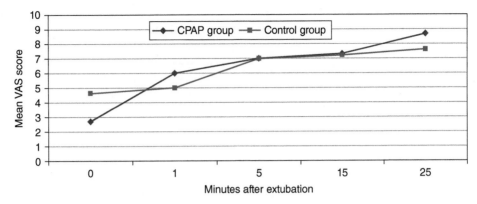

Figure 16.3 Analysis for visual analogue scale of demeanour by time point.

16.5 Tolerance and short-term effects of manual chest physiotherapy in dogs with aspiration pneumonia

Manual chest physiotherapy is often performed in veterinary hospitals, but staff members performing the treatments typically have little training in the safe or effective performance of the techniques and the techniques themselves often do not represent the true scope of chest physiotherapy. A pilot study was therefore designed to evaluate the tolerance and short-term effects of a manual chest physiotherapy protocol extrapolated from humans, designed by a qualified physiotherapist and based on an extensive literature search to maximise both the safety and efficacy of the treatment techniques chosen (Nicholson 2008).

Specific chest physiotherapy techniques include postural drainage, percussion, vibration and suction or cough stimulation. Postural drainage is a series of body positions that aim to use gravity to improve mucociliary transport and therefore remove retained secretions from various lobes of the lung (Humberstone 1990). The potential outcomes of postural drainage include increased volume of secretions expectorated; better clearance of tenacious secretions; reduced airway resistance; improved lung compliance; reduction in the work of breathing; and improved oxygenation and ventilation (Humberstone 1990).

Percussion (sometimes referred to as 'coupage') is both an inspiratory and expiratory technique that involves clapping the cupped hands on the chest wall in order to induce movement of secretions from the underlying lung lobes. It is the speed, not the intensity, of the percussion that makes it effective. Percussion may be indicated in the treatment of dogs with excessive secretions, such as aspiration pneumonia or other types of pneumonia that have consolidated.

Vibration differs from percussion in that vibration is an expiration-only technique and is thought to be less traumatic to the patient than percussion can be, especially postoperatively (Regan et al. 1990). Vibration is often used following percussion, and both are typically used with the patient in various postural drainage positions (Regan et al. 1990).

Once secretions have been moved closer to the mouth, suction or cough stimulation is typically used depending upon the level of consciousness, whether the patient is mechanically ventilated or not, and the volume of secretions requiring clearance (Regan et al. 1990). Suction may be nasopharyngeal, oropharyngeal or via an airway tube (Regan et al. 1990), whilst cough stimulation or augmentation techniques potentially applicable to dogs

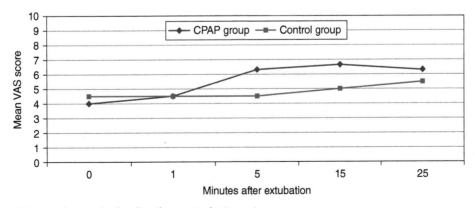

Figure 16.4 Analysis of visual analogue scale of quality of respiration by time point.

include tracheal rub, pressure applied at the third tracheal ring and manual support (Harden 2004; Manning 2004; Regan *et al.* 1990).

16.5.1 Manual chest physiotherapy protocol

The manual chest physiotherapy protocol the author prefers is three sets of percussion and vibration followed by manual facilitation of cough. Percussion is defined in this protocol as the fast clapping movement of the cupped hands on the aspects of the chest wall over the lungs that are able to be reached without moving critically ill dogs. Percussion is performed for 30 seconds, in keeping with safety recommendations for humans (Pryor 1999; Pryor *et al.* 1990), and is followed immediately by three expiratory vibrations, defined as the application of a shaking and gentle compression movement of the open hands on the chest wall over the lungs during the expiration phase of respiration. Three expiratory vibrations are used in an effort to mimic the active cycle of breathing technique, the gold standard for human expectorant physiotherapy (Pryor *et al.* 1994). The cough reflex is facilitated by rubbing the third tracheal cartilage, as described by Manning (2004).

16.5.2 Results of manual chest physiotherapy protocol in dogs with aspiration pneumonia

In a pilot study (Nicholson 2008), physiotherapy was performed on sequential days when the veterinarian determined that aspiration pneumonia was the main remaining problem keeping the subject dogs in hospital. None of the dogs had returned home since initial presentation and the mean length of stay in hospital that the first physiotherapy treatment was performed on was 6.50 ± 1.87 days. The overall mean length of stay in hospital was 7.83 ± 2.14 days.

The data for the dogs who participated in this pilot study were compared to determine if a clinical improvement could be detected from day 1 to day 2. The data sets after physiotherapy on day 1 were therefore compared to the data sets immediately prior to physiotherapy on day 2. The results of this analysis were that there was no change in most of the outcome measures from postphysiotherapy day 1 to prephysiotherapy day 2: heart rate $P = 0.452$; respiratory rate $P = 0.152$; VAS of demeanour $P = 0.232$; SpO_2 $P = 0.068$; auscultation score $P = 0.007$. Therefore, the dogs maintained most of their clinical improvements from one day to the next (Nicholson 2008).

16.5.3 Summary of manual chest physiotherapy in dogs with aspiration pneumonia

The manual chest physiotherapy protocol used in this pilot study caused a significant improvement in oxygen saturation and auscultation scores, demonstrating a short-term clinical benefit of the application of manual chest physiotherapy by a qualified physiotherapist to dogs with aspiration pneumonia (Nicholson 2008).

Although it was found that the dogs tolerated the protocol well, the most important finding was that the protocol was effective in improving the signs of respiratory failure associated with pneumonia, i.e. by removing secretions from the lungs, as evidenced by improved auscultation, more alveolar surface area was available for gas exchange, leading to an improved ventilation-perfusion ratio, as evidenced by the improvement in oxygen saturation.

Research into previous investigations in an animal model (Wong *et al.* 2003) enabled a manual chest physiotherapy protocol to be developed for this study that was most likely to be well tolerated by critically ill dogs and to have positive short-term effects. The results of this study agree with the previous animal model study (Wong *et al.* 2003) finding that there was no change in heart rate, and the previous canine study (Chopra *et al.* 1977) finding that percussion can be used without postural drainage, with improved auscultation in this study comparative to the findings of increased mean tracheal transport velocity in that study (Chopra *et al.* 1977).

The significant improvement in oxygen saturation as a result of physiotherapy on day 1 demonstrates the immediate effectiveness of a short intervention, as reflected in the improved auscultation score post physiotherapy on both days of the study. The importance of the improvement in SpO_2 is not just statistically significant, however; it demonstrates a reversal of respiratory failure. At a mean SpO_2 of 93% (day 1 and day 2 time point 1), PO_2 is approximately 70 mmHg; however, at an SpO_2 of 94.8 (day 2 time point 3), PO_2 is approximately 80 mmHg, whilst an SpO_2 of 98.7% (day 1 time point 3) is equivalent to a PO_2 of approximately 100 mmHg (Sherwood 1993). This vast improvement in PO_2 in comparison to a small improvement in SpO_2 is due to the plateau effect in the oxygen-haemoglobin dissociation curve, reflecting the extent to which oxygen is loaded onto haemoglobin in the pulmonary capillaries (Sherwood 1993). Therefore, by clearing secretions from the lungs, physiotherapy led to an improvement in gas exchange (Nicholson 2008).

The significantly improved demeanour scores from before to after physiotherapy on day 1 (Nicholson 2008) reflect the dogs' increased comfort afforded by being able to breathe more easily as a result of the secretions being shifted in their lungs to allow improved air entry and oxygenation. This therefore reflects both tolerance and effect of the physiotherapy protocol applied.

The author hypothesised that fewer significant improvements were demonstrated on day 2 for two reasons. The first is that the dogs maintained most of their improvements in the outcome measures from time point 3 of day 1 to time point 1 of day 2, and therefore it was not possible to make as much of an improvement as they had the previous day. Auscultation score, however, deteriorated overnight, which is to be expected given the sedentary nature of such critically ill dogs. The second hypothesised reason that there were fewer improvements on day 2 is that the dogs were clinically better than they were on day 1, as supported by the fact that some of the dogs in the pilot study were well enough to be discharged before receiving physiotherapy on day 3 (Nicholson 2008).

Therefore, this pilot study demonstrated the tolerance and short-term effect of a manual chest physiotherapy programme consisting of percussion, vibration and cough stimulation for dogs with aspiration pneumonia (Nicholson 2008).

16.6 Conclusion

Cardiorespiratory conditions are treated by physiotherapists every day in human hospitals, with an extensive evidence base of Level 1 research. Dogs can suffer from the same or very similar pathophysiologies as humans, rendering them critically unwell and receiving veterinary intensive care. However, the use of respiratory physiotherapy techniques in veterinary intensive care has been largely overlooked. This chapter has therefore discussed how physiotherapy can augment the veterinary care of dogs in intensive care, including discussion of the tolerance and effects of CPAP and manual chest physiotherapy in two common canine populations. Readers are therefore encouraged to research the cardiorespiratory conditions common to the dogs in their local area and apply evidence-based physiotherapy to assist the veterinary team in improving the quality of life of critically ill dogs.

References

Allen, C., Glasziou, P., del Mar, C. 1999, Bed rest: a potentially harmful treatment needing more careful evaluation. *Lancet* 354: 1229–1233.

Ambrosino, N., Nava, S., Bertone, P. *et al.* 1992, Physiologic evaluation of pressure support ventilation by nasal mask in patients with stable COPD. *Chest* 101(2): 385–387.

Aron, D.N., Crowe, D.T. 1985, Upper airway obstruction. *Vet. Clin. North Am. Small Anim. Pract.* 15(5): 891–917.

Atwell, R.B. 2002, Laryngeal paresis caused by I. holocyclus. *Aust. Vet. Pract.* 32(1): 41.

Atwell, R.B., Campbell, F.E., Evans, E.A. 2001, Prospective survey of tick paralysis in dogs. *Aust. Vet. J.* 79(6): 412–418.

Baker, G.D. 2004, Trans-tracheal oxygen therapy in dogs with severe respiratory compromise due to tick (I. holocyclus) toxicity. *Aust. Vet. Pract.* 34(2): 83.

Bersten, A.D., Holt, A.W., Vedig, A.E. *et al.* 1991, Treatment of severe cardiogenic pulmonary edema with continuous positive airway pressure delivered by face mask. *N. Engl. J. Med.* 325(26): 1825–1830.

Beveridge, J. 1991, Ixodes holocyclus in the Melbourne metropolitan area. *Aust. Vet. J.* 68(6): 214.

Boots, R.J., Lipman, J., Bellomo, R. *et al.* 2005, Disease risk and mortality prediction in intensive care patients with pneumonia. *Anaesth. Intens. Care* 33(1): 101–111.

Bray, J.P., Burbidge, H.M. 1998a, The canine intervertebral disk: Part one: Structure and function. *J. Am. Anim. Hosp. Assoc.* 34: 55–63.

Bray, J.P., Burbidge, H.M. 1998b, The canine intervertebral disk: Part two: Degenerative changes – Nonchondrodystrophoid versus chondrodystrophoid disks. *J. Am. Anim. Hosp. Assoc.* 34: 135–144.

Brochard, L., Isabey, D., Piquet, J. *et al.* 1990, Reversal of acute exacerbations of chronic obstructive lung disease by inspiratory assistanve with a face mask. *N. Engl. J. Med.* 323(22): 1523–1530.

Brochard, L., Mancebo, J., Wysocki, M. *et al.* 1995, Noninvasive ventilation for acute exacerbations of chronic obstructive pulmonary disease. *N. Engl. J. Med.* 333(13): 817–822.

Caldini, P., Leith, J.D., Brennan, M.J. 1975, Effect of continuous positive-pressure ventilation (CPPV) on edema formation in dog lung. *J. Appl. Physiol.* 39(4): 672–679.

Campbell, F.E., Atwell, R.B. 2001, Megaoesophagus in dogs with tick paralysis (Ixodes holocyclus). *Aust. Vet. Pract.* 31: 75.

Campbell, F.E., Atwell, R.B. 2002, Update on the management of tick toxicity (Ixodes holocyclus) in dogs and cats. Claws and Paws in Crisis: A Valentine Charlton Refresher Course for Veterinarians, ANA Hotel, Surfers Paradise, Post Graduate Foundation in Veterinary Science University of Sydney.

Campbell, F.E., Atwell, R.B. 2003, Heart failure in dogs with tick paralysis caused by the Australian paralysis tick, Ixodes holocyclus. *J. Appl. Res. Vet. Med.* 1(2): 148–162.

Canapp, D.A. 2007a, Select modalities. *Clin. Techn. Small Anim. Pract.* 22(4): 160–165.

Canapp, S.O. Jr. 2007b, The canine stifle. *Clin. Techn. Small Anim. Pract.* 22(4): 195–205.

Cassidy, S.S., Robertson, C., Pierce, A. *et al.* 1978, Cardiovascular effects of positive end-expiratory pressure in dogs. *J. Appl. Physiol.* 44: 743–750.

Chopra, S.K., Taplin, G.V., Simmons, D.H., Robinson, G.D. Jr, Elam, D., Coulson, A. 1977, Effects of hydration and physical therapy on tracheal transport velocity. *Am. Rev. Respir. Dis.* 115(6): 1009–1114.

Claman, D.M., Piper, A., Sanders, M. *et al.* 1996, Nocturnal noninvasive positive pressure ventilatory assistance. *Chest* 110(6): 1581–1588.

Collins, S.P., Mielniczuk, L., Whittingham, H. *et al.* 2006, The use of noninvasive ventilation in emergency department patients with acute cardiogenic pulmonary edema: a systematic review. *Ann. Emerg. Med.* 48(3): 260–269.

Council, T.A.N.K. 1998, *Illustrated Breed Standards.* Australian National Kennel Council, Australia.

Cullum, N., McInnes, E., Bell-Syer, S.E., Legood, R. 2004, Support surfaces for pressure ulcer prevention (Cochrane Review) [with consumer summary]. *Cochrane Database Syst. Rev.*, Issue 3.

Davis, P.G., Henderson-Smart, D. 2003, Nasal continuous positive airways pressure immediately after extubation for preventing morbidity in preterm infants. *Cochrane Database Syst. Rev.* 2: CD000143.

Denehy, L., Carroll, S., Ntoumenopoulos, G. *et al.* 2001, A randomized controlled trial comparing periodic mask CPAP with physiotherapy after abdominal surgery. *Physiother. Res. Int.* 6(4): 236–250.

Dolder, L.K. 2003, Metaldehyde toxicosis. *Vet. Med.* 98(3): 213–215.

Evans, H.E. 1993, *Miller's Anatomy of the Dog.* W.B. Saunders, Philadelphia, PA.

Fearnley, A. 2002, The importance of body temperature in the treatment of tick paralysis. *Aust. Vet. Pract.* 32(3): 137–138.

Fewell, J.E., Abendschein, D., Carlson, C. *et al.* 1980, Continuous positive-pressure ventilation decreases right and left ventricular end-diastolic volumes in the dog. *Circ. Res.* 46: 125–132.

Fitzgerald, M.P. 1998, Ixodes holocyclus poisoning. Clinical Toxicology, Stephen Roberts Lecture Theatre, Postgraduate Foundation in Veterinary Science, University of Sydney.

Frazier, S.K., Stone, K., Schertel, E.R., Moser, D.K., Pratt, J.W. 2000, Comparison of hemodynamic changes during the transition from mechanical ventilation to T-piece, pressure support, and continuous positive airway pressure in canines. *Biol. Res. Nurs.* 1(4): 253–264.

Frazier, S.K., Moser, D., Stone, K. 2001, Heart rate variability and hemodynamic alterations in canines with normal cardiac function during exposure to pressure support, continuous positive airway pressure, and a combination of pressure support and continuous positive airway pressure. *Biol. Res. Nurs.* 2(3): 167–174.

Gandini, G., Cizinauskas, S., Lang, J. *et al.* 2003, Fibrocartilagenous embolism in 75 dogs: clinical findings and factors influencing recovery rate. *J. Small Anim. Pract.* 44: 76–80.

Gaon, P., Lee, S., Hannan, S. *et al.* 1999, Assessment of effect of nasal continuous positive pressure on laryngeal opening using fibre optic laryngoscopy. *Arch. Dis. Child. Fetal Neonatal Ed.* 80: 230–232.

Giles, T.L., Lasserson, T., *et al.* 2006, Continuous positive airways pressure for obstructive sleep apnoea in adults. *Cochrane Database Syst. Rev.* 3: CD001106.

Halliday, H.L. 2004, What interventions facilitate weaning from the ventilator? A review of the evidence from systematic reviews. *Paediatr. Respir. Rev.* 5(suppl A): S347–S352.

Hansen, H.J. 1952, A pathologic-anatomical study on disk degeneration in the dog. *Acta Orthop. Scand. Suppl.* 11: 1–117.

Harden, B. 2004, *Emergency Physiotherapy: an on-call survival guide.* Churchill Livingstone, Edinburgh.

Hendricks, J.C. 1992, Brachycephalic airway syndrome. *Vet. Clin. North Am. Small Anim. Pract.* 22(5): 1145–1153.

Hielm-Bjorkman, A.K., Kuusela, E., *et al.* 2003, Evaluation of methods for assessment of pain associated with chronic osteoarthritis in dogs. *J. Am. Vet. Med. Assoc.* 222(11): 1552–1558.

Hill, N.S. 1993, Noninvasive ventilation: does it work, for whom, and how? *Am. Rev. Respir. Dis.* 147: 1050–1055.

Hobson, H.P. 1995, Brachycephalic syndrome. *Semin. Vet. Med Surg. (Small Anim.)* 10(2): 109–114.

Hollis, M. 1987, *Massage for Therapists.* Blackwell Scientific Publications, Oxford, UK.

Holton, L., Reid, J., Scott, E.M., Pawson, P., Nolan A. 2001, Development of a behaviour-based scale to measure acute pain in dogs. *Vet. Rec.* 148: 525–531.

Hubmayr, R. D., Rodarte, J., Walter, B. *et al.* 1987, Regional ventilation during spontaneous breathing and mechanical ventilation in dogs. *J. Appl. Physiol.* 63(6): 2467–2475.

Hudson, J.T., Slater, M., Taylor, L. *et al.* 2004, Assessing repeatability and validity of a visual analogue scale questionnaire for use in assessing pain and lameness in dogs. *Am. J. Vet. Res.* 65(12): 1634–1643.

Humberstone, N. 1990, Respiratory assessment and treatment. In: Irwin, S., Tecklin, J.S. (eds), *Cardiopulmonary Physical Therapy.* C.V. Mosby, St Louis, MO, pp. 283–321.

Ilkiw, J.E. 1979, *A Study of the Effects in the Dog of Ixodes holocyclus.* University of Sydney, Sydney, Australia.

Ilkiw, J.E. 1980, Tick paralysis in Australia. *Curr. Ther. Small Anim. Pract.* 7: 777–779.

Ilkiw, J.E., Turner, D.M. 1987a, Infestation in the dog by the paralysis tick Ixodes holocyclus. 2. Blood-gas and pH, haematological and biochemical findings. *Aust. Vet. J.* 64(5): 139–142.

Ilkiw, J.E., Turner, D.M. 1987b, Infestation in the dog by the paralysis tick Ixodes holocyclus. 3. Respiratory effects. *Aust. Vet. J.* 64(5): 142–144.

Ilkiw, J.E., Turner, D.M. 1988, Infestation in the dog by the paralysis tick Ixodes holocyclus. 5. Treatment. *Aust. Vet. J.* 65(8): 236–238.

Ilkiw, J.E., Turner, D.M., Howlett, C.R. 1987, Infestation in the dog by the paralysis tick Ixodes holocyclus. 1. Clinical and histological findings. *Aust. Vet. J.* 64(5): 137–139.

Ilkiw, J.E., Turner, D.M., Goodman, A.H. 1988, Infestation in the dog by the paralysis tick Ixodes holocyclus. 4. Cardiovascular effects. *Aust. Vet. J.* 65(8): 232–235.

Johnston, W.E., Vinten-Johansen, J., Santamore, W. *et al.* 1989, Mechanism of reduced cardiac output during positive end-expiratory pressure in the dog. *Am. Rev. Respir. Dis.* 140(5): 1257–1264.

Kathmann, I., Demierre, S., Jaggy, A. 2001, [Rehabilitation methods in small animal neurology] [German – English abstract]. *Schweiz. Arch. Tierheilkd.* 143(10): 495–502.

Kathmann, I., Cizinauskas, S., Doherr, M.G., Steffen, F., Jaggy, A. 2006, Daily controlled physiotherapy increases survival time in dogs with suspected degenerative myelopathy. *J. Vet. Intern. Med.* 20: 927–932.

Katz, J.A., Marks, J. 1985, Inspiratory work with and without continuous positive airway pressure in patients with acute respiratory failure. *Anesthesiology* 63: 598–607.

Kramer, N., Meyer, T., Meharg, J. *et al.* 1995, Randomized, prospective trial of noninvasive positive pressure ventilation in acute respiratory failure. *Am. J. Respir. Crit. Care Med.* 151: 1799–1806.

Levine, J.M., Levine, G., Johnson, S. *et al.* 2007, Evaluation of the succes of medical management for presumptive thoracolumbar intervertebral disk herniation in dogs. *Vet. Surg.* 36: 482–491.

Lin, M., Yang, Y.F., Chiang, H. *et al.* 1995, Reappraisal of continuous positive airway pressure therapy in acute cardiogenic pulmonary edema. Short-term results and long-term follow-up. *Chest* 107(5): 1379–1386.

Lorinson, D., Bright, R.M., White, R.A.S. 1997, Brachycephalic airway obstruction syndrome – a review of 118 cases. *Canine Pract.* 22(5-6): 18–21.

Low, J., Reed, A. 1994, *Electrotherapy Explained: principles and practice.* Butterworth-Heinemann, Oxford, UK.

Manning, A.M. 2004, Physical rehabilitation for the critically injured veterinary patient. In: Millis, D.L., Levine, D., Taylor, R.A. (eds), *Canine Rehabilitation & Physical Therapy.* W.B. Saunders, St Louis, MO, pp. 404–410.

Marcellin-Little, D.J., Levine, D., Canapp, S.O. Jr. 2007, The canine shoulder: selected disorders and their management with physical therapy. *Clin. Techn. Small Anim. Pract.* 22(4): 171–182.

Martin-Du Pan, R., Benoit, R., Girardier, L. 2004, The role of body position and gravity in the symptoms and treatment of various medical diseases. *Swiss Med. Weekly* 134: 543–551.

Mathru, M., Esch, O., Lang, J. *et al.* 1996, Magnetic resonance imaging of the upper airway: effects of propofol anesthesia and nasal continuous positive airway pressure in humans. *Anesthesiology* 84(2): 273–279.

McMillan, F.D. 2003, Maximising quality of life in ill animals. *J. Am. Anim. Hosp. Assoc.* 39: 227–234.

McNicholas, W.T., Ryan, S. 2006, Obstructive sleep apnoea syndrome: translating science to clinical practice. *Respirology* 11: 136–144.

Mehta, S., Jay, G.D., Woolard, L. *et al.* 1997, Randomized, prospective trial of bilevel versus continuous positive airway pressure in acute pulmonary edema. *Crit. Care Med.* 25(4): 620–628.

Miller, R.F., Semple, S. 1991, Continuous positive airway pressure ventilation for respiratory failure associated with Pneumocystis carinii pneumonia. *Respir. Med.* 85(2): 133–138.

Mlacnik, E., Bockstahler, B., Muller, M. *et al.* 2006, Effects of caloric restriction and a moderate or intense physiotherapy program for treatment of lameness in overweight dogs with osteoarthritis. *J. Am. Vet. Med. Assoc.* 229(11): 1756–1760.

Monk, M.L., Preston, C.A., McGowan, C.M. 2006, Effects of early intensive postoperative physiotherapy on limb function after tibial plateau leveling osteotomy in dogs with deficiency of the cranial cruciate ligament. *Am. J. Vet. Res.* 67(3): 529–536.

Monnet, E. 2003, Brachycephalic airway syndrome. In: Slatter, D.H. (ed), *Textbook of Small Animal Surgery*. W.B. Saunders, St Louis, MO, pp. 808–813.

Morton, C.M., Reid, J., Scott, E. *et al.* 2005, Application of a scaling model to establish and validate an interval level pain scale for assessment of acute pain in dogs. *Am. J. Vet. Res.* 66(12): 2154–2166.

Nakano, T., Ochi, T., Ito, N., Cahalin, L.P. 2003, Breathing assist techniques from Japan. *Cardiopul. Phys. Ther.* 14(2): 19–23.

Naughton, M.T., Liu, P., Bernard, D. *et al.* 1995, Treatment of congestive heart failure and cheyne-stokes respiration during sleep by continuous positive airway pressure. *Am. J. Respir. Crit. Care Med.* 151: 92–97.

Nicholson, H.L. 2008 Physiotherapy in the canine intensive care setting: with focus on the effects of recumbency, the post-operative management of dogs with brachycephalic airway obstructive syndrome, and aspiration pneumonia following tick (Ixodes holocyclus) poisoning. Doctoral thesis, University of Queensland, Australia. Retrieved from http://espace.library.uq.edu.au/view/UQ:179224

Nout, Y.S., Reed, S.M. 2005, Management and treatment of the recumbent horse. *Equine Vet. Educ.* 17(6): 324–336.

Pang, D., Keenan, S., Cook, D. *et al.* 1998, The effect of positive pressure airway support on mortality and the need for intubation in cardiogenic pulmonary edema: a systematic review. *Chest* 114(4): 1185–1192.

Pare, P.D., Warriner, B., Baile, E. *et al.* 1983, Redistribution of pulmonary extravascular water with positive end-expiratory pressure in canine pulmonary edema. *Am. Rev. Respir. Dis.* 127(5): 590–593.

Perel, A., Downs, J., Crawford, C. *et al.* 1983, Continuous positive airway pressure improves oxygenation in dogs after the aspiration of blood. *Crit. Care Med.* 11(11): 868–871.

Platt, S.R., Olby, N.J. 2004, *BSAVA Manual of Canine and Feline Neurology*. British Small Animal Veterinary Association, Quedgeley, UK, pp. 243–247.

Provet.co.uk 2008, Metaldehyde.

Pryor, J.A. 1999, Physiotherapy for airway clearance in adults. *Eur. Respir. J.* 14: 1418–1424.

Pryor, J.A., Prasad, S.A. 2002, *Physiotherapy for Respiratory and Cardiac Problems*, 4th edn. Churchill Livingstone, London.

Pryor, J.A., Webber, B.A., Hodson, M.E. 1990, Effect of chest physiotherapy on oxygen saturation in patients with cystic fibrosis. *Thorax* 45(1): 77.

Pryor, J.A., Webber, B.A., Hodson, M.E., Warner, J.O. 1994, The flutter VRP1 as an adjunct to chest physiotherapy in cystic fibrosis. *Respir. Med.* 88(9): 677–681.

Rasanen, J., Heikkila, J., Downs, J. *et al.* 1985, Continuous positive airway pressure by face mask in acute cardiogenic pulmonary edema. *Am. J. Cardiol.* 55: 296–300.

Regan, K., Kleinfeld, M.E., Erik, P.C. 1990, Physical therapy for patients with abdominal or thoracic surgery. In: Irwin, S., Tecklin, J.S. (eds), *Cardiopulmonary Physical Therapy*, 2nd edn. C.V. Mosby, St Louis, MO, pp. 323–350.

Ricksten, S.E., Bengtsson, A., Soderberg, C. *et al.* 1986, Effects of periodic positive airway pressure by mask on postoperative pulmonary function. *Chest* 89(6): 774–781.

Road, J.D., Leevers, A. 1990, Inspiratory and expiratory muscle function during continuous positive airway pressure in dogs. *J. Appl. Physiol.* 68(3): 1092–1100.

Scott, A., Hill, A.E., Chakrabarti, M.K., Carruthers, B. 1978, A comparison of the cardiorespiratory effects of continuous positive airway pressure breathing and continuous positive pressure ventilation in dogs. *Br. J. Anaesth.* 50: 331–338.

Shade, E., Kawagoe, Y., Brower, R.G., Permutt, S., Fessler, H.E. 1994, Effects of hyperinflation and CPAP on work of breathing and respiratory failure in dogs. *J. Appl. Physiol.* 77(2): 819–827.

Sherwood, L. 1993, *Human Physiology: from cells to systems*. West Publishing Company, St Paul, MN.

Shumway, R. 2007, Rehabilitation in the first 48 hours after surgery. *Clin. Techn. Small Anim. Pract.* 22(4): 166–170.

Smidt, N., de Vet, H.C., Bouter, L.M. *et al.* 2005, Effectiveness of exercise therapy: a best-evidence summary of systematic reviews. *Aust. J. Physiother.* 51(2): 71–85.

Stock, M.C., Downs, J., Gauer, P. *et al.* 1985, Prevention of postoperative pulmonary complications with CPAP, incentive spirometry, and conservative therapy. *Chest* 87(2): 151–157.

Stone, B.F. 1988, Tick paralysis, particularly involving Ixodes holocyclus and other Ixodes species. *Adv. Dis. Vector Res.* 5: 61–85.

Stone, B.F., Neish, A.L., Wright, I.G. 1983, Tick (*Ixodes holocyclus*) paralysis in the dog: quantitative studies on immunity following artifical infestation with the tick. *Aust. Vet. J.* 60(3): 65–68.

Wiseman-Orr, M.L., Scott, M., Reid, J. *et al.* 2006, Validation of a structured questionnaire as an instrument to measure chronic pain in dogs on the basis of effects on health-related quality of life. *Am. J. Vet. Res.* 67(11): 1826–1836.

Wojciechowska, J.I., Hewson, C., Stryhn, H. *et al.* 2005, Development of a discriminative questionnaire to assess nonphysical aspects of quality of life of dogs. *Am. J. Vet. Res.* 66(8): 1453–1460.

Wong, W.P., Paratz, J.D., Wilson, K., Burns, Y.R. 2003, Hemodynamic and ventilatory effects of manual respiratory physiotherapy techniques of chest clapping, vibration, and shaking in an animal model. *J. Appl. Physiol.* 95: 991–998.

Wykes, P.M. 1991, Brachycephalic airway obstructive syndrome. *Probl. Vet. Med.* 3(2): 188–197.

Wysocki, M., Antonelli, M. 2001, Noninvasive mechanical ventilation in acute hypoxaemic respiratory failure. *Eur. Respir. J.* 18: 209–220.

Yas-Natan, E., Segev, G., Aroch, I. 2007, Clinical, neurological and clinicopathological signs, treatment and outcome of metaldehyde intoxication in 18 dogs. *J. Small Anim. Pract.* 48(8): 438–443.

Xu, F.S., Zhou, Z., Zhang, X. *et al.* 2003, [Effects of a novel CPAP device on breathing and blood gases in newborns with pneumonia]. *Zhonghua Erke Zazhi* [*Chinese Journal of Pediatrics*] 41(10): 782–784.

CHAPTER 17

Small animal treatment and rehabilitation for neurological conditions*

Heli Hyytiäinen
Veterinary Teaching Hospital, University of Helsinki, Finland

Summary

Physiotherapy has gained a prominent position as part of treatment of small animals with neurological disease. This chapter introduces basic principles of neurological physiotherapy, and the application to small animals. Both a clinical approach and current evidence base for physiotherapy intervention are presented, aiming to provide the reader with an inclusive general view on the topic.

17.1 Introduction

Neurological rehabilitation is one of the largest areas of animal physiotherapy, especially in small animals. There are several factors in animal physiotherapy that are more important than in human neurological physiotherapy that should be considered at all times. In particular are cost and time used in treatment and rehabilitation, and the consideration of the welfare of the animal. In some cases, this may lead to a limitation in treatment options or even the possibility of euthanasia of the animal. Rehabilitation of an animal patient is always a multidisciplinary effort (see also Chapter 9), and the owner of the animal also plays a major role in the physiotherapy process. Owners must be carefully advised throughout the whole process, with discussions about the effort and commitment that rehabilitating their animal requires, and how to manage the ever-changing situation.

Although publications on neurological veterinary physiotherapy are scarce, some still do exist, and many of the methods used in rehabilitating neurological patients are derived from human neurological physiotherapy. The corollary is that many of the methods used in rehabilitating humans originally derived from animal models, with the cat and dog still frequently represented in the basic science literature. However, when wanting to implement human methods for animals, the differences in both the anatomy and the pathologies between species should always be remembered, as well as the effect of behavioural and communication aspects.

---

*Adapted from the first edition section, which was written by Helen Nicholson

---

Animal Physiotherapy: Assessment, Treatment and Rehabilitation of Animals, Second Edition. Edited by Catherine M. McGowan and Lesley Goff.
© 2016 John Wiley & Sons, Ltd. Published 2016 by John Wiley & Sons, Ltd.

17.2 Principles of neurological rehabilitation

Many of the principles of neurological rehabilitation in humans have focused on rehabilitation of the stroke, head or spinal cord-injured patient and/or development or redevelopment of finely adjusted movements and skills characteristic of the pyramidal system, which is the predominant descending upper motor neuron system in the human spinal cord. However, it should be remembered that the pyramidal system in dogs, for example, is far less important and it reduces by half after the cervical spine. This means the focus of neurological rehabilitation should be on functional gait retraining and development of the stereotypical patterns of gait and coarse movements compared with fine movements in humans. The following information on motor learning has been derived from work in humans (Carr & Shepherd 1987; Magill 1989; Marteniuk 1979).

17.2.1 Principles of skill acquisition and the stages of motor control
Phases of motor learning
- Cognitive (elementary) phase: a large number of errors occur with variable performance and slow reaction time. The patient's full attention is required.
- Associative (intermediate) phase: fewer errors occur as components of the task become more integrated and performance becomes more consistent and efficient.
- Autonomous (advanced) phase: movement becomes habitual with fast reaction times. Attention is released for other tasks.

Practice schedules
Motor learning is enhanced by practice schedules that include the following.

Motivation
The use of positive reinforcement and owner involvement keeps motivation levels high in most dogs, although different forms of positive reinforcements work with different patients, such as food rewards; vocal encouragement; familiar toys or fetch items; environmental stimulus or familiarity (outside, grass surfaces, own home); other household animals being present; owner's touch and sensory stimulation (scratching or tickling); smells and sounds. When working with food-motivated but overweight dogs, subtract rewards from daily rations and encourage patients to work for meals to reduce exacerbating the weight problem.

Specificity
Goals must be attainable and appropriate in order for rehabilitation to be effective – discuss treatment goals with the owners from the outset. Break complex tasks into parts, but always include practice of the whole task (with assistance as required to ensure successful performance). Owners must be made aware of the smaller goals or components of the task that make up the larger goal or functional activity. For example, if the dog is able to stand for 1 min with one person's light assistance of the pelvis following a thoracolumbar upper motor neuron disc lesion, this does not mean it is able to coordinate or has the strength to get into standing or walk under its own volition.

Meaningful context
Relevance is important – many dogs find food lures make motor learning exercises meaningful. In people, mental practice alone has been proven to help improve motor performance – it is therefore possible that using familiar verbal commands may help dogs mentally 'rehearse' the commands that they are as yet unable to perform, although this has not been studied objectively.

Contiguity
The patient must be able to perceive the relationship of events that occur together in time – instead of practising exercises in isolation, practise them in sequence. For example, once a tetraplegic dog has lifted the head, assist it into sternal recumbency, sitting and then standing so that the total task gives the dog feedback from the outcome of the initial head lifting task, even if the dog has to be fully supported by a sling in standing.

Reinforcement
To maintain and enhance motivation, the use of positive reinforcement is vital – excited tones of verbal praise and prompt delivery of food or other rewards both help to reinforce that the correct movement has just been performed and encourage the animal to remain motivated.

Feedback
Feedback is essential if skill acquisition is to be maximally enhanced and must be positive and motivating, specific and accurate. Extrinsic feedback – food rewards, verbal praise or luring the dog into position – can provide feedback about the desired position to be attained. Intrinsic feedback is derived from sensory receptors, e.g. tactile input can be used to help provide proprioceptive feedback. Feedback must be instantaneous after each attempt for the animal to understand best what it is that the physiotherapist is trying to teach.

Activation
Try to relate learning to past function, e.g. if a dog habitually trotted preinjury, teach stepping in the same sequence. Reduce distractions to enable selective attention to the task.

Repetition
Repetition of tasks is vital, but the physiotherapist should be aware of rapid development of fatigue in many neurological cases. Fatigue interferes with the performance of a task and the physiotherapist must always aim to work 'to' not 'through' fatigue. Prolonged or too frequent practice sessions do not significantly improve learning. Rest is important and should

be emphasised to overenthusiastic owners. For example, when practising sit to stand with a dog recovering from paresis of its pelvic limbs, have it start by sitting on a block to raise its pelvic position from the ground, thus making the task easier and more repetitions possible. Include rehabilitation exercises designed to improve cardiovascular fitness and discuss the pathophysiology of the diagnosis with the veterinarian to reduce the risk of muscle injury, e.g. delayed-onset muscle soreness occurring as a result of overexertion.

Stages of motor control

Stages of motor control are just as important to small animals as they are to humans.

Mobility

Requires adequate range of motion and motor unit activity to make use of that range of motion.

Stability

Requires ability to co-contract agonist and antagonist muscles to allow maintenance of antigravity weight-bearing postures.

Controlled mobility

Requires at least one of the weight-bearing limbs to be lifted while the animal continues to control posture.

Skill

This is the highest level of motor control and requires proximal stability so that distal body segments can undertake free skilled movement.

17.2.2 Therapeutic approaches to neurological rehabilitation

As for the above information on skill acquisition and the stages of motor control, information on the various therapeutic approaches to neurological rehabilitation is briefly included below to direct the reader to the relevant area of human physiotherapy. The use of a variety of principles from the following approaches is necessary when working with canine patients, to compensate for their inability to speak and perform various key components of movements on command. The reader is encouraged to refer to the cited literature to learn more about specific approaches with respect to central and peripheral neural plasticity along with sensory and motor integration and retraining.

The Bobath approach

The Bobath approach (Bobath 1990) is based on the concept that abnormal posture and movement 'shunt' sensation so that the abnormal patterns begin to feel normal to the patient. Treatment therefore aims to facilitate normal movement and posture so the patient experiences the sensation of normal movement patterns. Selective, isolated control is developed by the reduction of hypertonus, dissociation of mass patterns, avoidance of associated reactions and prevention of effort. Functional skills are built upon selective isolated control.

Bobath techniques include:
- handling of 'key points' (regions of the body where movement is centred or initiated from)
- awareness and active correction of differences between positions and postures
- reflex inhibition of patterns and control of associated reactions
- tapping and joint compression or weight bearing
- accurate feedback
- repetition of normal movement as often as possible throughout the day
- sensorimotor reeducation.

Although none of these techniques has been defined in small animals, it can be seen clinically that some of these techniques may lend themselves better than others to small animal neurological physiotherapy, with great variability expected between individual dogs' and cats' acceptance of these techniques.

The Rood approach

The Rood approach (Rood 1956) is the concept of using very specific sensory stimuli to facilitate specific responses.

Rood advocated the following sensory stimuli.
- Cutaneous – fast brushing, light touch, stroking
- Thermal – ice, warmth
- Proprioception – stretch, tapping, resistance, joint compression
- Labyrinthine – rocking, rolling
- Visual
- Auditory
- Olfactory
- Taste

In the Rood approach, the initial reflex muscular response is used in developmental sequences before being incorporated into purposeful skilled movement. Rood's developmental sequence components can be modified for dogs to include:
- prone (drop)
- sitting
- standing
- walking.

Rood considered feedback and repetition crucial for learning to occur.

Proprioceptive neuromuscular facilitation

Proprioceptive neuromuscular facilitation (PNF) (Voss *et al.* 1985) aims to use specific proprioceptive stimulation to reeducate the neuromuscular system. The spiral and diagonal movement patterns used in PNF are considered to be characteristic of mature movement.

Specific PNF techniques include the following.
- Hold relax – an isometric contraction of the muscle limiting motion.
- Contract relax – a concentric contraction of the muscle limiting motion.
- Slow reversal – alternating slow rhythmical concentric isotonic contraction of first the agonist then the antagonist muscle.

- Rhythmic stabilisation – uses simultaneous isometric contraction of agonist and antagonist to encourage co-contraction, stability or even relaxation. Clinically, this tends to be the easiest technique used with dogs, working with the obedience command 'stay'; the technique can be progressed from four-point stance to three- and then diagonal two-point stance.

The Brunnstrom approach

Brunnstrom advocated that movement recovery occurs through six successive stages (Sawner 1992).

1 Flaccidity.
2 Synergies developing with increasing spasticity.
3 Synergies performed voluntarily with spasticity at its peak.
4 Some movement out of synergy as spasticity decreases.
5 Independence from basic synergies develops as spasticity decreases further.
6 Isolated coordinated movements performed at will.

In early treatment with the Brunnstrom approach, synergies are facilitated through the use of postural reactions and proprioceptive and other stimuli as precursors to normal movement. A clinical example of this application is for a dog with a central lumbar disc herniation and postsurgical bilateral pelvic limb flaccid paresis: with the dog supported in standing, the head can be lured to one side with a food treat, stimulating the asymmetrical tonic neck reflex, which increases the extensor tone of the ipsilateral limbs and the flexor tone of the contralateral limbs. By alternating food treats to the left and right, the physiotherapist stimulates the precursors of normal extension tone for stance phase and flexion tone of swing phase of gait.

The motor relearning programme

Carr and Shepherd have turned the focus of the inductive neurofacilitation models developed by Bobath, Brunnstrom and colleagues towards the deductive motor relearning model. In a motor relearning programme for stroke (Carr & Shepherd 1992), the (human) patient's performance is compared with normal movement, based upon knowledge of the essential components of that task. The physiotherapist then assists the patient to activate the required muscles and practise so that selective control over those muscles is improved. The physiotherapist teaches the patient how to perform that motor task while concentrating on those task components that are both critical to the successful performance of the task and difficult to perform. The patient is therefore encouraged to become an active learner and problem solver and as such, one might expect difficulties in applying this cognitive strategy to dogs. In practice, however, most dogs are easily motivated and easily taught a motor skill in much the same way that positive reinforcement, shaping and operant conditioning are used to teach puppies the basic motor tasks of 'sit', 'drop', 'come' and 'stay'. Clinically, it has, however, often been the case that dogs that have previously been taught motor tasks, such as the basic obedience commands, adapt more easily to the motor relearning approach.

17.3 Physiotherapy for small animals with neurological disease

After neurological insult, spontaneous recovery of function may occur as a result of reduction in swelling or reabsorption of haemorrhage, due to remyelination in the case of demyelinating disorders or due to collateral circulation in the case of infarcts (Stephenson 1993). Alternatively, neuroplasticity, defined as the reorganisation or adaptation of neural tissue after insult, and Wallerian degeneration, via regeneration of axons or dendrites, the collateral sprouting of remaining nerve fibres or the unmasking of latent synapses, may be responsible for recovery (de Lahunta 1983). Physiotherapy therefore aims to take advantage of spontaneous recovery; manipulate neuroplasticity to assist functional return; prevent or minimise complications; and implement compensatory strategies when poor prognosis results in the threat of euthanasia.

17.3.1 Potential indications for physiotherapy in neurological small animal patient

Potential indications for neurological physiotherapy include the following.

- Spinal cord disease, cervical, thoracolumbar and cauda equine, e.g. caudal cervical vertebral malformation (CCVM), Hansen's type I and type II intervertebral disc disease, fibrocartilaginous embolism, chronic degenerative radicular myelopathy (CDRM), inflammatory diseases involving central nervous system, and neurological signs related to surgical treatment of dermoid sinus.
- Peripheral nerve disease, e.g. traumatic peripheral nerve paralysis.
- Generalised neuromuscular disease, e.g. polymyositis, tick paralysis, polyradiculoneuritis (also known as 'coonhound paralysis'), tetanus.
- Cranial nerve disease, e.g. trigeminal neuralgia, facial nerve dysfunction, which may be localised after tick poisoning, traumatic vestibular disease or post surgical, e.g. after ear canal ablation.
- Vestibular disease.
- Pain.

The approach to neurological small animal patients should be based on an understanding of layered factors, primarily the localisation of the lesion and therefore therapy based on either upper or lower motor neuron signs. The phases of rehabilitation alter according to the patient's functional and neurological status; whether the animal is plegic with no deep pain sensation, plegic with deep pain sensation, paretic non-ambulatory, paretic ambulatory or normal. Functionally, there are descriptive substages to these, for example ambulatory supported, facilitated, with strong/mild assistance, etc. Other aspects affecting therapy are whether the patient is in the acute or chronic phase, an inpatient or outpatient, and whether surgically or conservatively treated.

17.3.2 Therapy methods in neurological small animal physiotherapy

Therapy methods commonly used in small animal neurological therapy include active therapeutic exercises (including the previously mentioned basic principles), passive range of motion (PROM), massage, and in some cases electrical muscle stimulation (NMES). Another important part of therapy is the therapeutic handling, and breed typical and functional positioning during resting periods.

Frequently, aggressive physiotherapy is introduced at the beginning of the neurological episode, usually starting from the first day postoperatively. Therapy is commenced several times per day by the therapist for the hospitalised patient, and by either the therapist or the owner for the outpatient. Therapy is often performed in various forms, in short periods at a time, according to the character of the disease or injury and the endurance level of the dog, with emphasis on quality of the movement during the exercises.

The exercises are progressive in nature, changing continuously according to the level of patient rehabilitation. Functionality is of the essence, and is taken into account in every stage of the combined actions, as well as in all positions – lying, sitting, standing, during walking – and other gaits, activities of daily living as well as working or sporting tasks.

17.3.3 Measuring the level of rehabilitation and outcome of therapy

As in any field of physiotherapy, measuring the effect of our interventions and the status of the patient is important. Especially so with the neurological patient, where the progression of rehabilitation is of the utmost importance, as euthanasia is often an option for these patients, especially if the progression is slow or if severe relapses occur. Also, since visits to the veterinarian tend to become less frequent as time progresses after the original insult, but regular physiotherapy rehabilitation can persist for months, it can be the physiotherapist who has the first opportunity to notice causes for concern (red flags). Reevaluation is important, as problems or set-backs in a rehabilitation programme can be detected, and the animal promptly referred back to the veterinarian. It should be ensured that if the patient no longer fits the pattern of the condition they were referred for, urgent veterinary review is sought.

The results of therapy and treatment outcome should be quantified with reliable and valid evaluation methods (see also Chapter 22). There are several validated evaluation methods that have been used to evaluate the functionality of dogs with neurological dysfunctions. In 2001 Olby *et al.* presented a reliability tested hindlimb functional scoring system for dogs with acute spinal cord injuries. In this method, the recovery was divided into five stages, which are further divided into 14 subdivisions based on recovery patterns (Olby *et al.* 2001). Another method of evaluation for neurological patients is the Texas Spinal Cord Injury Score, giving a numerical score (0–10 per limb) on gait, postural reactions and nociception of the limbs (Levine *et al.* 2009).

In addition, the Finnish neurological function test battery (FINFUN) has been validated and reliability tested to be used for evaluating the functional level of neurological canine patients (Boström *et al.* 2014). The testing battery evaluates functional tasks other than walking, such as position changes, different gaits and ambulating on stairs. It consists of 11 items, and provides a numerical score ranging between 0 and 44.

Pain can be an important part of the clinical signs and responses of neurological patients, and there are several methods used to evaluate pain in small animals; however, none of them has been validated specifically for neurological patients. Quality of life has been suggested to be measured through a weighted owner questionnaire, in the case of spinal cord-injured dogs (Budke *et al.* 2008). The score in such an owner-assigned questionnaire system is higher in ambulatory than in non-ambulatory dogs (Levine *et al.* 2008) and, as such, may be a useful outcome measure.

17.3.4 Assistive aids

Various versions of several different assistive aids from external prosthesis to orthosis and carts are available, especially for dogs. Providing and advising on appropriate assistive aids for the neurologically dysfunctional patient is one aspect of physiotherapy services. It should be emphasised that to ensure ethical and appropriate use of equipment, acquiring such aids should only be contemplated after a veterinary evaluation of the animal's condition. It is of the utmost importance that assistive aids are used only if it is acceptable to both the veterinarian and physiotherapist. It must be emphasised that the primary criterion for acquiring such devices is that the animal is pain free either due to the equipment or despite the equipment.

In addition to providing the animal with a method of ambulating, assistive aids also take into account the owner's ergonomics whilst handling a neurologically dysfunctional animal. For example, with a paraplegic giant sized dog, a cart can save the owner from carrying the dog's hind part around, therefore effectively saving the owner's musculoskeletal system from a lot of unnecessary stress.

When the acquiring of assistive aid is considered, some basic factors should be taken into account, such as the living environment of the animal (e.g. stairs in the house, block house with no lift, house in the forest), and the owner's ability to use the aid. The fit of the assistive aid should be under constant supervision as ill-fitting equipment is more of a hazard for further injuries rather than a help. Also the owner needs to be trained about the equipment and its use very carefully.

- Owners need to be able to 'read' their dogs in carts, in order to recognise when the dog is tired, and needs to be taken from the cart as they cannot lie down with it.
- Carts should be custom made for each dog, and fitted carefully to avoid secondary injuries due to cart use.
- It is important to carefully check skin and soft tissues daily for any pressure or friction injuries.

- Limb range of motion needs to be uninhibited enough for the dog to get into and out of, as well as use, the cart.
- As the dog's musculoskeletal system changes (for example, via atrophy, gaining or losing weight, contractures), the cart's fit needs to be constantly reevaluated.

17.3.5 Problems related to neurological patients

Skin lesions in affected limbs must be rapidly detected and treated. In the case of a low arc in the swing phase of gait due to neurological deficits, the animal may drag its toes to the degree that either a nail or the skin gets injured, and this may cause several problems for physiotherapy. Risk of infection may limit therapy options (hydrotherapy may be contraindicated due to hygiene issues) and, of course, possible pain due to the lesion may require suspension of the rehabilitation programme. Therefore, skin health should always be closely monitored, and owners instructed to take necessary measures to prevent such lesions from occurring, by using appropriate protective gear, such as taping, bandaging or boots.

Skin care and lesion prevention are also important if the patient is recumbent. Soft, possibly heat- or pressure-reactive material bedding and frequent position changes and mobilisation should be provided, to avoid any bedsores. Constant monitoring of the surgery site is also important; any signs of infection in the area should be acted upon immediately.

A urinary tract infection in a neurological patient is a medical emergency and veterinary treatment should not be delayed under any circumstances. It is not uncommon for animals to be discharged from hospital before developing full bladder control and owners may not be able to competently manage their bladder care at home. Owners often confuse overflow incontinence and voluntary urinating. The physiotherapist should evaluate the bladder function during therapy sessions. If any problems are noted, the dog needs to be referred to the treating veterinarian immediately. Incontinence is also a common issue with neurological patients, and may cause significant burden to the life of the dog and the owner (Olby *et al.* 2003).

The weight of the dog and deep pain sensation have both been reported to have a significant impact on the prognosis of dogs with intervertebral disc disease (Bull *et al.* 2008). Weight, along with age, has also been shown to affect the speed of recovery to ambulation in dogs with thoracolumbar spinal cord injury (Olby *et al.* 2003). Hence, obesity is a serious problem in rehabilitation of neurological patients. Also, as part of a long-term rehabilitation plan for neurological patients, secondary issues should be taken into account, such as spondylosis or spondyloarthrosis at the site of removed intervertebral disc (Bull *et al.* 2008). Another example might include biceps tendinitis in a paraplegic patient that overloads the front limbs, or some underlying musculoskeletal issues, provoked by the ambulation-related compensatory systems of a neurological patient. The possibility of overlapping signs of orthopaedic and neurological issues should never be overlooked.

The mental status of the patient should always be taken into account. In particular, the acute phase of the neurological episode may be challenging for the animal, due to possible pain, medication, hospitalisation, limited motion or separation from family and pack. Mental status should be supported as much as possible, by frequent owner visits at the hospital, familiar food and toys, and home visitation during weekends if possible.

Costs of treatment and rehabilitation are often high, and should be made clear to the owner at all times, as it may affect the therapy plan through time limits set for the rehabilitation. However, it should also be clear that in most neurological cases physiotherapy needs to be aggressive, especially in the early stages of the episode. Many patients require hospitalisation, where physiotherapy can be provided several times per day for short periods at a time, or the patient can be taken into rehabilitation units for a day for the purpose. However, if there are financial restraints, therapy can also be performed using a home-based approach, through careful instructions from the physiotherapists based on regular reevaluation. If the owners are well informed about the demands of home care of a paraplegic dog and are dedicated to the task, home care will be successful, and owners can manage with a paraplegic dog at the home environment (Bauer *et al.* 1992).

17.4 Current evidence base for neurological small animal physiotherapy

Currently physiotherapy is considered as an important part of the treatment in small animal neurological patients, such as dogs with intervertebral disc disease (Bach *et al.* 2014). Although intervertebral disc disease may be one of the most common reasons for a dog to be referred for physiotherapy, reports of other diseases involving various types of physiotherapy also do exist. For example, physiotherapy consisting of passive range of motion exercises, neuromuscular stimulation and functional weight-bearing exercises as part of treatment in a case of a traumatic cervical myelopathy dog has been reported (Smarick *et al.* 2007).

Early physiotherapy has been shown to be beneficial for the recovery rate in dogs with fibrocartilaginous embolism (Gandini *et al.* 2003). Physiotherapy in this report consisted of joint passive range of motion, massage, positional exercises, electrical stimulation, physiological positions, gait training with support and hydrotherapy. The effect of intensive physiotherapy on the survival time of dogs with suspected degenerative myelopathy (DM) is also signifigant (Kathman *et al.* 2006). Dogs who received intensive physiotherapy had almost double the survival time (255 days) of dogs that received a moderate physiotherapy protocol (130 days). Also the time that the dogs remained ambulatory was longer in those receiving intensive therapy. When DM dogs with an intensive therapy programme were compared to dogs who received no physiotherapy, the difference in survival time was 200 days. The physiotherapy administered in this study consisted of various active therapeutic exercises, passive joint range of motion exercises, massage and hydrotherapy (either walking in water or swimming) (Kathman *et al.* 2006). A rehabilitation programme with an intensity of approximately one session during 6 weeks for dogs with thoracolumbar intervertebral disc disease and surgical treatment (hemilaminectomy) has also been described (Ruddle *et al.* 2006). The programme consisted of varying protocols including balance, range of motion and strengthening exercises as well as hydrotherapy (swimming or underwater treadmill). As a result, 17 out of 22 preoperatively non-ambulatory paraparetic dogs with or without deep pain sensation were rehabilitated to be ambulatory (Ruddle *et al.* 2006).

Although most of the techniques used in small animal neurological physiotherapy are not yet studied, some are. For example, global postural techniques in dogs with both orthopaedic and neurological issues have been reported, and suggested to be beneficial when used as part of therapy (Vallani *et al.* 2004). Techniques used consist of coordination, static-dynamic and functional balance exercises, which are done in a manner of normal movements, based on the action-repetition principle, always putting emphasis on correct postural and motor patterns during the exercises (Vallani *et al.* 2004). Posture and its relation to lesion type has been studied in rabbits (Lyalka 2009; Lyalka *et al.* 2005). Both postural corrective movements and body control as well as the hindlimb postural control decrease distal to spinal cord lesions, and depending on the lesion type and severity, postural reflexes may be restored but the limb and trunk configuration not (Lyalka 2009; Lyalka *et al.* 2005).

Another, more thoroughly studied therapy method is hydrotherapy. Non-weight-bearing performance in water, swimming, is considered to be a good therapy method as it results in large step repetition amounts with high frequency. Swimming as an exercise method has been shown to improve hindlimb function in rats with a contusion injury at the caudal thoracic spine, in comparison to rats with similar injury and no training (Smith *et al.* 2006). The importance of sensory feedback and cutaneous afferent feedback in therapeutic training is emphasised in several studies (Kuerzi *et al.* 2010; Rossignol *et al.* 2004; Smith *et al.* 2006), hence manual facilitation as part of hydrotherapy of the neurological patients should always be taken into account.

One of the most important benefits of water in neurological rehabilitation is the buoyancy. Partial unloading has been shown to be beneficial in activating spinal locomotor centres in cats with complete and incomplete paraplegia (Dietz *et al.* 1997; Kuerzi *et al.* 2010). The ability of rats with moderate thoracic spinal cord contusion to bear their own bodyweight has been shown to decrease, although the lesion does not affect the capacity for movement pattern generation. In cases of more severe contusion, the animals also lose the locomotor pattern generation ability (Kuerzi *et al.* 2010). However, the training effect in water may not be functional as such, as although the effect is seen while walking in water, in locomotion on dry land there may be no effect. This has been shown to be the case in spinal cord-injured rats (Kuerzi *et al.* 2010). Training rats with severe but incomplete caudal thoracic spinal cord contusion partially supported on a dry treadmill for a period of time results in partial weight-bearing steps, and patterns of movements restored close to normal in comparison to untrained animals. The untrained animals can also produce movements, but the step cycle's trajectories are not as fine-tuned and controlled as in trained animals (Heng & de Leon 2009).

The repetitive activation of selected neural pathways in the spinal cord, i.e. training specific motor learning, be it stepping or standing, is an important part of neurological rehabilitation (de Leon *et al.* 1998a). When cats with spinal cord injury were studied, weight bearing of both trained and untrained cats recovered to pretrauma level, although the cats that were trained were able to stand five times longer than the cats with no training. In addition, unilateral training resulted in unilateral results in standing performance (de Leon *et al.* 1998a).

When step training was performed by cats with spinal injury, it was shown that trained cats performed three times better than the untrained, spontaneously recovered cats, when measured by the amplitude of electromyographic bursts of certain muscles, the amount of extension during stride, and in the arch of swing phase (de Leon *et al.* 1998b). The emphasis of functional adaptations in response to training has been stated in relation to step training. Training activates appropriate neurons, and may reinforce the function of extant sensorimotor pathways (de Leon *et al.* 1998b). Locomotion recovery of the hindlimbs in a moving treadmill in cats with caudal thoracic spine spinalisation has been reported (Rossignol *et al.* 2004).

The ceiling effect has also been discussed in animal studies; it is mentioned as a limiting factor for the training effect in cases of rats with spinal cord injury. With rats, the animal's spontaneous movement in cage has been mentioned as a part of 'training' and the effect of training possibly being limited due to the ceiling effect (Kuerzi *et al.* 2010).

17.5 Physiotherapy for horses with neurological disease

Today referrals to physiotherapy for neurological equine patients are not rare. The variety of disease or neurology-based dysfunction is wide, from monoparetic radial paresis to ataxic cervical vertebral malformation and tetraplegic tetanus patients. The same principles apply as for small animal neurology. However, obviously, due to the size and handleability of the patients, many therapy methods used in humans or small animals can only be used in small foals or only to an extent with adult horses, although many of the methods can be adjusted accordingly (Mykkänen *et al.* 2011). An example might be the idea of a walking frame/cart modified to a 'foal-walker', built for a foal rehabilitating from tetanus (Figure 17.1).

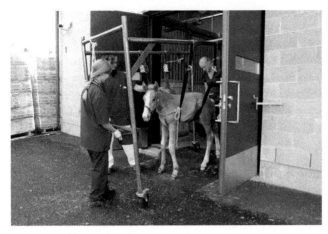

Figure 17.1 Modified walking frame/cart used as a 'foal-walker', built for a foal rehabilitating from tetanus.

For a physiotherapist, it is important to recognise the neurological signs when they are present (see Chapter 10). One should be aware of species differences in the presentation of signs. Safety is a big issue with neurological horse patients. It is critically important to maintain close communication with the treating veterinarian with regard to the status of the patient, and any possible changes in it. Safety has to come first when planning rehabilitation programmes for these patients, and when instructing the owner, for example about whether the horse is safe to ride or not, and what type of work can be done with the horse. A few case reports relating to horses with neurological disease and their physiotherapy have been published (Gracia Calvo *et al.* 2011; Mykkänen *et al.* 2011).

17.6 Case studies

17.6.1 Case 1

Signalment: Irish Wolfhound, male, 4 years old, 80 kg.

Veterinary diagnosis: fibrocartilaginous embolism, non-ambulatory paraparesis, right hindlimb paretic, left hindlimb plegic. Deep pain sensation intact bilaterally. Referral to physiotherapy within 24 h from the onset of clinical signs.

Physiotherapy assessment: functional problems: unable to get up from lying or from sitting position, unable to stand without support. Remained in lateral recumbency with no voluntary movements in left hindlimb, voluntary movements in right hindlimb. Needs two people to assist in standing.

The inpatient phase lasted for 11 days. Physiotherapy treatment 2–6 times per day for nine of the 11 days.

- Passive range of motion exercises to maintain the range in the joints and soft tissues of the left hindlimb, and to stimulate muscle activity.
- Manual stimulation of the left hindlimb: brushing, tapping, scratching – both in passive state and functionally during walking or sitting or lying positions.

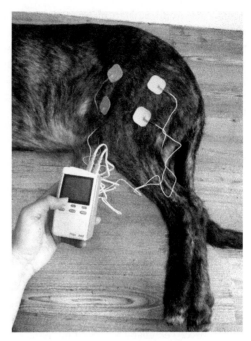

Figure 17.2 Neuromuscular electrical muscle stimulation of quadriceps, biceps femoris and tibialis cranialis of Irish Wolfhound with fibrocartilaginous embolism and paraparesis.

- Neuromuscular electrical muscle stimulation (30 Hz/300 msec $1^{\text{contract}}/3^{\text{relax}}$) in quadriceps, biceps femoris and tibialis cranialis daily during the first 4 days (Figure 17.2).
- Positioning during resting periods in breed-typical, functional positions.
- Weight-bearing exercises in different positions: lying, sitting, standing, walking.
- Functional exercises to teach the dog techniques of getting up and down from lying to sitting, sitting to standing, etc.
- Walking exercise with weight supported in any amount needed, including also manual assistance and facilitation of the left hindlimb.
- Massage of the back muscles which had tensed up by the eighth day of hospitalisation, corresponding to an increase in independent mobility (and with that the secondary muscle splinting at the same time).
- Amount of repetitions, times or intensity of each method used varied, and depended on the current situation and status of the dog at the time, including his attitude, behaviour and levels of fatigue. Constant reevaluation of functional ability and response to physiotherapy was undertaken.

By the third day from the onset of the clinical signs, there were clear voluntary movements in the left hindlimb. However, functionally, there remained the problems in the left hindlimb of overknuckling, inability to protract sufficiently with high enough swing arch, as well as an inability to bear weight on the limb. The dog still needed support and manual assistance of two people when walking.

By the sixth day from the start of physiotherapy, the dog was able to get up independently from lying and sitting positions with verbal reinforcement and needed only minor weight-bearing support when walking. He still needed strong manual assistance in the movement of the left hindlimb when walking.

Other issues to be noted during the hospitalised rehabilitation period included the following.

- A urinary catheter was set immediately at the initial contact and it remained through the whole inpatient period.
- Due to the size and immobility of the dog, a soft bedding was provided at all times to prevent pressure sores.
- A set of 'carrying pants' was used, and at some point the skin around the penis was irritated due to pressure from the pants. Attention was paid to the use of the assistive aid, and skin was treated appropriately.
- Nursing was rehabilitative in nature, based on instructions by the physiotherapists.
- Special attention was paid to the ergonomic aspects of the people treating and taking care of the dog, due to its size and level of independent mobility.
- Assistive aids used: Theraband to aid left hindlimb clearance during swing and protraction (Figure 17.3), or manual pull with a bandage material set the same way. Carrying pants to provide for weight-bearing support and ensure safe mobility during the whole inpatient period.

The dog was discharged on the 12th day after the onset of clinical signs. By this time, the dog did not need weight-bearing support but for safety reasons the owner was instructed to use a minimal, assuring support just in case of sudden falling or other unexpected situation when walking. The dog was fully able to perform independently all position changes, but it still needed some facilitation of the left hindlimb through a pulley system built of Theraband.

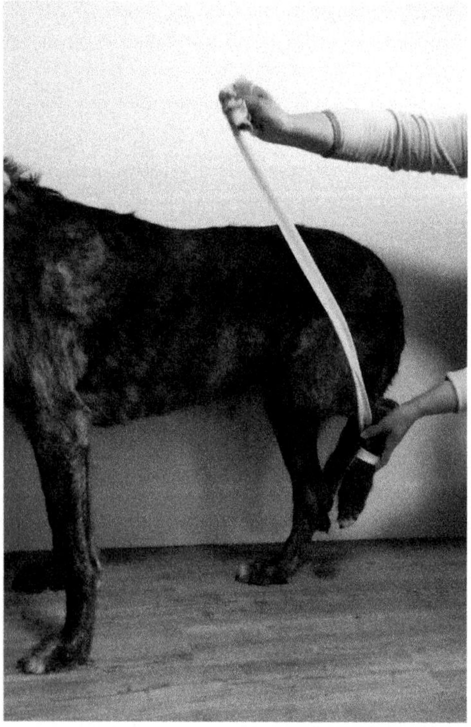

Rehabilitation was continued at home by the owner, based on the instructions received from the physiotherapists at discharge, including the following.

- Controlling the dog's home environment: no slippery surfaces, no stairs or other obstacles, no playing with other dogs or high-impact exercises until he is functional and confident with his movement.
- Ensuring the dog did not gain weight.
- Walking exercises: walking with a Theraband tied from his harness to the left hindlimb, or held by the owner to assist protraction and slightly resist retraction, and to provide clearance to the swing phase.
- Standing; weight shift and weight-bearing exercises.
- Sitting and sit to stand exercises.
- Lying exercises.
- Passive range of motion exercises to the left hindlimb.
- Activation of the left hindlimb through the flexor reflex.
- The owner was instructed about the correct amount of weight-bearing support and left hindlimb manual assistance.

After 3 days at home, the owner reported that the support for walking was no longer required, only the manual facilitation of the left hindlimb was still needed. After 3–4 weeks following discharge, the pulley system in the left hindlimb at home environment was no longer needed except for on longer walks in rough terrain. After 2 months, the dog was fully independently mobile.

After 3 years, the dog was still pain free, fully functional and independently mobile with a high quality of life and no ambulatory limitations (Figure 17.4). The owner reported that the affected limb developed fatigue following prolonged high-level

Figure 17.3 Theraband being used to aid left hindlimb clearance during swing and protraction for Irish Wolfhound with fibrocartilaginous embolism.

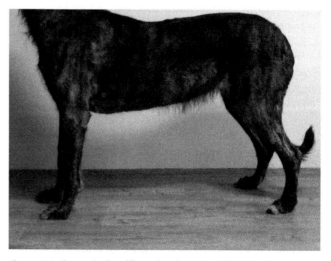

Figure 17.4 Case 1. Irish wolfhound, male, 4 years old, 80 kg, 3 years post fibrocartilaginous embolism showing a balanced stance.

physical exercise, and sometimes following such activities a soft bandage support was used. Fatigue was quickly resolved by the dog sitting in a good position, so could be managed by owner.

17.6.2 Case 2

Signalment: American Bulldog, female, 2.5 years old, 31.5 kg.

History: fell down a cliff, after which she was hit by at least one car on a highway.

Veterinary diagnosis: brachial plexus injury. Left front limb monoplegia, no deep pain sensation. Mild neurological deficits in right forelimb (resolved to normal within a week). Prognosis for the left forelimb motor function recovery hopeless, as no deep pain sensation at all.

Treatment choices: left forelimb amputation or physiotherapy.

The owner chose physiotherapy. Due to the poor prognosis, the aim of therapy and treatment was not the full recovery of the motor function, but management of situation.

Physiotherapy started at the third day after the trauma. During the following 3 months, there were eight physiotherapy visits. The amount of physiotherapy was limited due to the owner's life situation and logistical reasons. The dog also received acupuncture treatment performed by a veterinarian.

Physiotherapy plan
Acute phase

- Neuromuscular electrical stimulation (NMES) to activate the muscles in the left scapular area (supraspinatus, infraspinatus, triceps, deltoideus, biceps, extensor carpi radialis, extensors of the carpus); the owner was instructed in the use of the NMES equipment and the equipment was loaned to the owner to be used independently at home daily.
- Mobilisation (massage and stretching) of the soft tissues due to overload in the intact three quarters and back.
- Cold therapy of the left front quarter scapular, thoracic and chest area (mm. trapezius pars thoracica, rhomboids area) due to acute soft tissue injury-related swelling and pain.
- Positional treatment at all positions to the left front limb.
- Sensory stimulation of the left front limb: brushing, tickling, petting, tapping.
- Environment control: limit trauma possibilities by eliminating other dogs, slippery surfaces, any levels where the dog may fall from, stairs, etc. from the dog's environment.
- Instructions for restricted movement.
- Preparation for weight control as mobility level suddenly limited.
- Instructions for the owner regarding proper ergonomics, as the dog needs to be supported from her harness when moving about.

Subacute and chronic phase

- Weight-bearing exercises.
- Stretching and mobilisation of the joints and soft tissues involved with the carpus and distal joints to prevent contractures.
- Proprioceptive taping on the proximal limb area, stabilising taping to the carpus. (Neither of the two were feasible in the home environment and therefore were not used continuously.)
- Supportive bandaging for the carpus.
- As the limb was flaccid, it was at constant risk of further injury and also inhibited the dog's mobility to an extent. Therefore, a sling was built to stabilise the limb to as physiological a position as possible and fixed to the body.
- After 2 months, a contracture had developed to the distal parts of the left forelimb, especially in the carpus. Underwater treadmill was added to the programme.

Follow-up

After 3 months, the rehabilitation was continued by the owner through swimming and home exercises. At this point, the dog was functional on three limbs, left front limb plegic with contractures in carpus and distally (Figure 17.5, Figure 17.6). Muscles at the proximal left quarter were markedly atrophied. The owner decided against amputation, and various assistive aids were discussed.

Ten months after the trauma to the left front limb, the left hindlimb underwent a cranial cruciate ligament operation. Six months later, the same stifle was operated on again. No rehabilitation by a physiotherapist was administered due to the owner's life situation and logistical reasons.

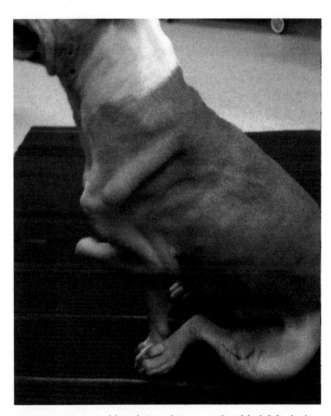

Figure 17.5 Case 2. Left lateral view: obvious atrophy of the left forelimb following traumatic brachial plexus injury.

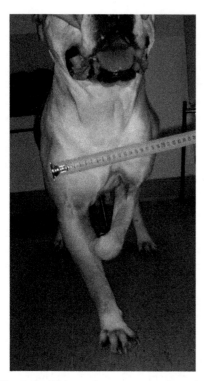

Figure 17.6 Case 2. In addition to the contracture and atrophy of the left front limb, the compensatory position of a three-legged stance is seen.

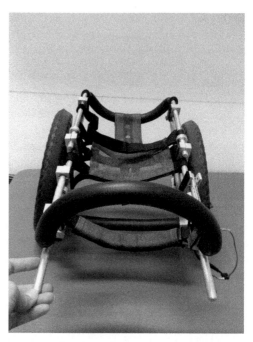

Figure 17.7 Case 2. The assistive device, a cart, used for the American Bulldog with brachial plexus injury.

17.7 Conclusion

In conclusion, neurological physiotherapy is an important part of physiotherapy practice with a growing evidence base as well as support from the basic science literature where animal models are used. In clinical practice, maintaining an excellent

Three years and 5 months after the trauma, physiotherapy consultation was sought for acquiring an assistive aid to support the front part of the dog. At that point, the dog was unwilling to move and would not stand on its feet but lay down frequently; when outside, it only walked a maximum of 20–100 meters before lying down again. Physiotherapeutic assessment revealed an apparent overload situation of the musculoskeletal system due to the inability of the left front limb to bear weight. Axial structures as well as the three limbs, especially the right front limb, were strained due to excessive weight and altered movement patterns. A custom-made cart was acquired for the dog and following its implementation, the dog's quality of life level was reported by its owner to have been remarkably improved. It was happy, playful, went for long walks, and the overall result due to the assistive aid was remarkable not only for the dog but also for the owner's quality of life (Figure 17.7, Figure 17.8).

Four years and 5 months from the trauma, unwillingness to move was again noted. On veterinarian examination, there were osteoarthritic findings in the right hip, left stifle and right elbow joint. Three months later, the dog was euthanased at the owner's request.

After a disabling neurological injury to the left front limb, the dog continued its life for over 4.5 years, with the help of an active and dedicated owner. Amount of therapy performed by a physiotherapist was limited and the rehabilitation was mainly based on a home exercise programme and specific instructions for the owner by the therapist. By use of an assistive aid, both the quality and quantity of life were increased remarkably.

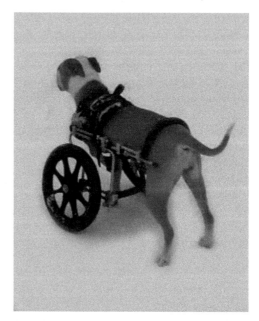

Figure 17.8 Case 2. Use of an assistive device. The dog is in a stable and balanced stance with a front cart. Independently and actively mobile, not overloading the musculoskeletal system.

veterinarian-physiotherapist relationship as well as an excellent relationship with the animal owner is vital to ensuring success.

References

Bach, F., Willems, N., Penning, L., Ito, K., Meij, B., Tryfonidou, M. 2014, Potential regenerative treatment strategies for intervertebral disc degeneration in dogs. *BMC Vet. Res.* 4: 3–14.

Bauer, M., Glickman, N., Glickman, L., Toombs, J., Golden, S., Skiwrinek, C. 1992, Follow-up study of owner attitudes toward home care of paraplegic dogs. *J. Am. Vet. Med. Assoc.* 200: 1809–1816.

Bobath, B. 1990, *Adult Hemiplegia Evaluation and Treatment*. Butterworth Heinemann, Oxford, UK.

Boström, A.F., Hyytiäinen, H.K., Koho, P., Cizinauskas, S., Hielm-Björkman, A.K. 2014, The Finnish neurological function test-battery for dogs, intra- and inter-rater reliability. Proceedings of the 8th International Symposium on Veterinary Rehabilitation/Physical Therapy and Sports Medicine, University of Helsinki, Finland.

Budke, C.M., Levine, J.M., Kerwin, S.C., Levine, G.J., Hettlich, B.F., Slater, M.R. 2008, Evaluation of a questionnaire for obtaining owner-perceived, weighted quality-of-life assessments for dogs with spinal cord injuries. *J. Am. Vet. Med. Assoc.* 233: 925–930.

Bull, C., Fehr, M., Tipold, A. 2008, Canine intervertebral disk disease: a retrospective study of clinical outcome in 238 dogs (2003–2004). *Berl. Munch. Tierarztl. Wochenschr.* 121: 159–170.

Carr, J., Shepherd, R. (eds) 1987, *Movement Sciences: foundations for physical therapy in rehabilitation*. Aspen Publishers, Rockville, MD.

Carr, J.H., Shepherd, R.B. 1992, *A Motor Relearning Programme for Stroke*. Butterworth-Heinemann, Oxford, UK.

De Lahunta, A. (ed.), 1983, *Veterinary Neuroanatomy and Clinical Neurology*. W.B. Saunders, Philadelphia, PA.

De Leon, R., Hodgson, J., Roy, R., Edgerton, V. 1998a Full weight-bearing hindlimb standing following stand training in the adult spinal cat. *J. Neurophysiol.* 80: 83–91.

De Leon, R., Hodgson, J., Roy, R., Edgerton, V. 1998b, Locomotor capacity attributable to step training versus spontaneous recovery after spinalization in adult cats. *J. Neurophysiol.* 79: 1329–1340.

Dietz, V., Wirz, M., Jensen, L. 1997, Locomotion in patients with spinal cord injuries. *Phys. Ther.* 77: 508–516.

Gandini, G., Cizinauskas, S., Lang, J., Fatzer, R., Jaggy, A. 2003, Fibrocartilaginous embolism in 75 dogs: clinical findings and factors influencing the recoccery rate. *J. Small Anim. Pract.* 44: 76–80.

Gracia Calvo, L.A., Tapio, H., Hyytiäinen, H., Paananen, T., Tulamo, R.-M. 2011, Distal physeal radius fracture in a colt. *Suomen Eläinlääkärilehti* 8: 499–503.

Heng, C., de Leon, R. 2009, Treadmill training enhances the recovery of normal stepping patterns in spinal cord contused rats. *Exp. Neurol.* 216: 139–147.

Kathmann, I., Cizinauskas, S., Doherr, M. 2006, Daily controlled physiotherapy increases survival time in dogs with suspected degenerative myelopathy. *J. Vet. Intern. Med.* 20: 927–932.

Kuerzi, J., Brown, E., Shum-Siu, A. et al. 2010, Task-specificity vs. ceiling-effect: step-training in shallow water after spinal cord injury. *Exp. Neurol.* 224: 178–187.

Levine, G.J., Levine, J.M., Budke, D.M. et al. 2009, Description and repeatability of a newly developed spinal cord injury scale for dogs. *Prev. Vet. Med.* 89: 121–127.

Levine, J.M., Budke, C.M., Levine, G.J., Kerwin, S.C., Hettlich, B.F., Slater, M.R. 2008, Owner-perceived, weighted quality-of-life assessment in dogs with spinal cord injuries. *J. Am. Vet. Med. Assoc.* 233: 931–935.

Lyalka, V. 2009, Impairment of postural control in rabbits with extensive spinal lesions. *J. Neurophysiol.* 101: 1932–1040.

Lyalka, V., Zelenin, P., Karayannidou, A., Orlovsky, G., Grillner, S., Deliagina, T. 2005, Impairment and recovery of postural control in rabbits with spinal cord lesions. *J. Neurophysiol.* 94: 3677–3690.

Magill, R. 1989, *Motor Learning Concepts and Applications*. W.M.C. Brown Publishers, Dubuque, IA.

Marteniuk, R. 1979, Motor skill performance and learning: considerations for rehabilitation. *Physiother. Can.* 31; 187–202.

Mykkänen, A.K., Hyytiäinen, H.K., McGowan, C.M. 2011, Generalised tetanus in a 2-week-old foal: use of physiotherapy to aid recovery. *Aust. Vet. J.* 11: 447–451.

Olby, N., de Risio, L., Muñana, K. et al. 2001, Development of a functional scoring system in dogs with acute spinal cord injuries. *Am. J. Vet. Res.* 62: 1624–1628.

Olby, N., Levine, J., Harris, T., Munana, K., Skeen, T., Sharp, N. 2003, Long-term functional outcome of dogs with severe injuries of the thoracolumbar spinal cord: 87 cases (1996–2001). *J. Am. Vet. Med. Assoc.* 222: 762–769.

Rood, M. 1956, Neurophysiological mechanisms utilised in the treatment of neuromuscular dysfunction. *Am. J. Occup. Ther.* 10: 220–225.

Rossignol, S., Bouyer, L., Langlet, C. et al. 2004, Determinants of locomotor recovery after spinal injury in the cat. *Prog. Brain Res.* 43; 163–172.

Ruddle, T.L., Allen, D.A., Schertel, E.R. et al. 2006, Outcome ad prognostic factors in non-ambulatory Hansen type I intervertebral disc extrusions: 308 cases. *Vet. Comp. Orthop. Traumatol.* 19: 29–34.

Sawner, K. 1992, *Brunnstrom's Movement Therapy in Hemiplegia: a neurophysiological approach*. Lippincott, Philadelphia, PA.

Smarick, S., Rylander, H., Burkitt, J. et al. 2007, Treatment of traumatic cervical myelopathy with surgery, prolonged positive-pressure ventilation and physical therapy in a dog. *J. Am. Vet. Med. Assoc.* 230: 370–374.

Smith, R., Shum-Siu, A., Baltzley, R. et al. 2006, Effects of swimming on functional recovery after incomplete spinal cord injury in rats. *J. Neurotrauma* 23: 908–919.

Stephenson, R. 1993, A review of neuroplasticity: some implications for physiotherapy in the treatment of lesions in the brain. *Physiotherapy* 79: 699–704.

Vallani, C. Carcano, C. Piccolo, G. et al. 2004, Postural pattern alterations in orthopaedics and neurological canine patients: postural evaluation and postural rehabilitation techniques. *Vet. Res. Commun.* 28(suppl 1): 389–391.

Voss, D.E., Ionta, M.K., Myers, B.J. 1985, *Proprioceptive Neuromuscular Facilitation: patterns and techniques*. Harper & Row, Philadelphia, PA.

CHAPTER 18

Canine treatment and rehabilitation for orthopaedic conditions*

Laurie Edge-Hughes

Canine Fitness Centre Ltd, Calgary, Canada; Four Leg Rehab Inc., Cochrane, Canada

Summary

Orthopaedic conditions are a mainstay of canine physiotherapy and rehabilitative practices. This chapter will provide information on common conditions and a therapeutic approach to each. Soft tissue lesions, osteoarthritis, postoperative rehabilitation, fracture healing, hip dysplasia and conditioning of canine athletes will be covered in detail. Concepts, strategies and techniques garnered in this section will be applicable on a broader spectrum to conditions not covered within the chapter.

18.1 Introduction

It is clearly impossible in this textbook to cover all potential small animal physiotherapy applications. However, this book is intended to support physiotherapists in translating their human physiotherapy skills to animals, not to provide generic recipe-based treatment and rehabilitation. Therefore, principles and clinical reasoning will be the focus of this chapter with clinical case studies to illustrate this approach.

Physiotherapy for orthopaedic conditions has a strong scientific background in human medicine. The canine physiotherapist should be aware of and rely on what is known to be effective in human practice and apply many of the same therapeutic goals, strategies and techniques to the animal patient when at all possible. Crucial to the success of application to small animals is knowledge of the differences in canine anatomy, biomechanics, disease processes and surgical interventions. Many of the techniques are simple to apply, but it is the clinical reasoning as to when each should be applied that takes professional judgement and skill.

---

*Adapted from the first edition chapter, which was written by Laurie Edge-Hughes and Helen Nicholson

---

Animal Physiotherapy: Assessment, Treatment and Rehabilitation of Animals, Second Edition. Edited by Catherine M. McGowan and Lesley Goff.
© 2016 John Wiley & Sons, Ltd. Published 2016 by John Wiley & Sons, Ltd.

18.2 Soft tissue lesions: muscle, tendon and ligament

Soft tissue injuries are an often underdiagnosed source of canine lameness (Breur & Bevins 1997; Fitch *et al.* 1997; Steiss 2002). Sporting and working dogs may be particularly at risk of suffering acute traumatic muscle strains, ligamentous sprains or chronic overuse degenerative tendinosis lesions resulting from poor healing of repetitive strain injuries. Less conditioned animals may also be at risk when performing infrequent burst activities or endurance tasks, much like the phenomenon known as weekend warrior syndrome in humans. Physical therapy skills and knowledge lend the ability to systematically assess, diagnose and conservatively treat soft tissue injuries in the canine patient.

Muscle strains may be caused by poor flexibility, inadequate warm-up, fatigue, sudden forceful contraction or forced extension/flexion, strength imbalances, intense interval training, insufficient breaks and overtraining (Steiss 2002). The potential for certain muscles to be strained or torn is greater for some muscles than others. Multi-joint muscles are those that cross two or more joints and are at greatest risk for strain because they can be stretched by the movement at more than one joint (Fitch *et al.* 1997; Neilsen & Pluhar 2005; Steiss 2002). A strain may also occur when high forces are put through tendons and muscles, as occurs during eccentric muscle contractions (where a muscle is contracted during a stretch), when forces are applied quickly and obliquely, or during an explosive burst of movement (Fitch *et al.* 1997; Neilsen & Pluhar 2005; Sharma & Maffulli 2005; Steiss 2002). Muscle strains most often affect the muscle origin or insertion, typically at the musculotendinous and teno-osseous junctions, but can occur within the muscle belly as well (Maganaris *et al.* 2004; Nielsen & Pluhar 2005; Steiss 2002).

Tendon injuries may be secondary to acute trauma or repetitive loading (Wilson & Best 2005). The designation of tendon pain as 'tendonitis' is often a misnomer as it implies an inflammatory process (Wilson & Best 2005). Tendinopathy is a better generic descriptor that can be used to include all pathologies that arise in and around tendons (i.e. tendonitis, tendinosis or paratenonitis) (Khan *et al.* 1999).

There is a lack of good-quality histological data from symptomatic tendon disorders of short duration to unequivocally state that tendon lesions are actually inflammatory in nature (Rees *et al.* 2006). Marr *et al.* (1993) described an inflammatory reaction in superficial digital flexor tendon injuries in horses, but only within the first 2 weeks. Other animal models suggest that an inflammatory reaction is present in acute situations but that a degenerative process soon supersedes this (Rees *et al.* 2006). Classic inflammatory changes are not frequently seen in chronic athletic tendon conditions, and it has been suggested that the time at which the tendon becomes symptomatic for pain does not coincide with onset of pathology (Maganaris *et al.* 2004; Rees

et al. 2006; Wilson & Best 2005). On a practical note, in clinical practice most tendinopathies are chronic (tendinosis lesions) by the time the patient (or animal owner) seeks medical attention (Khan *et al.* 1999; Wilson & Best 2005). So perhaps, the clinician should place only minimal, if any, focus on inflammation for tendon pain conditions.

Paratenonitis occurs when a tendon rubs over a bony protuberance and is alternatively known as peritendinitis, tenosynovitis and tenovaginitis (Khan *et al.* 1999). It is clinically characterised by acute oedema and hyperaemia of the paratenon with infiltration of inflammatory cells and within hours or days, fibrinous exudate fills the tendon sheath (Khan *et al.* 1999). Despite these results, pathologists and scientists in this field argue that inflammation of the paratenon is a rare occurrence (Khan *et al.* 1999).

Tendinosis describes intratendinous degeneration without clinical or histological signs of an inflammatory response (Khan *et al.* 1999). This form of tendinopathy is typically considered an overuse injury that involves excessive loading of the tendons, frequent cumulative microtrauma and subsequent mechanical breakdown of the loaded tendon (Khan *et al.* 1999; Rees *et al.* 2006; Sharma & Maffulli 2005; Wang *et al.* 2006; Wilson & Best 2005). In order to mediate the repair process, local tenocytes must maintain a fine balance between extracellular matrix network production and degradation, and unless fatigue damage is actively repaired, tendons will weaken and eventually rupture (Sharma & Maffulli 2005). In humans, tendinosis is a common problem that is characterised by persistent, localised, activity-related pain and swelling associated with common Achilles, patellar and supraspinatus tendons (Fransson *et al.* 2005). The histological appearance of tendinosis is that of collagen disorientation, disorganisation and fibre separation with an increase in mucoid ground substance, increased prominence of cells and vascular spaces with or without neovascularisation and focal necrosis or calcification (Sharma & Maffulli 2005). Additionally, affected tendons are characterised by fibrocartilaginous metaplasia of tenocytes and hypercellularity (Fransson *et al.* 2005).

On visual inspection of affected portions of a tendon, they are lacking their normal glistening-white appearance and have been reported to have a grey-brown or pink-yellow appearance (Fransson *et al.* 2005; Sharma & Maffulli 2005). Pain in these cases can be attributable to both mechanical and biochemical factors but not necessarily due to inflammation alone (Sharma & Maffulli 2005). Inflammatory lesions are infrequent and most commonly associated with partial ruptures (Khan *et al.* 1999). It has been hypothesised that the neovascularisation in the regain of nerve endings accounts for the pain and swelling in the tendon (Langberg *et al.* 2007).

Barring a direct trauma or muscle strain, it is more likely that a soft tissue injury is a tendinosis lesion, and the practitioner should be aware of the pathology.

Ligamentous injuries are usually caused by traumatic overloads in atypical joint movements (i.e. lateral shearing or rotation of the stifle) or an overextension of a normal physiological motion (i.e. hyperextension of the carpus or stifle). However, overuse degenerative lesions may also occur in ligamentous structures such as the cranial cruciate ligament in dogs (Jerram & Walker 2003).

18.2.1 Grading of soft tissue injuries (ligamentous sprains, muscle strains and partial tendon ruptures)

Utilising a grading system of sprains and strains and healing stages greatly enhances the practitioner's ability to successfully rehabilitate muscles, ligament or tendon lesions. When ligaments or tendons are sprained or strained, micro- or macro-tearing (partial rupture) has occurred at the level of the fibres with a predictable damage pattern (Kujala *et al.* 1997; Magee 2008; Steiss 2002).

- *Grade one*: micro-tearing of the inner fibres within the structure, with the surrounding sheath intact.
- *Grade two*: both micro- and macro-tearing of the inner fibres and the sheath occurs. Grade two lesions can vary in degrees of fibre damage.
- *Grade three*: complete rupture of the fibres. Non-surgical healing of the structure is impossible, because no fibres are left intact. Nerve fibres within the structure are also ruptured, therefore animals may exhibit less pain than those with a partial lesion. However, the associated joint(s) may be unstable or functionally compromised as a result of a complete lesion (Kujala *et al.* 1997), an example being a ruptured calcaneal tendon in the dog.

18.2.2 Assessment of soft tissue injuries

Assessment of the injury requires an in-depth knowledge of anatomy and exceptional palpation skills, because animals cannot verbalise where and when pain occurs or understand verbal instructions, such as voluntary muscle contractions or resisting motion. Assessment relies on palpation of the specific muscle structure, including its entire length, while targeting the musculotendinous and teno-osseous junctions where structural failure most commonly occurs (Maganaris *et al.* 2004). A cross-fibre, deep palpation can be utilised to determine tenderness or tissue irritability. Irritability on palpation can be correlated with specific muscle stretching of that structure. A strained muscle or tendon will be painful to stretch (Edge-Hughes 2004, 2005). Ligament injuries are assessed similarly, utilising direct palpation of the entire length of the ligament and ligamentous stress/provocation test (i.e. gap testing). As in human orthopaedic medicine practices, the intracapsular ligaments, although non-palpable, can be examined using both functional assessment and provocation tests, such as the cranial drawer and tibial thrust tests for the cranial cruciate ligament in the dog (see Chapter 6).

18.2.3 Healing stages and treatment of acute or traumatic soft tissue injuries (ligament sprains/muscle strains)

The treatment goals are to first relieve the signs and facilitate healing and then, if possible, identify and correct the causative factor(s) (Wang *et al.* 2006).

Stages of connective tissue repair are sequential and predictable; the following phases occur in the healing process.

Early stage 1

This is the *haemorrhagic phase* (24–48 h). Cellular changes and swelling occur as erythrocytes and inflammatory cells (i.e. neutrophils) enter the area (Sharma & Maffulli 2005). The treatment goals are to minimise the initial bleeding, control swelling, prevent stress and tension, control inflammation and reduce pain, therefore following the PRICE principles: *Protect, Rest, Ice, Compression* and *Elevation*. Depending on the severity of the lesion, generally rest is beneficial only in the first 24–48 h to allow the active bleeding to stop. After 48 h, it is counterproductive to healing, so controlled, pain-free movements should be initiated while considering the lesion's vulnerability (Geffen 2003; Kerkhoffs *et al.* 2002). Ice assists in the reduction of swelling and pain by promoting vasoconstriction, decreasing inflammation and reducing nerve conduction velocity (Rees *et al.* 2006). As a general rule, ice should only be applied for 10–15 min per application. However, clinical trials on the efficacy of RICE (Rest, Ice, Compression, Elevation) have supported the use of compression but have found no value in icing, other than a temporary numbing effect (Hubbard & Denegar 2004), and other studies have noted that icing an acute injury may actually delay healing (Takagi *et al.* 2011). A compression or elastic bandage should be used around the affected joint, especially in lesions where the animal is predominantly recumbent. Care should be taken to avoid impairing the circulation distal to the compression bandage by wrapping a limb too tight, so the animal must be supervised and circulation monitored. Elevation, while good in theory, is not always practical for the canine or feline patient.

Environmental considerations, such as providing the animal with non-slip surfaces, adequate confinement and sleeping surfaces, are vital. Use of inexpensive rugs to create a pathway over hardwood or linoleum flooring can aid in avoiding slip-related reinjury and gaining animal confidence in ambulation with early use of the affected limb (Edge-Hughes 2005).

Late stage 1

This is the *substrate phase* (days 3–5). Dead cells and damaged collagen are removed or broken down. Monocytes and macrophages predominate and phagocytosis of necrotic material occurs. Vascular permeability is increased. Granulation tissue, which needs oxygen and nutrients begins to form, so capillaries divide and grow in the area (Sharma & Maffulli 2005). The goal here is to assist in removal of traumatic inflammatory exudates so that healing may begin. At this point, you can still choose compression, but also consider physiotherapy modalities such as pulsed (non-thermal) ultrasound, low-dose laser or pulsed electromagnetic field therapy (PEMF) at the lowest setting (Green *et al.* 2003; Lee *et al.* 1997; Michlovitz 1990; Saini *et al.* 2002). Grade one Maitland mobilisations have been utilised in resolving joint pain and inflammation, and may be useful in addressing adjacent or intraarticular ligament sprains (Gross-Saunders *et al.* 2005; Maitland 1966).

Stage 2

This is the *regeneration phase*, which usually occurs during days 5–21 but can last for up to 15 weeks, depending upon the severity of the injury or the body's ability or opportunity to heal. Formation of new collagen fibres commences by *fibroblasts*, *tenoblasts* or *myofibroblasts* (depending upon the structure). These cells lay down new, small, weak fibres in a disorganised fashion. The tensile strength of the muscle, tendon or ligament has the chance to increase during this time as long as appropriate stimulus is applied (Sharma & Maffulli 2005). In this stage of healing, treatment should be directed toward the following.

1 The aim of this phase is to *help the new fibres to align* in the strongest format possible, organised and parallel to each other in the best direction to withstand force, and to reduce adhesion formation. Within the first 2 weeks following injury (severity dependent), it is best to adhere to relative rest incorporating pain-free activity and range of motion (ROM) (Wilson & Best 2005). In a canine model, passive stretching of repaired flexor digitorum profundus tendons was shown to be an effective therapy to lessen adhesions and improve tensile strength (Zhao *et al.* 2002). This can be done with progressive walking, balancing or weight-shifting exercises, passive or active motion of the joint/limb in pain-free ranges. At 2 weeks post injury, collagen synthesis is at its greatest (Sharma & Maffulli 2005). This is the most crucial time to start adding a small degree of stress to the injured tendon or ligament in order to promote collagen alignment. This may create a stronger wound and ultimately a faster return to function. Treatments in this stage can incorporate regaining lost ROM or flexibility by stretching into a small amount of discomfort (but not pain) and beginning strengthening (Sharma & Maffulli 2005; Wilson & Best 2005). Early strengthening for the dog could include three-leg or two-leg static standing balance and easy concentric muscle contractions, which might be achieved by flat land walking, pawing action or stepping over obstacles.

2 *Strengthening*: once pain has subsided, advanced strengthening should be considered (Wilson & Best 2005). Eccentric strength training can be particularly effective in treating tendinopathies and may help promote the formation of new collagen or reverse degenerative changes if present (Khan *et al.* 1999; La Stayo *et al.* 2003; Wilson & Best 2005; Rees *et al.* 2006). Mechanical loading accelerates tenocyte metabolism and may speed repair (Khan *et al.* 1999). Eccentric strengthening in the dog may include walking backwards or sideways,

use of hills or stairs, trotting or even small jumps, depending upon the target muscle group or ligament. Exercising with neuromuscular electrical stimulation (NMES) may also aid in healing (Khan *et al.* 1999). For dogs, a functional application of NMES is very effective while encouraging weight shifting or static balancing on two legs (i.e. cross-leg standing with NMES on the gluteal muscles or quadriceps complex).

3 *Enhancing circulation to the affected area.* Circulation allows for the delivery of oxygen and nutrients to the healing area and takes away the products of inflammation. Promotion of circulation can be accomplished in several ways, including many therapeutic modalities as described in Chapter 13; heat, cyclical hot/cold, laser, ultrasound, PEMF and NMES (Michlovitz 1990; Nelson & Currier 1987). Other circulatory enhancing methods include prescription exercises, deeper transverse frictions and stimulating active muscle contractions (Cyriax 1982; Michlovitz 1990; Nelson & Currier 1987).

4 *Encourage tissue regeneration and metabolism.* Physiotherapy modalities such as laser, ultrasound and PEMF encourage collagen synthesis and metabolism of tenocytes and myocytes (Green *et al.* 2003; Khan *et al.* 1999; Lee *et al.* 1997; Sharma & Maffulli 2005). Use of ultrasound has been shown to speed up the production of more normal fibre matrix, and parallel bundle formation within the fibres, thereby accelerating the time to achieve normal tendon tissue status in severed and repaired Achilles tendons in dogs (Saini *et al.* 2002).

5 *Restoring coordination and body awareness.* A widely researched phenomenon in humans following an injury or surgery is a diminished sense of proprioception (Lephart *et al.* 1997), leading to altered neuromotor control owing to a compromised feedback mechanism. Therefore sensory facilitation techniques should be used to retrain proprioception and neuromotor control to avoid reinjury and secondary dysfunction and hasten return of an athletic animal to full performance. Retraining proprioception allows for a much more responsive musculoskeletal system which is needed for any high-end athletic venture (Lephart *et al.* 1997). This may include running off-leash in a park through to agility sports. Some techniques may include joint compressions, postural facilitation balancing activities, and coordination training that is not so challenging as to reinjure the area (i.e. walking over poles, walking on uneven surfaces, agility training, etc.).

Stage 3

This is the *remodelling phase*, which commences at approximately 6 weeks and can take up to a year. It is further divided into a *consolidation stage* and a *maturation stage* (Magee 2008). The *consolidation stage* may take from 6 to 10 weeks and is marked by the change of the repair tissue from cellular to fibrous. Fibroblast (tenoblast or myofibroblast) activity remains high and the fibres become aligned in the direction of stress. At 10 weeks, the *maturation stage* occurs and is characterised by a change of the fibrous tissue to scar-like tissue. Vascularity is decreased and metabolism of repair tissue gradually ceases (Sharma & Maffulli 2005).

Treatment targets building up muscular strength, maintaining ligament or musculotendinous extensibility, enhancing joint mobility and improvement of the proprioceptive system and neuromotor control. Treatments can include prescribed exercises that allow for a gradual return to function. This may include leash walks followed by short allowances of off-leash running with a gradual increase of the off-leash time. Destination jumping (onto something like a bed or over a small jump), trotting up or down hills and zigzag trotting in the other direction, and gaiting exercises (specific techniques to address any gait adaptations) are useful at this stage. Gradual return to sport could include modified activity with more rest periods, specific turning directions and lower jump heights. Joint ROM may be gained simply by continuing to range the joint, therapeutic joint mobilisations (Grades 3 or 4; see Chapter 12) (Maitland 1966; Gross-Saunders et al. 2005) and exercises that target full joint ROM. Stretching should continue during this stage of rehabilitation to avoid scar tissue contracture and to promote collagen orientation. Proprioceptive exercises can progress to include more difficult balancing or displacement exercises (i.e. use of a wobble board or mini-trampoline), walking on different surfaces or over sporadically spaced objects of varying heights, walking on a narrow plank of wood, backing up or walking sideways over poles and destination jumping.

18.2.4 Healing and treatment of chronic tendinopathy lesions

Treatments for tendinosis would utilise alternative treatment strategies to those of traumatic or acute tendon lesions or muscle strains.

Prolonged immobilisation may have detrimental effects such as a tendon atrophy, decrease in tensile strength and strain at failure, decreased water and proteoglycan content of tendons and an increase in number of reducible collagen cross-links (Sharma & Maffulli 2005). Therefore a proper balance between guided activity and relative rest is imperative.

Hands-on manual therapy treatments, such as deep transverse frictions, have been proposed for soft tissue lesions (Cyriax 1982). Studies have been unable to show a consistent benefit over control groups for improvement of pain (Rees et al. 2006). Massage, which is thought to increase blood supply and therefore promote healing, is another form of manual therapy that has not been adequately studied in these cases. Therefore, neither of these treatment methods has proven efficacy as a therapy of choice for tendinosis.

Cryotherapy is believed to decrease blood flow and tendon metabolic rate and hence reduce swelling and inflammation (Rees et al. 2006). While tendinosis lesions are not inflamed, this therapy could help if paratenonitis is present or for its analgesic effects (Khan et al. 1999; Rees et al. 2006).

Prescription antiinflammatories or cortisone injections are of little benefit since a chronic injury is a non-inflammatory condition (Khan et al. 1999; Paavola et al. 2002). Animal model studies have revealed that NSAID administration or corticosteroid injections inhibit or delay collagen repair of muscles/tendons (Almekinders & Gilbert 1986; Fransson et al. 2005; Obremsky et al. 1994).

The use of modalities such as ultrasound, laser, pulsed electromagnetic field or extracorporeal shockwave therapy may be beneficial in the treatment of muscle and tendon lesions. Both laser and ultrasound have been proven to have a beneficial effect for tendon healing (Demir et al. 2004). Effective laser dosages for tendinopathy lesions have been compiled in a metaanalysis study (Tumilty et al. 2010).

- Epicondylitis: 3.5 J/cm^2 using a 904 nm laser; 150 J/cm^2 with a 1064 nm laser
- Rotator cuff: 4.3–42 J/cm^2 with a 904 nm or 820 nm laser respectively
- Achilles tendinopathy: 1.8–3.6 J/cm^2 with a 904 nm or 820 nm laser respectively
- de Quervain's tendinopathy: 4 J/cm^2 with an 830 nm laser

Pulsed magnetic field therapy (at 17 Hz) has been shown to improve collagen fibre alignment and increase the force to breakage, yet other studies failed to find improvement in adhesion formation with use in lacerated tendons (Sharma & Maffulli 2005).

Perhaps the strongest evidence for treatment of tendinosis lesions lies in eccentric strength training protocols. Mechanical loading has been identified as an accelerant of tenocyte metabolism (Khan et al. 1999). Eccentric muscular training is described as an event where the muscle contraction is purposely less than the opposing outside force, hence allowing for a slow controlled lengthening of the muscle or musculotendinous unit (Magee 1988). Eccentric training consisting of twice-daily exercises of several repetitions for 12 weeks was able to produce a decrease in tendon thickening, resolution of neovascularisation and an increase in patient satisfaction in the Achilles tendons as well as showing similar improvement with patellar tendinopathy and supraspinatus lesions (Alfredson et al. 1998; Ohberg et al. 2004; Rees et al. 2006). Gravare Silbernagel et al. (2001) used a 12-week programme aimed at increasing local blood circulation, improving ROM, plus balancing and gait exercises and specific eccentric exercises, which graduated in intensity to eventually incorporate quick rebounding exercises to address an Achilles tendinopathy. This programme was shown to provide subjective improvement in symptoms over a training program that utilised concentric exercise training.

An additional study for patellar tendinopathy utilised eccentric squats on a decline board, doing three sets of 15 reps, twice a day for 12 weeks, while adding 5 kg increments of weighting to progress the exercise (Bahr et al. 2006). This study did allow for a resumption of cycling, jogging on a flat surface, or exercise in water at the 8-week mark if pain was not involved in the exercise. Yet another study of Achilles tendinosis in soccer players utilised 12 weeks of heavy resistance eccentric training while allowing the participants to continue with their regular soccer training so long as the pain did not increase in doing so (Langberg *et al.* 2007). This study did find an increase in collagen synthesis rate with this protocol despite the lack of relative rest prescribed in many other protocols. A few of the studies cited above mentioned the importance of acceptance of pain during eccentric loading in order to obtain excellent results with this therapy (Bahr *et al.* 2006; Langberg *et al.* 2007; Norregaard *et al.* 2007). With this information, all muscular and tendinous lesions should undergo eccentric training at some point in time during their rehabilitation.

Extracorporeal shockwave therapy (ESWT) has been shown to create neovascularisation and nitric oxide synthase and may promote healing of experimentally induced Achilles tendinopathy lesions in rats (Sharma & Maffulli 2005). Both high- and low-energy ESWT have been shown to improve pain and function, and aid in the resorption of calcific deposits within tendons (Ioppolo *et al.* 2013; Verstrelen *et al.* 2014). Users of ESWT should be warned that there may be the possibility of dose-dependent tendon damage, including fibrinoid necrosis, fibrosis and inflammation (Rees *et al.* 2006).

Stretching has been shown to increase collagen synthesis and improve collagen fibre alignment, resulting in higher tensile strength (Sharma & Maffulli 2005). One study compared eccentric exercise training with a stretching regime for Achilles tendon pain and found that both groups exhibited marked improvement in symptoms and there was no significant difference between the groups (Norregaard *et al.* 2007).

Prolotherapy can be an effective treatment for tendinosis. It has been shown to be beneficial in Achilles tendinosis lesions, its use when combined with eccentric exercise providing more rapid improvements (Yelland *et al.* 2011). Stem cell therapy may also be an effective option. This technique has been used in both small and large animal models; for example, mesenchymal stem cells do promote healing in a rabbit Achilles tendon, and using autologous bone marrow-derived stromal cells, researchers have developed a treatment for the management of injuries to the digital flexor tendons in horses (Rees *et al.* 2009).

18.2.5 Prevention of soft tissue injuries

Numerous cases of lameness may be undiagnosed in veterinary medicine and many are probably associated with muscle injury (Fitch *et al.* 1997).

Stretching has been shown to be effective in increasing joint and muscle flexibility (Davis *et al.* 2005; Decoster *et al.* 2005; Knudson 1999; Magnusson *et al.* 1998; Power *et al.* 2004; Thacker *et al.* 2004). Regular stretching has been shown to improve eccentric and concentric force production, velocity of contractions, maximal volitional contractions, counter-movement jump height, 50-metre dash and athletic performance (Hunter & Marshall 2002; Shrier 2004). One study found that regular stretching can induce hypertrophy in immobilised muscles and another speculated that this effect

might improve performance in the long term (Coutinho *et al.* 2004; Shrier 2004).

However, studies have shown that implementing stretching 'pre-event' or immediately before exercise or testing decreases:
- isokinetic performance
- velocity of contraction
- muscle force produced with contractions
- musculotendinous unit compliance
- ability to store elastic energy in the eccentric phase (Behm *et al.* 2004; Fletcher & Jones 2004; Power *et al.* 2004; Shrier 2004; Thacker *et al.* 2004).

These negative effects have been reported to last for up to 1 h after stretching (Thacker *et al.* 2004). An effective recommendation for regular stretching can be made for daily or every second day after a training session, but not before competition or a training bout. Stretches are effective for muscle elongation when utilised this often, holding 15–30 sec and at as little as one repetition (Bandy & Irion 1994; Davis *et al.* 2005; Decoster *et al.* 2005; Thacker *et al.* 2004).

Warming up the animal before racing or exercise is of great importance to achieve superior performance and prevent injuries (Strickler *et al.* 1990). A warm-up of 5–10 min is more beneficial for improving oxygen kinetics than a shorter warm-up period (de Vries 1986; Tyler *et al.* 1996). There are conflicting findings, however, as to whether warming up has any effect on performance in speed activities (de Vries 1986). Some literature also suggests that endurance athletes perform better with 5 min of vigorous high-intensity warm-ups that include some sprinting (de Vries 1986). Essentially, heating of muscle tissues by 1–2°C can improve musculotendinous extensibility and may thereby reduce its susceptibility to strain injury (Steiss 2002). The cooldown should be at least 15–20 min of walking after an especially strenuous session (de Vries 1986; Skinner 1987).

Attention to skill training, training on different surfaces or in adverse conditions can aid in avoiding injuries on 'race day' (Evans 2000). Human studies have cited the need to enhance neuromuscular control and proprioception in athletes as prevention against soft tissue injuries or as part of an advanced rehabilitation programme (de Vries 1986; Lephart *et al.* 1997). Consistent and regular repetitive training utilising balance training and joint repositioning should be implemented in a progressive manner in respect to difficulty (Lephart *et al.* 1997).

The training targets:
- joint mechanoreceptors
- Ruffini endings
- Pacinian corpuscles
- unmyelinated free nerve endings
- Golgi tendon organs
- muscle spindles in order to target the central nervous system (CNS).

The CNS receives input from these sensory receptors and responds accordingly via spinal cord reflexes, the brainstem and cognitive programming to promote dynamic joint stability and functional stability (Lephart *et al.* 1997). Human endurance athletes have utilised variable-intensity training to enhance performance, and sprint training should incorporate mandatory rest periods to avoid muscular fatigue (Esteve-Lanao *et al.* 2005; Paavola *et al.* 2002). Recommendations for conditioning in canine athletics have been made but have yet to be studied (Blythe *et al.* 1994; Zink 1997; Zink & Daniels 1996).

18.2.6 Rehabilitation example for grade one cranial cruciate ligament injuries

Characteristics of a grade one cranial cruciate ligament (CCL) injury:

- mild swelling detectable at the parapatellar tendon
- mild discomfort on stress testing (unanaesthetised)
- partial weight-bearing use of limb.

The following treatment protocol can be used in dogs with partial cruciate tears.

- Keep the dog on a leash for 2–3 months without exception.
- Modalities that may encourage circulation to the cruciate ligament (i.e. PEMF or laser) on a regular basis (see also Chapter 10).
- Joint proprioception techniques such as joint compressions and cross-leg standing (Figure 18.1).
- Strengthening of the adjacent musculature: up-hill walking (steep going up and gradual coming down).
- Balancing/coordination: walking on different terrain (i.e. to cause high stepping or somewhere with uneven footing), rocker boards, mini-trampolines, obstacle course and cushions off the couch, etc.
- At 2–3 months (individually based): add some 'destination jumping' (i.e. onto a bed or couch or over a small jump) and/or tug-of-war exercises if the dog is safe doing so.
- Supplementation: glucosamine HCl and methylsulphonyl methane (MSM) have been found to be useful for joint protection and soft tissue healing respectively (Holt 1998).

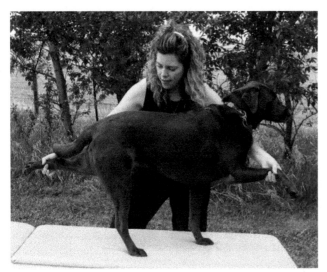

Figure 18.1 Cross-leg/diagonal-leg standing exercise.

- Owners must be educated to avoid throwing balls or playing 'Frisbee' with their dog for 4–6 months, and they need to be educated on the mechanics of injury – how the cruciate was injured in the first place and what to avoid (i.e. hyperextension or 'pivot-shift').
- Return to normal off-leash activity should be addressed with advanced-level neuromuscular retraining (see section 18.8.2 for further recommendations).

18.2.7 Conservative management of full cruciate tears

All practitioners involved in small animal healthcare are well aware of the fact that some animals are not surgical candidates, due to age, poor health, an inadequate state of fitness, and/or because of financial constraints or owners' beliefs. This subset of patients deserves a chance at optimal function as much as those that are prime surgical candidates with owners willing and able to bear the financial burden of surgery.

The cruciate-deficient canine stifle

In the case of cruciate deficiency (CCL-D), the stifle of the canine patient exhibits an increase in synovial macrophage density and synovial fluid biomarkers of cartilage disease (i.e. osteoarthritis) (Innes *et al.* 1999; Johnson *et al.* 2002; Klocke *et al.* 2005; Spreng *et al.* 2000). The chronology of degenerative events in the cruciate deficiency follows through the stages of cartilage fibrillation, periarticular hypervascularity, osteophyte development, medial joint swelling, periarticular fibrosis (restabilisation), meniscal injury, peak osteophyte formation and synovitis, settling synovitis, articular cartilage erosion, collagen fibril network breakdown, and finally, slowing of osteophyte formation (Johnson & Johnson 1993). However, following RCCL reconstruction, there is an increase in the global progression of the osteoarthritis disease process, proliferation of osteophytes and joint effusion as well as notable quadriceps atrophy at 7 and 13 months postoperatively (Innes & Barr 1998; Innes *et al.* 2004). Contralateral stifle joint osteoarthritis has also been detected following a unilateral cranial cruciate ligament rupture (de Bruin *et al.* 2007).

DeCamp *et al.* (1996) described gait alteration in CCL-D dogs. The stifle joint angle was more flexed throughout stance and early swing phase of stride and failed to extend in late stance. In contrast, the hip and tarsus were more extended during stance phase, and there was an overall loss of propulsion. The authors of this study noted that meniscal injury occurred in several of the study dogs by 3 months and commented that fibrosis of the joint is insufficient in 6 months to result in joint stability and significant improvement in gait.

The cruciate-deficient human knee

A scant amount of literature has been published specifically dedicated to conservative rehabilitation of canine cruciate deficiency (Vasseur 1979). While some studies have used cruciate-deficient dogs as control animals, evidence-based rehabilitation

Table 18.1 EMG activity in muscles of ACL-D knees compared to normal and reconstructed knees in humans

Muscle activation	Implication
Increase in vastus lateralis activity at loading	Vastus lateralis resists internal rotation of the tibia
Increase in rectus femoris activity at preswing	This may indicate a decrease in knee flexion
Increase in biceps femoris activity at terminal swing	This may be to prevent anterior tibial translation with quadriceps contraction at loading
Increase in tibialis anterior activity at terminal stance	Tibialis anterior creates a dorsiflexion and inversion which also externally rotates the tibia (hence resisting internal rotation forces)

programmes are not generally part of standard management protocols for a comparable evaluation of this option. Human literature has attempted to make comparisons between surgical and conservative management of the cruciate-deficient knee and to study specific treatments and outcomes pertaining to the rehabilitation of the non-operative knee joint.

Ciccotti *et al.* (1994) studied the EMG activity of anterior cruciate ligament-deficient (ACL-D) knees as compared to normal and reconstructed knees at a walk. The same muscle activity was found in other movements as well. The findings are described in Table 18.1.

The authors concluded that rehabilitation does not restore normal EMG patterns, yet surgery does. They further postulated that there is probably a reduction in performance in ACL-D knees in more strenuous sports. These results also suggest that neuropathways other than those mediated by ACL mechanoreceptors exist to coordinate muscle activity. Other studies have shown a greater flexion angle in ACL-D knees during certain periods of stance (Wexler 1998). Quadriceps weakness has been identified as a common problem after ACL injury, and this weakness was persistent in patients with poor functioning knees (Tagesson *et al.* 2008). Prior to rehabilitation strengthening, these patients did not extend the injured knee to the same extent as the uninjured knee. While a certain amount of tibial translation is important to good functioning after ACL injury (Tagesson *et al.* 2008), symptomatic ACL-D patients exhibited more anterior displacement than those who were asymptomatic during weight bearing (Friden *et al.* 1993). Yet, static tibial translation has not been found to correlate with functional outcome (Tagesson *et al.* 2008). Several studies have shown significant proprioceptive deficits to affect

both the cruciate-deficient or surgically reconstructed knee as well as the contralateral normal knee (Friden *et al.* 1999, 2001; Roberts *et al.* 1999, 2000; Zatterstrom *et al.* 1994). There is a correlation between proprioceptive deficits and subjective knee function in patients with symptomatic ACL deficiency (Friden *et al.* 2001; Roberts *et al.* 1999). There is also a relation between the patient's ability to detect passive motion and morphological lesions (chondral or meniscal lesions) (Friden *et al.* 1999).

Rehabilitation of the cruciate-deficient human knee

Some papers report conservative treatment of human anterior cruciate ligament deficiency to be unsuccessful or only successful in older or inactive patients (Buss *et al.* 1995; Scavenius *et al.* 1999; Strehl & Eggli 2007; Zysk & Refior 2000). However, successful treatment of the non-surgical ACL-deficient knee has been shown to be possible with specifically targeted rehabilitation programmes. Noyes *et al.* (1983) proposed the rule of thirds for chronic ACL injuries treated with rehabilitation: one-third of patients can resume previous recreation activities without reconstruction; one-third manage without reconstruction by modifying or lowering their activity level; and one-third require reconstruction because of recurring giving way episodes even in activities of daily living, thus creating three groups of patients: copers, compensators and non-copers (Noyes *et al.* 1983). Comparison of rehabilitated ACL-D and normal knees for function (using the single leg hop test) resulted in 77% of the subjects having normal function at 1 year post injury, 89% normal at 3 years, and 85% normal at 15 years of follow-up (Ageberg *et al.* 2001, 2007). Strength (isometric and concentric) as measured by the Biodex dynamometer was shown to be normal in 42–56% of the subjects at 1 year, 54–68% at 3 years and 69–82% at 15 years follow-up (Ageberg *et al.* 2001, 2007).

Activity levels change with rehabilitation management and surgical management of the ACL-injured knee (Kostogiannis *et al.* 2007). Table 18.2 reflects the decline in activity levels regardless of the intervention using the Tegner activity level scoring system.

The same study also collected data on subjective knee function scoring/quality of life (QOL) scoring. Patients scored the highest 1 and 3 years following injury in the rehab-only group, with patients injured in contact sports scoring the lowest compared to those injured in non-contact sports (Kostogiannis *et al.* 2007). Interestingly, at the15-year follow-up, those patients with reconstruction surgery scored lower in the QOL scores than the non-reconstructed patients (Kostogiannis *et al.* 2007). This same cohort of patients was also evaluated for evidence of

Table 18.2 Tegner activity level scoring following unilateral ACL injury (median)

Treatment	Pre injury	One-year follow-up	Three-year follow-up	Fifteen-year follow-up
Rehabilitation only	7	6	6	4
Reconstruction and rehabilitation	7	5	6	5

radiographic osteoarthritis at the 15-year mark following injury (Neuman *et al.* 2008). Sixteen percent of the rehabilitated patients developed radiographic osteoarthritis (OA). All of the patients with OA had undergone a meniscectomy. None of the non-meniscetomised patients developed OA. Sixty-eight percent of the patients reported an asymptomatic knee, while 23% reported having reconstructive surgery at an average of 4 years after injury (Neuman *et al.* 2008). Myklebust *et al.* (2003) found that 91% of competitive handball players treated without reconstruction could return to preinjury activity level, whereas only 58% in the reconstructed group were able to do the same. A review of literature by Casteleyn (1999) concluded that while ACL reconstruction yielded the least amount of secondary meniscal surgery, osteoarthritic morbidity was higher compared with a conservatively managed group. Sports participation tended to be higher in the reconstructed group as well (Casteleyn 1999).

Conservative rehabilitation of cruciate deficiency

Successful management of the ACL-D knee in humans centres on some common goals: early activity modification, neuromuscular knee rehabilitation and strength training (Ageberg *et al.* 2007; Brotzman & Wilk 2007; Kostogiannis *et al.* 2007; Neuman *et al.* 2008; Tagesson *et al.* 2008). It is appropriate to stage the rehabilitation goals and activities through rehabilitation. Time alone is not the signal for advancement from one programme to another, and attention should be paid to ROM, strength, fluidity of performance of functional activities as well as functional

Table 18.3 Goals and treatment suggestions for phase 1 (protection) of the canine CCL-D stifle (weeks 1–4)

Goal	Suggestion
Increase ROM	PROM flexion and extension; tummy rubs into extension; 'square' sitting practice
Increase muscle function using movement synergies and motor learning transfer	Active sitting down to a stool (guiding rear legs for symmetry of movement); toe pinches (alternating and simultaneous) in side lying; leash walking to toilet, progressing to 5 min and increasing time by 3–5 min per week (if no increase in joint inflammation); weight-shifting exercises; balance board exercises (front legs on the board); standing on soft surfaces and balance; 3-leg standing; walking in circles or figure-of-eight patterns
Increase proprioception	Joint compressions; Grades 1–2 joint mobilisations
Decrease pain and effusion	Icing; PROM & AROM within pain tolerance; joint compressions; Grades 1–2 joint mobilisations; NMES; modalities

Table 18.4 Goals and treatment suggestions for phase 2 (early strengthening) of the canine CCL-D stifle (weeks 5–8)

Goal	Suggestion
Full ROM	As above; may add toe-touch hanging, or extension on the stairs; may add sitting practice on a stool or platform
Normal gait	Walking with a 'disturbance' on the unaffected foot; obstacle walking or trotting; steep uphill walking or trotting
Increase motor control (neuromuscular training) and strength	Underwater treadmill or swimming exercise; NMES or manual tapping on quadriceps or gluteals with 3-leg standing; NMES or manual facilitation on/of hamstrings with sitting practice; step-ups (Figure 18.2); side stepping or back stepping over a pole; stepping up backwards; walking backwards; any of the above land exercises on a soft surface; hill walking; stair walking
Load: 50–60% of uninjured limb	Increase time and duration of exercises above

testing (Markey 1991). Using the goals for each phase of rehabilitation of an ACL-D human knee, treatment regimes can be proposed. Tables 18.3–18.6 illustrate the goals and this author's suggestions for rehab of the canine patient in each phase.

The regimen described above may be considered gradual in its progressions. More recent human literature has suggested that progressive rehabilitation conducted within a mean timeframe of 5 weeks with emphasis on heavy resistance training and challenging neuromuscular exercises significantly improves knee function in the early stages after ACL injury in people (Eitzen *et al.* 2010). This group started a conditioning programme when no swelling or ROM deficits were detectable. They then carried out their exercise programme, with the primary aim being to restore muscle strength and adequate neuromuscular responses. This phase emphasised intensive muscle strength training, plyometric exercises and advanced neuromuscular exercises. Both

Table 18.5 Goals and treatment suggestions for phase 3 (intense strengthening) of the canine CCL-D stifle (weeks 9–12)

Goal	Suggestion
Increased strength, and motor control (neuromuscular training)	Continue most challenging exercises from previous tables; walking with a weight on the affected leg (open kinetic chain training); trotting up/down hills; walking on uneven surfaces; recall running between two people
Increase load: 70–80% of uninjured limb (increasing by 10% nearer end of stage)	Increase time and duration of exercises from previous tables; perform them with a weight pack

Table 18.6 Goals and treatment suggestions for phase 4 (intensive strength training and return to sports) of the canine CCL-D stifle (weeks 13–16)

Goal	Suggestion
Increased strength	Continue most challenging exercises from previous tables; destination jumping exercises from a stand (plyometrics)
Increased coordination	Agility-type training
Increased ability in sport-specific activities	Short distance ball retrieves; 1 or 2 agility-type pieces of equipment; avoid play with other dogs until closer to 6 months or longer and start with only short intervals
Load 80% of uninjured leg (increasing by 10% nearer end of stage)	Increase time and duration of exercises from previous tables; perform them with a weight pack

single and multiple joint exercises, open and closed kinetic chain exercises, as well as concentric, eccentric and isometric strength exercises were utilised. Following 5 weeks of these types of exercises, participants were then retested and decisions were made regarding reconstructive surgery or a continuation of exercise-based therapy.

While natural healing of a meniscal tear has been reportedly possible (Ihara *et al.* 1994), a meniscal injury may inhibit success of this regimen. Preventing osteoarthritis should be an important goal for all animals that have suffered a joint trauma. Human studies have found a correlation with glucosamine use and a reduction in joint space narrowing and erosive effects of OA over a period of 3 years (Bruyere *et al.* 2003; Verbruggen *et al.* 2002). Canine studies have found that the use of a glucosamine/chondroitin sulphate mixture can enhance synthesis and turn-over of the matrix of proteoglycans and collagen and hence can have a protective effect against synovitis and associated bone remodelling (Canapp *et al.* 1999; Johnson *et al.* 2001). Cetylated fatty acids have also been shown in both human and animal studies to modulate the immune response and inflammatory process of osteoarthritis and in turn improve ROM and overall function (Curtis *et al.* 2002; Hesslink *et al.* 2002; Richardson *et al.* 1997). Advice on nutritional supplementation should be considered just as important as physical management of the condition.

Additionally, excessive weight can affect the stresses on articular cartilage. A human study found that each pound of weight lost will result in a four-fold reduction in the load exerted on the knee per step during daily activities (Messier *et al.* 2005). A canine study found that dogs with hip OA that were fed 60% of their current calorie intake lost 11–18% of their bodyweight and experienced a significant decrease in hindlimb lameness (Impellizeri *et al.* 2000). Weight management should be an integral part of rehabilitation of the cruciate-deficient dog.

Summary
Good functional recovery following a cruciate ligament injury is possible with conservative management. Older animals and those not engaged in high-energy sporting activities might have an acceptable outcome with conservative care. Additionally, animals who are not surgical candidates for whatever reason may benefit from this evidence-based proposal for the conservative management of cruciate deficiency in dogs.

18.3 Additional concepts regarding soft tissue injury

18.3.1 Potential indications
Animals may present with similar conditions to those in humans, including but not limited to (see also Chapter 9):
* delayed-onset muscle soreness
* muscle weakness, shortening or overlengthening
* myofascial trigger points
* ossifying or fibrotic myopathies, e.g. semitendinosus fibrotic myopathy, myositis ossificans
* contractures, e.g. infraspinatus contracture, quadriceps contracture.

Grade of soft tissue injury, stages of healing and management of soft tissue injuries have been covered earlier in this chapter. Special note will be made here regarding contractures, with a relevant case study included.

18.3.2 Ossifying or fibrotic myopathies and contractures
Conditions such as myositis ossificans and fibrotic myopathy of the semitendinosus and other muscles (such as gracilis, biceps femoris or semimembranosus) are uncommon in dogs (Steiss 2002; see also Chapter 9). Muscle contractures may occur acutely after injury, more chronically after periods of recumbency or postoperatively due to tethering to a fracture site (Chapter 9).

Case study: Cat quadriceps contracture. Courtesy of Lindsey Connell, MAnimSt (Animal Physiotherapy)
The cat had sustained an injury to her right hindlimb (RHL), causing a grade 4 medially luxating patella and subluxation of the calcaneoquartal joint (between the calcaneus and the fourth tarsal bone), resulting in non-weight-bearing (NWB) lameness. Veterinary management of the injury included casting the limb for 3–4 weeks. Initially the cat was weight bearing (WB) on the cast limb. However, on its removal she was again NWB lame on her RHL. At 5 weeks post injury the cat was referred to a specialist veterinary hospital. Surgical stabilisation of the stifle and hock joints was performed and included right medial patellar luxation repair and calcaneoquartal arthrodesis using cancellous bone graft taken from the right proximal humerus and stabilised with a pin and tension wire. The limb was then placed in a Robert Jones bandage and splint postoperatively. Postoperative instructions were to keep the cat confined in a small room for 4–6 weeks. Antibiotic and antiinflammatory medications were initiated and follow-up radiographs planned for 4 weeks after surgery.

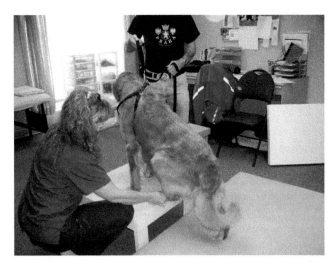

Figure 18.2 Step-up exercise.

The Robert Jones bandage was removed at 2 weeks and at 3 weeks after surgery, the cat was still not using the leg at all. Although the arthrodesis was stable, it was evident that there were marked hip and stifle contractures. The case was referred to the physiotherapist and a plan made to assess and treat the cat under sedation or general anaesthetic (GA), as the veterinarian felt that the stability and position of patella and tarsus were sufficient for physiotherapy to commence.

Physiotherapy consultation under GA: the RHL passive extension ROM at the hip was 90° pretreatment; stifle flexion ROM 75° and extension 145° (Figure 18.3). Manual physiotherapy techniques performed on the RHL hip and stifle included passive accessory and physiological joint mobilisations including mobilisation with passive movement, soft tissue myofascial release techniques, passive joint and whole-limb ROM exercises into flexion–extension; and hip rotation, flexion and extension

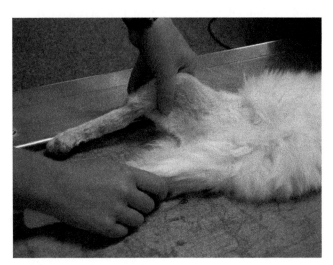

Figure 18.3 A cat with contracture after right hindlimb immobilisation and surgery showing reduced hip and stifle range of motion under general anaesthetic.

sustained stretches (Figure 18.4). The hip ROM post treatment was 110° with the stifle remaining unchanged. The owner was instructed on how to perform the passive stretches and ROM exercises (4 × a day). Weight-bearing exercises were given to the owner as able, i.e. three-point standing by lifting a forelimb to encourage right hind toe touch (4 × a day). These were demonstrated to the owner and the nursing staff by the physiotherapist, before and after the GA.

After 2 weeks of in-hospital physiotherapy treatments under GA three times per week, a review of the cat showed much improved hip ROM, but the stifle was still very flexed and extremely restricted, especially involving semimembranosus, semitendinosus and biceps femoris. However, the cat was beginning to WB on the limb. The cat was discharged to continue with home exercise and physiotherapy.

After 3 weeks of physiotherapy, it was evident that the cat did not require GA for treatment, which continued with hip and stifle mobilisations and soft tissue manipulation including trigger-point therapy and myofascial release techniques to the aforementioned musculature.

Six weeks after surgery, radiography revealed a good tarsal fusion and the pin was removed. There were still moderate hip and tarsal contractures, although the cat was now WB with the musculature noticeably beginning to return. Physiotherapy was to continue along with the owner's home treatment programme.

Two months after surgery, the cat had regained full hip and stifle extension with minimal pain, and she was increasing in strength and muscle bulk. The owner was instructed to continue with her home exercise programme and allow the cat freedom to exercise outside the room, to progress to outdoor exercise after three more weeks.

Three months after surgery, the cat was doing extremely well and returned to her normal functional activities both inside and outdoors. There was no visible RHL lameness with full ROM at hip and stifle, but still some visible and palpable reduction of muscle mass, which with her normal activity was expected to return.

18.4 Osteoarthritis

Osteoarthritis is characterised by progressive loss of articular cartilage, reactive changes at the margins of the joints and bones, and chronic joint inflammation (Ray & Ray 2008; Schumacher 1988). Clinical manifestations include aching discomfort that worsens with activity and is relieved by rest, a restriction of activity level, a limitation in the ability to perform, poorer proprioception, pain and discomfort, joint stiffness, effusion and enlargement, and loss of strength and flexibility (Buckwalter 2003; Millis & Levine 1997; Schumacher 1988; Shrier 2004; Snibbe & Gambardella 2005).

The causes of OA are unfavourable genetics and poor conformation, joint incongruity, uneven load-bearing, as well as obesity, repetitive stress and joint trauma (such as subchondral bone damage, intraarticular derangement, instability or surgical

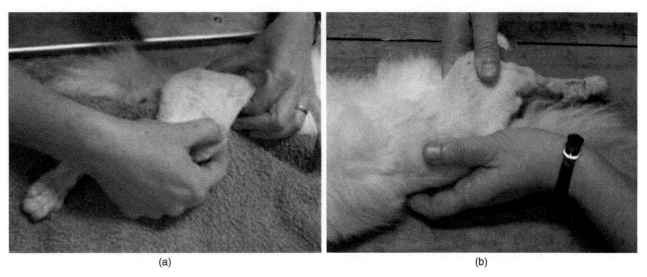

(a)   (b)

Figure 18.4 Same cat as Figure 18.3 showing (a) myofascial release, (b) passive extension of hip, performed under general anaesthesia.

interventions) (Johnson & Johnson 1993; Lahm *et al.* 2004; Millis 2004; Olmstead 1995; Ray & Ray 2008; Schumacher 1988). Physiotherapy can prove useful in both the treatment of OA and in attempting to prevent or delay its onset and progression.

18.4.1 Assessment of osteoarthritis

Early detection and subsequent treatment of OA will yield the most favourable outcomes. Radiographic or MRI imaging that reveals evidence of OA does not correlate well with clinical signs of pain or dysfunction (Bockstahler *et al.* 2007; Gordon *et al.* 2003). Physiotherapists have long used manual testing techniques and clinical reasoning to diagnose early-onset joint OA (Cibulka & Threlkeld 2004; Magee 2008). If there is a joint capsule lesion or a total joint reaction present (OA lesions), a characteristic pattern of restriction in the passive ROM will occur (Cibulka & Threlkeld 2004; Magee 2008). This is called a capsular pattern, and in humans, the common capsular patterns for all joints are documented (Gross-Saunders *et al.* 2005; Magee 2008). The same is not true for animals but extrapolation can be made from clinical practice as to common patterns of restriction, i.e. hip extension is commonly restricted in OA at the canine hip joint (Gross-Saunders *et al.* 2005). Pain and a loss of end-range extension is a frequent finding in early OA of many canine joints (Olmstead 1995). Additionally, physiotherapists utilise 'joint end-feel' to assist in determining the pathology at the joint (Magee 2008). This practice can also be transferred to the canine patient by a practitioner skilled in manual therapy (see Chapter 12).

18.4.2 Treatment of osteoarthritis

The goals for the treatment of OA are to improve the joint and overall function and quality of life of the animal, relieve pain and associated muscle spasm, maintain and regain joint ROM, improve joint health, strengthen supporting muscles, address proprioceptive deficits and advise on lifestyle modifications.

Relief of pain may be accomplished by use of modalities (ultrasound, laser, PEMF, shockwave therapy and NMES; see Chapter 13) (Gur *et al.* 2003; Michlovitz 1990; Millis & Levine 1997; Mueller *et al.* 2007; Nelson & Currier 1987; Sutbeyaz *et al.* 2005). Massage has been shown to reduce pain, increase pain tolerance and stimulate a release of endorphins, so long as regular massage sessions are administered (Corbin 2005; Plews-Ogan *et al.* 2005; Tappan 1988). For this reason, owners could be instructed in how to perform massage techniques properly as a regular home-based intervention. Thermal agents such as heat or cold are both reported to have pain-relieving effects and application of each should be taught to owners and/or utilised as part of a therapy session (Michlovitz 1990; Millis & Levine 1997; Steiss & Levine 2005). Additionally, isokinetic muscle-strengthening exercises are capable of significantly reducing pain (Huang *et al.* 2005). Many other forms of manual therapy techniques can also be utilised to reduce pain as described in Chapter 12.

The goals of improving joint ROM, joint health, muscular strength, functioning and proprioception can be accomplished by case-specific strengthening and exercise (Brosseau *et al.* 1997; Buckwalter 2003; Millis & Levine 1997; Roddy 2005; Roos & Dahlberg 2005; Stitik *et al.* 2005). Strengthening the supporting muscles aids in shock absorption, with the increase in strength minimising fatigue-related injuries in general conditions (Bement 2009; Buckwalter 2003; Millis & Levine 1997). Both aerobic walking and quadriceps-strengthening exercises have been shown to reduce pain, increase joint ROM and improve function in human knee OA patients, thus reducing disability (Roddy *et al.* 2005; Roos & Dahlberg 2005; Snibbe & Gambardella 2005). Strengthening exercises specifically have been shown to be efficacious for hip OA (Hernandez-Molina *et al.* 2008). Moderate exercise has also been shown to improve knee cartilage glycosaminoglycan content in humans at risk of developing OA (Roos & Dahlberg 2005). Articular cartilage can be stressed and damaged with repetitive impact loads, blows to the joint or torsional loads (Buckwalter 2003). Thus, aquatic exercises have been praised for OA patients because of the buoyancy effect of the water which allows exercise without significant joint impact (Cochrane *et al.* 2005; Stitik *et al.* 2005). The use of an underwater treadmill or swim therapy can be very beneficial and utilised as a cross-training tool (Hamilton 2002; Huang *et al.* 2005; Millis & Levine 1997).

Cross-training has been proposed as a method to reduce the repetition of the same patterns of joint loading and motion (Buckwalter 2003). This information can be translated to the care of dogs with OA. Regular exercise (walks or trotting) on a softer surface (grassy areas) should be encouraged. Walking on hilly terrain could also alter joint loading and build different muscle groups (Edge-Hughes 2002), and may decrease the risk of developing radiographically detectable hip dysplasia (Krontveit *et al.* 2012). Competitive athletics should be discouraged or modified, however, as canine sports such as agility, fly ball and racing could impart excessive joint loading or torsional forces.

Manual physiotherapy techniques such as joint mobilisations, stretching and joint traction/distraction have been found to be effective in improving function, walking tolerance and quality of life in humans and ROM in dogs (Crook 2004; Hoeksma *et al.* 2004). Manual therapy as an adjunct to exercise therapy has been shown to have a greater effect than exercise therapy alone on OA of the human hip (Deyle *et al.* 2005; Hoeksma *et al.* 2004). A physiotherapist trained in manual therapy is superbly qualified to apply mobilisation treatments, as a keen appreciation of arthrokinematics and end-feel and an ability to grade the mobilisation are required (see Chapter 12). Owners can be instructed in muscle stretching and joint traction if deemed safe to perform these manoeuvres.

Joint health, cartilage regeneration and slowing of the progression of OA lesions can be targeted with use of modalities and nutritional supplementation. PEMF has been shown to increase chondrocyte matrix synthesis and proliferation *in vitro* and *in vivo* and has been shown to preserve the morphology of articular cartilage and retard the development of OA lesions in the knee of aged osteoarthritic guinea pigs (Fini *et al.* 2005; Fioravanti *et al.* 2002; Sutbeyaz *et al.* 2005). Laser therapy (Chapter 13) is able to enhance the biosynthesis of arthritic cartilage, and results in the improvement of arthritic histopathological changes (Cho *et al.* 2004; Lin *et al.* 2005). Medium-intensity extracorporeal shockwave treatment may have a chondroprotective effect if aimed at the subchondral bone adjacent to a joint and may improve bone remodelling and aid in prevention or regression of OA (Figure 18.5) (Wang *et al.* 2011a,b, 2012). Additionally, human studies have found a correlation with glucosamine use and a reduction in joint space narrowing and erosive effects of OA over a period of 3 years (Bruyere *et al.* 2003; Verbruggen *et al.* 2002). Canine studies have found that the use of a glucosamine/chondroitin sulphate mixture can enhance synthesis and turnover of the

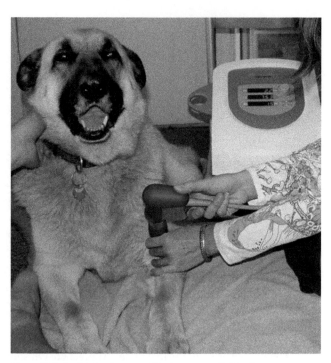

Figure 18.5 Radial shockwave application to an arthritic elbow.

matrix of proteoglycans and collagen and hence can have a protective effect against synovitis and associated bone remodelling (Canapp *et al.* 1999; Johnson *et al.* 2001). Cetylated fatty acids have been shown in both human and animal studies to modulate the immune response and inflammatory process of OA and in turn improve ROM and overall function (Curtis *et al.* 2002; Hunter & Marshall 2002; Kraemer *et al.* 2005; Richardson *et al.* 1997). Advice regarding nutritional supplementation should be considered just as important as physical management of the disease.

Overall improvement in functioning and quality of life is the ultimate treatment goal for OA. Excessive bodyweight can increase the stresses on articular cartilage. In a human study, each pound of bodyweight lost resulted in a four-fold reduction in the load exerted on the knee per step during daily activities (Messier *et al.* 2005). A canine study found that dogs with hip OA that were fed 60% of their current calorie intake lost 11–18% of their bodyweight and experienced a significant decrease in hindlimb lameness (Impellizeri *et al.* 2000). A review of the correlation between OA and obesity in dogs concluded that weight loss can be an effective treatment for OS, and may reduce the incidence or severity of OA depending upon the joint (Marshall *et al.* 2009). Thus weight management should be an integral part of rehabilitation of the osteoarthritic dog.

18.4.3 Prevention of osteoarthritis

Preventing OA should be an important goal for all ageing animals or animals that have suffered a joint trauma (including surgical interventions). One canine study found that lifelong exercise did not cause cartilage erosion, osteophytes or meniscal injuries (Newton *et al.* 1997). In fact, a separate study found that dogs exercised 4 km/day × 5 days/week × 40 weeks had increased cartilage thickness, proteoglycan content and indentation stiffness; dogs exercised 20 km/day × 5 days/week × 15 weeks had a decrease in cartilage thickness and proteoglycan content but no degeneration; and dogs exercised 40 km/day × 1 year had a decrease in proteoglycan concentration and indentation stiffness and stimulated remodelling of subchondral bone but no degeneration (Buckwalter 2003). The authors commented that increasing exercise causes changes in cartilage composition and mechanical properties but does not accelerate joint degeneration. So, given that muscle strengthening aids in shock absorption capabilities for joints (Buckwalter 2003), exercising to strengthen muscles may help to prevent the development of OA (Berend *et al.* 2004). Lifelong weight management is also an excellent prevention aid. The results of a 14-year-long study suggest that a 25% restriction in food intake can increase median lifespan and delay the onset of signs of chronic disease in dogs (Kealy *et al.* 2002).

In summary, to prevent or delay the onset of OA, dogs should be kept lean, exercised regularly on surfaces which reduce joint impact and torsions, and owners advised on nutritional supplementation as the animal ages or should joint injuries/surgical procedures arise.

18.5 Postoperative rehabilitation

Stringent protocols for postoperative rehabilitation may be unnecessary when the physiotherapist utilises clinical reasoning skills, creates problem lists, sets rehabilitation goals and is cognisant of healing times. ACL surgeries are common in both humans and dogs. Postoperative rehabilitation has been studied more thoroughly for this condition than any other orthopaedic surgery and can be used as a model for postoperative rehabilitative care in general.

First, it is important to understand what happens to soft tissues and articular structures after joint irritation, surgical intervention and/or a period of immobilisation or disuse. The effects of disuse on muscle include a loss of lean tissue mass; atrophy of type I slow-twitch muscle fibres (generally the extensor muscle groups) and associated tendons; biochemical conversion of slow-twitch muscle fibres to fast twitch and changes in the sarcoplasmic reticulum within muscles which decrease strength (Francis *et al.* 2002; Taylor & Adamson 2002; Uhthoff *et al.* 1985). In human ACL-deficient knees, the sartorius, gracilis and vastus medialis muscles exhibit a small decrease in power, while there is a significant decrease in power of the semitendinosus, rectus femoris, tensor fascia lata, vastus lateralis and lateral head of gastrocnemius (Williams *et al.* 2003). Muscle firing patterns were also altered and displayed a greater magnitude of co-contractions than in normal legs (Williams *et al.* 2003). Ligaments were affected by immobilisation in that it lead to ligament

atrophy, a decrease in maximum load to failure and decreased biochemical, structural and mechanical properties (Taylor & Adamson 2002; Uhthoff *et al.* 1985).

Cartilage can also be affected by immobilisation; degenerative changes occur via a gradual reduction in proteoglycan content and production, a thinning or loss of articular cartilage, a decrease in cartilage matrix and cellular components, and a decrease in synovial fluid, thus reducing cartilage nutrition (Taylor & Adamson 2002; Uhthoff *et al.* 1985). Loss of subchondral bone, osteoporosis, osteopenia, osteophytes and periarticular fibrosis are problems with immobilisation which affect bone (Francis *et al.* 2002; Taylor & Adamson 2002; Uhthoff *et al.* 1985). Proprioception is compromised; the ability to receive input from muscles, tendons and joints, and to process information in a meaningful way in the central nervous system and assist in the knowledge of where the limb is in space is affected, thus ultimately reducing the regulation of reflexes and neuromotor control (Hewett *et al.* 2002). Human ACL reconstruction results in proprioception deficits in both the involved and non-involved limbs at 3, 6, 9 and 12 months after surgery (Hewett *et al.* 2002).

18.5.1 Treatment of postoperative joints

Rehabilitation can allow the salvaging and acceleration of recovery time of some patients and it can make either the best or worst surgical procedure better (Taylor & Adamson 2002). The goals for any postoperative case are to reduce pain; promote healing; maintain muscle mass and promote muscular development and joint stability; maintain joint flexibility; retrain proprioception, balance and coordination; facilitate early return to function; prevent degenerative joint disease; and rebuild cardiovascular endurance (Francis *et al.* 2002; Hewett *et al.* 2002; Nwadike & Hesback 2004; Taylor & Adamson 2002). Physiotherapy is also important for addressing complications that can ensue with any postoperative case, such as identification of infections or surgical failure, treatment of secondary tendinitis/tendinopathies and/or soft tissue adhesions (Nwadike & Hesbach 2004).

The general goals for all postoperative rehabilitation will be very similar and can be categorised into stages of healing. A two-part division of physiotherapy goals has been documented for dogs (Clark & McLaughlin 2001).

- *Phase one*: immediately following surgery and in the initial inflammatory stage of tissue healing through to the end of the reparative stage, which could last approximately 3–4 weeks. Goals in this stage are to:
  - resolve pain and inflammation
  - stimulate early tissue healing
  - preserve muscle mass
  - joint ROM and articular homeostasis
  - prevent mechanically dysfunctional compensatory postures and movement strategies by the patient.
- *Phase two*: targets challenging the healing tissues during remodelling and maturation stages of healing to improve

strength and mobility, mobilise scar tissue and enhance functional return (Clark & McLaughlin 2001; Nwadike & Hesbach 2004; Taylor & Adamson 2002).

From clinical observations it may be more appropriate to divide the postoperative rehabilitation into four stages:

- acute phase
- subacute phase
- mid-stage
- end-stage.

Human postoperative protocols for athletes recovering from ACL reconstruction recognise six stages/phases to a postoperative strengthening programme (Hewett *et al.* 2002). A combination of goals, theories and suggestions is presented below (Berend *et al.* 2004; Bocobo *et al.* 1991; Clark & McLaughlin 2001; Davidson *et al.* 2005; Delitto *et al.* 1988; Edge-Hughes 2006; Fitzgerald *et al.* 2000, 2003; Hewett *et al.* 2002; Johnson & Johnson 1993; Johnson *et al.* 1997; Kvist 2004; Lephart *et al.* 1997; Marsolais *et al.* 2002; Perry *et al.* 2005; Ross *et al.* 2001; Shaw *et al.* 2005; Zink 1997).

Acute stage (weeks 1–3)
Lifestyle management
To reduce the risk of reinjury, it is imperative to educate the owners about avoiding rough play; toileting on leash only; short 5-min leash walks building up to 10 min by the end of week 3; no excessive stair negotiations; no jumping; and promotion of non-slip flooring (i.e. rubber-backed slip-rugs). In very early stages after surgery, slings may be necessary to help the dog ambulate to perform toileting tasks.

Manage inflammation
Low doses of modalities (ultrasound, laser or PEMF) can be useful to reduce inflammation after the first 24–48 h after surgery. Cryotherapy can also be used on a regular basis for home management. Grade 1 Maitland's mobilisations for the joint/s (joint glides, joint distraction or joint compression) may also assist in settling the joint. NMES to the surrounding musculature may also have a positive effect on joint inflammation and adjacent soft tissue swelling.

Enhance or maintain ROM
Passive ROM, avoiding pain at end ranges, can help to maintain normal joint ROM, and may also improve circulation and, via stimulation of proprioceptive mechanoreceptors, may aid in sensory awareness. Active ROM may be accomplished through easy weight-shifting activities to regain some extension in the elbow, carpus, stifle or hock. Easy, active hip extension may be accomplished by 'tummy rubs' at this stage. Gentle active flexion could be accomplished by 'shake-a-paw' activity in the forelimbs or stimulating a 'scratching' reflex for the hind end or by gently pinching the toes in either the front or hind legs to stimulate a reflexive pulling away response. Additionally, active hindlimb flexion can be accomplished by proper 'sit' training – having the owners give a verbal command to sit, correct any improper postures such as side sitting (which avoids flexing the hindlimb) by tapping on the offending limb or reverbalising the command until a proper 'sit' is given before giving a treat reward. Forelimb elbow and shoulder flexion may be accomplished similarly by asking for a 'down' (sternal recumbency position) and correcting any offending limb compensations before rewarding with a treat.

Proprioception
At this stage, ROM and grade 1 Maitland's mobilisations may stimulate Ruffini ending or Pacinian corpuscles within the joint capsule that can reawaken the central nervous system's awareness of the body, which is necessary after any surgical intervention. Massage to the affected limb may stimulate Golgi tendon organs and muscle spindles. Weight-shifting activities and the allowance of partial weight bearing will not only aid in return to normal function, but is also a proprioceptive stimulus. The use of NMES with the weight-shifting activities may target both early strengthening and proprioception.

Address axial skeleton issues
Clinically, physiotherapists have reported finding spinal or sacroiliac joint dysfunctions subsequent to prolonged lameness issues (Edge-Hughes 2001; Kerfoot 1997). A study of a population of horses with orthopaedic problems found that 74% of horses with back problems had lameness and that back problems were diagnosed in 32% of the lame horses; these findings were significantly higher than those recorded in a control population (Landman *et al.* 2004). This would mean that the postoperative animal could be at risk of developing back pain secondary to postural alterations following surgery. Therefore, clinically it is recommended that the entire animal is evaluated, especially the spine and pelvis, on a regular basis throughout the rehabilitation process.

Subacute phase (4–6 weeks)
Strengthening
In this stage, the animal must start to build its muscular support surrounding the affected joint. Both closed-chain and open-chain exercises are of benefit when combined in a postoperative exercise programme. The therapist may prescribe slowly, beginning to challenge the weight-bearing status of the limb with activities such as static balancing by lifting one or two of the unaffected limbs off the ground (with or without the additional use of NMES) (Figure 18.6), walking up or down gradually sloping hills, or stepping over poles or objects (closed-chain). Muscular endurance should also be targeted and increasing walking times/distances should begin, gradually increasing to 20 min by the end of this stage. Use of a hydrotreadmill or pool swimming may be effective for strengthening at this stage as well (open-chain).

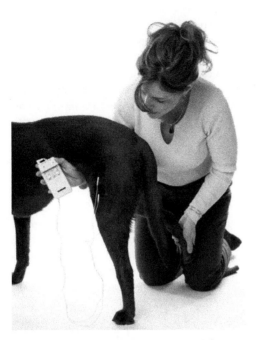

Figure 18.6 Use of NMES on the quadriceps muscles while concurrently lifting the unaffected leg off the ground.

Soft tissue stretching and ROM

Care should be taken not only to address ROM deficits of the affected joint, but also to manage ROM of uninvolved joints, as compensatory gait alteration may have affected them. Muscle stretching of two-joint muscles should also be undertaken, as they will not be stretched with simple ROM (e.g. with any elbow joint surgery, the long head of triceps should be stretched, which is accomplished by combined simultaneous shoulder extension and elbow flexion).

Proprioception

Proprioception can be challenged to a greater extent in this phase. Use of balance boards, slow walking on uneven or unstable surfaces, or walking over obstacles may target this goal. Near the end of this stage, the static balancing exercises described above can be progressed to include small manual balance perturbations while holding positions.

Mid-stage (7–9 weeks)
Strengthening and proprioception

Increasing time, distances, speed or terrain traversed during leashed walks will aid in strengthening. Steeper hill and/or stairs at walk may aid in advanced strengthening. Trotting exercises may be appropriate. Static balancing on two legs should be introduced, such as making the animal balance on the surgical leg and its opposite thoracic limb by holding the other diagonal pair off the ground. This may include manual displacement or while on a novel surface (i.e. foam or mini-trampoline) to challenge both strength and proprioception. Stepping-over exercises

in all planes of motion, including lateral, rotational or backwards, assist in increasing the complexity of the neuromotor task. Walking on a plank of wood elevated a few inches above the ground will address coordination issues, and may be combined with volitional balance disturbances (e.g. such as making the dog turn to take treats from side to side).

Gait retraining

Often dogs will develop compensatory postural or movement strategies following surgery. Many of the exercise and proprioceptive techniques described above can address these issues, but other therapeutic interventions might include taping or bandaging techniques or the use of mild, noxious mechanoreceptive stimuli to promote proper limb usage.

End-stage (10 weeks)
Strengthening and proprioception

If healing has occurred appropriately and according to schedule, then advanced strengthening techniques can be encouraged, such as destination jumping (i.e. on to a bed or over a jump). Longer trotting sessions may be necessary to build up muscular and cardiovascular endurance. A gradual return to off-leash activities may begin after 12 weeks, depending on safety issues, e.g. time of the year, condition of the ground for non-slip footing, only when not near other dogs that might initiate rough play, etc. Owners need to be instructed to allow for a long warm-up (10 min or more) before allowing a short off-leash run (consisting of just 5 min off leash to start) or that the initiation of the off-leash time should occur in the middle of the dog's walk. Straight line running can be attempted (i.e. asking the animal to run back and forth between two people).

Return to sports (14 weeks)
Advanced strengthening and proprioception

As mentioned above, if healing has not been compromised during the postoperative period and the owners are determined to return the animal to sporting activities, then advanced training and intensive rehabilitation must be accomplished. Plyometrics, jumping, agility training, sport-specific training, sprints, training using greater balance perturbations, quick directional changes/pivoting/figure-of-eight exercises at submaximal effort at first, then progressing to greater speeds, cardiovascular endurance and a continuation of strength training should be targeted.

Important note for postoperative rehabilitation

Not all surgical interventions will progress at the same rate, although they will go through the same healing stages. It is important to make the postoperative rehabilitation specific to the extent of the surgery and the animal's rate of healing. The physiotherapist should regularly assess when it is appropriate to progress through the various stages/phases of rehabilitation or to determine if a referral back to the surgeon is required.

18.6 Fracture healing

Successful healing of a fracture is not only determined by complete bony union on radiographs, but also by the functional use of the limb thereafter. Physiotherapy following veterinary management of a fracture can be beneficial to fracture healing and is just as important as the corrective procedure itself in determining long-term outcome (Nwadike & Hesback 2004; Olmstead 1995). Comprehension of healing stages and times is required for the implementation of an appropriate rehabilitation plan.

18.6.1 Stages of fracture healing
- *Stage 1*: haematoma formation.
- *Stage 2*: traumatic inflammation (vasodilation, local swelling and loosening of attachment of periosteum to bone).
- *Stage 3*: demolition (macrophages remove red blood cells, debris and fibrin. Detached bone fragments necrose and are attacked by macrophages and osteoclasts).
- *Stage 4*: granulation (tissue formation, capillary loops form).
- *Stage 5*: formation of woven bone and cartilage (woven bone is made of collagen ground substance called osteoid, a process which is known as callus formation). Cartilage eventually dies and calcifies.
- *Stage 6*: lamellar bone formation: woven bone or cartilage is invaded by capillaries, and osteoblasts create osteoid.
- *Stage 7*: remodelling: osteoclastic removal and osteoblastic formation occur simultaneously until bone is close to its pre-fracture state. Callus is slowly removed and becomes lamellar bone. The internal callus hollows and forms the marrow cavity (Magee 2008).

18.6.2 Expected bone healing times
Time to clinical union for a fracture may be dependent upon age along with fracture type, severity and site (Nwadike & Hesback 2004; Olmstead 1995). In canine patients younger than 3 months, bone healing takes roughly 2–4 weeks while for animals 3–6 months of age, healing is 4 weeks to 3 months. When animals are between 6 and 12 months, healing can take 5 weeks to 5 months and if the dog is more than 1 year old, then one might expect 7 weeks or up to 1 year for healing. There are known factors in human medicine that can contribute to delayed healing times such as insufficient frame stability, smoking (in the case of the canine patient, perhaps owner smoking could retard healing), poor weight bearing (perhaps due to pain), poor vascularisation, diabetes and poor nutrition (Gebauer 2002; Gebauer & Correll 2005; Steim & Lerner 2005).

18.6.3 Physiotherapy management of fractures
Physiotherapy management of fractures is very similar to postoperative joint surgery rehabilitation. Treatments can begin when the area is accessible (i.e. when a bandage or cast is off) or immediately if an internal fixation has been used. See section 18.5.1 to determine goals for different stages of healing. The goals of physiotherapy in the postoperative treatment of patients with fractures consist of pain management, aerobic fitness, avoidance of complications related to immobility or reduced muscle mass, and strengthening and retraining functional activities (Carneiro *et al.* 2013).

Additional physiotherapeutic interventions and electromodalities (see Chapter 13) have been recommended specifically for fracture management and may warrant consideration.

Ultrasound (US)
Low-intensity, pulsed US (0.03–0.05 W/cm^2 with a 1.0 MHz or 1.5 MHz or 3.3 MHz sound head used for 10–20 min per session daily, beginning day 1 post operative fracture repair) has been shown to stimulate endochondral ossification due to stimulation of bone cell differentiation and calcified matrix production by intracellular calcium signalling and incorporation in chondrocytes (Gebauer 2002; Korstjens *et al.* 2004; Parvizi *et al.* 2002; Santa-Rodriguez *et al.* 2010). US has been shown to be useful in increasing the stiffness of bone and speeding healing in diabetic rats (Gebauer 2002), and may be effective by stimulation of angioneogenesis (Childs 2003; Steim & Lerner 2005). Additionally, US has been shown to be effective on delayed unions and non-unions in children and did not have any effect on the growth plates (Gebauer & Correll 2005). Santa-Rodriquez *et al.* (2010) also showed benefit with use of 0.1 and 0.25 W/cm^2 settings to increase messenger RNA expression of insulin-like growth factor 1, suppressor of cytokine signalling-2 and -3, and vascular endothelial growth factor and decrease monocyte chemoattractant protein-1 and collagen type II-alpha 1.

Laser
The use of laser has been reported to increase osteoblastic proliferation, collagen deposition and new bone formation, and increase bone stiffness by forming a smaller, stronger callus, with an increased amount of well-organised bone trabeculae (Gerbi *et al.* 2005; Lirani-Galvao *et al.* 2006; Luger *et al.* 1998; Pinheiro & Gerbi 2006; Weber *et al.* 2006). Laser therapy is more effective if the treatment is carried out at early stages when high cellular proliferation occurs (Pinheiro & Gerbi 2006). Laser dosages for bone healing are as follows.
- GaAlAs laser, 780 nm, 30 mW, 112.5 J/cm^2 –cumulative over 12 sessions (approximately 4.5 J/cm^2 per day over 2 spots) (Lirani-Galvao *et al.* 2006).
- 830 nm, 40 mW, continuous wave × 16 J/cm^2/session, divided into 4 points around the defect (4 J/cm^2) – starting immediately after surgery and repeated 7 times, Q48 h (Gerbi *et al.* 2005).
- 830 nm, 0.5 cm^2 area × 50 mW x 10 J/cm^2 (fractioned into 4 points), Q48 h (Weber *et al.* 2006).
- 632.8 nm laser, 35 mW, for 30 min, delivering 892 J/cm^2 cumulative over 14 days (63 J/cm^2 per day. Note direct penetration is only 1.5 cm) (Luger *et al.* 1998).

Pulsed electromagnetic field

Pulsed electromagnetic field (PEMF) has been reported to stimulate osteoblasts and chondroblasts (Childs 2003), but in the literature there are contradictory findings over the effectiveness of PEMF in bone healing. For this reason, particular attention should be paid to the parameters utilised in the studies that found this technique to be efficacious.

Utilising a dog model, one study found that use of a PEMF setting of 1.5 Hz for 1 h/day at 4 weeks postoperatively and lasting for 8 weeks significantly increased stiffness and promoted greater new bone formation (Inoue *et al.* 2002). This study also found an increase in mineral apposition rate and reduced porosity in the cortex adjacent to an osteotomy site. Delayed unions and non-unions have been shown to improve with electrical stimulation and PEMF versus placebo and were comparable to bone grafting (Aaron *et al.* 2004). Preservation of bone mass was demonstrated in animals with osteotomy gaps and a significantly reduced size of gap was noted versus controls using 15 Hz for 3 h a day (Ibiwoye *et al.* 2004). The prevention of osteoporosis following ovariectomy was demonstrated with PEMF at 7.5 Hz, for 8 h/day, for 30 days versus controls. This same setting was utilised in an earlier study, which demonstrated its ability to heal fracture non-union (Yang *et al.* 1994). However, one study found that PEMF at 100 Hz for 4–8 h/day for 2–4 weeks was effective in promoting bone formation around a rough-surfaced implant (Matsumoto *et al.* 2000). A study looking at the combined use of PEMF, ice and exercise following fractures found that the combination group had better pain reduction and joint ROM than an ice and exercise group or a PEMF and exercise group (Cheing *et al.* 2005). This study utilised 50 Hz for 30 min/day. Other studies have found no effect with PEMF on healing of fractures, using similar settings. Clearly, more research needs to be conducted on different types and settings of PEMF machines to improve their role in clinical decision making for practitioners.

Electrical stimulation

Some studies utilise implantable electrodes (Clark 1987), but as this is not generally considered standard physiotherapy practice, this section will address use of surface neuromuscular electrical stimulation (NMES).

An NMES protocol used in rabbits (surface electrode placed 3 cm proximal to the fracture site and the other proximal to the first electrode) involved 25 mA of current, at a pulse width of 50 μs, at 4 Hz with an on cycle of 20 sec, and an off cycle of 15 sec and a ramp of 5 sec. This was performed for 1 h daily, beginning on day 4 after surgery, for 25 days, and resulted in an increase in mineralised callus by 2 weeks, and a significant increase in callus mineral content and mineralised callus compared with controls by 8 weeks (Park & Silva 2004). Bone had greater torsional parameters for stiffness, maximum torque withstood, and required a greater amount of energy to create failure (Park & Silva 2004). It is reported that the cathode should be placed closest to the site of the fracture and the anode near the first electrode for proper application (Childs 2003).

Shockwave therapy

Shockwave therapy (SWT) is a relatively new modality that could be utilised to treat disorders of the bone. SWT seems to produce its effects on bone by upregulating proteins critical for angiogenesis, accentuating the release of growth factors important in osteogenesis and stimulating the production of osteoblasts (Furia *et al.* 2010; Zelle *et al.* 2010).

Two review papers report that treatment of non-unions with SWT seems to yield promising results (Furia *et al.* 2010; Zelle *et al.* 2010). The overall union rate in patients with delayed union/non-union was 73–79% (mean was 76%) with the use of shockwave therapy. Hypertrophic non-unions showed a better response to SWT than atrophic non-unions. Non-unions are usually treated with 2000–6000 shocks using an energy flux density between 0.3 mJ/mm^2 and 0.6 mJ/mm^2. The total number of impulses is usually divided along the proximal and distal margins of the non-union. The total number of treatments (ranging between 1 and 4) and interval between treatments (ranging from 1 to 4 weeks) varies from paper to paper, centre to centre. It was noted that the success rate for treatment of non-unions via SWT was as effective as surgery in these cases.

Weight bearing and early mobilisation

A study of the effects of weight bearing on healing of cortical defects in the canine tibia (Meadows *et al.* 1990) found significantly less woven bone formed in the defects in the non-weight-bearing tibia than in the weight-bearing tibia. This was determined to be due to the disuse response in the underloaded tibia, in which less bone formed, rather than to the formation of more bone in the weight-bearing tibia. In one review paper, it was found consistently that early mobilisation was preferable over rest in human patients and the authors recommended that mobilisation could be employed more often and perhaps more vigorously (Nash *et al.* 2004). They did, however, caution that it would also be naïve to assume that mobilisation is better than immobilisation in all circumstances. Other studies on humans and animals have had similar findings and have reported that early mobilisation has the potential to result in earlier recovery of mobility and strength, facilitation of an earlier return to activities and did not affect fracture alignment (Cheing *et al.* 2005; Davidson *et al.* 2005; Feehan & Bassett 2004; Kamel *et al.* 2003; Meadows *et al.* 1990; Nash *et al.* 2004). Patel *et al.* (2007) wrote that in humans, the first step in reconditioning post fracture should be a non-weight-bearing activity such as swimming, followed by cycling and non-impact weight bearing such as an elliptical machine or stair climber. Final activities would be more impact exercises such as walking, jogging and finally running. Progressions should always be pain free and progress from low intensity, short duration to high intensity long duration, and take 6–8 weeks to return to normal activity. In dogs, aquatic therapy (swimming and/or underwater treadmill) could be utilised to provide the low-impact, reduced or graduated weight-bearing exercise programme (see Chapter 14), progressing to use of a land treadmill and various land-based therapeutic exercises for strength, balance and coordination.

Case study: Postoperative rehabilitation after internal femoral fracture stabilisation. Courtesy of Lindsey Connell, MAnimSt (Animal Physiotherapy)

A 6-month-old female Belgian Shepherd was diagnosed with a fractured femur by her veterinarian, who referred her to a specialist veterinary hospital for surgery. The surgeon found a Salter–Harris Type II fracture of her medial distal femoral condyle (Figure 18.7). The fracture was stabilised via internal fixation by reconstructing the medial ridge of the femoral condyle with lag screws via a medial approach to the distal femur. Following this, a 90/90 bandage was applied and the dog medicated with non-steroidal antiinflammatory medication. The veterinarian's instructions for postoperative care were to keep the dog confined in a cage, with toileting privileges only, and for physiotherapy review and removal of the 90/90 bandage 7 days postoperatively. Follow-up radiographs were scheduled for 4–5 weeks postoperatively.

Initial physiotherapy consultation (7 days postoperatively)

After removal of the 90/90 bandage, the dog was non-weight bearing (NWB) on right hindlimb (RHL). Examination

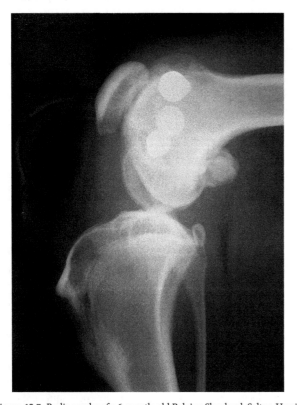

Figure 18.7 Radiographs of a 6-month-old Belgian Shepherd, Salter–Harris Type II fracture of her medial distal femoral condyle. The fracture was internally fixed by reconstructing the medial ridge of the femoral condyle with three lag screws via a medial approach to the distal femur.

findings: right stifle ROM was measured using goniometry and found to be reduced (flexion 80%, extension 50% normal), as was the right hip (flexion 90%, extension 50% normal) and right tarsus (flexion 70%, extension 80% normal).

Soft tissue manipulative techniques were implemented to treat the loss of soft tissue extensibility and joint ROM treatment, for the hip flexors (iliopsoas complex and cranial sartorius) and quadriceps complex, along with stifle flexors and the medial thigh musculature. The stifle and hip were gently mobilised through the available ROM into extension passively.

The owner was shown passive ROM exercises to all joints of the RHL and given advice about confining the dog as well as a slow leash-walking programme for toileting 3–4 times a day to encourage toe-touch weight bearing. Antiinflammatory medication prescribed by the veterinary surgeon was continued.

Physiotherapy consultation (2 weeks postoperatively)

The owner was concerned about the dog's lack of progress and that she was having difficulty doing the home physiotherapy programme. Dog was NWB on her RHL with it held up, into flexion. Right stifle, hip and tarsal ROM were unchanged. Dog was very 'tense' and with marked tissue irritability throughout iliopsoas, quadriceps, sartorius and hamstring musculature.

After discussing the case with the consulting veterinarian and owner, it was decided to treat the dog three times per week as a minimum owing to the fear of a flexion contracture developing.

Treatment sessions included soft tissue manual therapy of the hip, including myofascial release techniques and trigger-point therapy, combined with gentle, slow, sustained passive stretches through the entire available length of the associated tissues, i.e. iliopsoas complex, sartorius and quadriceps into hip and stifle extension and stifle flexion. The coxofemoral joint was mobilised via passive accessory joint manual therapy techniques, i.e. cranial glides to the femoral head and passive physiological motions to encourage extension through the entire available ROM, combined with passive stretches. The tibiofemoral joint was treated by soft tissue techniques as described above to semimembranosus, semitendinosus, biceps femoris and gracilis, followed by gentle tibiofemoral passive physiological joint extension mobilisations via caudal glide to proximal tibia on femur. The tarsal joints were also mobilised into extension via passive physiological extension mobilisations and soft tissue structures passively stretched into extension. Repeated functional ROM exercises into flexion and extension and sustained passive stretches for the whole limb were performed gently.

Hydrotherapy/physiotherapy consultation (2.5 weeks postoperatively)

The dog was still NWB RHL. Assessment and treatment consisted of swimming with buoyancy vest with assistance by the physiotherapist, as she required facilitation of right hindlimb to obtain any active motion of this limb while swimming (see Chapter 14). The dog completed 24 m swimming (two lengths), with rest periods to minimise posttreatment soreness.

Physiotherapy consultation (3 weeks postoperatively)

Weight bearing starting with toe touching evident in RHL. ROM improving: hip and stifle extension now 70% with treatment continuing. Veterinary and physiotherapy plan: the dog is to continue to be caged and only walk on lead 3–4 times a day for 5 min and to continue physiotherapy three times a week and hydrotherapy twice a week. Treatment progression guided by the clinical findings at each session.

Physiotherapy consultation (4 weeks postoperatively)

Consistent partial WB on RHL, although limb was still held in excessive flexion and lameness graded 3.5/5. ROM of hip extension now 90% with a tight 'restrictive capsular end-feel' but full flexion, abduction and rotation were now possible. The stifle could be fully flexed, but extension remained at 70% with some crepitus noted during and into end of ROM. The tarsus was now full ROM. Thigh circumference reduced (29 cm affected versus 34 cm unaffected limb).

Due to the nature of the fracture and surgery to the tibiofemoral joint, the veterinarian needed to reexamine the dog before progressing with the intensity of the stifle treatment to regain extension of the joint.

Follow-up radiographs (5 weeks postoperatively)

Follow-up radiographs demonstrated good healing of fracture. Assessment and treatment by the physiotherapist were then performed under anaesthetic to gauge the joint integrity without muscle tone altering available joint ROM. Techniques used: passive accessory physiological joint manual therapy techniques to the hip, stifle and tarsus; sustained stretching into end-of-range hip and stifle extension. During treatment, full hip ROM was attained and 70% stifle extension. N.B. the stifle was not 'overpressed' due to the fracture. Plan to continue with current physiotherapy and hydrotherapy treatment.

Physiotherapy consultation (8 weeks postoperatively)

Reduced lameness (2/5 at walk). Marked improvement in RHL thigh circumference 32 cm (left 34 cm) and ROM improved with full hip extension and 85% stifle extension. As the dog was much more functionally active, the treatment frequency was reduced to twice a week, while continuing to attend hydrotherapy twice a week, consistently using RHL in the water.

Physiotherapy consultation (3 months postoperatively)

A structured walking programme was commenced and graduated to include exercise from a bike at trot. Physiotherapy treatment was reduced to one session per week, and hydrotherapy kept at two sessions per week.

Physiotherapy consultation (4 months postoperatively)

Dog was no longer lame at walk and minimally intermittently lame at trot 0.5–1/5. Thigh circumference was now 32.5 cm and

stifle extension 90% with no pain on end-of-range joint overpressure, with minimal irritability and 'tightness' in the stifle flexors and gracilis. Exercise programme included leash walking and trotting for 30 min twice a day and hydrotherapy (swimming twice weekly). Dog was now allowed to be off lead and live with other dogs normally again and has returned to a successful showing career.

18.7 Hip dysplasia

Even though affected puppies are born with normal hips, by 2 weeks changes have already occurred that predispose to excessive joint laxity and alterations in the shape of the femoral and pelvic components of the joint (Read 2000). The joint incongruity leads to osteoarthritis and varying degrees of dysfunction and pain (Read 2000).

Environmental factors, including diet, have been shown to have significant effects on the incidence and severity of degenerative joint disease (DJD) in dogs with canine hip dysplasia (CHD) (Smith *et al.* 2001, 2006). Lifelong diet restriction (at 75% of the volume of control dogs) was shown to result in fewer radiographic signs of OA that, when present, showed up on average 6 years later (Smith *et al.* 2006). Month of birth may affect rates of CHD. Puppies born from July to October in England, spring and summer in Norway, and autumn in New Zealand tended to be least likely to develop CHD (Krontveit *et al.* 2012; Wood & Lakhani 2003; Worth *et al.* 2012). Theories as to why this would be found revolve around opportunity for outdoor exercise. Cardinet *et al.* (1997) reported that reduced pelvic muscle mass at a young age predisposes dogs to development of CHD. Krontveit *et al.* (2012) found that puppies allowed outdoor exercise on soft ground in moderately rough terrain had a reduced risk for developing radiographically detectable CHD, but that access to stairs at an early age (between birth and 3 months) could be a contributing factor to CHD development. Thus exercising could be beneficial for puppies and could be what increases pelvic muscle mass and therefore contribute to normal modelling forces around the hip during development. Additionally, a delay in neutering male Golden Retrievers (after 1 year of age) showed a reduction of CHD development by 50% (Torres de la Riva *et al.* 2013). There is a natural tendency for many immature dysplastic dogs to overcome acute hip pain as they mature (Black 2000). This may be due to fibrosis of the joint capsule and acetabular remodelling which increases stability and healing of microfractures (Black 2000).

There are several surgical options to treat the condition (total hip replacement, triple pelvic osteotomy, femoral head and neck ostectomy, or capsular denervation to name a few) (Moses 2000; Olmstead 1995; Read 2000). Postoperative physiotherapy goals and treatments can be addressed according to stages of healing (see section 18.5).

Conservative measures may provide a specific role for physiotherapists. A long-term study followed 68 dogs diagnosed with

CHD which were managed conservatively for 10 years (Barr *et al.* 1987), with 76% of the animals evaluated at the end of this time. Of these, 63% had no discomfort with forced hip extension, 79% had normal ROM, and 72% had normal exercise tolerance. Another paper discussed the rationale for conservative management that included controlled exercise, prevention of obesity and use of heat (Johnston 1992). Physiotherapy management of the non-surgical CHD patient aims to create the best possible musculoskeletal environment for pain-free hip functioning and to slow down the process of DJD.

Treatments should include controlled gross motor strengthening (general exercise and conditioning) and fine neuromotor control (balance and proprioception activities). ROM and stretching should focus on hip extension and rotation. Greene *et al.* (2013) found that longer daily exercise duration was associated with lower lameness scores in dogs with hip dysplasia. Joint nutrition may be addressed by exercise, joint compressions, ROM and nutritional advisement (see Chapter 3). Polysulphated glucosaminoglycans have been shown to significantly decrease lameness and histological evidence of cartilage reparative markers (Fujiki *et al.* 2007).

Impellizeri *et al.* (2000) studied overweight dogs and lameness attributable to CHD and implemented a calorie restriction diet which yielded at least a 10% reduction of initial bodyweight. They found a decrease in lameness during the mid-point and end of the study period. When pain is symptomatic, pain management can be assisted by manual therapy techniques and electrotherapy (see Chapters 12, 13). Radial shockwave has also been shown to improve gait in dogs with hip OA (Mueller *et al.* 2007). Additional factors to consider are secondary and compensatory movement patterns and neuromuscular dysfunctions that may ensue, such as spinal management to address facet joint dysfunctions or DJD elsewhere.

18.8 Conditioning canine athletes

Research on training and conditioning for the canine athlete is not readily available, but there is much to be extrapolated from horse and human research and literature. Fitness for sport is of the utmost importance. Fitness should encompass cardiorespiratory function, muscle strength, endurance, flexibility and coordination (de Vries 1986; Marcellin-Little *et al.* 2005; Zink 1997; Zink & Daniels 1996). Athletes training for sport-specific fitness need to also consider aerobic power and capacity, anaerobic power and capacity, muscular power, muscular endurance, balance, and body composition values that will optimise performance (Butcher & Webber 2012).

A full conditioning programme should not be implemented until the dog is skeletally mature and physeal closure has occurred (Marcellin-Little *et al.* 2005; Zink 1997; Zink & Daniels 1996). Generally, the epiphyseal plates close at 10 months in large dogs, a few months earlier in small dogs and a few months later

in giant breed dogs (Marcellin-Little *et al.* 2005). Before engaging in a training regime, animals should be examined for medical and musculoskeletal health by a veterinarian. A physiotherapist trained in animal physiotherapy can assess musculoskeletal function.

The physical requirements and physiological adaptations required to perform a sprint race (Greyhound), endurance race (sled dog) or sporting event (agility dog) are very different. The Greyhound is required to sprint at speeds up to 45 mph (72 km/h) (Geffen 2003). The distance can vary from 5/16, 3/8, 7/16, or 9/16 of a mile (500 metres, 600 metres, 700 metres, 900 metres) (Greyhound Racing Association of America website: www.gra-amerifca.org/). In the Iditarod, the sled dog must race for distances up to 1150 miles (1840 km) (Ultimate Iditarod website: www.ultimateiditarod.com/), and often will run continuously for 10–12 h at speeds of 10–12 mph (16–19.2 km/h) between rests (Topham 2005, personal communication). Shorter races usually see mushers running their dogs for only 6 or 7 h continuously (Topham 2005, personal communication). Agility competitions require competitors to sprint in one or several trials daily, going over, under, through or around all kinds of equipment (Zink & Daniels 1996). The agility athlete is like a football, basketball or rugby player, needing to possess coordination, strength, speed and the ability to recuperate quickly between runs.

Training programmes aim principally to improve cardiorespiratory and musculoskeletal responses, including strengthening (see also Chapter 6). Bone density and the thickness of the calcified cartilage layer of articular cartilage can both be increased to strengthen and improve overall load-bearing capabilities (Marlin 2003). Proprioception and exceptional body awareness are important for all animals, but are of critical importance for agility dogs.

A training programme that can promote dynamic joint and functional stability is desirable and should incorporate the following three levels of motor control:

- spinal reflexes
- cognitive programming
- brainstem activity (Lephart *et al.* 1997).

When a joint is placed under mechanical loading, reflex muscular stabilisation is stimulated through the spinal reflexes (Lephart *et al.* 1997). Voluntary movements that are repeated and stored as central commands are considered cognitive programming (utilising the highest level of CNS functioning) (Lephart *et al.* 1997). Brainstem reflexes include righting reactions and displacement reactions (Umphred & McCormack 1990).

18.8.1 Injury prevention
Stretching
In sprinting, muscle and fascial flexibility should be adequate to allow full ROM required for the activity (de Vries 1986) but not be overly flexible, which could impede the immediate transference of musculotendinous forces to the bones and potentially

reduce the speed of movement (Witvrouw *et al.* 2004). Stretching related to performance and injury prevention is very sports specific and a contentious issue in the literature. Some studies have shown there to be a negative impact on immediate athletic performance following stretching, so stretching needs to be appropriately applied in a sports-specific manner during or after competition or training sessions (Behm *et al.* 2004; Power *et al.* 2004; Shrier 2004; Thacker *et al.* 2004) (see section 18.2.6).

The racing Greyhound requires flexibility in the multiple-joint muscles, such as gracilis, biceps femoris, semitendinosus, semimembranosus, gastrocnemius and the calcaneal tendon, as well as the long head of triceps and latissimus dorsi that act in propulsion of both the fore- and hindlegs. The goal for implementing a stretching programme for the racing Greyhound is to ensure adequate muscle length in order to achieve the exaggerated ROMs and eccentric muscle contractions in those ranges. A stretching programme should be implemented only after training sessions for these athletes as a warm-up period is essential, and should include all the muscles/muscle groups (bilaterally) mentioned above, consisting of one 30-sec stretch every second day excluding race days.

Stretching to gain flexibility may not be essential for injury prevention in the sled dog as the gait and speed at which an endurance race is run only utilise the mid-ranges of the extremity joints (Witvrouw *et al.* 2004). The sled dog may be required to traverse (at a trot) over land or snow for several hours. End-of-range flexibility is not a requirement or an asset for this athlete and there is little need in this sport to utilise the energy-absorbing capacity of the muscle–tendon unit. No studies found reported any performance enhancement in endurance athletes with stretching. The current literature does not support a static end-of-range stretching regime in endurance animals as part of a regular or pre- or postevent activity.

The agility dog utilises its body in a very ballistic manner with rapid 'bursts' of power: jumping, changing directions and performing agile feats. This dog relies on kinetic/potential energy from elastic recoil of its musculotendinous apparatus as well as muscle power in jumping performance. A regular stretching programme may assist with this athlete, targeting the biceps brachii, long head of triceps and the carpal and digit flexors of the forelimbs (bilaterally) as well as the gluteals, hamstrings, quadriceps and the calcaneal tendon of the hindlimbs (bilaterally). One 30-sec stretch every second day to all the muscles/muscle groups mentioned should be utilised for these athletes.

Avoiding overtraining

Overtraining and overreaching should be avoided (see Chapter 6) (Feehan & Bassett 2004). During any training programme, an animal should be allowed adequate rest and recovery periods between exercise bouts to avoid overtraining and overreaching. Monitoring appetite, bodyweight, recovery of bodyweight after racing, behavioural changes, reluctance to exercise, muscle soreness, reduction in performance and slow recovery following exercise may be advised (Evans 2000).

Warming up and cooldown

It has been stated that warming up before competition is important for warming muscular tissues, enhancing muscle extensibility and improving oxygen kinetics (de Vries 1986; Steiss 2002; Tyler *et al.* 1996). The cooldown should be at least 20 min of walking after an especially strenuous session (Evans 2000) (see section 18.2.6).

Skill training

Attention to skill training, training on different surfaces or in adverse conditions can aid in avoiding injuries on 'race day' or 'trial weekend' (Evans 2000). Appropriate racing paces for sled dogs should be trialled to resist fatigue in both normal conditions and adverse weather (i.e. excessive heat) (Evans 2000; www.ultijmateiditarod.com). Racing Greyhounds should practise on different tracks, course styles or course lengths. Sled dogs should train with varying sled weights, and over variable terrain in different kinds of weather. Agility dogs should train on different surfaces, with different pieces of equipment arranged in different orders.

Health checks

All dogs should be regularly evaluated for signs of overtraining during a conditioning or training programme. The owner/trainer should be instructed to monitor for signs of overtraining, and be advised that monthly or bimonthly veterinary and physiotherapy evaluation should be conducted to monitor the medical and musculoskeletal well-being of the dog in training, so that treatment can be provided as needed.

18.8.2 Treatment of athletic injuries

The main difference in treating injuries in athletic dogs is the owner's expectations and desire to return to sport. Trauma to tissues or joints may result in a partial deafferentation and can lead to proprioceptive deficits (Lephart *et al.* 1997). Regaining neuromuscular control after injury or surgery is a necessary prerequisite for athletes wishing to return to competition (Lephart *et al.* 1997). Additionally, because these animals are more highly conditioned before injury, they may be able to tolerate a faster progression through the rehabilitation phases and most certainly will require advanced proprioception training and eccentric muscle strengthening exercises to make a safe return to sport (La Stayo *et al.* 2003; Lephart *et al.* 1997).

End-stage athletic rehabilitation

An end-stage or advanced level of rehabilitation may include the following (Edge-Hughes 2002, 2004; Steiss 2003; Zink 1997; Zink & Daniels 1996).

1 Exercises up and down hills
  • Varying hill steepness
  • May incorporate retrieving
  • Using different gaits and speeds

2 Trotting exercises
- In straight lines
- In serpentine, circular or figure-of-eight directions
- On different surfaces

3 Acceleration/deceleration activities
- Retrieving
- Short burst sprints (such as practising racing starts or recall exercises with the owner a distance away from the dog)
- Jumping (gradually increasing the jump height or breadth)

4 Cutting or rapid turning exercises
- Playing games of chase or keep away
- Running a mock agility course (starting with easy turns and low jumps and progressing to more difficult turns and manoeuvres)

5 Jumping exercises
- In different directions (circles, serpentine, figure-of-eight)
- Over varying heights
- Over jumps raised at odd angles

6 Concentric strengthening
- Pulling exercises (attaching a weight to a pulling harness)
- Mushing or skijoring
- Swimming
- Treadmills (land or water)

7 Endurance
- Gradual increases in duration of exercise
- Gradual increases in distances travelled
- Gradual increases in intensity of exercise

8 Static balancing
- Using wobble boards or mini-trampolines
- Standing on narrow planks of wood or small stools
- Standing on a physio ball

9 Dynamic balancing
- Walking on different surfaces (on foam, in sand, in tall grass, on uneven ground, in shallow water or in the woods)
- Walking across narrow planks of wood
- Walking across a seesaw
- Weave poles
- Jumping and recall exercises
- A-frame training
- Walking through ladders
- Walking through an obstacle course with poles spaced unevenly apart (forwards, backwards and sideways)

10 Power training
- Step-ups onto a platform or stool
- Squats: raising and lowering using one rear leg on a stool while the front feet are elevated (Figure 18.8)
- Jumping up onto a platform
- Tug of war
- Sit to stand facing up hill
- Exercises using a weighted vest

11 Return to sport

As people develop expertise, their motor control becomes less susceptible to interference from other tasks (Helton 2007b). In agility dogs, it has been shown that a statistically significant

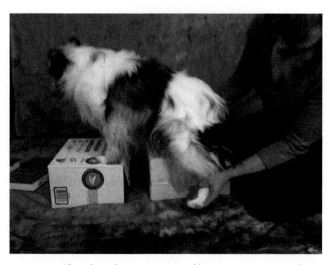

Figure 18.8 Three-legged squats: raising and lowering using one rear leg on a step.stool while the front feet are elevated.

relationship exists between the amount of deliberate practice and measured performance (Helton 2007a). Racing Greyhounds show marked improvement in skill development with increasing race experience (Helton 2009). Given this information, one could argue that utilisation of advanced level skills, known to the dog through years of training and skill acquisition, could be incorporated into end-stage rehabilitation programmes. This author has found that use of sport-specific activities has ameliorated lingering learned non-use or limb off-loading when traditional physiotherapy strengthening exercises have faltered in making end-stage gains.

Physiotherapists should be aware of canine sports and work with owners/handlers to incorporate sport-specific training into prescriptive therapy at this terminal stage of rehabilitation.

18.8.3 Summary

All rehabilitation, regardless of the species of patient, should be undertaken from a critical analysis perspective. A detailed physical diagnosis or at minimum a working diagnosis, presumption or problem list is required before proceeding with treatment. Communication between veterinarians and physiotherapists is essential to accomplish this goal. Treatment selection should be approached with a clear understanding of the mechanism of injury or surgical technique, healing times and physiological effects of each treatment modality or therapy chosen. Physiotherapy clearly has an expanding role in the health management of the dog.

References

Aaron, R.K., Ciombor, D.M., Simon, B.J. 2004, Treatment of non-unions with electric and electromagnetic field. *Clin. Orthop. Relat. Res.* 419: 21–29.

Ageberg, E., Zatterstrom, R., Moritz, U. *et al.* 2001, Influence of supervised and nonsupervised training on postural control after an acute anterior cruciate ligament rupture: a three-year longitudinal prospective study. *J. Orthop. Sports Phys. Ther.* 31(11): 632–644.

Ageberg, E., Pettersson, A., Friden, T. *et al.* 2007, 15-year followup of neuromuscular function in patients with unilateral nonreconstructed anterior cruciate ligament injury initially treated with rehabilitation and activity modification: a longitudinal prospective study. *Am. J. Sports Med.* 35(12): 2109–2117.

Alfredson, H., Pietila, T., Jonsson, P. *et al.* 1998, Heavy-load eccentric calf muscle training for the treatment of chronic Achilles tendinosis. *Am. J. Sports Med.* 26: 360–366.

Almekinders, L.C., Gilbert, J.A. 1986, Healing of experimental muscle strains and the effects of non-sterioidal anti-inflammatory medication. *Am. J. Sports Med.* 14: 303–308.

Bahr, R., Fossan, B., Loken, S., Engerbretsen, L. 2006, Surgical treatment compared with eccentric training for patellar tendinopathy (Jumper's Knee). *J. Bone Joint Surg. Am.* 88-A(8): 1689–1698.

Bandy, W.D., Irion, J.M. 1994, The effect of time on static stretch on the flexibility of the hamstring muscles. *Phys. Ther.* 74(9): 845–850.

Barr, A.R., Denny, H.R., Gibbs, C. 1987, Clinical hip dysplasia in growing dogs: the long-term results of conservative management. *J. Small Anim. Pract.* 28: 243–252.

Behm, D.G., Bambury, A., Cahill, F. *et al.* 2004, Effects of acute static stretching on force, balance, reaction time and movement time: *Med. Sci. Sports Exer.* 36(8): 1397–1402.

Bement, M.H. 2009, Exercise-induced hypoalgesia: an evidence-based review. In: Sluka, K.A. (ed), *Mechanisms and Management of Pain for the Physical Therapist*. IASP Press, Seattle, WA, pp. 143–166.

Berend, K.R., Lombardi, A.V., Mallory, T.H. 2004, Rapid recovery protocol for peri-operative care of total hip and total knee arthroplasty patients. *Surg. Technol. Int.* 13: 239–247.

Black, A.P. 2000, Triple pelvic osteotomy for juvenile canine hip dysplasia. *Aust. Vet. J.* 78(12): 820–821.

Blythe, L., Gannon, J.R., Craig, A.M. 1994, *Care of the Racing Greyhound*. American Greyhound Council, Abilene, KS.

Bockstahler, B.A., Henninger, W., Müller, M. *et al.* 2007, Influence of borderline hip dysplasia on joint kinematics of clinically sound Belgian Shepherd dogs. *Am. J. Vet. Res.* 68: 271–276.

Bocobo, C., Fast, A., Kingery, W. *et al.* 1991, The effect of ice on intra-articular temperature in the knee of the dog. *Am. J. Phys. Med. Rehab.* 70(4): 181–185.

Boddy, K.N., Roche, B.M., Schwartz, D.S. *et al.* 2004, Evaluation of the six-minute walk test in dogs. *Am. J. Vet. Res.* 65(3): 311–313.

Breur, G.J., Blevins W.E. 1997, Traumatic injury of the iliopsoas muscle in three dogs. *J. Am. Vet. Med. Assoc.* 210(11): 1631–1634.

Brosseau, L., MacLeay, L., Robinson, V., Wells, G., Tugwell, P. 2003, Intensity of exercise for the treatment of osteoarthritis (Review). *Cochrane Database Syst. Rev.* 2: CD004259.

Brotzman, S.B., Wilk, K.E. 2007, *Handbook of Orthopedic Rehabilitation*, 2nd edn. Mosby Elsevier, Philadelphia, PA.

Bruyere, O., Honore, A., Ethgen, O. *et al.* 2003, Correlation between radiographic severity of knee osteoarthritis and future disease progression – results from a 3-year prospective, placebo-controlled study evaluating the effect of glucosamine sulphate. *Osteoarthr. Cartil.* 11(1): 1–5.

Buckwalter, J.A. 2003, Sports, joint injury and post-traumatic osteoarthritis. *J. Orthop. Sports. Phys. Ther.* 33: 578–588.

Buss, D.D., Min, R., Skyhar, M. *et al.* 1995, Non-operative treatment of acute anterior cruciate ligament injuries in a selected group of patients. *Am. J. Sports Med.* 23(2): 160–165.

Butcher, S., Webber, S. 2012, Revolutionizing rehabilitation and healthy aging: bringing exercise 'Taboos' into the mainstream of care. *Physiother. Can.* 64(suppl 1): 52–53.

Canapp, S.O. Jr, McLaughlin, R.M. Jr, Hoskinson, J.J. *et al.* 1999, Scintigraphic evaluation of dogs with acute synovitis after treatment with glucosamine hydrochloride and chondroitin. *Am. J. Vet. Res.* 60(12): 1552–1557.

Cardinet, G.H. 3rd, Kass, P.H., Wallace, L.J. *et al.* 1997, Association between pelvic muscle mass and canine hip dysplasia. *J. Am. Vet. Med. Assoc.* 210(10): 1417–1418.

Carneiro, M.B., Alves, D.P., Mercadante, M.T. 2013, Physical therapy in the postoperative of proximal femur fracture in elderly. Literature review. *Acta Orthop. Bras.* 21(3): 175–178.

Casteleyn, P.P. 1999, Management of anterior cruciate ligament lesions: surgical fashion, personal whim or scientific evidence? Study of medium- and long-term results. *Acta Orthop. Belg.* 65(3): 327–339.

Cheing, G.L., Wan, J.W., Lo, S.K. 2005, Ice and pulsed electromagnetic field to reduce pain and swelling after distal radius fractures. *J. Rehabil. Med.* 37: 372–377.

Childs, S.G. 2003, Stimulators of bone healing. *Orthop. Nurs.* 22(6): 421–428.

Cho, H.J., Lim, S.C., Kim, S.G., *et al.* 2004, Effect of low-level laser therapy on osteoarthropathy in the rabbit. *In Vivo* 18(5): 585–591.

Cibulka, M.T., Threlkeld, J. 2004, The early clinical diagnosis of osteoarthritis of the hip. *J. Orthop. Sports Phys. Ther.* 34(8): 461–467.

Ciccotti, M.G., Kerlan, R.K., Perry, J. *et al.* 1994, An electromyographic analysis of the knee during functional activities: II. The anterior cruciate ligament-deficient and -reconstructed profiles. *Am. J. Sports Med.* 22(5): 651–658.

Clark, B., McLaughlin, R.M. 2001, Physical rehabilitation in small-animal orthopaedic patients. *Vet. Med.* 96(3): 234–247.

Clark, D.M. 1987, The use of electrical current in the treatment of non-unions. *Vet. Clin. North Am. Small Anim. Pract.* 17(4): 793–798.

Cochrane, T., Davey, R.C., Matthes-Edwards, S.M. 2005, Randomised controlled trial of the cost-effectiveness of water-based therapy for lower limb osteoarthritis. *Health Technol. Assess.* 9(31): iii–iv, ix–xi, 1–114.

Corbin, L. 2005, Safety and efficacy of massage therapy for patients with cancer. *Cancer Control* 12(3): 158–164.

Coutinho, E.L., Gomes, A.R., Franca, C.N. *et al.* 2004, Effect of passive stretching on the immobilized soleus muscle fibre morphology. *Braz. J. Med. Biol. Res.* 37(12): 1853–1861.

Crook, T.C. 2004, The effects of passive stretching on canine joint motion restricted by osteoarthritis *in vivo*. *Proc. 3rd Int. Symp. Rehabil. Phys. Ther. Vet. Med.* North Carolina State College of Veterinary Medicine, Raleigh, NC, p. 207.

Curtis, C.L., Rees, S.G., Cramp, J. *et al.* 2002, Effects of n-3 fatty acids on cartilage metabolism. *Proc. Nutr. Soc.* 61(3): 381–389.

Cyriax, J. 1982, *Textbook of Orthopaedic Medicine – diagnosis of soft tissue lesions*, 8th edn. Baillière Tindale, London.

Davidson, J.R., Kerwin, S.C., Millis, D.L. 2005, Rehabilitation for the orthopaedic patient. *Vet. Clin. Small Anim. Pract.* 35(6): 1357–1388.

Davis, D.S., Ashby, P.E., McCale, K.L. *et al.* 2005, The effectiveness of three stretching techniques on hamstring flexibility using consistent stretching parameters. *J. Strength Cond. Res.* 19(1): 27–32.

de Bruin, T., de Rooster, H., Bosmans, T. *et al.* 2007, Radiographic assessment of the progression of osteoarthrosis in the contralateral stifle joint of dogs with a ruptured cranial cruciate ligament. *Vet. Rec.* 161(22): 745–750.

DeCamp, C.E., Riggs, C.M., Olivier, N.B. *et al.* 1996, Kenematic evaluation of gait in dogs with cranial cruciate ligament rupture. *Am. J. Vet. Res.* 57(1): 120–126.

Decoster, L.C., Cleland, J., Altieri, C. *et al.* 2005, The effects of hamstring stretching on range of motion: a systematic literature review. *J. Orthop. Sports Phys. Ther.* 35: 377–387.

de Lahunta, A. (ed) 1983, *Veterinary Neuroanatomy and Clinical Neurology.* W.B. Saunders, Philadelphia, PA.

Delitto, A., Rose, S.J., McKowan, J.M. *et al.* 1988, Electrical stimulation versus voluntary exercise in strengthening thigh musculature after anterior cruciate ligament surgery. *Phys. Ther.* 68(5): 660–663.

Demir, H., Menku, P., Kirnap, M. *et al.* 2004, Comparison of the effects of laser, ultrasound, and combined laser + ultrasound treatments in experimental tendon healing. *Lasers Surg. Med.* 35(1): 84–89.

de Vries, H.A. 1986, *Physiology of Exercise for Physical Education and Athletics,* 4th edn. W.C. Brown, Dubuque, IA.

Deyle, G.D., Allison, S.C., Matekel, R.L. *et al.* 2005, Physical therapy treatment effectiveness for osteoarthritis of the knee: a randomised comparison of supervised clinical exercise and manual therapy procedures versus a home exercise program. *Phys. Ther.* 85(12): 1301–1317.

Edge-Hughes, L.M. 2001, Check out that pelvis. *CHAP Newsletter* Summer/Fall: 4–5.

Edge-Hughes, L.M. 2002, Therapeutic exercise for the canine patient. *Proc. 2nd Int. Symp. Rehabil. Phys. Ther. Vet. Med.* Knoxville, TN, pp. 59–62.

Edge-Hughes, L.M. 2004, Anatomy, biomechanics, physiology, diagnosis and treatment of teres major strains in the canine. *Proc. 3rd Int. Symp. Rehabil. Phys. Ther. Vet. Med.* North Carolina State College of Veterinary Medicine, Raleigh, NC, p. 229.

Edge-Hughes, L.M. 2005, Treatment of STI in the canine patient. *Proc. 3rd Ann. RVC Vet. Physiother. Con.* Royal Veterinary College, Hatfield, UK, pp. 10–17.

Edge-Hughes, L.M. 2006, *Introduction to Canine Rehabilitation. Course Manual.* Available at: www.animalrehabinstitute.com

Eitzen, I., Moksnes, H., Snyder-Mackler, L., *et al.* 2010, A progressive 5-week exercise therapy program leads to significant improvement in knee function early after anterior cruciate ligament injury. *J. Orthop. Sports Phys. Ther.* 40(11): 705–721.

Esteve-Lanao, J., San Juan, A.F., Earnest, C.P. *et al.* 2005, How do endurance runners actually train? Relationship with competition performance. *Med. Sci. Sports Exerc.* 37(3): 496–509.

Ettinger, S.J., Feldman, E.C. 2002, *Textbook of Veterinary Internal Medicine: diseases of the dog and cat,* 6th edn. Elsevier Saunders, St Louis, MO.

Evans, D. 2000, *Training and Fitness in Athletic Horses.* Rural Industries Research and Development Corporation, Barton, ACT.

Feehan, L.M., Bassett, K. 2004, Is there evidence for early mobilization following an extra-articular hand fracture? *J. Hand. Ther.* 17(2): 300–308.

Fini, M., Giavaresi, G., Torricelli, P. *et al.* 2005, Pulsed electromagnetic fields reduce knee osteoarthritic lesion progression in the aged Dunkin Hartley guinea pig. *J. Orthop. Res.* 23: 899–908.

Fioravanti, A., Nerucci, F., Collodel, G. 2002, Biochemical and morphological study of human articular chondrocytes cultivated in the presence of pulsed signal therapy. *Ann. Rheum. Dis.* 61: 1032–1033.

Fitch, R.B., Jaffe, M.H., Montgomery, R.D. 1997, Muscle injuries in dogs. *Comp. Cont. Ed. Pract. Vet.* 19(8): 947–956.

Fitzgerald, G.K., Axe, M.J., Snyder-Mackler, L. 2000, Proposed practice guidelines for non-operative anterior cruciate ligament rehabilitation of physically active individuals. *J. Orthop. Sports Phys. Ther.* 30(4): 194–203.

Fitzgerald, G.K., Piva, S.R., Irrgang, J.J. 2003, A modified neuromuscular electrical stimulation protocol for quadriceps strength training following anterior cruciate ligament reconstruction. *J. Orthop. Sports Phys. Ther.* 33: 492–501.

Fletcher, I.M., Jones, B. 2004, The effect of different warm-up stretch protocols on a 20-metre sprint performance in trained rugby union players. *J. Strength. Cond. Res* 18(4): 885–888.

Francis, D.A., Millis, D.L., Stevens, M. *et al.* 2002, Bone and muscle loss from disuse following cranial cruciate ligament transaction and stifle stabilization surgery. *Proc. 2nd Int. Symp. Rehabil. Phys. Ther. Vet. Med.* Knoxville, TN, pp. 203–204.

Fransson, B.A., Gavin, P.R., Lahmers, K.K. 2005, Supraspinatus tendinosis associated with biceps brachii tendon displacement in a dog. *J. Am. Vet. Med. Assoc.* 227(9): 1429–1432.

Friden, T., Egund, N., Lindstrand, A. 1993, Comparison of symptomatic versus nonsymptomatic patients with chronic anterior cruciate ligament insufficiency. Radiographic sagittal displacement during weightbearing. *Am. J. Sports Med.* 21(3): 389–393.

Friden, T., Roberts, D., Zatterstrom, R. *et al.* 1999, Proprioceptive defects after an anterior cruciate ligament rupture – the relation to associated anatomical lesion s and subjective knee function. *Knee Surg. Sports Traumatol. Arthrosc.* 7(4): 226–231.

Friden, T., Roberts, D., Ageberg, E. *et al.* 2001, Review of knee proprioception and the relation to extremity function after an anterior cruciate ligament rupture. *J. Orthop. Sports Phys. Ther.* 31(10): 567–576.

Fujiki, M., Shineaha, J., Yamanokuchi, K. *et al.* 2007, Effects of treatment with polysulfated glycosaminoglycan on serum cartilage oligomeric matrix protein and C-reactive protein concentrations, serum matrix metalloproteinases 2 and 9 activities, and lameness in dogs with arthritis. *Am. J. Vet. Res.* 68: 827–833.

Furia, J.P., Rompe, J.D., Cacchio, A., Maffulli, N. 2010, Shock wave therapy as a treatment of nonunions, avascular necrosis, and delayed healing of stress fractures. *Foot Ankle Clin. North Am.* 15(4): 651–662.

Gebauer, G.P. 2002, Low intensity pulsed ultrasound increases the fracture callus strength in diabetic *BB Wistar* rats but does affect cellular proliferation. *J. Orthop. Res.* 20: 587–592.

Gebauer, D., Correll, J. 2005, Pulsed low-intensity ultrasound. A new salvage procedure for delayed unions and non-unions after leg lengthening in children. *J. Pediatr. Orthop.* 25(6): 750–754.

Geffen, S.J. 2003, Rehabilitation principles for treating chronic musculoskeletal injuries. *Med. J. Aust.* 178(3): 238–242.

Gerbi, M.E., Pinheiro, A.L., Marzola, C. *et al.* 2005. Assessment of bone repair associated with the use of organic bovine bone and membrane irradiated at 830nm. *Photomed. Laser Surg.* 23(4): 382–388.

Gordon, W.J., Conzemius, M.G., Riedsel, F. et al. 2003, The relationship between limb function and radiographic osteoarthrosis in dogs with stifle osteoarthrosis. *Vet. Surg.* 32: 451–454.

Gravare Silbernagel K., Thomee R., Thomee P. *et al.* 2001, Eccentric overload training for patients with chronic Achilles tendon pain – a randomized controlled study with reliability testing of the evaluation methods. *Scand. J. Med. Sci. Sports* 11: 197–206.

Green, S., Buchbinder, R., Hetrick, S. 2003, Physiotherapy interventions for shoulder pain (Review). *Cochrane Database Syst. Rev.* 2: CD004258.

Greene, L.M., Marcellin-Little, D.J., Lascelles, B.D. 2013, Associations among exercise duration, lameness severity, and hip joint range of motion in Labrador Retrievers with hip dysplasia. *J. Am. Vet. Med. Assoc.* 242(11): 1528–1533.

Gross-Saunders, D., Walker, J.R., Levine, D. 2005, Joint mobilization. *Vet. Clin. Small Anim. Pract.* 35(6): 1287–1316.

Gur, A., Cosut, A., Sarac, A.J. *et al.* 2003, Efficacy of different therapy regimes of low-power laser in painful osteoarthritis of the knee: a double blind and randomised-controlled trial. *Lasers Surg. Med.* 33(5): 330–338.

Hamilton, S.A. 2002, Rehabilitation of osteoarthritis in a dog. *Proc. 2nd Int. Symp. Rehabil. Phys. Ther. Vet. Med.* Knoxville, TN, p. 127.

Helton, W.S. 2007a, Deliberate practice in dogs: a canine model of expertise. *J. Gen. Psychol.* 134(2): 247–257.

Helton, W.S. 2007b, Skill in expert dogs. *J. Exp. Psychol. Appl.* 13(3): 171–178.

Helton, W.S. 2009, Exceptional running skill in dogs requires extensive experience. *J. Gen. Psychol.* 136(3): 323–332.

Hernandez-Molina, G., Reichenbach, S., Zhang, B. *et al.* 2008, Effect of therapeutic exercise for hip osteoarthritis pain: results of a meta-analysis. *Arthritis Rheum.* 59(9): 1221–1228.

Hesslink, R., Armstrong, D. 3rd, Nagendran, M.V. *et al.* 2002, Cetylated fatty acids improve knee function in patients with osteoarthritis. *J. Rheumatol.* 29(8): 1708–1712.

Hewett, T.E., Paterno, M.V., Myer, G.D. 2002, Strategies for enhancing proprioception and neuromuscular control of the knee. *Clin. Orthop. Rel. Res.* 402: 76–94.

Hoeksma, H., Dekker, J., Ronday, H. *et al.* 2004, Comparison of manual therapy and exercise therapy in osteoarthritis of the hip: a randomised clinical trial. *Arthritis Rheum.* 51: 722–729.

Holt, S. 1998, Bone and Joint Health: Part 2 – Dietary Supplements. *Alt. Compl. Ther.* 4(3): 195–205.

Huang, M.H., Lin, Y.S., Lee, C.L. *et al.* 2005, Use of ultrasound to increase effectiveness of isokinetic exercise for knee osteoarthritis. *Arch. Phys. Med. Rehabil.* 86(8): 1545–1551.

Hubbard, T.J., Denegar, C.R. 2004, Does cryotherapy improve outcomes with soft tissue injury? *J. Athl. Train.* 39(1): 88–94.

Hunter, J.P., Marshall, R.N. 2002, Effects of power and flexibility training on vertical jump technique. *Med. Sci. Sports Exerc.* 34(3): 478–486.

Ibiwoye, M.O., Powell, K.A., Grabiner, M.D. *et al.* 2004, Bone mass is preserved in a critical-sized osteotomy by low energy pulsed electromagnetic fields as quantitated by *in vivo* micro-computed tomography. *J. Orthop. Res.* 22: 1086–1093.

Ihara, H., Miwa, M., Takayanagi, K. *et al.* 1994, Acute torn meniscus combined with acute cruciate ligament injury. Second-look arthroscopy after 3-month conservative treatment. *Clin. Orthop. Relat. Res.* 307: 146–154.

Impellizeri, J.A., Tetrick, M.A., Muir, P. 2000, Effect of weight reduction on clinical signs of lameness in dogs with hip osteoarthritis. *J. Am. Vet Med. Assoc.* 216(7): 1089–1091.

Innes, J.F., Barr, A.R. 1998, Clinical natural history of the post surgical cruciate deficient canine stifle joint: year 1. *J. Small Anim. Pract.* 39(7): 325–332.

Innes, J.F., Costello, M., Barr, F.J. *et al.* 2004, Radiographic progression of osteoarthritis of the canine stifle joint: a prospective study. *Vet. Radiol. Ultrasound.* 45(2): 143–148.

Innes, J.F., Sharif, M., Barr, A.R. 1999, Changes in concentrations of biochemical markers of osteoarthritis following surgical repair of ruptured cranial cruciate ligaments in dogs. *Am. J. Vet. Res.* 60(9): 1164–1168.

Inoue, N., Ohnishi, I., Chen, D. *et al.* 2002, Effect of pulsed electromagnetic fields (PEMF) on late-phase osteotomy gap healing in a canine tibial model. *J. Orthop. Res.* 20: 1106–1114.

Iopollo, F., Tattoli, M, Di Sante, L. *et al.* 2013, Clinical improvement and resorption of calcifications in calcific tendinitis of the shoulder after shock wave therapy at 6 months' follow up: a systematic review and meta-analysis. *Arch. Phys. Med. Rehabil.* 94(9): 1699–1706.

Jerram, R.M., Walker, A.M. 2003, Cranial cruciate ligament injury in the dog: pathophysiology, diagnosis and treatment, *N. Z. Vet. J.* 51(4): 149–158.

Johnson, J.M., Johnson, A.L. 1993, Cranial cruciate ligament rupture – pathogenesis, diagnosis and post-operative rehabilitation. *Vet. Clin. North Am. Small Anim. Pract.* 23(4): 717–733.

Johnson, J.M., Johnson, A.L., Pijanowski, G.J. *et al.* 1997, Rehabilitation of dogs with surgically treated cranial cruciate ligament-deficient stifles by use of electrical stimulation of muscles. *Am. J. Vet. Res.* 58(12): 1473–1478.

Johnson, K.A., Hulse, D.A., Hart, R.C. *et al.* 2001, Effects of an orally administered mixture of chondroitin sulphate, glucosamine hydrochloride and manganese ascorbate on synovial fluid chondroitin sulphate 3B3 and 7D4 epitope in a canine cruciate ligament transaction model of osteoarthritis. *Osteoarthr. Cartil.* 9: 14–21.

Johnson, K.A., Hay, C.W., Chu, Q. *et al.* 2002, Cartilage-derived biomarkers of osteoarthritis in synovial fluid of dogs with naturally acquired rupture of the cranial cruciate ligament. *Am. J. Vet. Res.* 63(6): 775–781.

Johnston, S.A. 1992, Conservative and medical management of hip dysplasia. *Vet. Clin. North Am. Small Anim. Pract.* 22(3): 595–606.

Kamel, H.K., Iqbal, M.A., Mogallapu, R. *et al.* 2003, Time to ambulation after hip fracture surgery: relation to hospitalisation outcomes. *J. Gerontol.* 58A(11): 1042–1045.

Kealy, R.D., Lawler, D.F., Ballam, J.M. *et al.* 2002, Effects of diet restriction on life span and age-related changes in dogs. *J. Am. Vet. Med. Assoc.* 220(9): 1315–1320.

Kerfoot, L. 1997, An introduction to topline dysfunction in the equine athlete. *CHAP Newsletter* Fall: 8–10.

Kerkhoffs, G.M., Rowe, B.H., Assendelft, W.J., Kelly, K., Struijs, P.A., van Dijk, C.N. 2002, Immobilisation and functional treatment for acute lateral ankle ligament injuries in adults (Review). *Cochrane Database Syst. Rev.* 3: CD003762.

Khan, K.M., Cook, J.L., Bonar, G. *et al.* 1999, Histopathology of common tendinopathies: update and clinical management. *Sports Med.* 27(6): 393–408.

Klock, N.W., Snyder, P.W., Widmer, W.R. *et al.* 2005, Detection of synovial macrophages in the joint capsule of dogs with naturally occurring rupture of the cranial cruciate ligament. *Am. J. Vet. Res.* 66(3): 493–499.

Knudson, D. 1999, Stretching during warm-up: do we have enough evidence? *J. Phys. Ed. Rec. Dance* 70(7): 24–26.

Korstjens, C.M., Nolte, P.A., Burger, E.H. *et al.* 2004, Stimulation of bone cell differentiation by low-intensity ultrasound – a histomorphometric *in vitro* study. *J. Orthop Res.* 22: 495–500.

Kostogiannis, I., Ageberg, E., Neuman, P. *et al.* 2007, Activity level and subjective knee function 15 years after anteiro cruciate ligament injury. A prospective, longitudinal study of nonreconstructed patients. *Am. J. Sports Med.* 35(7): 1135–1143.

Kraemer, W.J., Ratamess, N.A., Maresh, C.M. *et al.* 2005, A cetylated fatty acid topical cream with menthol reduces pain and improves functional performance in individuals with arthritis. *J. Strength. Cond. Res.* 19(2): 475–480.

Krontveit, R.I., Nodtvedt, A., Saevik, B.K. *et al.* 2012, Housing- and exercise-related risk factors associated with the development of hip dysplasia as determined by radiographic evaluation in a prospective cohort of Newfoundlands, Labrador Retrievers, Leonbergers, and Irish Wolfhounds in Norway. *Am. J. Vet. Res.* 73(6): 838–846.

Kujala, U.M., Orava, S., Jarvinen, M. 1997, Hamstring injuries: current trends in treatment and prevention. *Sports Med.* 23: 397–404.

Kvist, J. 2004, Rehabilitation following anterior cruciate ligament injury – current recommendations for sports participation. *Sports Med.* 34(4): 269–280.

Lahm, A., Uhl, M., Erggelet, C. *et al.* 2004, Articular cartilage degeneration after acute subchondral bone damage: an experimental study in dogs with histopathological grading. *Acta Orthop. Scand.* 75(6): 762–767.

Landman, M.A., de Blaauw, J.A., van Weeren, P.R. *et al.* 2004, Field study of the prevalence of lameness in horses with back problems. *Vet. Rec.* 155(6): 165–168.

Langberg H., Ellingsgaard H., Madsen T. *et al.* 2007, Eccentric rehabilitation exercise increases peritendinous type I collagen synthesis in humans with Achilles tendinosis. *Scand. J. Med. Sci. Sports* 17(1): 61–66.

La Stayo, P.C., Woolf, J.M., Lewek, M.D. *et al.* 2003, Eccentric muscle contractions: their contribution to injury, prevention, rehabilitation and sport. *J. Orthop. Sports Phys. Ther.* 33: 557–571.

Lee, E.W., Maffulli, N., Li, C.K. *et al.* 1997, Pulsed magnetic and electromagnetic fields in experimental Achilles tendonitis in the rat: a prospective randomised study. *Arch. Phys. Med. Rehabil.* 78: 399–404.

Lephart, S.M., Pincivero, D.M., Giraldo, J.L. *et al.* 1997, The role of proprioception in the management and rehabilitation of athletic injuries. *Am. J. Sports Med.* 25(1): 130–137.

Lin, Y.S., Huang, M.H., Chai, C.Y. 2005, Effects of helium-neon laser on the mucopolysaccharide induction in experimental osteoarthritic cartilage. *Osteoarthr. Cartil.* 14(4): 377–383.

Lirani-Galvao, A.P., Jorgetti, V., da Silva, O.L. 2006, Comparative study of how low-level laser therapy and low-intensity pulsed ultrasound affect bone repair in rats. *Photomed. Laser Surg.* 24(6): 735–740.

Luger, E.J., Rochkind, S., Wollman, Y. *et al.* 1998, Effect of flow-power laser irradiation on the mechanical properties of bone fracture healing in rats. *Lasers Surg. Med.* 22(2): 97–102.

Lumb, A.B. 2000, *Nunn's Applied Respiratory Physiology.* Butterworth-Heinemann, Edinburgh, Scotland.

Maganaris, C.N., Narici, M.V., Almekinders, L.C. *et al.* 2004, Biomechanics and pathophysiology of overuse tendon injuries – ideas on insertional tendonopathy. *Sports Med.* 34(14): 1005–1017.

Magee, D.J. 2008, *Orthopedic Physical Assessment.* Saunders Elsevier, St Louis, MO.

Magnusson, S.P., Aagard, P., Simonsen, E. *et al.* 1998, A biomechanical evaluation of cyclic and static stretch in human skeletal muscle. *Int. J. Sports Med.* 19(5): 310–316.

Maitland, G.D. 1966, Manipulation – mobilisation. *Physiotherapy* 52(11): 382–385.

Marcellin-Little, D.J., Levine, D., Taylor, R. 2005, Rehabilitation and conditioning of sporting dogs. *Vet. Clin. North Am. Small Anim. Pract.* 35(6): 1427–1439.

Markey, K.L. 1991, Functional rehabilitation of the cruciate-deficient knee. *Sports Med.* 12(6): 407–417.

Marlin, D., Nankervis, K. (eds) 2003, Skeletal responses. In: *Equine Exercise Physiology.* Blackwell Science, Malden, MA, pp. 86–93.

Marr C.M., McMillan I., Boyd J.S. *et al.* 1993 Ultrasonographic and histopathological findings in equine superficial digital flexor tendon injury. *Equine Vet. J.* 25: 23–29.

Marshall, W.G., Bockstahler, B.A., Hulse, D.A., Carmichael, S. 2009, A review of osteoarthritis and obesity: current understanding of the relationship and benefit of obesity treatment and prevention in the dog. *Vet. Comp. Orthop. Traumatol.* 22(5): 339–345.

Marsolais, G.S., Dvorak, G., Conzemius, M.G. 2002, Effects of postoperative rehabilitation on limb function after cranial cruciate ligament repair in dogs. *J. Am. Vet. Med. Assoc.* 220(9): 1325–1330.

Marteniuk, R.G. 1979, Motor skill performance and learning: considerations for rehabilitation. *Physiother. Can.* 31: 187–202.

Matsumoto, H., Ochi, M., Abiko, Y. 2000, Pulsed electromagnetic fields promote bone formation around dental implants inserted into the femur of rabbits. *Clin. Oral Imp. Res.* 11: 354–360.

Meadows, T.H., Bronk, J.T., Chao, E.Y. *et al.* 1990, Effects of weight bearing on healing of cortical defects in the canine tibia. *J. Bone Joint Surg.* 72A(7): 1074–1080.

Messier, S.P., Gutekunst, D.J., Davis, C. *et al.* 2005, Weight loss reduces knee-joint loads in overweight and obese older adults with knee osteoarthritis. *Arthritis Rheum.* 52(7): 2026–2032.

Michlovitz, S.L. 1990, *Thermal Agents in Rehabilitation.* F.A. Davis, Philadelphia, PA.

Millis, D.L. 2004, Managing chronic osteoarthritis using physical rehabilitation. *Proc. 3rd Int. Symp. Rehabil. Phys. Ther. Vet. Med.* Research Triangle Park, Durham, NC, pp. 127–130.

Millis, D.L., Levine, D. 1997, The role of exercise and physical modalities in the treatment of osteoarthritis. *Vet. Clin. North Am. Small Anim. Pract.* 27(4): 913–930.

Mondejar, E.F., Mata, G.V., Cardenas, A. *et al.* 1996, Ventilation with positive end-expiratory pressure reduces extravascular lung water and increases lymphatic flow in hydrostatic pulmonary edema. *Crit. Care Med.* 24(9): 1562–1567.

Moses, P.A. 2000, Alternative surgical methods for treating juvenile canine hip dysplasia. *Aust. Vet. J.* 78(12): 822–824.

Mueller, M., Bockstahler, B., Skalicky, M. *et al.* 2007, Effects of radial shockwave therapy on the limb function of dogs with hip osteoarthritis. *Vet. Rec.* 160(22): 762–765.

Myklebust, G., Holm, I., Maehlum, S. *et al.* 2003, Clinical, functional, and radiologic outcome in team handball players 6–11 years after anterior cruciate ligament injury: a follow-up study. *Am. J. Sports Med.* 31: 981–989.

Nash, C.E., Mickan, S.M., Del Mar, C.B., Glasziou, P.P. 2004, Resting injured limbs delays recovery: a systematic review. *J. Fam. Pract.* 53(9): 706–712.

Nelson, R.M., Currier, D.P. 1987, *Clinical Electrotherapy*. Appleton & Lange, Norwalk, CT.

Neuman, P., Englund, M., Kostogiannis, I. *et al.* 2008, Prevalence of tibiofemoral osteoarthritis 15 years after nonoperative treatment of anterior cruciate ligament injury: a prospective cohort study. *Am. J. Sports Med.* 36(9): 1717–1725.

Newton, P.M., Mow, V.C., Gardner, T.R., Buckwalter, J.A., Albright, J.P. 1997, The effect of lifelong exercise on canine articular cartilage. *Am. J. Sports Med.* 25(3): 282–287.

Nielsen, C., Pluhar, C. 2005, Diagnosis and treatment of hind limb muscle strain injuries in 22 dogs. *Vet. Comp. Orthop. Traumatol* 18: 247–253.

Norregaard, J., Larsen, C.C., Bieler, T. *et al.* 2007, Eccentric exercise in treatment of Achilles tendinopathy. *Scand. J. Med. Sci. Sports.* 17(2): 133–138.

Noyes, F.R., Matthews, D.S., Mooar, P.A. *et al.* 1983, The symptomatic anterior cruciate-deficient knee. Part II: The results of rehabilitation, activity modification, and counselling on functional disability. *J. Bone Joint Surg. Am.* 65: 163–174.

Nwadike, B.S., Hesbach, A. 2004, Rehabilitation of fracture patients. *Proc. 3rd Int. Symp. Rehabil. Phys. Ther. Vet. Med.* Research Triangle Park, Durham, NC, pp. 141–144.

Obremsky, W.T., Seaber, A.V., Ribbeck, B.M. *et al.* 1994, Biomechanical and histologic assessment of a controlled muscle strain injury treated with piroxicam. *Am. J. Sports Med.* 22: 558–561.

Ohberg L., Lorentzon R., Alfredson H. 2004, Eccentric training in patients with chronic Achilles tendinosis: normalized tendon structure and decreased thickness at follow up. *Br. J. Sports Med.* 38:8–11.

Olmstead, M.L. 1995, *Small Animal Orthopedics*. Mosby, St Louis, MO.

Paavola, M., Kannus, P., Jarvinen, T.A. *et al.* 2002, Treatment of tendon disorders. Is there a reason for corticosteroid injections? *Foot Ankle Clin.* 7(3): 501–513.

Park, S.H., Silva, M. 2004, Neuromuscular electrical stimulation enhances fracture healing: results of an animal model. *J. Orthop. Res.* 22: 382–387.

Parvizi, J., Parpura, V., Greenleaf, J.F. *et al.* 2002, Calcium signalling is required for ultrasound-stimulated aggrecan synthesis by rat chondrocytes. *J. Orthop. Res.* 20: 51–57.

Patel, S.K., Dick, B.H., Busconi, B.D. 2007, Fracture management. In: Magee, D.J., Zachazewski, J.E., Quillen, W.S. (eds), *Scientific Foundations and Principles of Practice in Musculoskeletal Rehabilitation*. Saunders Elsevier, St Louis, MO, pp. 607–627.

Perry, M.C., Morrissey, M.C., King, J.B. *et al.* 2005, Effects of closed versus open kinetic chain knee extensor resistance training on knee laxity and leg function in patients during the 8- to 14-week post-operative period after anterior cruciate ligament reconstruction. *Knee Surg. Sports Traumatol. Arthrosc.* 13: 357–369.

Pinheiro, A.L., Gerbi, M.E. 2006, Photoengineering of bone repair. *Photomed. Laser Surg.* 24(2): 169–178.

Plews-Ogan, M., Owens, J.E., Goodman, M. *et al.* 2005, Brief report: a pilot study evaluating mindfulness-based stress reduction and massage for the management of chronic pain. *J. Gen. Intern. Med.* 20: 1136–1138.

Power, K., Behm, D., Cahill, F. *et al.* 2004, An acute bout of static stretching: effects on force and jumping performance. *Med. Sci. Sports Exerc.* 36(8): 1389–1396.

Ray, A., Ray BK. 2008, An inflammation-responsive transcription factor in the pathophysiology of osteoarthritis. *Biorheology.* 45(3): 399–409.

Read, R.A. 2000, Conservative management of juvenile canine hip dysplasia. *Aust. Vet. J.* 78(12): 818–819.

Rees, D.J., Wilson, A.M., Wolman, R.L. 2006, Current concepts in the management of tendon disorders. *Rheumatology* 45(5): 508–521.

Rees, J.D., Maffulli N., Cook J. 2009, Management of tendinopathy. *Am. J. Sports Med.* 37(9): 1855–1867.

Richardson, D.C., Schoeherr, W.D., Zicker, S.C. 1997, Nutritional management of osteoarthritis. *Vet. Clin. North Am. Small Anim. Pract.* 27(4): 883–911.

Roberts, D., Friden, T., Zatterstrom, R. *et al.* 1999, Proprioception in people with anterior cruciate ligament-deficient knees: comparison of symptomatic and asymptomatic patients. *J. Orthop. Sports Phys. Ther.* 29(10): 587–594.

Roberts, D., Friden, T., Stromberg, A. *et al.* 2000, Bilateral proprioceptive defects in patients with a unilateral anterior cruciate ligament reconstruction: a comparison between patients and healthy individual. *J. Orthop. Res.* 18(4): 565–571.

Roddy, E., Zhang, W., Doherty, M. 2005, Aerobic walking or strengthening exercise for osteoarthritis of the knee? A systematic review. *Ann. Rheum. Dis.* 64: 544–548.

Rood, M. 1956, Neurophysiological mechanisms utilised in the treatment of neuromuscular dysfunction. *Am. J. Occup. Ther.* 10: 220–225.

Roos, E.M., Dahlberg, L. 2005, Positive effects of moderate exercise on glycosaminoglycan content in knee cartilage: a four-month, randomised, controlled trial in patients at risk of osteoarthritis. *Arthritis Rheum.* 52(11): 3507–3514.

Ross, M.D., Denegar, C.R., Winzenried, J.A. 2001, Implementation of open and closed kinetic chain quadriceps strengthening exercises after anterior cruciate ligament reconstruction. *J. Strength. Cond. Res.* 15(4): 466–473.

Ruiz-Bailen, M., Fernandez-Mondejar, E., Hurtado-Ruiz, B. *et al.* 1999, Immediate application of positive-end expiratory pressure is more effective than delayed positive-end expiratory pressure to reduce extravascular lung water. *Crit. Care Med.* 27(2): 380–384.

Saini, N.S., Roy, K.S., Bansal, P.S. *et al.* 2002, A preliminary study on the effects of ultrasound therapy on the healing of surgically severed Achilles tendons in five dogs. *J. Vet. Med. Assoc.* 49: 321–328.

Santa-Rodriguez, N., Clavo, B., Fernandez-Perez, L. *et al.* 2010, Pulsed ultrasounds accelerate healing of rib fractures in an experimental animal model: an effective new thoracic therapy? *J. Thorac. Cardovasc. Surg.* 141(5): 125–128.

Sawner, K. 1992, *Brunnstrom's Movement Therapy in Hemiplegia: a neurophysiological approach*. Lippincott Williams & Wilkins, Philadelphia, PA.

Scavenius, M., Bak, K., Hansen, S. *et al.* 1999, Isolated total ruptures of the anterior cruciate ligament – a clinical study with long-term follow-up of 7 years. *Scand. J. Med. Sci. Sports.* 9(2): 114–119.

Schumacher, H.R. (ed.) 1988, *Primer on Rheumatic Diseases*, 9th edn. Arthritis Foundation, Atlanta, GA.

Sharma, P., Maffulli, N. 2005, Tendon injury and tendinopathy: healing and repair. *J. Bone Joint Surg.* 87(1): 187–202.

Shaw, T., Williams, M.T., Chipchase, L.S. 2005, Do early quads exercises affect the outcome of ACL reconstruction? A randomised controlled trial. *Aust. J. Physio.* 51(1): 9–17.

Shrier, I. 2004, Does stretching improve performance? A systematic and critical review of the literature. *Clin. J. Sports Med.* 14(5): 267–273.

Skinner, J. 1987, *Exercise Testing and Exercise Prescription for Special Cases.* Lea & Febiger, Philadelphia, PA.

Smith, G.K., Mayhew, P.D., Kapatkin, A.S. *et al.* 2001, Evaluation of risk factors for degenerative joint disease associated with hip dysplasia in German Shepherd Dogs, Golden Retrievers, Labrador Retrievers and Rottweilers. *J. Am. Vet. Med. Assoc.* 219(12): 1719–1724.

Smith, G.K., Paster, E.R., Powers, M.Y. *et al.* 2006, Lifelong diet restriction and radiographic evidence of osteoarthritis of the hip joint in dogs. *J. Am. Vet. Med. Assoc.* 229: 690–693.

Snibbe, J.C., Gambardella, R.A. 2005, Treatment options for osteoarthritis. *Orthopaedics* 28(2 suppl): S215–S220.

Spreng, D., Sigrist, N., Jungi, T. *et al.* 2000, Nitric oxide metabolite production in the cranial cruciate ligament, synovial membrane, and articular cartilage of dogs with cranial cruciate ligament rupture. *Am. J. Vet. Res.* 61(5): 530–536.

Steim, H., Lerner, A. 2005, How does pulsed low-intensity ultrasound enhance fracture healing? *Orthopaedics* 28(10): 1161–1163.

Steiss, J.E. 2002, Muscle disorders and rehabilitation in canine athletes. *Vet. Clin North Am. Small Anim. Pract.* 32(1): 267–285.

Steiss, J.E. 2003, Canine rehabilitation. In: Braund, K.G. (ed.), *Clinical Neurology in Small Animals – localization, diagnosis and treatment.* International Veterinary Information Service, Ithaca, NY.

Steiss, J.E., Levine, D. 2005, Physical agent modalities. *Vet. Clin. North Am. Small Anim. Pract.* 35(6): 1317–1333.

Stitik, T.P., Kaplan, R.J., Kamen, L.B. *et al.* 2005, Rehabilitation of orthopaedic and rheumatological disorders: 2. Osteoarthritis assessment, treatment and rehabilitation. *Arch. Phys. Med. Rehabil.* 86(suppl 1): S48–S55.

Strehl, A., Eggli, S. 2007, The value of conservative treatment in ruptures of the anterior cruciate ligament (ACL). *J. Trauma* 62(5): 1159–1162.

Strickler, T., Malone, T., Garrett, W.E. 1990, The effects of passive warming on muscle injury. *Am. J. Sports Med.* 18(2): 141–145.

Sullivan, P.E., Markos, P.D., Minor, M.A.D. 1982, *An Integrated Approach to Therapeutic Exercise: theory and clinical application.* Reston Publishing Company, Reston, VA.

Sutbeyaz, S.T., Sezer, N., Koseoglu, B.F. 2005, The effect of pulsed electromagnetic fields in the treatment of cervical osteoarthritis: a randomised, double-blind, sham-controlled trial. *Rheumatol. Int.* 26(4): 320–324.

Sutton, P.P., Pavia, D., Bateman, J.R., Clarke, S.W. 1982, Chest physiotherapy: a review. *Eur. J. Respir. Dis.* 63(3): 188–201.

Tagesson, S., Oberg, B., Good, L. *et al.* 2008, A comprehensive rehabilitation program with quadriceps strengthening in closed versus open kinetic chain exercise in patients with anterior cruciate ligament deficiency. A randomized clinical trial evaluating dynamic tibial translation and muscle function. *Am. J. Sports Med.* 36 (2): 298–307.

Tappan, F.M. 1988, *Healing Massage Techniques. Holistic, classic, and emerging methods,* 2nd edn. Appleton & Lange, Norwalk, CT.

Takagi, R, Fujita, N., Arakawa, T. *et al.* 2011, Influence of icing on muscle regeneration after crush injury to skeletal muscles in rats. *J. Appl. Physiol.* 110(2): 382–388.

Taylor, R.A., Adamson, C.P. 2002, Stifle surgery and rehabilitation. *Proc. 2nd Int. Symp. Rehabil. Phys. Ther. Vet. Med.* Knoxville, TN, pp. 143–146.

Taylor, R.S., Brown, A., Ebrahim, S. *et al.* 2004, Exercise-based rehabilitation for patients with coronary heart disease: systematic review and metaanalysis of randomized controlled trials. *Am. J. Med.* 116: 682–692.

Thacker, S.B., Gilchrist, J., Stroup, D.F. *et al.* 2004, The impact of stretching on sports injury wrist – a systematic review of the literature. *Med. Sci. Sports Exerc.* 36(3): 371–378.

Torres de la Riva, G., Hart, B.L., Farver, T.B. *et al.* 2013, Neutering dogs: effects on joint disorders and cancers in golden retrievers. *PLoS One* 8(2): e55937.

Tumilty, S., Munn, J., McDonough, S. *et al.* 2010, Low level laser treatment of tendinopahty: a systematic review with mata-analysis. *Photomed. Laser Surg.* 28(1): 3–16.

Tyler, C.M., Hodgson, D.R., Rose, R.J. 1996, Effect of a warm-up on energy supply during high intensity exercise in horses. *Equine Vet. J.* 28(2): 117–120.

Uhthoff, H.K., Sekaly, G., Jaworski, Z.F. 1985, Effect of long-term nontraumatic immobilization on metaphyseal spongiosa in young adult and old Beagle dogs. *Clin. Orthop.* 192: 278–284.

Umphred, D.A., McCormack, G.L. 1990, Classification of common facilitatory and inhibitory treatment technique. In: Umphred, D.A. (ed.), *Neurological Rehabilitation,* 2nd edn. Mosby, Philadelphia, PA, p. 152.

Vasseur, P.B. 1979, Clinical results following nonoperative management for rupture of the cranial cruciate ligament in dogs. *Vet. Surg.* 13: 283.

Verbruggen, G., Goemaere, S., Veys, E.M. 2002, Systems to assess the progression of finger joint osteoarthritis and the effects of disease-modifying osteoarthritis drugs. *Clin. Rheumatol.* 21: 231–243.

Verstraelen, F.U., In den Kleef, N.J., Jansen, L., Morrenhof, J.W. 2014, High-energy versus low-energy extracorporeal shock wave therapy for calcifying tendinitis of the shoulder: which is superior? A meta-analysis. *Clin. Orthop. Relat. Res.* 472(9): 2816–2825.

Voss, D.E., Ionta, M.K., Myers, B.J.1985, *Proprioceptive Neuromuscular Facilitation: patterns and techniques.* Harper & Row, Philadelphia, PA.

Wang, C.J., Weng, L.H. Ko, J.Y. *et al.* 2011a, Extracorporeal shockwave shows regression of osteoarthritis of the knee in rats. *J. Surg. Res.* 171(2): 601–608.

Wang, C.J., Weng, L.H., Ko, J.Y. *et al.* 2011b, Extracorporeal shockwave shows chondroprotective effects in osteoarthritic rat knee. *Arch. Orthop. Trauma Surg.* 131(8): 1547–1553.

Wang, C.J., Sun, Y.C., Wong, T. *et al.* 2012, Extracorporeal shockwave therapy shows time-dependent chondroprotective effects in osteoarthritis of the knee in rats. *J. Surg. Res.* 178(1): 196–205.

Wang, J.H.-C., Iosifidis, M.I., Fu, F.H. 2006, Biomechanical basis for tendonopathy. *Clin. Orthop. Rel. Res.* 443: 320–332.

Weber, J.B., Pinheiro, A.L., de Oliveira, M.G. *et al.* 2006, Laser therapy improves healing of bone defects submitted to autologous bone graft. *Photomed. Laser Surg.* 24(1): 38–44.

Wexler, G., Hurwitz, D.E., Bush-Joseph, C.A. *et al.* 1998, Functional gait adaptations in patient with anterior cruciate ligament deficiency over time. *Clin. Orthop. Rel. Res.* 248: 166–175.

Williams, G.N., Barrance, P.J., Snyder-Mackler, L. *et al.* 2003, Specificity of muscle action after anterior cruciate ligament injury. *J. Orthop. Res.* 21: 1131–1137.

Wilson, J.J., Best, T.M. 2005, Common overuse tendon problems: a review of recommendations for treatment. *Am. Fam. Phys.* 72(5): 811–818.

Witvrouw, E., Mahieu, N., Danneels, L. *et al.* 2004, Stretching and injury prevention, an obscure relationship. *Sports Med.* 34(7): 443–449.

Wood, J.L.N., Lakhani, K.H. 2003, Effect of month of birth on hip dysplasia in labrador retrievers and Gordon setters. *Vet. Rec.* 152: 69–72.

Worth, A.J., Bridges, J.P., Caves, N.J. *et al.* 2012, Seasonal variations in the hip score of dogs as assessed by the New Zealand Veterinary Association hip dysplasia scheme. *N. Z. Vet. J.* 60(2): 110–114.

Yang, R.S., Chang, W.H., Liu, T.K. *et al.* 1994, Clinical evaluation of nonunion and delayed union by a specific parameter electrical stimulation. *J. Japan. Bio-Electr. Res. Soc.* 8: 117–125.

Yelland, M.J., Sweeting, K.R., Lyftogt, J.A. *et al.* 2011, Prolotherapy injections and eccentric loading exercises for painful Achilles tedninosis: a randomised trial. *Br. J. Sports Med.* 45(5): 421–428.

Zatterstrom, R., Friden, T., Lindstrand, A. *et al.* 1994, The effect of physiotherapy on standing balance in chronic anterior cruciate ligament insufficiency. *Am. J. Sports Med.* 22(4): 531–536.

Zelle, B., Gollwitzer, H., Zlowodzki, M., Buhren, V. 2010, Extracorporeal shock wave therapy: current evidence. *J. Orthop. Trauma* 24(3) Suppl 1: S66–S70.

Zhao, C., Amadio, P.C., Momose, T. *et al.* 2002, Effects of synergistic wrist motion on adhesion formation after repair of partial *flexor digitorum profundus tendon* lacerations in a canine model *in vivo*. *J. Bone Joint Surg. Am.* 84(1): 78–84.

Zink, M.C. 1997, *Peak Performance – coaching the canine athlete*. Canine Sports Productions, Lutherville, MD.

Zink, M.C., Daniels, J. 1996, *Jumping from A to Z: teach your dog to soar*. Canine Sports Productions, Lutherville, MD.

Zysk, S.P., Refior, H.J. 2000, Operative or conservative treatment of the acutely torn anterior cruciate ligament in middle-aged patients. A follow-up study of 133 patients between the ages of 40–59 years. *Arch. Orthop. Trauma Surg.* 120 (1-2): 59–64.

CHAPTER 19

Assessment and treatment techniques of the equine head, neck and thoracic limb*

Emma Dainty

University of Liverpool, Liverpool, UK

Summary

This chapter further explores the earlier chapters' overview of this region with specific assessment and treatment techniques of the equine head, neck and thoracic limb, placing particular emphasis on region-specific variances of both articulations and soft tissue structures that may be affected. An overview of the multifaceted options available for treatment is outlined.

19.1 Introduction

The primary role of the veterinary physiotherapist is to assess and treat the horse under the umbrella of the Veterinary Surgeons Act (1966). Although a potentially outdated piece of legislation, it ensures that the animal receives appropriate and timely treatment and that the clinician maintains the chain of communication with the referring veterinarian, protecting all involved in the rehabilitation process.

At the initial assessment, a thorough, specific subjective assessment of all relevant history, including husbandry and training, is required. Time spent obtaining a clear picture of the level of management and fitness can help identify areas of inconsistency prior to palpation. The horse may have been referred by the primary treating veterinarian for a degenerative disorder or acute trauma, by a secondary referral hospital following investigations or surgery, or alternatively, the owner/rider may have requested an assessment to address loss of performance issues or to gain a baseline measure of the neuromusculoskeletal fitness at any one point in time. Treatment may address a primary problem or resolve underlying compensatory issues affecting locomotion (Porter 2005). The assessment process may be a multifaceted procedure including involvement from riders, trainers, farriers, saddlers and owners. Occasionally, an opinion is requested at pre-purchase by either the purchaser or a veterinarian requiring further information regarding the horse's current level of fitness, but care must be taken by the veterinary physiotherapist to ensure there is no undermining of the vetting procedure.

Although this chapter primarily identifies the thoracic limb and cranial axial skeleton, the principles are relevant to the whole horse and should be treated as such.

---

*Adapted from and expanded upon the following first edition chapters:
9: Manual therapy by Lesley Goff and Gwendolen Jull
14: Equine treatment and rehabilitation by Lesley Goff and Narelle Stubbs

---

Animal Physiotherapy: Assessment, Treatment and Rehabilitation of Animals, Second Edition. Edited by Catherine M. McGowan and Lesley Goff.
© 2016 John Wiley & Sons, Ltd. Published 2016 by John Wiley & Sons, Ltd.

Assessment, treatment and rehabilitation of the horse should follow the current human and veterinary evidence-based practice as described throughout this text. This encompasses not only orthopaedic and neuromuscular rehabilitation principles but also exercise physiology (Chapter 6), biomechanics (Chapter 5) and performance management (Chapter 21). Thus a 'neuromotor or neuromechanical control model' is encouraged for rehabilitation. Ironically, these neurophysiological terms describe the equine locomotive system – balance of stability and mobility (Chapter 5). However, clinically the majority of physiotherapeutic techniques, including manual therapy, soft tissue and skeletal mobilisation and manipulation, proprioceptive facilitation techniques, electrotherapy and exercise-based rehabilitation, can be adapted and successfully performed. These are all part of the multimodal approach to physiotherapy management of athletic, traumatic and degenerative injuries seen in the performance and pleasure horse. The lack of direct verbalisation with the animal necessitates quality veterinary and physiotherapy assessment, diagnosis and management in all levels of equine sport, from the child's aged pony to the elite athlete, with respect to injury prevention, treatment, rehabilitation, quality of life and performance enhancement.

As previously discussed in Chapter 12, physiotherapy for equine musculoskeletal and neurological conditions is based on a strong scientific background in human medicine. There are numerous professional and lay texts available to the reader in relation to equine treatment and rehabilitation. However, while there have been considerable advances in diagnostic methods and veterinary management, the current equine therapeutic literature often lacks a solid scientific evidence base. It is therefore a necessity that physiotherapists develop expert clinical reasoning skills and are able to apply the available evidence-based knowledge to treatment, rehabilitation and management of the equine, continually keeping abreast of new evidence-based advances. Denoix & Pailloux (2001) assimilate physiotherapy and sports medicine concepts with veterinary management, describing physiotherapy as being 'based on the understanding of, and respect for, biomechanical structures. It is however more than just a therapeutic technique through touch and gesture; it is also a means of sensory communication, of bridging the silence between horse and rider'.

The pathophysiology of injury and healing of the animal's body systems is presented elsewhere in this text, including information presented in the canine treatment and rehabilitation chapters (Chapter 18). These principles can be adapted for the horse's comparative anatomical and biomechanical differences. Unlike the dog and human, in the majority of circumstances the horse is treated in standing, so much of the musculoskeletal system is treated in the weight-bearing (WB) or partially weight-bearing (PWB) postures. This is due to the necessity to anaesthetise a horse to obtain and then maintain recumbency, although some professions use this to apply large and specifically directed forces for chronic high-velocity injury assessment and treatment (Pusey & Brooks 2010). Horses may be sedated by

veterinarians for manual examination, and even when sedated, the horse can remain standing due to the stay apparatus. As the postural muscles of the horse are active when standing, true passive accessory movement testing is not possible for some joints, such as those of the thoracolumbar region. Palpation of some soft tissues in a relaxed state may not be possible, for example the triceps group, although modified passive physiological joint movements can be carried out in standing.

Horses requiring physiotherapy are generally accustomed to being handled by owners, farriers and veterinarians, so are quite receptive to manual physiotherapy examination. Great care must be taken with regard to safety of the physiotherapist and the handler at all times. Even horses under sedation may deliver accurate kicks. Owner cooperation regarding handling of the equine patient is paramount to the safety of the physiotherapist and handler competency should be assessed as a matter of course prior to undertaking any assessment or treatment techniques.

19.2 Technical aspects of manual therapy

In Chapter 12, several types of articular assessment and treatment were discussed, including Maitland mobilisation, Mulligan mobilisation and neurodynamics. Additional soft tissue techniques can be utilised to either stimulate or relax muscle groups whilst either lengthening or shortening the structure – again depending on the nature and the direction of the force applied, and whether high amplitude or a slow sustained stretch. For example, reflex inhibition techniques apply a rapid flick or strike to stimulate the basic stretch reflex arc at longissimus dorsi and the cervical musculature including brachiocephalicus, longus capitis and rectus capitis. The technique is believed to relieve contralateral muscle activity via the myotactic reflex of the antagonistic pairs of muscles, releasing segmental tension and reducing raised muscle tone (Colborne et al. 2004). In comparison, myofascial release techniques use a localised, slow, sustained fascial stretch to release tightness and reduce pain, thus improving function. Proprioceptive taping techniques with products such as Kinesio tape have been utilised for additional effect post treatment to further enhance the effects although there is little research to promote this. These techniques are outlined further in Chapter 21. Following these specific manual techniques with appropriate stretching or strengthening can have a profound effect on biomechanics and function of the animal.

19.3 Anatomical regions – head

The head articulates with the vertebral column at the atlantooccipital joint (C0–1). It is essential that during the subjective assessment, all aspects of interventions involving the cervical spine be questioned, including types of bitting, use of additional training aids such as chambon or de Gogue (Figure 19.1), types

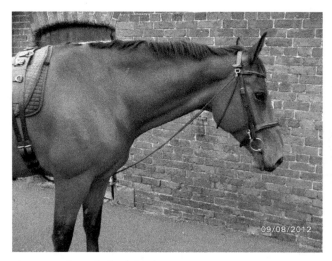

Figure 19.1 Correctly fitted chambon.

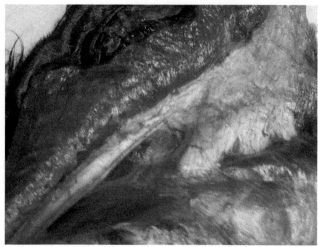

Figure 19.2 Dissection of the nuchal ligament showing the lamellar attachment at C2.

of nosebands, potential loss of performance issues including contact issues such as leaning on the bit, head tilt, tooth grinding or evasions such as sticking the tongue out to the side. Careful initial observation of head posture at rest may identify subtle dysfunctions such as head tilt, and other cranial nerve signs such as asymmetries of nostril size and tone or altered ear posture. Additionally, head shaking, tossing or facial twitching may be observed. Muscular asymmetries of the facial muscles and/or restriction within the myofascial tissues of temporalis, buccinator and masseter muscles may be observed, including overdevelopment in the upper cervical spine of rectus capitis in horses that crib-bite or from chronic overuse of long lever bits (gags, pelhams and weymouths) causing upper cervical hyperflexion. Another concern is poor training where the horse is forced into upper cervical flexion incorrectly, causing the head to sit behind the vertical (Lashley *et al.* 2014) which creates a caudal 'break' or hyperflexion with nuchal ligament loading at C2 (Elgersma *et al.* 2010), rather than the poll being maintained at the most elevated and cranial point.

All these observations can highlight significant dysfunction of atlantooccipital and upper cervical joints and may be symptomatic of systemic or idiopathic issues, for example head shaking, cranial nerve dysfunction and dental pathology.

19.3.1 The nuchal ligament

The nuchal ligament is a specific, specialised structure crucial to equine head and neck mobility and stability. With the head raised and alert, the ligament is off stretch but it allows lowering of the head to the ground to graze. This highly elastic ligamentous structure contains 80% elastin with collagen fibre content to stiffen the matrix of elastin (Gellman & Bertram 2002). Variations exist between the two defined regions; the cord-like funicular section is a continuation of the collagenous supraspinous ligament that contains increasing amounts of elastin between T8 and T4. At the cranial thoracic spinous process summit, this flat

band continues cranially to the skull. The additional flat, sheet-like lamellar section branches cranioventrally and attaches onto the spinous processes of the cervical vertebrae from C6 to C2. At C2 the longest and most robust attachment is found (Figure 19.2). This ligamentous structure can store and redistribute energy, although the mechanism is not fully understood in the horse, and possibly has a role in accelerating the head and neck during motion (Gellman & Bertram 2002). Pathology is limited in the structure although local trauma will cause damage to the overlying musculature, creating scar tissue – for example abscesses caused by vaccinations or microchips, pressure from rugs or bites that may cause localised pain and inflammation. At the origin of the ligament at C2, a bursa exists that can become inflamed; on palpation, there is a defined rigidity which, when mobilising the region, creates a clunky translation of the cranial soft tissues of the crest of the mane, especially cranial cervical lateral flexion.

Idiopathic head shaking is a poorly understood condition but has some clinical features in common with trigeminal neuralgia in humans (Newton *et al.* 2000). During assessment, it is crucial to ascertain the type of head shake – whether a twitch, sneeze, nose blow, wiping of nostrils on the thoracic limb or other structures; when and how it started; whether there are climatic variations such as deterioration of the condition in bright light or drizzly rain; whether trauma was the precursor to symptoms or if nose nets or full facial masks have any effect. Mills & Taylor (2003) investigated the use of nose nets during a field trial and established that nets had significant effects on reducing most behaviours associated with head shaking, especially if using a full face net as opposed to a dorsorostral nostril and muzzle net. However, side-to-side headshaking, rubbing the nose when stationary and shaking the head at rest were not significantly altered. Compensatory myofascial restrictions may be treated and upper cervical articular stiffness may be mobilised with beneficial effect, but outcome is variable and long-term medical management is crucial. Cranial nerve dysfunction is discussed in Chapter 10.

Questions regarding previous dental history should identify the type of practitioner used, whether a veterinarian or equine dental technician, the time since last routine dental assessment or treatment and whether wolf teeth have been removed, frequency of assessment and whether future treatment is required. Incongruency of the dental arcades may be conformational, or may be due to incisor and molar tooth occlusions or overgrowth such as hooks. Cheek ulceration may have been noted in horses with poor dental management. Dominant forage type feed can have implications for dental health – Bonin *et al.* (2007) found that horses fed hay had an increased range of mediolateral displacement of the mandible and this was sufficient to give full occlusal contact of the upper and lower dental arcades when chewing hay compared with chewing pellets.

Extreme care should be taken when palpating the upper molars by sliding the thumb lateral to the cheek teeth at the corners and between the soft tissues of the mouth. This may highlight sharp edges indicating potential dental problems.

19.3.2 Temporomandibular joint

As herbivores, the essential requirements are a good dental arcade and a lateral excursion to facilitate the grinding of foodstuffs over the tooth surfaces. The temporomandibular joint (TMJ) articulation predominantly allows this grinding of the lower molar surface on a fixed upper jaw (Bonin *et al.* 2006) as it articulates with the cranium at the dorsal end of the vertical ramus of the mandible, allowing opening of the oral cavity and lateral translation. Additionally, it is anatomically close to the external and middle ear. The presence of a horizontal intraarticular meniscus further promotes congruency of the joint, also affecting the relative protraction and extension of the mandible as the head is lowered to graze. As with any synovial joint, the TMJ is subject to wear and tear, and can be implicated in loss of performance where there may be unsteady head carriage, although head tilt can be consistent with either central or peripheral vestibular disease (Watrous 1987). The confirmation of vestibular disease is based on physical findings, including results of cranial nerve functional evaluation (described in Chapter 10) and observation of stance, posture and gait.

Lateral translation of the TMJ can be performed by carefully stabilising the maxilla and applying a lateral glide to the lower incisors relative to the upper jaw, to assess the effect of a passive assisted glide both left and right (Figure 19.3). Palpation of the TMJ itself may provide further information regarding pathology, including loss of congruency, hypersensitivity and facial pain along the line of the dental tables and along the facial nerve. If restriction is found unilaterally, a Maitland-type graded joint mobilisation into the restriction can be used. The treatment technique glides the mandibular teeth on the maxillary teeth, creating a long lever at the TMJ. Myofascial release can be very effective at altering tone in the dominant groups of balancing

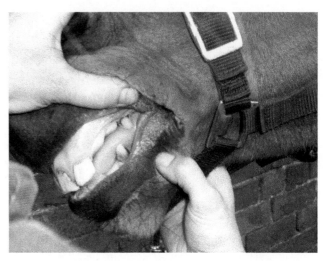

Figure 19.3 TMJ lateral translation. The left hand is fixing the nasal bones and exposing the incisors, the right hand glides the mandible laterally.

side and working side muscles of mastication (posterior temporalis, medial pterygoid, superficial and deep masseter). Asymmetry of muscular bulk can suggest a dominant chewing side and may imply dental pathology (Williams *et al.* 2007).

The hyoid bone and associated soft tissues play an intimate role in the stability of the airways during activity, providing a framework for the larynx and the tongue musculature. Although little research exists regarding treatment of this region, the fascia can be palpated in the intermandibular space. Chronic insidious otitis media or interna (ear infections) can present initially as headshaking and may cause temporohyoid joint osteoarthropathy that if left untreated could cause stress fractures of the petrous temporal bone, causing acute neurological signs including facial nerve paralysis and vestibular dysfunction (Blythe 1997).

19.4 Anatomical regions – cervical spinal joints

The joints of the equine vertebral column may be taken through passive physiological and translatory movements for both assessment and treatment. The orientation of the facet (zygapophyseal) joints directs the movements that can occur at each level of the vertebral column. Intervertebral discs are present segmentally throughout the axial skeleton but it is unclear what the absolute functional role is, compared with interspecies models. Ross & Dyson (2011) reported that at dissection of a large number of equine necks, the discs were found to be predominantly fibrocartilagenous without a nucleus pulposus, suggesting less of a shock-absorbing role with more resistance to shearing forces at the disc. Early work by Yovich *et al.* (1985) identified specific regions within equine cervical discs, including a fibrocartilagenous central part and a fibrous periphery but without the distinct margins of an annulus fibrosus or nucleus pulposus. In some specimens there was evidence of small regions of damage to the annulus, similar to that of a Hansen type II disc. Cases of disc herniation in the cervical spine have been reported, but rarely (Nappert *et al.* 1989). Although ataxia associated with cervical vertebral malformation is more often seen in thoroughbreds, true intervertebral disc protrusion is an extremely rare cause of ataxia in horses (Nappert *et al.* 1989).

Caudal vertebral body endplates increased in width and bone density with age, also suggestive of a response to shear rather than compression. Extensive work has been published (Clayton *et al.* 2010, 2012; Stubbs *et al.* 2009) regarding dynamic mobilising neck stretches as both an assessment and treatment tool. Indeed, often when assessing cervical range of motion, the combined movement patterns including upper cervical rotation with midcervical lateral flexion are already being performed by owners who routinely do 'carrot stretches' for well-being. During the assessment process, it is useful to try and isolate motion according to the regions being assessed although this is an active-assisted range of motion rather than a passive assessment and therefore difficult to truly isolate.

Clayton & Townsend (1989) assessed cervical range of motion segmentally throughout ranges of dorsoventral flexion and extension, axial rotation and lateral bending. Cervical lateral flexibility was found to be uniform throughout the cervical spine, ranging from 25° to 45° of motion per level except at C1-2 where the range was less than 4° of motion. Axial rotation occurred maximally at C1–2 with approximately 70% of range of motion (around 110° of motion) whereas at C0–1 less than 30° of total range occurred. Between C3 and C7 less than 3° of rotation occurred at each segment. Dorsoventral flexion and extension occurred maximally at C0–1 with 32% of motion occurring here. Clayton *et al.* (2010) concluded that the maximal dorsoventral range occurred at either extremity of the cervical spine and these areas were responsible for sagittal range of motion and head and neck orientation. Greater cervical ventral flexion also created increased intersegmental angles at T6–L1.

Lateral flexion motion of the horse's neck can be replicated during physiotherapeutic assessment and treatment by using a dynamic baited stretch into lateral flexion, progressing from cranial to caudal cervical spine. Increasingly caudal placement of the bait increases caudal lateral flexion gained with cumulative segmental range, especially at C6 (Clayton *et al.* 2012). To promote an effect at the upper cervical spine, baited rotation is produced with a nose-to-shoulder directed movement (Figure 19.4). To affect loading at the cervicothoracic (CT) junction, the baited motion is angled at stifles and hocks (Figure 19.5). This baited activity also affects segmental musculature, including cervical multifidus, longus colli and longus thoracis as dissected out by Rombach *et al.* (2014). These authors observed spinal regional variances with cervical multifidus present from C2 to the thoracic spine caudally, longus colli present from C1 to C5 (although laterally spanning up to four intervertebral joints to C6), and finally longus thoracis spanning C6–T6 ventrally.

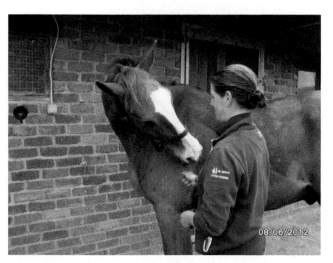

Figure 19.4 Upper cervical spine baited neck exercise – nose to shoulder.

This interlocking mesh of bundles provides a comprehensive scaffold to the highly mobile antigravity articulations making up the cervicothoracic spine. Segmentally, if muscle function is inhibited by pain following trauma or articular degeneration, the effect causes destabilisation of intersegmental levels throughout the vertebral column.

19.4.1 Techniques for C0–1, C1–2

Assessing the equine cranial cervical spine joint range of motion is a modified passive movement as the horse's cervical spine is not relaxed in standing. Passive extension can be achieved with dorsoventral extension of the head and upper cervical spine, balancing the rostral end of the mandible on the therapist's shoulder but taking care to minimise compression pressure from the weight of the horse's head. Padding may be used by the therapist to minimise risk of damage from impact and a step may be required for assessing larger horses. Additionally, this region can

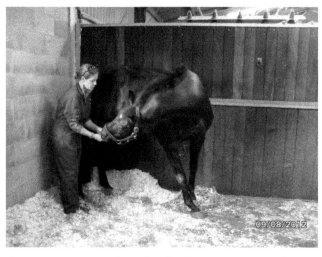

Figure 19.5 Lower cervical spine baited neck exercise – nose to stifle.

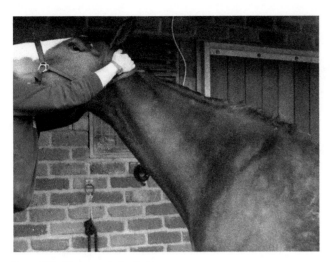

Figure 19.6 Upper cervical extension.

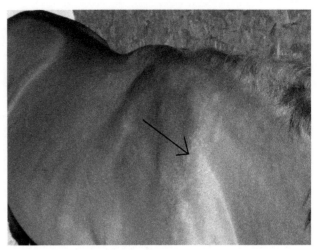

Figure 19.7 Fractured withers – note the patchy sweat (*arrow*) on the cranial aspect of the spine of scapula.

be further assessed and treated with a mild traction/distraction force applied at the occiput or dorsal rami of the mandible in a cranioventral direction to assist upper cervical extension (Figure 19.6).

With the horse's head in an extended posture, the therapist is able to guide the cranial cervical spine into physiological assisted rotation left and right with careful but firm pressure at C0–1 and the dorsorostral end of the nasal bones or even by guiding the motion from the wings of the atlas at C1. This becomes a useful assessment of range of motion at C1–2 where maximal axial rotation occurs. Application of mild overpressure rostrally in a sagittal direction will also increase passive cervical flexion.

C2–6 techniques are discussed further in Chapter 12, but predominantly address lateral flexion and segmental stiffness. Treatment involves a translatory accessory glide segmentally, using each hand to mobilise the contiguous joints, and can utilise a combined movement of the cervical spine being globally moved into lateral flexion as a mobilisation with movement (MWM).

19.4.2 Cervicothoracic (CT) junction

The caudal cervical joints articulate with the thoracic spine at the CT junction where various anatomical normal variances exist, depending on breed and gender (Santinelli *et al.* 2014). The palpable dorsal spinous processes (DSPs) of the cranial thoracic joints at the withers (T5, 6, 7, 8) provide a long lever for transverse translation, with some degree of accessory rotation at the CT junction. Otherwise this vertebral region is nearly impossible to palpate due to the inaccessibility of the joints as they are overlaid by the scapulohumeral joints and scapulae, and are positioned deep to musculature within the thoracic sling. Full retraction of the scapula and shoulder extension are required to access the lower cervical joints but palpation of the transverse processes of C7–T1 is nearly impossible.

Fractured withers may present as an altered wither profile, commonly caused by blunt force trauma at the withers, for example horses that have reared over backwards or jumped out over a stable door. The longest four thoracic spinous processes may no longer be palpable but a caudoventral bony mass slightly lateral to the midline or flattened and impacted into the wither region may be seen and can be described as 'knocked-off' withers. In the acute phase, the horse may be extremely tender to palpation around the scapulothoracic region, occasionally having localised effusion or haematoma, and may hold the head and neck stiffly into extension, resenting lowering the head to graze and walking with a marked shortened cranial phase of stride as if wearing a tight skirt! (Ross & Dyson 2011). The more chronic presentation may be of a flattened craniodorsal portion (Figure 19.7). This rarely causes a performance problem but does have implications for saddle fit and muscular symmetry. Physiotherapeutically, soft tissue compensations will exist, especially at the cranial scapula border. Limb protraction may be limited at end range and CT junction stiffness may be noted with alteration in head carriage in the acute phase.

19.5 Anatomical regions – thoracic limb proximal

19.5.1 Scapulothoracic region

The equine thorax is entirely slung within the musculature supporting the thoracic limb, acting as a shock absorption system, loading tendons and ligaments as well as musculoskeletal structures and fascia of the thoracic limb. Issues in this region may include discomfort when tacking up or biting at the girth region so awareness of the cutaneous trunci reflex around the girth (Essig *et al.* 2013) is essential, and ensure that gastric ulcers have been eliminated as a source of discomfort.

A thorough assessment of the scapula and its supporting structures is required. Cranial scapula glide is achieved via facilitating a lift of the thoracic limb into full elbow and shoulder

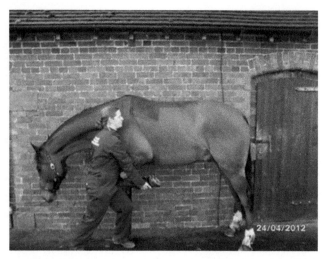

Figure 19.8 Scapula retractions to enhance thoracic flexion and pelvic limb load.

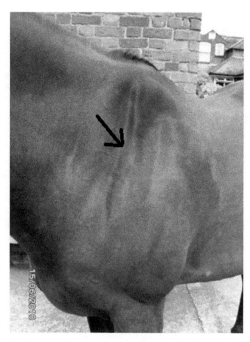

Figure 19.9 Suprascapular nerve palsy (Sweeney shoulder). Note atrophy of the supraspinatus muscle cranial to the spine of scapula (*arrow*).

flexion, envisaging the cartilage of the scapula levelling up with the DSPs of the withers. Additionally, thoracic limb protraction with the hoof capsule low to the ground will relatively depress this region at the withers, providing a long stretch throughout all the thoracic limb structures. To caudally glide and rotate the scapula in an anticlinal direction, the limb can be used as a long lever with a greater degree of elbow flexion and shoulder extension, therefore stretching the triceps surae and serratus ventralis (Figure 19.8). Scapular retraction is a useful assessment and treatment technique facilitating mid to caudal thoracic and lumbar dorsiflexion, loading the pelvic limbs and quarters, whilst creating an indirect mobilisation at the CT junction and scapulothoracic joint. The handler stands facing caudally with the carpus flexed approximately to 90° and approximating this with the handler's hip. Additionally, the handler's shoulder rests dorsocranial to the horse's shoulder and the combined compression into these regions facilitates a caudad offloading – creating a postural sway on the sagittal plane, increasing loading of the pelvic limb and facilitating abdominal lift.

Specific localised muscle wasting of the infraspinatus and supraspinatus is seen when the suprascapular nerve is subjected to direct trauma at the cranial aspect of the neck of the scapula or with subluxation of the scapulohumeral joint, often as a result of blunt force trauma (Dutton *et al.* 1999). Commonly named Sweeny shoulder (Figure 19.9), acute neuropraxia causes muscular wastage of infraspinatus and supraspinatus within days of injury, differentiating it from disuse atrophy. The key finding on assessment of the scapula is marked localised muscle wasting and a prominent spine of scapula. On gait assessment, especially down slopes, a moderate degree of lateral instability at the shoulder is noted on stance phase (Devine *et al.* 2006). Treatment using neuromuscular stimulation (Chapter 13), controlled postural exercise including weight transference, taping and the use of proprioceptive chains (Figure 19.10) will all enhance recovery.

19.5.2 Shoulder joint

Articulating with the humerus caudally and the scapula cranially, the shoulder joint is relatively uncommonly injured. Localised trauma to both the joint and soft tissue structures, including bursae and the muscles stabilising the joint that act as 'lively ligaments', is more commonly seen. Lameness is often

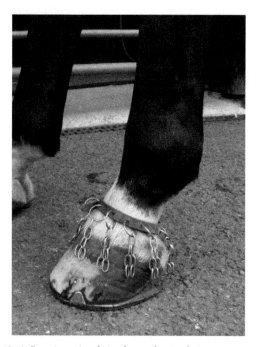

Figure 19.10 Proprioceptive chains for tactile stimulation.

more evident at walk than at trot with the affected limb on the outside of a circle where a shortened cranial phase of stride may be seen (Whitcomb *et al.* 2006). Biceps brachii has a dual joint attachment and function at the shoulder and elbow and has an intimate relationship with the shoulder joint and neck; the thick tendon branches to form the lacertus fibrosus as a thinner tendinous structure that plays a crucial role linking biceps and extensor carpi radialis, essential in the thoracic limb stay apparatus. Watson & Wilson (2007) examined biceps muscle and revealed the tendon had a greater isometric force generation capacity and a greater moment arm than supraspinatus, suggesting that biceps is more suited to power and movement and the latter to shoulder stabilisation. The strong biceps tendon is infrequently damaged although a fall at speed whilst jumping can cause rupture (Dyson 2011). However, ultrasonographic abnormalities have been described by Dyson (2011), including tendon enlargement, loss of definition, hypoechoic defects with altered fibre pattern, fibrosis, mineralisation and ossification with occasional adhesions of the tendon onto the bursa.

Implications for the physiotherapist include a thorough assessment of the joint articulation including end range combined movements. The tendon is assessed with the thoracic limb retracted and shoulder flexed – the radius is held behind the vertical and the elbow slowly extended, placing the musculotendinous structures on tension. The combined movement assessment retracts the limb and encourages the head and cervical spine into lateral flexion, away from the tested side (Figure 19.11). This loads biceps brachii, brachiocephalicus and the cervical myofascia and also applies tension to the radial nerve. Using a reverse-origin model, the limb can be retracted as the

primary or secondary motion, i.e. the thoracic limb is retracted and then the cervical spine is laterally flexed away from the limb or vice versa, where the cervical spine is laterally flexed away and then the thoracic limb retracted. Increased tension at the insertion of brachiocephalicus is often identified in horses with concurrent bilateral foot pain or chronic lameness, presenting as a shortened cranial phase of the stride. Tokuriki *et al.* (1999) found increased electromyographic activity of brachiocephalicus when swimming compared with water treadmill or dry land and this can be correlated in sport-specific training. For example, dressage horses working in high degrees of collection will adversely train topline musculature due to the extended head and neck posture required to swim, whereas use of a water treadmill to enhance carpal flexion with water at a much lower level will aid functional specificity and improve postural muscle strength, aiding core stability. Mendez-Angulo *et al.* (2013) looked at range of motion of carpal flexion whilst horses underwent exercise on a water treadmill and found that flexion and extension of the carpus specifically increased maximally when the water was at tarsal height and that stance phase reduced but swing phase increased the deeper the water.

19.5.3 Elbow joint

Predominantly, the joint moves in a sagittal plane, being stabilised by the very strong collateral ligaments and triceps group. With no pronation or supination (excluding physiological glide) due to the dominant radius and the vestigial ulna, a minor degree of accessory glide applied as a varus and valgus stress may be attempted, but due to the position required for handling the limb, the majority of shear occurs at the carpus.

To assess elbow range of motion, first the carpus is flexed (avoiding compressive articular overpressure) and the brachium is brought up into approximation with the humerus. The carpus can then be guided laterally or medially to affect the physiological end range of the elbow (and carpus) joints.

Although this joint is rarely injured, the effect can be considerable if trauma is induced; olecranon fractures from a kick or blunt force trauma around the elbow and forearm can be associated with radial nerve damage. Dysfunction is characterised by inability to flex the shoulder and extend the elbow, carpus, fetlock and interphalangeal joints, with the horse resting the toe pointing on the ground, producing a dropped elbow posture. Marked muscular atrophy of triceps and the digital extensors is noted in the acute phase due to denervation (Lopez *et al.* 1997).

19.5.4 Carpus

Observation of the carpus at stance phase may show conformational variations, such as 'back at the knee', 'over at the knee', 'offset' or 'bench knees', carpal valgus and carpal varus. These conformational variations may predispose the horse to thoracic limb lameness or primary osteoarthritis. Additionally, local trauma such as falling onto knees or a direct kick, running into fencing

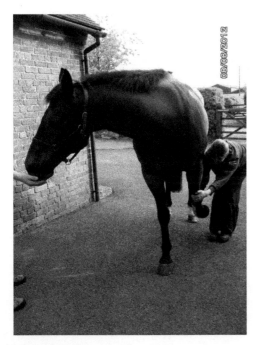

Figure 19.11 Combined biceps stretch.

and hyperextension of the joint can lead to carpal lameness and is often seen in sport horses (predominantly racehorses).

Assessment of the joint's ROM is achieved with soft tissue opposition of the metacarpus to radius/ulna, and when the distal phalanx is flexed at the hoof capsule towards the olecranon of the elbow, this creates further 'wind-up' of the soft tissues, including the common and lateral digital extensor tendons. With the carpus held at approximately 90° flexion, a caudad joint mobilisation can be applied with a relative distraction of the metacarpus by applying pressure at the proximal third of the cannon bone in a ventral direction. Accessory mobilisation can be made with a varus/valgus shearing in carpal flexion. The position in which to assess carpal accessory motion is also an effective way of assessing the soft tissue ligamentous and tendinous structures of the distal limb, including assessing the inferior check ligament (inferior accessory ligament) as it attaches proximally to the deep digital flexor tendon (DDFT). Other soft tissue structures of the metacarpophalangeal region include the superficial digital flexor tendon (SDFT) and the suspensory ligament (SL). Management and rehabilitation of tendon injuries are discussed in Chapter 21.

Degeneration of the carpal joints initially causes loss of end range flexion with few other limitations in function. Indeed, horses with mild loss of range of motion – for example, a loss of 20° end range flexion at the carpus – may not show lameness and may still lie down with ease. Carpal osteoarthritis is frequently seen in 2–3-year-old racehorses and other horses undergoing high-intensity training (Murray *et al.* 1999). Carpal articular cartilage in strenuously trained horses showed more fibrillation and chondrocyte clusters than cartilage from animals that underwent gentle exercise. Thus, strenuous training may lead to deterioration of cartilage at sites with a high clinical incidence of lesions such as dorsal radial carpal cartilage (Murray *et al.* 1999). Mendez-Angulo *et al.* (2013) looked at range of motion of carpal flexion whilst horses underwent exercise on a water treadmill and found that flexion and extension of the carpus specifically increased maximally when the water was at tarsal height and that stance phase reduced but swing phase increased the deeper the water.

Another common condition in performance horses, especially young racehorses, is sore or 'bucked' shins (third metacarpal bone) (Marlin & Nankervis 2003). This often interferes with the training programme. Management of bucked shins is discussed in Chapter 21.

Occasionally, assessment of the metacarpal III or cannon bone may identify new bony exostoses associated with either the lateral (fourth metacarpal bone) or medial (second metacarpal bone) splint bones of the thoracic limb (also seen in the pelvic limb metatarsal bones). These may be caused by direct blunt trauma, including kicks, and can present as a variable sized bony outgrowth at any point along the margin of the metacarpal III either medially or laterally, and although not a load-bearing bone and considered an accessory structure, the more proximal splints may interfere with the carpus articulation. Jeffcott

et al. (1986) assessed the contribution of the splint bones to the total bone mineral content proximally and distally, below the midpoint of the metacarpus. They identified that the proximal shaft of the splint contributed 12% to total bone mineral content whereas the distal splints only contributed 2% and that lame horses had reduced total bone mineral content in the affected limb, suggesting an offloading effect.

When non-traumatic splints are initially identified, there may be heat and tenderness to direct palpation although often the level of lameness is subtle and only noticeable on firm surfaces whilst turning or soft surfaces with the limb on the outside of a circle. Occasionally, the rider may report a loss of performance or a shorter striding horse without a definitive cause. Some young horses may present with a pair of splints after starting to work on firm surfaces and they are considered to be a symptom of concussion or altered foot biomechanics. Splint formation requires differentiation from splint bone fracture or suspensory ligament desmopathy. Fractures are commonly seen in polo ponies where swinging mallets hit the distal limb. Where splint formation has settled but subtle lameness persists, assessment of the suspensory ligaments should be made to exclude other pathology (Bertoni *et al.* 2001). The implication for physiotherapists is to ensure palpation of the distal limb anatomy during assessment if subtle lameness is suspected and to be confident at identifying changes to both osseous and soft tissue structures.

19.6 Anatomical regions – thoracic limb distal

19.6.1 Metacarpophalangeal (MCP) joint

The MCP joint of the metacarpus III articulates with the first phalanx (P1) and the accessory proximal sesamoid bones to create a highly mobile, intensely loaded joint that is subject to huge repetitive, compressive and shearing forces. Physiotherapeutically, the significance of injury relates both to the range of motion of the joint articulation and to the palpatory findings of the soft tissue structures, including the flexor tendons, tendon sheaths, suspensory ligaments and annular ligaments. Observation of the joint can help identify articular, tendinous and ligamentous health of the horse. The presence of significant articular or tendinous windgalls can suggest pathology and it is essential that a comparison of bilateral joints is made. This may indicate whether an effused digital tendon sheath is acute or chronic and can act as barometer for the horse's joint health. A markedly enlarged, turgid, effused unilateral tendinous windgall that occurs after running cross-country is more significant than a pair of soft, cold, mildly puffy fetlocks noted after standing in a stable for a length of time. The more cranially sited capsular distension of the articular 'windgall' or 'windpuff' may be seen in all four fetlocks in older horses. This may concurrently fit with slight end range stiffness on fetlock flexion when mobilising the toe of the hoof capsule towards the olecranon (ensuring there is no preexisting stiffness in the carpal joints). Although veterinarians may be required to treat the joint orthopaedically – be that with steroid injection, the use of glucosaminoglycans or surgical procedures for ligamentous or tendinous trauma – the role of the physiotherapist in the acute phase is to limit the inflammatory phase using all modalities available, whether that be electrotherapy (Chapter 13), the use of ice or gentle mobilisations.

19.6.2 Proximal interphalangeal (PIP) joint

An articulation between the long (P1) and short (P2) pastern bones, this joint predominantly moves in flexion and extension although small degrees of true passive accessory rotation, abduction and adduction are possible. It is a relatively low-motion joint compared with MCP joints. The distal end of P2 is closely approximated with the coronary band and therefore is partially enveloped within the hoof capsule, making individual isolation of joint range slightly difficult unless truly fixing the MCP joint and the hoof capsule to perform PIP passive and accessory mobilisations. Pathology in this region can have a marked effect on gait, and may include high to low ringbones, sidebone of the collateral cartilages, suspensory branch desmitis and degenerative joint disease of the PIP joint or simply raised digital pulses as a result of a foot abscess or laminitis.

19.6.3 Distal interphalangeal (DIP) joint

An articulation between P1 and P2 and commonly named the coffin joint, this articulates within the hoof capsule and isolation of the movement pattern is very difficult. The cranial aspect of the joint may be palpated at the most cranial portion of the coronet band and pastern intersection and when effused, may be felt as a soft crest above the coronet band. This is an unlikely joint to require physiotherapy techniques *per se*, but often early changes to function and gait may be noted by both the rider and physiotherapist and palpation in this region may be an indicator of early pathology and prompt further investigations. Hypomobility at the joint (tested by sagittal plane articular, accessory glides) may be assisted by utilising the same articular glides as a manual therapy treatment.

The navicular bone is closely approximated with the P2 and P3 bones, acting as an accessory bone – it is a fulcrum to the attachment of the DDFT to P3 caudally and prone to degeneration causing involutions within the bone as erosions. Historically, navicular syndrome was diagnosed in horses displaying palmar foot pain. However, with the advent of magnetic resonance imaging, several comparative diagnoses have been hypothesised for foot pain, including ligamentous damage to the collateral ligaments and the impar ligament, or localised damage to the DDFT within the hoof capsule, inflammation of the navicular bursa and specific joint degeneration.

The physiotherapist may be involved in rehabilitation of horses with chronic palmar foot pain or the compensatory soreness associated with pectoral and brachiocephalicus spasm off-loading the region. A careful lameness assessment may allude to foot pain, especially if assessing stride on the lunge on a firm surface. If raised digital pulses are associated with forelimb lameness and laminitis has been excluded, the use of crushed ice bowls to aid cooling of joints may become beneficial, regardless of whether the horse is barefoot or shod. Horses with chronic foot pain require routine corrective shoeing to aid heel support and reduce the break-over point by ensuring the toe does not become overlong. Often it is the physiotherapist who notices the subtle changes within the foot or as a result of shoeing.

19.6.4 Hoof capsule

Although discussed in greater detail in Chapter 5, it is essential that all physiotherapists have a good understanding of foot balance, conformation and correct shoeing. Often the physiotherapist is the first person to notice subtle changes in lameness levels or may be asked to see a pony with loss of performance issues with subclinical laminitis or a horse with a brewing foot abscess. It is necessary to be able to palpate normal and abnormal digital pulses and to locate areas of sensitivity with hoof testers so appropriate advice and further onward referral can be made.

In the competition environment, it is essential that the physiotherapist can appropriately assess any new, subtle lameness and its significance for performance. For example, during the cross-country phase, if a shoe is lost at high speed and under torsion, there may be localised soft tissue trauma or ligamentous damage within the hoof capsule that requires rest. Alternatively, some horses do not cope well with losing a shoe and solar bruising may be a problem. In this instance, it is appropriate to manage the foot with hourly tubbing in iced water to reduce the inflammatory component within the capsule that may allow further competition. It may not be the remit of the physiotherapist within the team to make a judgement as to whether the rider continues to compete but any reservations must be voiced and veterinary opinion sought.

19.7 Conclusion

Assessment of the head, neck and thoracic limb must not be made in isolation from the rest of the axial skeleton or pelvic limb. A good subjective assessment should create an excellent grounding for the manual assessment of the articular, myofascial and neuromuscular components and eventual treatment of these structures in combination with the axial skeleton and pelvic limb (Chapter 20).

References

Bertoni, L., Forresu, D., Coudry, V. *et al.* 2012, Exostoses on the palmar or plantar aspect of the diaphysis of the third metacarpal or metatarsal bone in horses: 16 cases (2001–2010). *J. Am. Vet. Med. Assoc.* 240(6): 740–747.

Blythe, L.L. 1997, Otitis media and interna and temporohyoid osteoarthropathy. *Vet. Clin. North Am. Equine Pract.* 13(1): 21–42.

Bonin, S.J., Clayton, H.M., Lanovaz, J.L. *et al.* 2007, Comparison of mandibular motion in horses chewing hay and pellets. *Equine Vet. J.* 39(3): 258–262.

Bonin, S.J., Clayton, H.M., Lanovaz, J.L. *et al.* 2006, Kinematics of the temporomandibular joint. *Am. J. Vet. Res* .67(3): 423–428

Clayton, H.M., Townsend, H.G. 1989, Kinematics of the cervical spine of the adult horse. *Equine Vet. J.* 21(3): 189–192.

Clayton, H.M., Kaiser, L.J., Lavagnino, M. *et al.* 2010, Dynamic mobilisations in cervical flexion: effects on intervertebral angulations. *Equine Vet. J.* 38(suppl): 688–694.

Clayton, H.M., Kaiser, L.J., Lavagnino, M. *et al.* 2012, Evaluation of intersegmental vertebral motion during performance of dynamic mobilization exercises in cervical lateral bending in horses. *Am. J. Vet. Res.* 73(8): 1153–1159.

Colborne, G.R., McDonald, C., Barratt, A. *et al.* 2004, Effect of reflex inhibition technique for muscular back pain. *Equine Compar. Exerc. Physiol.* 1(2): A8.

Denoix, J.M., Pailloux, J.M. 2001, *Physical Therapy and Massage for the Horse: biomechanics, exercise and treatment*, 2nd edn. Manson, London.

Devine, D.V., Jann, H.W., Payton, M.E. 2006, Gait abnormalities caused by selective anesthesia of the suprascapular nerve in horses. *Am. J. Vet. Res.* 67(5): 834–836.

Dutton, D.M., Honnas, C.M., Watkins, J.P. 1999. Nonsurgical treatment of suprascapular nerve injury in horses: 8 cases (1988–1998). *J. Am. Vet. Med. Assoc.* 214(11): 1657–1659.

Dyson, S. 2011, Unexplained lameness. In: Ross, M.W., Dyson, S.J. (eds), *Lameness in the Horse*, 2nd edn. Elsevier Saunders, St Louis, MO, pp. 145–159.

Elgersma, A.E., Wijnberg, I.D., Sleutjens, J. *et al.* 2010, A pilot study on objective quantification and anatomical modelling of in vivo head and neck positionscommonly applied in training and competition of sport horses. Equine Vet. J. 38(suppl): 436–443.

Essig, C.M., Merritt, J.S., Stubbs, N.C. *et al.* 2013, Localization of the cutaneus trunci muscle reflex in horses. *Am. J. Vet. Res.* 74(11): 1428–1432.

Gellman, K.S, Bertram, J.E. 2002, The equine nuchal ligament 1: structural and material properties. *Vet. Compend. Orthopaed. Traumatol.* 1: 1–6.

Jeffcott, L.B., McCartney, R.N., Speirs, V.C. 1986, Single photon absorptiometry for the measurement of bone mineral content in horses. *Vet. Rec.* 118(18): 499–505.

Lashley, M.J., Nauwelaerts, S., Vernooij, J.C. *et al.* 2014, Comparison of the head and neck position of elite dressage horses during top-level competitions in 1992 versus 2008. *Vet. J.* 202(3): 462–465.

Lopez, M.J., Nordberg, C., Trostle, S. 1997, Fracture of the 7th cervical and 1st thoracic vertebrae presenting as radial nerve paralysis in a horse. *Can. Vet. J.* 38(2): 112.

Marlin, D., Nankervis, K. (eds) 2003, Skeletal responses. In: *Equine Exercise Physiology.* Blackwell Science, Malden, MA, pp. 86–93.

Mendez-Angulo, J., Firshman, A., Groschen, D. *et al.* 2013, Effect of water depth on amount of felxion and extension of joints of the distal aspects of the limbs in healthy horses walking on an undrewater treadmill. *Am. J. Vet. Res.* 74(4): 557–566.

Mills, D.S., Taylor, K. 2003, Field study of the efficacy of three types of nose net for the treatment of headshaking in horses. *Vet. Rec.* 152(2): 41–44.

Murray, R.C., Whitton, R.C., Vedi, S. *et al.* 1999, The effect of training on the calcified zone of equine middle carpal articular cartilage. *Equine Vet. J.* 30(suppl): 274–278.

Nappert, G., Vrins, A., Breton, L. *et al.* 1989, A retrospective study of nineteen ataxic horses. *Can. Vet. J.* 30(10): 802–806.

Newton, S.A., Knottenbelt, D.C., Eldridge, P.R. 2000, Headshaking in horses: possible aetiopathogenesis suggested by the results of diagnostic tests and several treatment regimes used in 20 cases. *Equine Vet. J.* 32(2): 208–216.

Porter, M. 2005, Equine rehabilitation therapy for joint disease. *Vet. Clin. North Am. Equine Pract.* 21(3): 599–607.

Pusey, A., Brooks, J. 2010, Palpatory examination of the sedated horse. In: Pusey, A., Brooks, J., Jenks, A. (eds), *Osteopathy and the Treatment of Horses.* Wiley-Blackwell, Chichester, UK, pp. 91–99.

Rombach, N., Stubbs, N.C., Clayton, H.M. 2014, Gross anatomy of the deep perivertebral musculature in horses. *Am. J. Vet. Res.* 75(5): 433–440.

Ross, M.W., Dyson, S.J. 2011, *Lameness in the Horse*, 2nd edn. Elsevier Saunders, St Louis, MO, pp. 145–159.

Santinelli, I., Beccati, F., Arcelli, R. *et al.* 2014, Anatomical variation of the spinous and transverse processes in the caudal cervical vertebrae and the first thoracic vertebra in horses. *Equine Vet. J.* doi: 10.1111/evj.12397 (epub ahead of print).

Stubbs, N.C., Kaiser, L.J., Hauptman, J. *et al.* 2009, Dynamic mobilisation exercises increase cross-sectional area of musculus multifidus. *Equine Vet. J.* 43(5): 522–529.

Tokuriki, M., Ohtsuki, R., Kai, M. *et al.* 1999, EMG activity of the muscles of the neck and forelimbs during different forms of locomotion. *Equine Vet. J.* 30(suppl): 231–234.

Watrous, B.J. 1987, Head tilt in horses. *Vet. Clin. North Am. Equine Pract.* 3(2): 353–370.

Watson, J.C., Wilson, A.M. 2007, Muscle architecture of biceps brachii, triceps brachii and supraspinatus in the horse. *J. Anat.* 210(1): 32–40.

Whitcomb, M.B., le Jeune, S.S., MacDonald, M.M. *et al.* 2006, Disorders of the infraspinatus tendon and bursa in three horses. *J. Am. Vet. Med. Assoc.* 229(4): 549–556.

Williams, S.H., Vinyard, C.J., Wall, C.E. *et al.* 2007, Masticatory motor patterns in ungulates: a quantitative assessment of jaw–muscle coordination in goats, alpacas and horses. *J. Exp. Zool. A Ecol. Genet. Physiol.* 307(4): 226–240.

Yovich, J.V., Powers, B.E., Stashak, T.S. 1985, Morphologic features of the cervical intervertebral disks and adjacent vertebral bodies of horses. *Am. J. Vet. Res.* 46(11): 2372–2377.

CHAPTER 20

Assessment and treatment techniques of the equine thoracolumbar spine, pelvis and pelvic limb*

Emma Dainty

University of Liverpool, Liverpool, UK

Summary

This chapter further explores the earlier chapter's overview of this region with the specific assessment and treatment techniques of the equine thoracolumbar spine, pelvis and pelvic limb, with particular emphasis on region-specific variances of both articulations and soft tissue structures that may be affected. An overview of the multifaceted options available for treatment is outlined.

20.1 Introduction

Assessment of the equine thoracolumbar spine, pelvis and pelvic limb is done in conjunction with the head, neck and thoracic limb as outlined in Chapter 19. Appropriate subjective assessment prior to the physical examination should identify risk factors for handling the horse as well as areas of concern relating to

loss of performance from the owner's perspective. Physiotherapeutic management of orthopaedic and neurological conditions in horses is based largely on human research and an understanding of the principles can guide us in managing the injured equine and aid injury prevention.

In the horse, many musculoskeletal injuries are directly related to developing particular pathologies; these mechanisms have been discussed in previously in this publication. Acute conditions, for example muscle tears, may require initial interventions to reduce inflammatory response, so as not to compromise tissue-level healing, with mobilisation implemented in later treatments (Warden 2005). Chronic conditions, such as degenerative joint disease of the hocks or sacroiliac degenerative joint disease, which often result in poor performance (Jeffcott *et al.* 1985) may benefit from specific exercises aimed at facilitating normal neuromotor control at initial treatment.

Thoracic and pelvic limb gait abnormalities are not considered to be separate entities in physiotherapy assessment and treatment. Such is the genetic make-up of the quadruped that any dysfunction from the pelvic limb or pelvis may present with disuse atrophy and muscle wasting on either the same side or

---

*Adapted from and expanded upon the following first edition chapters:
9: Manual therapy by Lesley Goff and Gwendolen Jull
14: Equine treatment and rehabilitation by Lesley Goff and Narelle Stubbs

Animal Physiotherapy: Assessment, Treatment and Rehabilitation of Animals, Second Edition. Edited by Catherine M. McGowan and Lesley Goff.
© 2016 John Wiley & Sons, Ltd. Published 2016 by John Wiley & Sons, Ltd.

as an asymmetry associated with the diagonally opposite paired limb. A thorough assessment of the whole horse will help determine whether the axial skeleton suffers musculoskeletal dysfunction as a result of thoracic and/or pelvic limb gait abnormalities that may or may not be associated with primary pathology, or secondary compensations associated with an altered gait or movement pattern (Gómez Alvarez *et al.* 2007). Recent research by Maliye *et al.* (2015) assessed the effect forelimb lameness had on the hindlimb and pelvic movement in horses with clinical lameness. It identified compensatory load redistribution with reduced pelvic limb propulsion on the contralateral limb. In addition, it is necessary to consider that a horse may have lameness issues on more than one leg and therefore multiple issues must be assessed and addressed.

20.2 Assessment of the axial skeleton

The primary functions of the vertebral column include protection of the spinal cord, support for weight bearing and flexibility for locomotion (Haussler *et al.* 1999) and these are all crucial factors when assessing the axial skeleton for dysfunction and pathology. Assessment and treatment of the equine axial skeleton follow a thorough subjective assessment of multiple factors associated with day-to-day management and ridden issues, including fitness, level of workload and presenting symptoms. A careful and comprehensive subjective assessment can help identify potential spinal pathology ranging from subtle change in attitudes to work and apprehension when grooming or changing rugs, no longer rolling over, 'cold-backed' behaviour on mounting such as hyperflexing the thoracic spine on sitting onto the saddle or when moving off or a reluctance to move forwards off the leg. Loss of performance may be specific to a ridden exercise only; the rider may feel a loss of quality of step or asymmetry in certain aspects of lateral work or with a change of trot diagonal, suggesting a subtle pelvic limb lameness. More extreme behavioural changes such as rearing, bucking down hills and refusing to jump may also be noted.

Gait assessment is essential when assessing dysfunction (Dyson 2014). This may include walking and trotting in hand in straight lines on both hard and soft surfaces, turning in hand, backing up, lunging and ridden assessment. The horse may present with an obvious overt gait abnormality noted by the owner and seen at the first walk and trot on the hard in a straight line, for example stringhalt – the exaggerated upward flexion of one or two pelvic limbs at walk. This is differentiated from shivers or shivering which is observed as an episodic hyperflexion of the pelvic limb, exacerbated by picking up the limb and the horse involuntarily holding the limb into flexion/abduction for several seconds. Fibrotic myopathy displays the characteristic shortened cranial swing phase of the pelvic limb, snatch into retraction and slap of the foot down onto the ground (Dyson & Ross 2011b). Articular issues may be more evident, for example, when lunging in trot on a hard surface, but care must be taken that the

assessment process does not exacerbate the problem or cause injury. The handler must be given the opportunity to voice any concerns regarding assessment procedures and the therapist should always ask permission prior to undertaking any procedure. For example, if a horse routinely uses protective exercise boots for work, it would be foolish to omit using them to assess gait on the lunge.

The most qualified person present is responsible for managing the assessment process, whether that be a veterinarian or a physiotherapist. If there is an accident, the most senior person becomes accountable. The handler must be deemed confident and competent to lunge for assessment purposes and the area provided should be safe and suitable. Care must be taken when using expanses of concrete that may be slippery. When lunging on soft surfaces, the ligamentous and tendinous structures are loaded and soft tissue dysfunctions may be noted during transitions at walk, trot and canter.

Assessment of specific gaits and paces may identify regional pathology specific to a site and comparisons should be made for symmetry of movement on both reins, including assessment of head and neck posture and pelvic motion (Pfau *et al.* 2014). A horse presenting with a thoracic limb lameness associated with foot pain is commonly seen head nodding, with the head raised when weight bearing on the affected limb and exacerbated when it is on the inside of a lunge circle. The horse may also hold the head laterally flexed away from the affected limb and with the head to the outside of the circle. A horse may present with splinting of the dorsal thoracic musculature if the pelvic limb on the inside of a lunge circle is affected and loaded, but may not present with the visible head nod of a thoracic limb lameness.

Khumsap *et al.* (2003) assessed the kinematics of horses trotting over a force-plate before and after induction of a unilateral tarsal joint synovitis and concluded that whilst tarsal joint range of motion, peak vertical force and vertical impulses decreased, no compensatory changes in work were performed by other joints within the lame hindlimb during the stance phase. Vertical impulse in the diagonal forelimb decreased, but there were no significant changes in forces or impulses in the ipsilateral forelimb or contralateral hindlimb, indicating that horses are able to manage mild, unilateral hindlimb lameness by reducing the airborne phase of the stride rather than by increased loading of the compensating limbs. However, it is uncertain what effect this has on the axial skeleton. Pelvic limb toe drag on sand may suggest a loss of impulsion and poor swing phase clearance. The quality of the transitions, both upwards and downwards, on the lunge and when ridden, is necessary to distinguish whether the horse can canter on the correct lead and maintain a circle of canter without disuniting; the ability of the horse to load the pelvic limbs in the downwards transitions can be observed with the outside hind protracting on the first step down into trot.

Body condition scoring may identify the horse as obese and apart from potentially reflecting the general level of fitness, makes true assessment more difficult and affects the ability of the physiotherapist to palpate the horse's axial skeleton. Adams *et al.* (2009) examined obesity in older horses and found a correlation between age-related obesity and increased production of inflammatory cytokines, compared with thin old horses. This systemic inflammatory response may have implications for pain response but further work is required to substantiate this.

A generalised global observation of standing posture, including head and neck (see Chapter 19), may already highlight areas of concern. These areas may include global epaxial, postural and segmental muscle wasting of horses with chronic symptoms, kyphosis, lordosis or scoliosis, incongruence of thoracic and lumbar dorsal spinous processes (including the wither profile). The areas of concern may also include observed asymmetry of the pelvic bony architecture of the tuber coxae (TC), tuber sacrale (TS) and tuber ischii (TI) (Figure 20.1a) and the muscular bulk of the gluteals, biceps femoris, semimembranosus and semitendinosus (Figure 20.1b) and altered tail positioning, possibly held to one side or clamped down.

20.2.1 Thoracolumbar joint morphology

When assessing the axial skeleton, consideration should be given to the regional variances in joint morphology and the range of motion that results. Early work by Townsend *et al.* (1983) described the ranges of motion throughout the thoracolumbar spine and recorded degrees of dorsoventral (DV) flexion and extension, lateral bending and axial rotation occurring at all levels. These authors noted that most DV flexion and extension range occurred at the lumbosacral junction and first thoracic intervertebral joints. The greatest degree of axial rotation and lateral flexion occurred in the midthoracic spine at T11–12 with the caudal thoracic and lumbar spine least mobile. Lateral flexion was found to be coupled with axial rotation although the thoracic ribcage created stability which limited rotation. Townsend & Leach (1984) subsequently divided the thoracolumbar spine into four divisions relating to joint morphology: cranial T1–2; midthoracic spine (T2–16); caudal thoracic and lumbar (T16–L6); and the lumbosacral joint. Additionally, they observed frequent fusion of the lateral joints of the lumbar spine. Further work by Townsend *et al.* (1986) compared the spinal biomechanics of the thoracolumbar spine with the pathology identified. Ventrolateral vertebral body osteophytes were commonly seen between T10 and T17, most frequently seen at T11–13 where most axial rotation and lateral bending occurs. Impingement of dorsal spinous processes between T13 and T18 was seen but did not relate to regional spinal mobility. Degeneration of the intervertebral disc was present in three out of four specimens at T1–2 and the lumbosacral joints – both regions of highest DV flexion and extension.

Faber *et al.* (2001) assessed the three-dimensional reaction of the spine during canter on a treadmill and found that the greatest degree of DV flexion and extension occurred at the lumbosacral junction. During the single stance phase, there was segmental rotation throughout the lumbar spine coupled with the pelvic limb protraction and retraction. Recent work by Jones (2015) further assessed spinal biomechanics of the thoracolumbar

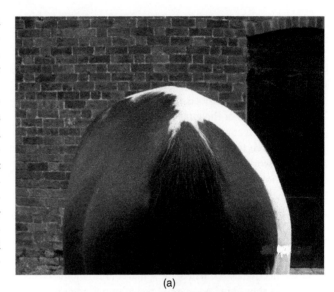

(a)

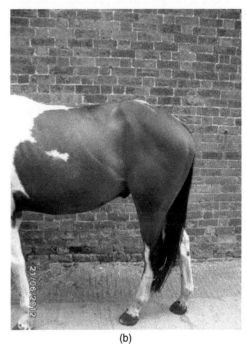

(b)

Figure 20.1 Pelvic asymmetry. (a) Caudal aspect, demonstrating asymmetry of tuber sacrale. (b) Lateral view. This demonstrates the poorly developed gluteal musculature in this horse with pelvic asymmetry.

vertebrae and identified that the four movement patterns (dorsiflexion (DF), ventroflexion (VF), lateral flexion (LF), axial rotation (AR)) were defined by bone morphology of the vertebral bodies and zygapophyseal joints in the caudal lumbar spine. DF and VF range of sagittal movement was limited by a tall heart-shaped vertebral body with increased restriction of DF due to bony interactions. Lateral flexion was associated with a narrow vertebral body with a short transverse process lever arm and the narrowly placed, horizontally oriented zygapophyseal joints. Caudal lumbar lateral flexion was restricted by the lateral joints.

Axial rotation in the lumbar spine relates to the shape of the lumbar zygaphophyseal joints.

Haussler *et al.* (1997) assessed morphological findings in thoroughbreds (TBs), revealing variations including transitional vertebra of the thoracolumbar and sacrococcygeal joints as well as asymmetry and ankylosis in pairs of intertransverse joints. They noted fusion of the lumbosacral vertebra and pelvic physeal closure both at approximately age 5, whereas the iliac crest and ischial arch fusion showed closure at ages 7 and 5 respectively. This work is the basis of the physiotherapist's assessment of spinal mobility and guides the assessment procedure, highlighting the normal variances in a population of apparently normal specimens.

20.2.2 Thoracic spine assessment
Palpation

Specific objective assessment of the spinal column should be systematic and should include careful palpation of the dorsal thoracic region centrally and laterally, noting any pain, heat, effusion, scarring or soft tissue oedema. The supraspinous ligament can be palpated with moderate ease, especially at the caudal portion of the withers when inflamed, which may give it a 'boggy' feel. Reaction at the dorsal spinous processes (DSPs) may be localised and palpation can reveal heat and superficial acute tenderness at a specific level. This may be associated with a generalised loss of epaxial topline musculature, segmental muscle wasting or specific osseous changes with regions of altered bony profiling that may indicate primary pathology. Pain response may vary from displays of extreme behaviour such as biting or kicking to overt flinching away or dropping into extension, to a more subtle twitch response on bony palpation or the placing on of a saddle.

The significance of localised pain on palpation of the DSPs may allude to the presence of overriding or impinging dorsal spinous processes of predominantly the thoracic regions and there is a correlation between the severity of impinging DSPs and vertebral laminar stress fractures in TBs (Haussler & Stover 1998). Much work relating to spinal pathology has used TBs as models because of the abundance of racehorse wastage off the track due to injury. In trying to determine the cause of impinging spinous processes (ISPs), genetic predisposition may be considered (Zimmerman *et al.* 2012). The effects of poor training may cause a horse to collect its frame in a more advanced outline than the core strength allows, creating false outline with poor ability to work over their back musculature or as a result of an underlying lameness such as sacroiliac pain, creating a weakened connection from the pelvis to the axial skeleton. The pathophysiology of impinging spinous processes is discussed later in this chapter, but the aim of all veterinarians and physiotherapists rehabilitating these horses is to create space between the affected spinous processes to allow gapping of the segments and thus unload the region. Berner *et al.* (2012) researched the effect of head and neck posture on radiographic changes in the amount of thoracic spinous process gapping. The lower the head and neck were positioned, the greater the gap between the thoracic dorsal spinous processes.

20.2.3 Assessment of the thoracic articulations

Direct palpation of the thoracic facet joints is not possible but the rib angles articulate dorsally at the costotransverse joints laterally to the midline, creating the 'shelf' upon which the epaxial muscles of the intercostals and serratus dorsalis caudalis may be palpated in fit horses. Palpation of the rib angles at the lateral aspect of the dorsal thorax corresponds with saddle placement and thus the region is predominantly loaded with DV pressure of the rider at these joints. It is thus a region susceptible to pain due to ill-fitting tack. Little research exists relating to rib pathology, although Dahlberg *et al.* (2011) observed cranial and caudal rib injuries, with cranial rib disorders eliciting severe acute lameness, presenting an abducted thoracic limb whilst protracting the leg. Caudal rib injury presented with resentment to tacking up. Costochondral junction disorders and costovertebral dysfunction dorsal to the sternal articulations were also identified.

Assessment of the articulations of the thoracic spine can be made with the physiotherapist standing lateral to the thorax and reaching down with the arms either side of the ribcage at a similar level and transversely gliding the pair of articulations of the facet and rib joints alternating from one arm to the other (Figure 20.2). The physiotherapist's own hip is used on the ipsilateral side to glide the thorax away; the most extended arm 'catches' the motion and pulls the thorax back toward the physiotherapist. This may be used segmentally as both an assessment and a treatment technique. Horses with DSP pathology may appear stiff or fixed at a particular segment and occasionally the crepitus of bone-on-bone spinous process movement may be either palpated or even heard during delivery of this technique. Some horses are extremely sensitive to the sensation of crepitus and this may elicit a pain response.

Greve & Dyson (2014) looked at thoracolumbar posture in a longitudinal study following 96 sport horses over a year, and measured the shape from the withers to the end of the thoracic spine using a flexicurve to measure the region every 2 months. They found that significant changes to posture and shape could occur even in the 2-month interval and that commonly, saddle fit was implicated with associated back pain.

20.3 Reflex motion to palpatory pressure

Most horses exhibit reflex movements to palpatory pressure. An example of such a reflex movement is the abdominal reflex (Figure 20.3) which assesses the ability of the horse to flex the thoracic spine. It is a demonstration of range of motion of the thoracic region and the ability of the horse to activate abdominal and trunk musculature. The abdominal reflex is provoked by the application of firm pressure at the ventral midline in a cranial direction just behind the elbow of the horse. This

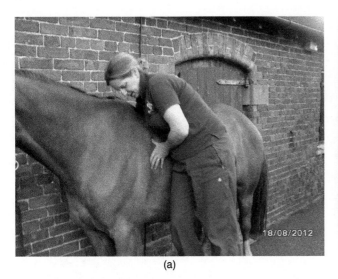

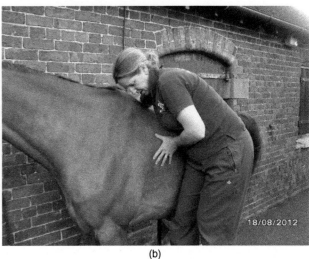

(a)

(b)

Figure 20.2 (a) Thoracic spine lateral translation away from the physiotherapist. The therapist's left hand and right hip are translating the thorax away, with the right hand 'catching' the lateral sway. (b) Thoracic spine lateral translation towards the physiotherapist. The therapist 'scoops' the thorax towards them with the right hand, supporting the translation with the left hand and right hip.

pressure should elicit some reflex dorsiflexion of the thoracic spine, but may also elicit a cow kick response or even compensatory forced ventroflexion or thoracic epaxial splinting to evade dorsal flexion.

Further assessment of thoracolumbar spinal mobility of dorsal and ventral flexion can be made using a pelvic rounding reflex (Figure 20.4). When combined with lateral flexion reflexes, eliciting a stimulation of the gluteals will cause a contralateral movement of the pelvis away from the physiotherapist, depending on the placement of the stimulus. When combined with lateral flexion movement of the thorax, it creates a combined lateral flexion of the whole thoracolumbar spine region. In combination with dynamic stability exercises associated with baited neck

stretches, the whole neuromuscular system of the axial skeleton can be stimulated. The reflex stimulus eliciting trunk flexion will exacerbate prominence of DSPs and can create a lumbar roach posture. Where lumbar segmental stiffness is the primary issue (which may arise from facet or spinous process ankylosis) (Haussler *et al.* 1997), rounding responses may have a limited effect, creating the appearance of a 'poker' back with little thoracic flexion but increased pelvic caudal flexion and gapping of the lumbosacral junction. Eliciting lateral flexion will create segmental gapping of rib angles on the convex side of the trunk. Gapping the segmental intercostal musculature on the contralateral side compresses the articulations on the ipsilateral side and vice versa.

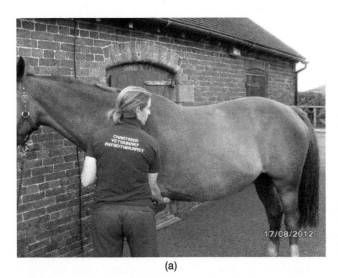

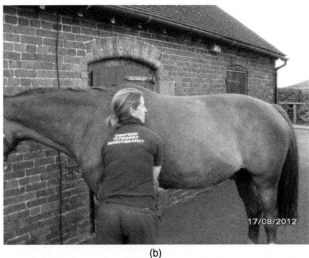

(a)

(b)

Figure 20.3 (a) Starting posture before abdominal stimulus. (b) Abdominal reflex into dorsal flexion – abdominal lift achieved.

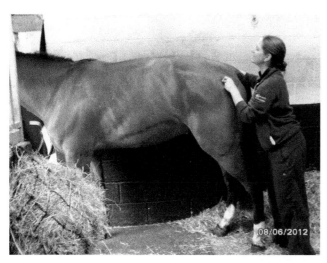

Figure 20.4 Pelvic rounding reflex showing thoracic, lumbar and pelvic dorsal flexion and activity of abdominals.

The use of reflex motion to palpatory pressure techniques is effective as both an assessment and a treatment technique in equine physiotherapy.

20.3.1 Thoracolumbar vertebral dorsal-flexion stretch

This utilises the rounding response via a noxious stimulus or pressure to palpation. In stoical horses, the use of the blunt end of a hoof pick may be required to elicit a response. This stretch, if performed repeatedly on a daily basis, may assist in preventing loss of spinal motion noted in the facet joints in all horses but especially those with an increased lordotic posture or conformation.

20.3.2 Equine baited slump stretch (neuromechanical)

This affects many structures including the nuchal and supraspinous ligaments, the entire epaxial myofascial system, thoracolumbar vertebral column and the neurological system (spinal cord and components of the brachial and lumbosacral plexuses and associated fascia). Figure 20.5a shows the winding up of these structures via flexion via head lowering between the carpus. To place neuromeningeal and myofascial structures on more stretch, unilateral hindlimb protraction may be added to the neck flexion. The protraction component is shown in Figure 20.5b.

20.4 Central core structures and associated pathology

Although a common diagnosis, specific 'kissing spine' primary pathology is implicated in a group of syndromes associated with spinal pathology and concurrent thoracic and/or pelvic limb involvement (Zimmerman *et al.* 2012). Rehabilitation is

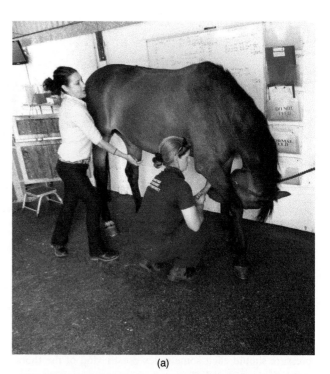

(a)

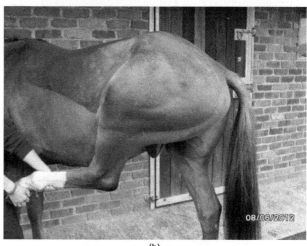

(b)

Figure 20.5 Equine slump test. (a) The horse takes a treat from between the carpus, to maximally flex the neck and thoracolumbar region. (b) Hindlimb protraction may be added to the neck flexion to further tension neuromechanical tissue and myofascia during the slump test.

required to promote correct use of spinal stabilisers to create a strong musculoskeletal bridge upon which the rider must balance. If pain inhibits the segmental muscles from appropriately stabilising individual segments, global mobilisers are inclined to take over and become overactive, further creating a relatively extended thoracolumbar spine and therefore a compressed vertebral bridge with potential for impinging dorsal spinous processes.

Conservative management is the primary aim for physiotherapists considering rehabilitating these clinical cases. The

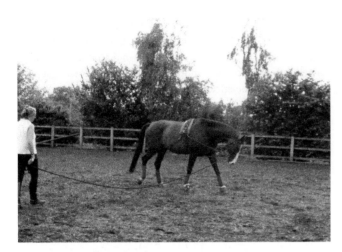

Figure 20.6 Use of training aids – Equiami in use.

principle involves creating a strong 'core' within both the epaxial spinal musculature including multifidus, sacrocaudalis dorsalis medialis, and the hypaxial abdominal musculature of the diaphragm, rectus abdominis and the external abdominal obliques to support the bony axial skeleton and the large abdominal content loading the horse ventrally. This becomes the basis from which the horse should work, as well as addressing muscle spasm and pain management by using electrotherapy, specific soft tissue techniques, taping techniques or exercise such as the appropriate use of the Pessoa training aid or an equivalent (Figure 20.6). Walker *et al.* (2013) evaluated the use of training aids for rehabilitation, finding the Pessoa beneficial for generalised rehabilitation work to stimulate activation of core musculature without increasing load on either the thoracic or pelvic limb structures.

Muscle fibre type is thought to reflect the role of muscle function – for example, a dominance of type I fibres suggests a role as a postural stabiliser. Hyytiainen *et al.* (2014) assessed the fibre types of the pelvic limb musculature and the thoracolumbar spine to identify those stabilisers which had a dominance of type I fibres. These were found in sacrocaudalis dorsalis and the diaphragm, whilst mixed fibre types existed in the locomotory groups of the pelvic limb including psoas major, iliocostalis and longissimus dorsi.

Additionally, Rombach *et al.* (2014) assessed the muscle fibres of longus thoracis in the cranial thoracic spine and found many intersegmental bands, suggesting a predominant role of this muscle as a postural stabiliser. Multifidus is known as the key human spinal intersegmental stabiliser (O'Sullivan 2000) and much work has been done to compare equine multifidus to the anatomy and function of multifidus in humans (Stubbs *et al.* 2006). Research by Stubbs *et al.* (2010) used ultrasonography to measure the cross-sectional area (CSA) of the multifidus muscle, which was found to have significantly reduced CSA, and sacrocaudalis dorsalis at or close to the level of pathology in horses with ipsilateral osseous pathology. Adaptations to the human equivalent of dynamic spinal stabilisation exercises were

developed to aid core stability of the equine thoracolumbar spine, by undertaking baited lateral cervical and ventroflexion stabilising exercises daily to stimulate activity of multifidus. Stubbs *et al.* (2011) created a dynamic exercise programme of baited exercises of five repetitions of each specific exercise performed daily five times weekly for 3 months. The CSA of multifidus was measured before and after the training regime and significant bilateral hypertrophy was noted in CSA multifidus, despite no other specific exercise being undertaken. Additionally, Clayton *et al.* (2012) utilised the dynamic baited stretches of the cervical spine to create increased thoracolumbar bending, to activate and strengthen the core stabilisers of the caudal thoracic spine.

Crook *et al.* (2008) compared the anatomy and muscle architecture of the pelvic limbs of Quarterhorses bred for speed and Arab horses bred for endurance, hypothesising a difference in muscle architecture associated with their differing breed specialties. The main finding was a greater muscle mass in the Quarterhorse, potentially enhancing the acceleration of the quarters. Further work by Crook *et al.* (2010) assessed pelvic limb muscle activity during walking on a treadmill, and noted that, with increased gradient, the mean electromyographic activity increased for all pelvic muscle groups, but specifically gluteus medius when trotting. This implied that slope work may be beneficial for rehabilitating pelvic limb injury and enhancing recruitment of muscle groups, aiding strengthening. Similarly, declining gradient, mirroring walking down a slope, maintained biceps femoris activity at walk, similarly to eccentric loading.

The use of trotting poles during the rehabilitation process can enhance core strength, increase joint range of motion and promote abdominal muscle recruitment (Figure 20.7). Clayton *et al.* (2015) hypothesised that increasing the height of raised poles may increase the ground reaction forces and thus load the limb increasingly; however, this was not the case and the forces involved were similar to those of trotting on flat ground. Brown *et al.* (2015) assessed the use of trotting poles and identified that

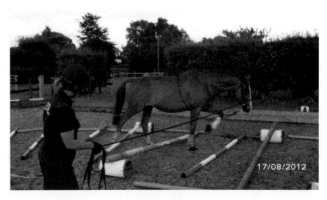

Figure 20.7 Horse going over raised walk poles.

the hooves cleared the poles due to increased joint flexion rather than by raising the body higher during the suspension phases of the stride and there was no habituation unlike the use of tactile stimulation.

There may be several reasons why failure to rehabilitate the core musculature appropriately occurs, including lack of experience of the owner/handler to work the horse appropriately, unsuitable facilities to undertake the rehabilitation process, unreasonable expectations of the owner/handler relating to the time required to rehabilitate prior to competition dates or underlying and/or concurrent pathology and lameness. In this event, the multidisciplinary team may feel that medical management is warranted, although it must be highlighted to the client that further rehabilitation will be necessary beyond this to maximise athletic potential and minimise poor outcome. Onward medical and surgical management of overriding or impinging dorsal spinous processes has evolved from intralesional corticosteroid medication and/or spinous process resection (Jeffcott & Hickman 1975) – both under anaesthetic and standing (Walmsley *et al.* 2002) – to interspinous ligament resection (ISLR) (Coomer *et al.* 2012) and subtotal ostectomy (Brink 2014) or cranial wedge osteotomy techniques (Jacklin *et al.* 2014). Improvements in surgical technique and the fact that the majority of this surgery is now done as standing surgery under local anaesthetic make it achievable for many more veterinary practices to perform (O'Brien & Hunt 2014). A surge in diagnoses of impinging DSP also correlates with improved imaging techniques, improved rider awareness of loss of performance and better surgical techniques, as well as an increase in the number of thoroughbred horses being retrained as riding horses following the end of their racing careers (Figure 20.8).

The cutaneous trunci skin muscle reflex is found to have maximal deformation in the thoracic region (Essig *et al.* 2013) and along with serratus ventralis spasm at the girth, must be considered a cause of sensitivity in the tense horse. Reluctance to lift cranially through stimulation of the abdominals may also be indicative of systemic pathology such as gastric ulcers (Sykes & Jokisalo 2014), and may require further investigation to exclude

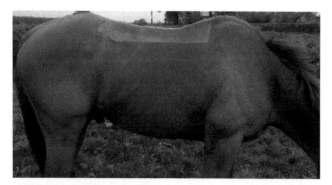

Figure 20.8 A 14-year-old thoroughbred gelding, 2 weeks following dorsal spinous process resection surgery of four levels (T10–18), after removal of stitches.

pathology. Some horses may display this altered behaviour on girthing up with sensitivity behind the elbows around the dorsolateral aspect of the thorax for no known reason. Use of scapular retractions to create a more cranial thoracic dorsal gapping into flexion can be effective both for assessment and treatment techniques as an alternative to abdominal reflex stretches, as it encourages gapping of the cranial thoracic DSPs and creates lift through the abdominals. Additionally, thoracic limb protraction stretches may aid release of myofascial tension and can be used as an exercise prior to girthing up.

It is also important to consider the intrinsic interfaces between horse and rider, including saddles and bits/bridles as additional factors affecting the horse–rider interface. Recent research into saddle stability (Greve & Dyson 2013) has correlated a direct link between saddle slippage and hindlimb lameness and suggests that slippage can be a potential indicator of a hindlimb lameness issue, easily identified by the physiotherapist from the subjective to objective assessment. Riders must be questioned about straightness in the saddle and their own orthopaedic issues that could potentially impact the horse–rider interface (see Chapter 21).

20.5 Lumbar spine

Although it is nearly impossible to isolate the lumbar intersegmental motion, the lumbar spine can be assessed similarly with addition of a lateral flexion reflex movement of the quarters both towards and away from the handler. This is done by fixing the thoracolumbar region carefully at the caudal rib angles with one hand and performing the reflex by stimulating the superficial gluteal muscle unilaterally, either on the ipsilateral or contralateral side, depending on the effect required. Further investigation of the degree of lumbar flexion and rotation can be made using the pelvic limb as a lever. Pelvic limb protraction with the hind toe reaching the carpus or elbow of the thoracic limb will create lumbosacral flexion predominantly coupled with thoracolumbar flexion (see Figure 20.5b). Abducting the pelvic limb at an angle of approximately 45° creates segmental rotation throughout the thoracolumbar spine but is difficult to isolate to a specific region. However, when assessing the symmetry of rotation on both sides, observation of the rib angles and both the costal cartilages and costal arch throughout the thorax will indicate relative segmental gapping. Abduction of the pelvic limb additionally loads the contralateral sacroiliac joint. Pelvic limb retraction will close down the lumbosacral interspinous space, creating a relative cranial tilt or nutated position of the pelvis, whilst additionally loading the trochlear groove at the stifle and moving the hip into extension.

20.6 Lumbosacral junction

The greatest amount of intersegmental flexion-extension in the thoracolumbar spine occurs at the lumbosacral junction. This sagittal motion is noted to increase with increasing velocity of stride (Johnson & Moore-Coyler 2009). The joint at the lumbosacral junction is demarcated by a large mobile intervertebral disc. This and the lack of supraspinous ligament at the lumbosacral junction has an effect on stability at this level (Henson *et al.* 2007).

On palpation of the lumbosacral junction, the therapist is aware of a dip which can be felt just cranial to the tuber sacrale and caudal to L6. This region may be sensitive to palpation. Nagy *et al.* (2010) assessed this articulation using ultrasonography and found no significant variances relating to breed, gender, age or size. However, Stubbs *et al.* (2006) found variances in anatomy at postmortem, including sacralisation of L6, affecting range of motion at this joint. Haussler *et al.* (1997) also found numerous vertebral variations including asymmetry in articulations of the articular processes in TBs. Assessment and treatment of this region should include assessing range of pelvic tilt with combined range at the thoracolumbar spine. Pelvic rounding response can be used to assess both cranial (nutation) and caudal pelvic rotation (counternutation) by both flexing and extending the lumbosacral junction relatively. Cranial pelvic tilt or nutation will close down the lumbosacral junction and increase compression of the lumbosacral disc, although it is unsubstantiated whether this creates a painful stimulus if pathology is present.

Pelvic limb protraction, whereby the hoof is taken cranially to the palmar aspect of the carpus or elbow, will create a degree of thoracolumbar and lumbosacral flexion and is a useful adjunct to assess unilateral pelvic range of nutation and combined thoracic, lumbar and lumbosacral flexibility (see Figure 20.5). Additionally, the use of scapular retractions of the thoracic limb (see Chapter 19, Figure 19.8) can increase pelvic limb loading and relative counternutation of the pelvis and load the axial structures.

20.7 Sacroiliac joint

Sacroiliac joint (SIJ) degenerative joint disease is a very common cause of wastage in dressage horses (Dyson 2000). Degenerative changes are often seen in the tarsal joints of performance horses, the vertebral column facet joints and sacroiliac joint surfaces collectively. In one study of 36 racehorses, all had degenerative or adaptive changes in the articular facet joints of the vertebral column and the sacroiliac joints (Haussler *et al.* 1999). Research suggests this is also the case for joints subjected to shear forces, such as the sacroiliac joint (Eckstein *et al.* 1999; Frank *et al.* 2001). In a population of horses studied for sacroiliac joint degeneration (SID), dressage horses and show jumpers were considered to be most at risk (Dyson & Murray 2003). Other factors that may contribute to SID included older, taller, heavier warmbloods than the normal clinic population, and those with poor epaxial musculature or pelvic muscle asymmetry. Riders complained of stiffness in the horse with an inability for the horse to work on the bit and/or having poor canter quality,

including disunited canter. Subjectively the farrier may struggle to shoe the horse's pelvic limb(s). Additionally, Dyson & Murray (2003) identified issues with an exaggerated response to palpation directly over the TS, resistance to standing on a single pelvic limb for protracted periods and lack of flexibility of the thoracolumbar spine.

It is thought that the equine musculoligamentous 'sling' and fascial system surrounding the vertebral column and SIJ may be under proprioceptive control of neural elements within the tissue, as is the case in humans and pigs (Brolinson *et al.* 2003; Indahl *et al.* 1999). Any cause of altered proprioception or altered load transfer through the SIJ or vertebral column through trauma or lameness may be a reason for development of joint surface changes in horses. Exercise designed to improve the neuromotor control around this musculoligamentous sling may therefore be required for articular cartilage health in this area.

Early work by Jeffcott *et al.* (1985) identified a larger surface area of the SIJ in horses with pathology of that joint, with increased extension of the joint at the caudomedial aspect. This may suggest a situation of chronic instability in horses with sacroiliac pathology related to a loss of this neuromotor control of the area and therefore impulsion. Direct palpation of the SIJ is not possible and veterinarians assess this joint using diagnostic ultrasonography or scintigraphy. Goff *et al.* (2008) reviewed the assessment and management of sacroiliac dysfunction, broadly dividing the pathology into two groups, those with pain, poor performance and poorly identified pathology and those with bony pathological changes and chronic instability. Assessment and treatment have been expanded from human research using pain provocation tests and assessment of neuromotor control.

For accurate assessment of the pelvic region, and to aid differentiation between a pelvic issue and primary hindlimb pathology, both movement analysis and static assessment should be undertaken. The horse should be stood four-square on a flat firm surface, noting whether the horse stands with legs camped under or camped out. The use of markers on bony prominences can assist the therapist in identifying subtle alterations in bony landmarks, in particular, differentiating asymmetry of TS, TC and TI (see Figure 20.1a). For example, ilial wing asymmetry seen at the TC may be due to stress fractures or direct pelvic trauma.

Muscular wasting or unilateral asymmetry of the gluteals, hamstrings and biceps femoris muscle groups (see Figure 20.1b) may suggest underlying articular pathology or chronic lameness. Scar tissue is occasionally identified at the TI associated with relative flattening of the semitendinosus or hypertrophy of the opposing side and may correlate with cranial bony asymmetry of the TS or TC, suggestive of chronic pelvic stress or trauma. Further palpation of the sacrum and its DSPs can help identify issues with the dorsal sacroiliac ligament (DSIL) and is a common site of ligamentous desmitis, associated with normal ageing. The DSIL may be palpated as it runs caudomedially from each tubera sacrale to the DSPs of the sacrum. Engeli *et al.* (2006) assessed this region ultrasonographically and noted that the

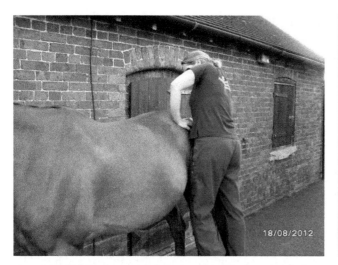

Figure 20.9 Mobilisation over the left tuber coxae. The force is applied in a dorsoventral direction, here via the therapist's left hand.

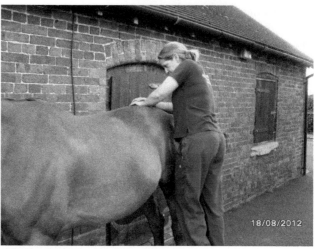

Figure 20.10 Tuber sacrale lateral transverse glide.

caudal portion of the thoracolumbar fascia joined the dorsal part of the DSIL and although two configurations were noted, caudally these structures combined to form a single structure that inserted onto the sacral spinous processes. Palpation of the tail base and coccygeal segments can prove useful, with the tail acting as a fulcrum to transmit forces through the pelvis and aiding assessment of pelvic stability. Under the tail base laterally to the anus, the caudal insertion of the broad sacrotuberous (ST) pelvic ligament can be palpated onto the ischium for symmetry. Further, palpation of this fascia-like ligamentous structure can result in contraction of adjacent soft tissue attachments of semitendinosus, biceps femoris and gluteal superficialis.

Dynamic testing of the structures supporting the sacroiliac joint includes direct dorsoventral palpation of the bony landmarks including the TC, TS and ischial compressions of the TI. Goff *et al.* (2006) identified a relative lengthening of the DSIL and reduction in the CSA of the fibres associated with direct force applied to the TS and TC. The greatest amount of motion was noted when pressure was applied transversely in a lateral or oblique direction. Resection of the DSIL and ST ligament further increased instability of the pelvis sagittally.

The physiotherapist stands lateral to the pelvis and preferably on a step to enable loading in a caudad direction from above. Firm pressure applied on the TC dorsally will elicit a subtle bounce or springing effect and end-range stiffness or hypermobility may be exhibited (Figure 20.9). This progressive loading involves a dorsoventral shear on the TC, with some concurrent movement at the sacrum laterally. The physiotherapist is assessing range and quality of the motion, comparing left and right sides. This direction of force also creates a relative cranial rotation of the pelvis relative to the sacrum.

Palpation caudally over the TS may elicit a pain response. Transverse pressure directly axially and applied to both TCs at the same time may produce a sense of instability or evoke a pain response in the horse (Figure 20.10).

Functional testing includes single hindleg stance, noting how easy it is to pick up the hindlimb into flexion and flexion/abduction to load the opposite side (Figure 20.11). This test may indicate how well the horse can load the stance leg. Obviously, this test is not specific for the SIJ. Relative loading of the contralateral limb and palpation of the TS on both the unloaded and loaded sides concurrently may identify any SIJ laxity that may exist. Relative motion between the TS and the sacral DSPs can be palpated on the loaded side and the unloaded side, like a modified stork test in human manual therapy (Goff *et al.* 2008).

Assessment of available protraction (flexion) and retraction (extension) of the coxofemoral joints will create a relative nutation and counternutation of the pelvis on the ipsilateral and contralateral sides, and variation in range of motion may be noted. Some horses may become unstable with pelvic limb

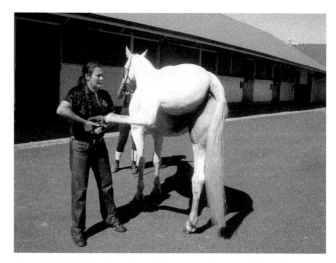

Figure 20.11 Testing the ability of the horse to functionally load-bear in unilateral hindlimb stance. Relative motion of the tuber coxae compared to the sacral DSPs may be palpated during this test.

retraction, suggesting SIJ instability, and static stability testing should include the ability of the horse to stand on the contralateral pelvic limb whilst a mediolateral glide is applied to the TS, by leaning onto the horse in a careful graded response, as if a rhythmic stabilisation exercise. Tail traction laterally and caudally will also create pelvic motion and assist assessment of relative pelvic stability, mimicking muscular contraction of the gluteals and the powerful global mobilising muscle groups including biceps femoris and the hamstrings.

Treatment of this region is dependent on accurate assessment of the whole horse and by identifying regions of instability and pain, most assessment techniques can be adapted to a treatment technique. For example, sensitivity to palpation of the sacrotuberous ligament may elicit myofascial spasm of the gluteals and hamstring complex, but sustaining pressure as a myofascial release technique is extremely effective to reduce compensatory overcontraction.

Manipulation of the SIJ may utilise the pelvic limb as a long lever when pressure is applied locally at the TC. There is much discussion regarding manipulation and whether a cranial force is applied to the lower side or a caudal compression is applied to the higher side. A thorough assessment of all the structures involved in pelvic stability, including muscle, tendon, ligaments, bone and myofascial components, in combination with a gait assessment, is the only way to comprehensively guide the treatment technique of choice.

20.8 Sacrococcygeal segments

Despite the relatively small region associated with the tail and sacrococcygeal anatomy, the tail is an important structure relating to balance of the horse, especially when jumping. Restricted motion in this region may limit function, especially after trauma, including rearing over backwards and landing on an extended tail or the overtightening of tail bandages leading to localised soft tissue trauma. Subjectively, an owner may notice altered tail posture during movement and it has been hypothesised (but not substantiated) that the tail held to one side may suggest hindlimb pain, and that it is held away from the lame limb (Ross 2011).

Assessment of the sacrococcygeal segments is easily made using the tail as a fulcrum and assessing range of relative extension, lateral flexion and individual segmental glide as an accessory movement. The use of caudal traction force at the tail can be applied to assess relative pelvic stability, including gluteal isometric contractions. When standing behind the horse, a sustained pull in a caudad direction is applied on the tail. Applying a caudad pull should create a counterpull cranially via the horse and the gluteals should contract concurrently. Where pelvic asymmetry exists and gluteal wasting is evident, there may be a time delay in the contractile reactions on the affected side. Tail traction can also be useful as a gapping release technique to the coccygeal segments and application will have a mild effect throughout the axial skeleton articulations. A lateral tail pull is

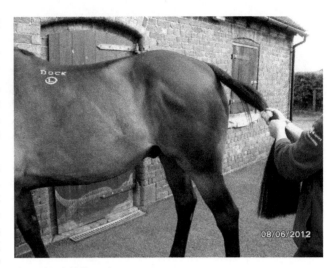

Figure 20.12 Tail traction.

used to assess proprioceptive deficit in neurological cases (see Chapter 10), but can also be used to assess pelvic and stifle stability. The handler stands to the side of the horse's pelvis and takes hold of the tail below the coccygeal segments and leans away from the pelvis, allowing the horse to take up the strain slowly – the horse should take a counterpull, recruit abdominals and load the opposite hind without stepping away or failing to 'lock' the patellofemoral joint on the opposite side (Figure 20.12). The release after approximately 10 sec from pulling is informative – where a horse has poor pelvic or stifle stability, the amount of postural sway or stepping out is marked. This technique is a useful home exercise for owners and in conjunction with dynamic stability exercises for the neck, can help with thoracolumbar stability.

20.9 Peripheral joints

20.9.1 Hip (coxofemoral) joint

The equine coxofemoral or hip joint is a large, load-bearing and relatively stable articulation and injuries are rarely seen. Rankin & Diesem (1976) dissected the nerves responsible for the innervation of the joint capsule and capsular ligaments, observing innervation from the femoral, obturator, cranial gluteal and sciatic nerves. This suggests a highly innervated structure that may have significant proprioceptive qualities. Clayton et al. (2001) identified that the hip joint musculature is the main source of energy generation at the walk, throughout the stride. Assessment of range of motion is difficult to isolate because much of the movement is coupled with the sacroiliac joint, stifle and lumbar flexion/extension. Gait assessment may identify non-specific pelvic limb lameness or global restrictions of range of motion. Assessment of passive range of motion is necessary to identify specific restrictions to each joint but the reciprocal apparatus will limit coupled movements between the stifle and tarsal joints, affecting the synchronous flexion and extension between these joints, making true end-range motion of the hip and its accessory or physiological movements near impossible.

Clayton *et al.* (2010, 2011a,b) assessed the use of both tactile stimulators and weights applied to the hind pasterns, assessing stride length, limb flight and muscle activity of the pelvic limb. The use of a tactile stimulator of 55 g attached to the pelvic limb pastern reduced stance phase duration but did not increase the concentric muscle activity of the hip flexors, whereas the stifle and hock did show increased range of motion and concentric activity. Later work researching the use of a weighted pastern boot of 700 g noted both increased height of flight arc in the distal articulations and increased concentric work of the hip flexors. Implications in rehabilitation suggest that different articulations and muscle groups may require different stimulation to effectively strengthen and mobilise. Bockstahler *et al.* (2012) assessed pelvic limb kinematics in arthritic dogs whilst walking up and down slopes and over small obstacles and concluded that complex gait changes occurred in several joints bilaterally and that each exercise created specific effects pertaining to planning rehabilitation programmes.

Associated soft tissue injury can occur, including trochanteric bursitis (Hawkins 2011) and gluteal strain, secondary to an altered gait associated with lameness in other regions. This may present as moderate-to-severe lameness and pain on palpation. Avulsion fracture of the third trochanter may rarely be seen and is associated with the massive torsional load of its attaching superficial gluteals. Palpation of the greater trochanter and third trochanter may elicit pain with hip pathology, but restriction of the associated muscle groups may be the only indicator.

Treatment of the hip region will depend on the soft tissue structures involved and awareness of any underlying concurrent pathology. Manual techniques to treat muscular soreness, including massage and myofascial release, and localised electrotherapy, including ultrasound and neuromuscular stimulation, may be applied beneficially, and stretching regimes and rehabilitation of associated pelvic limb stability may also be necessary.

Hill & Crook (2010) identified that massage of the caudal pelvic musculature, including semitendinosus, semimembranosus, biceps femoris and superficial gluteals, had a positive effect on soft tissue length, increasing both hindlimb protraction passively and stride length actively. This suggests benefits both in a rehabilitative field and during competition to enhance performance.

To effectively stretch the semimembranosus, the hock must be kept in flexion to wind up the calcaneal tendon or insertion. The limb then needs to be abducted. Biceps femoris would be stretched by adducting the limb from this position. It is important to note any cheating strategies the horse may implement to prevent a true stretch of middle gluteal; the muscle is unloaded by pelvic rotation, hitching thoracolumbar extension and raising of the head and neck. Due to the lumbar attachment of middle gluteal onto longissimus and the thoracolumbar fascia as far

cranially as the first lumbar vertebra, the thoracolumbar and cervical spine must be dorsally flexed (due to longissimus cervicus) as well as the limb.

20.9.2 Stifle

The equine stifle has similar anatomy and cartilage thickness to those of the human knee (Brehm *et al.* 2014). Assessment of intraarticular components of the stifle joint in horses is difficult due to the relatively large size and difficulty isolating movement, unlike the canine model where cruciate ligaments and meniscal testing can be applied. Rankin & Diesem (1976) identified a highly innervated joint that included the femoral, saphenous, obturator, common peroneal and tibial nerves, all supplying the joint capsule, fat pad, patellar and collateral ligaments and the meniscal and cruciate ligaments. This suggests a highly specialised joint with a specific role in limb mechanics and essential proprioceptive feedback requirements.

The primary finding of gait assessment when intraarticular structures are involved may be severe lameness, or more generalised subtle signs of loss of muscle bulk around biceps femoris and fascia lata with a wide, basey stance phase and relative weakness in eccentric loading through downwards transitions and seen as an occasional 'give' as if falling off the joint, particularly on turning. This can be exacerbated using tail pulls to assess pelvic limb stability. Localised effusion may be easily felt at the patellofemoral joint although care must be taken as many horses dislike palpation of this region. Flexion of the pelvic limb may be resented in a close-packed position, creating the feel of the limb being abducted to evade joint closure into this position, and subtle crepitus may be heard or felt throughout flexion.

In the competitive field, localised stifle injury is relatively common, especially during the cross-country phase if the limb is caught on a solid fence. Injuries may vary from superficial cuts and grazes to intraarticular damage of cruciate ligaments and/or menisci or extracapsular ligamentous damage including collateral ligament damage and patellar fracture, all of which can cause severe lameness. Peroni & Stick (2002) undertook a retrospective study to assess the arthroscopic findings of horses with stifle injuries, and assessed their return to function and outcome. The pathology noted included subchondral bone cysts of the medial femoral compartment, cruciate desmitis, degenerative joint disease and meniscal damage. They concluded that return to function was guarded for meniscal damage, although a good recovery was made with other conditions in isolation. Fowlie *et al.* (2012) further assessed the mechanics of the attachments of the cranial horn of the medial meniscus at the craniomeniscotibial ligament, and noted that full extension of the stifle increased the tensile forces at that region, predisposing the structure to damage with hyperextension of the stifle. Implications for physiotherapists suggest that great care should be taken when assessing the stifle if suspicious of meniscal damage, so as not to further damage the joint during the assessment process. As a common site of osteochondral defects, Lepeule *et al.* (2008) investigated breed variances and distribution of developmental orthopaedic disease in weanling foals, identifying prevalence in femoropatellar and hock joints, predominantly in warmblood and thoroughbred foals.

Cases of upward fixation of the patella (UFP) display specific signs including sudden-onset non-weight bearing with the limb held in retraction, most easily resolved by reversing the horse. Horses with unresolving or deteriorating UFP signs may undergo medial patellar desmotomy surgery.

Treatment of the stifle specifically relates to the pathology seen. In cases of intraarticular damage, veterinary intervention may include arthroscopy and protracted periods of confined rest. The role of the physiotherapist is therefore to maintain muscle bulk as able, without aggravating specific pathology. In cases of weakness and UFP, the aim is to strengthen the specific muscle groups associated with patellofemoral control. Taping techniques, muscle stimulation and rehabilitation using exercise to enhance pelvic stability including poles, slopes, appropriate concentric and eccentric loading will be essential (see Chapter 21).

20.9.3 Tarsus

The tarsus or hock joint, although a complex articulation involving several individual bony interfaces, is a relatively low motion joint and thus a common site of arthritic degeneration, known as bone spavin. During a drug trial, Orsini *et al.* (2012) evaluated the efficacy of a non-steroidal antiinflammatory drug (NSAID) on horses with both single and multiple joints affected by osteoarthritis and found the tarsus to be the most commonly affected single joint in over 40% of horses selected.

On initial observation, soft tissue swellings may be commonly seen around the joint, including thoroughpins (tarsal sheath tenosynovitis) and capped hocks (bursa of gastrocnemius). These may be idiopathic, a result of local trauma, a sign of mild concussive stress or degenerative in origin. Considered conformational defects in the showing ring, they are often associated with straight hocks. Often there is no associated lameness. Bog spavins (distension of the tarsocrural joint capsule) may also be observed at the hock and can be caused by osteochondral defects, arthritic changes or trauma. Lameness is dependent on the underlying cause but if the effusion is large enough, there may be a mechanical lameness due to physical restriction of flexion (Dyson & Ross 2011a).

Gait assessment may show altered limb mechanics with altered limb flight on swing phase – either abducting or adducting into protraction, toe drag or a relative pivot seen occurring at the hock joint. Farriers often notice increased lateral quarter hind shoe wear in horses with tarsal degenerative joint disease (DJD) and appropriate shoeing is crucial to stabilising the joints effectively (see Chapter 7). Khumsap *et al.* (2004) assessed the three-dimensional kinematics of horses with induced synovitis in the distal intertarsal (DIT) and tarsometatarsal (TMT) joints, identifying significantly reduced ranges of flexion in the tarsal joint and cranial translation of the metatarsus relative to the tibia during stance phase, and proximal translation of the metatarsus during swing phase, suggestive of reduced nutrition at these joints, further exacerbating the degenerative process. During the objective assessment, flexion of the hock joints may elicit a mild pain response to closing down the articulations or a reduction in range of motion with a sense of stiffness or bony block. Occasionally after releasing the distal pelvic limb from the flexed position, the horse is reluctant to relatively extend the joint to bear weight, exhibiting a hesitation in limb placement.

Due to the relative low motion rows of tarsal joints, it is difficult to identify which joints are affected although the presence of large bony spavins medially is suggestive of chronic osteoarthritis of the proximal intertarsal, centrodistal and/or tarsometatarsal joints of the tarsus. Physiotherapists assessing horses with mild loss of performance or loss of propulsion should always consider the relative reduction in limb flight associated with this and whether compensatory back pain is associated with this or secondary issues.

Ligamentous pathology is commonly observed in the pelvic limb and includes proximal suspensory desmopathy (PSD), a common condition in sport horses displaying poor performance, lack of propulsion or inability to 'sit' on the hindquarters, demonstrating toe drag or poor downwards transitions. It is also exacerbated in horses with a straight hindlimb conformation and hyperextending fetlocks – both considered risk factors for poor outcome (Dyson & Murray 2012). It is commonly seen in elite and non-elite dressage horses (Murray *et al.* 2006), especially when being asked to collect and when worked on soft surfaces excessively. Although a similar aetiology to the suspensory ligament desmopathy seen in the forelimb, the origin of the suspensory ligament in the distal pelvic limb is deep seated and fascially enveloped within the tarsal canal, predisposing the region to compression, especially if excessive strain causes relative hypertrophy of this ligament.

Whereas rest, timely judicious use of NSAIDs and controlled exercise may improve issues of thoracic limb suspensory desmitis, pelvic limb PSD responds poorly to this management protocol and so adjunctive extracorporeal shockwave therapy (ESWT) may be utilised. Lischer *et al.* (2006) assessed the outcome following ESWT, identifying that PSD was more likely to reoccur in the pelvic limb than the thoracic limb at long-term follow-up. Further intervention may include neurectomy of the deep branch of the lateral plantar nerve and plantar fasciotomy to address compressive factors.

Dyson & Murray (2012) investigated the outcome following surgery in three groups of horses, identifying that the best outcome occurred in horses with a diagnosis of PSD alone. A lower percentage of horses with additional secondary lameness issues recovered although those with poor conformational factors did not recover and remained lame a year after surgery.

The physiotherapist may become involved in any or all of these groups of cases postoperatively. There is a necessity to maintain core stability and proprioceptive awareness immediately postoperatively when the horse may undergo a period of box rest.

20.9.4 Metatarsophalangeal (MTP) joints

The pelvic limb fetlock joint or metatarsophalangeal joint is similar anatomically to that of the thoracic limb joints and during stance phase extension of the fetlock joint and stance flexion of the stifle, tarsal and coffin joints act as shock absorbers for the pelvic limb.

Articular and tendinous windgalls are commonly seen. Occasionally, the relative size of a tendon sheath effusion related to constriction of the flexor structures creates a golf ball-type convex swelling on the plantar aspect of the joint associated with annular ligament desmitis, so-called plantar (or palmar) annular ligament desmopathy (PAL) injury. Owen et al. (2008) retrospectively assessed cases with bilateral and unilateral lameness associated with PAL injury, identifying middle-aged or older general riding horses as more often affected and commonly seen in the hind fetlocks bilaterally although unilateral lameness was often identified. The physiotherapist can be effective in managing the PAL injury, provided they are given early access to reduce the effusion using electrotherapy modalities (see Chapter 13). Objective assessment of the amount of effusion is difficult, but simplistic measurement of the fetlock circumference or even the relative length of the tendinous windgall can be helpful. Controlled walking is required after an initial period of rest to allow the flexor structures to mobilise and reduce the risk of developing adhesions. Chronic annular ligament desmitis may require surgical intervention and physiotherapy can be useful post desmotomy for both mobilising scar tissue and preventing further adhesions. Owen et al. (2008) also identified that post-surgical outcome was a less than 50% return to former function. Mid to late stage postoperative rehabilitation requires the joint to be mobilised in functional ranges and over various surfaces to reestablish proprioceptive feedback (see Chapter 21).

Proximal interphalangeal (PIP) and distal interphalangeal (DIP) joints are generally discussed in Chapter 19. Despite subtle differences in the loading of these joints between the thoracic and pelvic limbs and the relative difference in hoof wall angle and hoof pastern axes (being more acute in the hind foot) (Clayton 1990a,b), the pathology remains the same and thus the assessment process of the accessory glide at these joints is similar.

Hoof capsule

It is essential that all physiotherapists have a good understanding of foot balance, conformation and correct shoeing. Often the physiotherapist is the first person to notice subtle changes in foot balance or identify mild lameness. They may be asked to see a pony with loss of performance issues with a subclinical laminitis or a horse with a brewing foot abscess. It is necessary to be able to palate normal and abnormal digital pulses and to locate areas of sensitivity with hoof testers so appropriate advice and further onward referral can be made.

20.10 Conclusion

Assessment of the thoracolumbar spine, pelvis and pelvic limb must not be made in isolation from the rest of the axial skeleton or thoracic limb. A good subjective assessment should create an excellent grounding for the objective assessment of the articular, myofascial and neuromuscular components and eventual manual treatment of these structures in combination with the cervical spine and thoracic limb (see Chapter 19).

References

Adams, A.A., Katepalli, M.P., Kohler, F. et al. 2009, Effect of body condition, body weight and adiposity on inflammatory cytokine responses in old horses. Vet. Immunol. Immunopathol. 127(3–4): 286–294.

Berner, D., Winter, K., Brehm, W. et al. 2012, Influence of head and neck position on radiographic measurement of intervertebral distances between thoracic dorsal spinous processes in clinically sound horses. Equine Vet. J. 43(supp): 21–26.

Bockstahler, B.A., Prickler, B., Lewy, E. et al. 2012, Hind limb kinematics during therapeutic exercises in dogs with osteoarthritis of the hip joints. Am. J. Vet. Res. 73(9): 1371–1376.

Brehm, W., Burk, J., Delling, U. 2014, Application of stem cells for the treatment of joint disease in horses. Methods Mol. Biol. 1213: 215–228.

Brink, P. 2014, Subtotal ostectomy of impinging dorsal spinous processes in 23 standing horses. Vet. Surg. 43(1): 95–98.

Brolinson, P.G., Kozar, A.J., Cibor, G. 2003, Sacroiliac joint dysfunction in athletes. Curr. Sports Med. Rep. 2(1): 47–56.

Brown, S., Stubbs, N.C., Kaiser, L.J. et al. 2015, Swing phase kinematics of horses trotting over poles. Equine Vet. J. 47(1): 107–112.

Clayton, H.M. 1990a, The effect of an acute hoof wall angulation on the stride kinematics of trotting horses. Equine Vet. J. 9(suppl): 86–90.

Clayton HM. 1990b, The effect of an acute angulation of the hind hooves on diagonal synchrony of trotting horses. Equine Vet. J. 9(suppl): 91–94.

Clayton, H.M., Hodson, E., Lanovaz, J.L. et al. 2001. The hindlimb in walking horses: 2. Net joint moments and joint powers. Equine Vet. J. 33(1): 44–48.

Clayton, H.M., White, A.D., Kaiser, L.J. et al. 2010, Hindlimb response to tactile stimulation of the pastern and coronet. Equine Vet. J. 42(3): 227–233.

Clayton, H.M., Lavagnino, M., Kaiser, L.J. et al. 2011a, Evaluation of biomechanical effects of four stimulation devices placed on the hind feet of trotting horses. Am. J. Vet. Res. 72(11): 1489–1495.

Clayton, H.M., Lavagnino, M., Kaiser, L.J. et al. 2011b, Swing phase kinematic and kinetic response to weighting the hind pasterns. Equine Vet. J. 43(2): 210–215.

Clayton, H.M., Kaiser, L.J., Lavagnino, M. et al. 2012, Evaluation of intersegmental vertebral motion during performance of dynamic mobilization exercises in cervical lateral bending in horses. Am. J. Vet. Res. 73(8): 1153–1159.

Clayton, H.M., Stubbs, N.C., Lavagnino, M. 2015, Stance phase kinematics and kinetics of horses trotting over poles. Equine Vet. J. 47(1): 113–118.

Coomer, R.P., McKane, S.A., Smith, N. *et al.* 2012, A controlled study evaluating a novel surgical treatment for kissing spines in standing sedated horses. *Vet. Surg.* 41(7): 890–897.

Crook, T.C., Cruickshank, S.E., McGowan, C.M. *et al.* 2008, Comparative anatomy and muscle architecture of selected hind limb muscles in the Quarter Horse and Arab. *J. Anat.* 212(2): 144–152.

Crook, T.C., Wilson, A., Hodson-Tole, E. 2010, The effect of treadmill speed and gradient on equine hindlimb muscle activity. *Equine Vet. J.* 38(suppl): 412–416.

Dahlberg, J.A., Ross, M.W., Martin, B.B. *et al.* 2011, Clinical relevance of abnormal scintigraphic findings of adult equine ribs. *Vet. Radiol. Ultrasound* 52(5): 573–579.

Dyson, S. 2000, Lameness and poor performance in the performance horse: dressage, show jumping and horse trials (eventing). *Am. Assoc. Equine Pract.* 46: 308–315.

Dyson, S. 2014, Recognition of lameness: man versus machine. *Vet. J.* 201(3): 245–248.

Dyson, S., Murray, R. 2003, Pain associated with the sacroiliac joint region: a clinical study of 74 horses. *Equine Vet. J.* 35: 240–245.

Dyson, S., Murray, R. 2012, Management of hindlimb proximal suspensory desmopathy by neurectomy of the deep branch of the lateral plantar nerve and plantar fasciotomy: 155 horses (2003–2008). *Equine Vet. J.* 44(3): 361–367.

Dyson, S., Ross, M. 2011a, The tarsus. In: Ross, M.W., Dyson, S.J. (eds), *Lameness in the Horse*, 2nd edn. Elsevier Saunders, St Louis, MO, pp. 508–532.

Dyson, S., Ross, M. 2011b, Mechanical and neurological lameness. In: Ross, M.W., Dyson, S.J. (eds), *Lameness in the Horse*, 2nd edn. Elsevier Saunders, St Louis, MO, pp. 558–559.

Eckstein, F., Tieschky, M., Faber, S. *et al.* 1999, Functional analysis of articular cartilage deformation, recovery and fluid flow following dynamic exercise in vivo. *Anat. Embryol.* 200: 419–424.

Engeli, E., Yeager, A.E., Erb, H.N. *et al.* 2006, Ultrasonographic technique and normal anatomic features of the sacroiliac region in horses. *Vet. Radiol. Ultrasound* 47(4): 391–403.

Essig, C.M., Merritt, J.S., Stubbs, N.C. *et al.* 2013, Localization of the cutaneus trunci muscle reflex in horses. *Am. J. Vet. Res.* 74(11): 1428–1432.

Faber, M., Johnston, C., Schamhardt, H.C. *et al.* 2001, Three-dimensional kinematics of the equine spine during canter. *Equine Vet. J.* 33(suppl): 145–149.

Fowlie, J.G., Arnoczky, S.P., Lavagnino, M. *et al.* 2012, Stifle extension results in differential tensile forces developing between abaxial and axial components of the cranial meniscotibial ligament of the equine medial meniscus: a mechanistic explanation for meniscal tear patterns. *Equine Vet. J.* 44(5): 554–558.

Frank, J., Quinn, T., Hunizer, E. *et al.* 2001, Tissue shear formation stimulates proteoglycan and protein biosynthesis in bovine cartilage explants. *Arch. Biochem. Biophys.* 395(1): 41–48.

Goff, L.M., Jasiewicz, J., Jeffcott, L.B. *et al.* 2006, Movement between the equine ilium and sacrum: in vivo and in vitro studies. *Equine Vet. J.* 36(suppl): 457–461.

Goff, L.M., Jeffcott, L.B., Jasiewicz, J. *et al.* 2008, Structural and biomechanical aspects of equine sacroiliac joint function and their relationship to clinical disease. *Vet. J.* 176(3): 281–293.

Gómez Alvarez, C.B., Wennerstrand, J., Bobbert, M.F. *et al.* 2007, The effect of induced forelimb lameness on thoracolumbar kinematics during treadmill locomotion. *Equine Vet. J.* 39(3): 197–201.

Greve, L., Dyson, S.J. 2013, An investigation of the relationship between hindlimb lameness and saddle slip. *Equine Vet. J.* 45: 570–577.

Greve, L., Dyson, S. 2014, Back shape changes in sports horses. *Equine Vet. J.* 46: 53.

Haussler, K.K., Stover, S.M. 1998, Stress fractures of the vertebral lamina and pelvis in Thoroughbred racehorses. *Equine Vet. J.* 30(5): 374–381.

Haussler, KK., Stover, S.,Willits, N. 1999, Pathological changes in the lumbosacral vertebrae and pelvis in Thoroughbred racehorses. *Am. J. Vet. Res.* 60: 143–153.

Haussler, KK., Stover, S.,Willits, N. 1997, Developmental variation in lumbosacropelvic anatomy of thoroughbred racehorses. *Am. J. Vet. Res.* 58(10): 1083–1091.

Hawkins, D.L. 2011, The thigh. In: Ross, M.W., Dyson, S.J. (eds), *Lameness in the Horse*, 2nd edn. Elsevier Saunders, St Louis, MO, pp. 552–555.

Henson, F.M., Lamas, L., Knezevic, S. *et al.* 2007, Ultrasonographic evaluation of the supraspinous ligament in a series of ridden and unridden horses and horses with unrelated back pathology. *BMC Vet. Res.* 1(3): 3.

Hill, C., Crook, T. 2010, The relationship between massage to the equine caudal hindlimb muscles and hindlimb protraction. *Equine Vet. J.* 38(suppl): 683–687.

Hyytiäinen, H.K., Mykkänen, A.K., Hielm-Björkman, A.K. *et al.* 2014, Muscle fibre type distribution of the thoracolumbar and hindlimb regions of horses: relating fibre type and functional role. *Acta Vet. Scand.* 56: 8.

Indahl, A., Kaigle, A., Reikeras, O., Holm, S. 1999, Sacroiliac joint involvement in activation of the porcine spinal and gluteal musculature. *J. Spinal Disord.* 12: 325–330.

Jacklin, B.D., Minshall, G.J., Wright, I.M.A. 2014, A new technique for subtotal (cranial wedge, ostectomy in the treatment of impinging/overriding spinous processes: description of technique and outcome of 25 cases. *Equine Vet. J.* 46(3): 339–344.

Jeffcott, L., Dalin, G., Ekman, S. *et al.* 1985, Sacroiliac lesions as a cause of chronic poor performance in competitive horses. *Equine Vet. J.* 17: 111–118.

Jeffcott. L.B., Hickman, J. 1975, The treatment of horses with chronic back pain by resecting the summits of the impinging dorsal spinous processes. *Equine Vet. J.* 7(3): 115–119.

Johnson, J.L., Moore-Colyer, M. 2009, The relationship between range of motion of lumbosacral flexion–extension and canter velocity of horses on a treadmill. *Equine Vet. J.* 41(3): 301–303.

Jones, K.E. 2015, Preliminary data on the effect of osseous anatomy on ex vivo joint mobility in the equine thoracolumbar region. *Equine Vet. J.* doi: 10.1111/evj.12461 (epub ahead of print).

Khumsap, S., Lanovaz, J.L., Rosenstein, D.S. *et al.* 2003, Effect of induced unilateral synovitis of distal intertarsal and tarsometatarsal joints on sagittal plane kinematics and kinetics of trotting horses. *Am. J. Vet. Res.* 64(12): 1491–1495.

Khumsap, S., Lanovaz, J.L., Clayton, H.M. 2004, Three-dimensional kinematic analysis of horses with induced tarsal synovitis. *Equine Vet. J.* 36(8): 659–663.

Lepeule, J., Bareille, N., Valette, J.P. *et al.* 2008, Developmental orthopaedic disease in limbs of foals: between–breed variations in the prevalence, location and severity at weaning. *Animal* 2(2): 284–291.

Lischer, C.J., Ringer, S.K., Schnewlin, M. *et al.* 2006, Treatment of chronic proximal suspensory desmitis in horses using focused electrohydraulic shockwave therapy. *Schweiz. Arch. Tierheilkd.* 148(10): 561–568.

Maliye, S., Voute, L.C., Marshall, J.F. *et al.* 2015, Naturally-occurring forelimb lameness in the horse results in significant compensatory load redistribution during trotting. Vet J. 204(2): 208–213.

Murray, R.C., Dyson, S.J., Tranquille, C. *et al.* 2006, Association of type of sport and performance level with anatomical site of orthopaedic injury diagnosis. *Equine Vet. J.* 36(suppl): 411–416.

Nagy, A., Dyson, S., Barr, A. 2010, Ultrasonographic findings in the lumbosacral joint of 43 horses with no clinical signs of back pain or hindlimb lameness. *Vet. Radiol. Ultrasound* 51(5): 533–539.

O'Brien, T., Hunt, R.J. 2014, Recent advances in standing equine orthopedic surgery. *Vet. Clin. North Am. Equine Pract.* 30(1): 221–237.

Orsini, J.A., Ryan, W.G., Carithers, D.S. *et al.* 2012, Evaluation of oral administration of firocoxib for the management of musculoskeletal pain and lameness associated with osteoarthritis in horses. *Am. J. Vet. Res.* 73(5): 664–671.

O'Sullivan, P.B. 2000, Lumbar segmental 'instability': clinical presentation and specific stabilizing exercise management. *Man. Ther.* 5(1): 2–12.

Owen, K.R., Dyson, S.J., Parkin, T.D. *et al.* 2008, Retrospective study of palmar/plantar annular ligament injury in 71 horses: 2001–2006. *Equine Vet. J.* 40(3): 237–244.

Peroni, J.F., Stick, J.A. 2002, Evaluation of a cranial arthroscopic approach to the stifle joint for the treatment of femorotibial joint disease in horses: 23 cases (1998–1999). *J. Am. Vet. Med. Assoc.* 220(7): 1046–1052.

Pfau, T., Jennings, C., Mitchell, H. *et al.* 2014, Lungeing on hard and soft surfaces: movement symmetry of trotting horses considered sound by their owners. *Equine Vet. J.* doi: 10.1111/evj.12374 (epub ahead of print).

Rankin, J.S., Diesem, C.D. 1976, Innervation of the equine hip and stifle joint capsules. *J. Am. Vet. Med. Assoc.* 169(6): 614–619.

Rombach, N., Stubbs, N.C., Clayton, H.M. 2014, Gross anatomy of the deep perivertebral musculature in horses. *Am. J. Vet. Res.* 75(5): 433–440.

Ross, M. 2011, Observation: symmetry and posture. In: Ross, M.W., Dyson, S.J. (eds), *Lameness in the Horse*, 2nd edn. Elsevier Saunders, St Louis, MO, pp. 32–43.

Stubbs, N.C., Hodges, P.W., Jeffcott, L.B. *et al.* 2006, Functional anatomy of the caudal thoracolumbar and lumbosacral spine in the horse. *Equine Vet. J.* 36(suppl): 393–399.

Stubbs, N.C., Riggs, C.M., Hodges, P.W. *et al.* 2010, Osseous spinal pathology and epaxial muscle ultrasonography in Thoroughbred racehorses. *Equine Vet. J.* 38(suppl): 654–661.

Stubbs, N.C., Kaiser, L.J., Hauptman, J. *et al.* 2011, Dynamic mobilisation exercises increase cross sectional area of musculus multifidus. *Equine Vet. J.* 43(5): 522–529.

Sykes, B.W., Jokisalo, J.M. 2014, Rethinking equine gastric ulcer syndrome: Part 1 - Terminology, clinical signs and diagnosis. *Equine Vet. Educ.* 26(10): 543–547.

Townsend, H.G., Leach, D.H. 1984, Relationship between intervertebral joint morphology and mobility in the equine thoracolumbar spine. *Equine Vet. J.* 16(5): 461–465.

Townsend, H.G., Leach, D.H., Fretz, P.B. 1983, Kinematics of the equine thoracolumbar spine. *Equine Vet. J.* 15(2): 117–122.

Townsend, H.G., Leach, D.H., Doige, C.E. *et al.* 1986, Relationship between spinal biomechanics and pathological changes in the equine thoracolumbar spine. *Equine Vet. J.* 18(2): 107–112.

Walker, V.A., Dyson, S.J., Murray, R.C. 2013, Effect of a Pessoa training aid on temporal, linear and angular variables of the working trot. *Vet. J.* 198(2): 404–411.

Walmsley, J.P., Pettersson, H., Winberg, F. *et al.* 2002, Impingement of the dorsal spinous processes in two hundred and fifteen horses: case selection, surgical technique and results. *Equine Vet. J.* 34(1): 23–28.

Warden, S.J. 2005, Cyclo-oxygenase-2 inhibitors: beneficial or detrimental for athletes with acute musculoskeletal injuries? *Sports Med.* 35(4): 271–283.

Zimmerman, M., Dyson, S., Murray, R. 2012, Close, impinging and overriding spinous processes in the thoracolumbar spine: the relationship between radiological and scintigraphic findings and clinical signs. *Equine Vet. J.* 44(2): 178–184.

CHAPTER 21

Equine sports medicine and performance management*

Lesley Goff

Lecturer, Equine Science, School of Agriculture & Food Sciences, The University of Queensland, Gatton, Australia; Director, Active Animal Physiotherapy, Toowoomba, Australia

Summary

Horses are extraordinary athletes, from the pony club horse to the racing Thoroughbred. As athletes, horses develop injuries and conditions related to their sport. Physiotherapists have a pivotal role as part of the equine sport medicine team, from assisting to manage the acute stage of injury to ongoing rehabilitation to ensure return to optimal performance.

21.1 Introduction

Physiotherapists are well known for their role in sports medicine, in management of injuries and performance in many types of athletes, including the equestrian athlete. Performance management in equestrian sports also involves assessment and treatment of the rider, as part of the horse–rider unit. This is where physiotherapists, with their initial qualification in human physiotherapy, offer the ultimate solution in equestrian performance.

Horses are extraordinary athletes, and optimal equine athletic performance is determined by the integration of the species' physiological and anatomical features (Hinchcliff *et al.* 2014). In many forms of equitation, the horse is often performing to the limit of its physiology or close to its physiological limits and in many cases loading the body systems in a repetitive or cyclical way. The equine physiotherapist should have an awareness of the physiology of training, and the adaptive responses of the horse's physiological and anatomical systems. The equine physiotherapist should also develop an understanding of the requirements of the rider, specific to different equestrian sports.

This chapter will discuss how the equine athlete's musculoskeletal system adapts to loading, with reference to the development of some common sporting injuries. The role of the equine physiotherapists will be discussed, with relation to these injuries. In addition, there is a section on assessment of the horse and rider unit.

---

*Adapted from Chapter 14 in the first edition, which was written by Lesley Goff and Narelle Stubbs

---

21.2 Physiotherapy in equine sports medicine

Assessment, treatment and rehabilitation of the horse should follow the current human and veterinary evidence-based practice as described throughout this text. This not only encompasses both orthopaedic and neuromuscular principles (see Chapters 7–11) but also exercise physiology (Chapter 6), biomechanics (Chapters 4 and 5) and performance enhancement. As physiotherapists work closely with veterinarians in the field of equine sports medicine and performance management, a grasp of veterinary management of the performance horse is recommended. Thus the reader is referred to publications such as *Equine Sports Medicine and Surgery: basic and clinical sciences of the equine athlete* (Hinchcliff *et al.* 2014) for detailed coverage of the veterinary management of equine sports.

The pathophysiology of injury and healing of the animal's body systems is presented elsewhere in this text, including that presented in the canine treatment and rehabilitation chapter (Chapter 18). These principles can be adapted to the horse's comparative anatomical and biomechanical differences. Unlike the dog and human, in the majority of circumstances, the horse is treated in standing; thus much of the musculoskeletal system is treated in the weight-bearing (WB) or partially weight-bearing (PWB) postures. This is because the horse can only be made recumbent via analgesia, i.e. you can't make them lie down! However, clinically, the majority of physiotherapeutic techniques, including manual therapy, soft tissue and skeletal mobilisation and manipulation, proprioceptive facilitation techniques, electrotherapy and exercise-based rehabilitation can be adapted and performed successfully. These are all part of the multimodal approach to physiotherapy management of athletic, traumatic and degenerative injuries seen in the performance and pleasure horse.

21.2.1 Exercise-based rehabilitation

Exercise therapy is not unique to physiotherapy. It is utilised by many practitioners, individuals and trainers in the rehabilitation and training of the sporting horse. The concept of neuromotor control, however, is a branch of exercise therapy, rehabilitation and overall management that has been investigated quite extensively in physiotherapy research, using both human and animal models. This concept is very well established in the management of back and neck pain (Hodges & Richardson 1996; Treleaven *et al.* 2011) and is becoming more important in the management of sporting injuries (Franettovich Smith *et al.* 2014; Wyndow *et al.* 2013). The introduction of exercise-based rehabilitation to the physiotherapy management of orthopaedic and neurological conditions in horses is based largely on human research; however, understanding the responses to exercise of injured and non-injured soft tissue, cartilage and bone can guide us in exercise prescription for rehabilitation, and possibly injury prevention.

Exercise-based rehabilitation should be introduced at a stage of physiotherapy management that is appropriate for the injury. It is a broad concept, encompassing strengthening, specific training regimes, facilitation of neuromotor control systems (including influencing proprioceptive systems) and stretching. Acute conditions may require initial interventions to reduce inflammatory response, so as not to compromise tissue-level healing, with mobilisation implemented in later treatments (Warden 2005). Chronic conditions, such as chronic sacroiliac joint injury or sacroiliac degenerative joint disease, which often result in poor performance (Jeffcott *et al.* 1985), may benefit from specific exercises aimed at facilitating normal neuromotor control at initial treatment.

In the horse, many musculoskeletal injuries are directly related to locomotion. Locomotion involves cyclical loading of both soft tissue and bone, in the vertebral column and extremities. There are some mechanisms in the horse, such as the passive stay apparatus, that predispose the horse to developing particular pathologies; these mechanisms have been discussed in Chapter 5. Prevention or management of musculoskeletal injuries thus relies on an understanding of the mechanical properties of bone, tendon, ligament, muscle and cartilage and how they respond to repetitive loading and unique equine locomotion.

21.2.2 Tendon

According to Birch *et al.* (2014), strain-induced tendon injury of the tendons and ligaments is the most common injury in the equestrian athlete. It is also the most common orthopaedic injury in human athletes. The equine superficial digital flexor tendon (SDFT) injury is one of the most common causes of lameness in Thoroughbred racehorses, as well as elite eventers and showjumpers (Patterson-Kane & Firth 2009). Less commonly injured are the deep digital flexor tendon, the interosseous tendon and accessory ligament of the deep digital flexor tendon (Batson *et al.* 2003; Meershoek *et al.* 2001). These tendons contribute to locomotor efficiency by storing energy; that is, they act like springs, returning 93–95% of stored energy, as a result of elastic deformation (Wilson *et al.* 2000). See also section 5.5 in Chapter 5.

Tendons that store energy during locomotion have a low safety margin – the tendon operates close to the level of gross tensile failure and therefore has a correspondingly high rate of injury (Batson *et al.* 2003). Such tendons are described as having conflicting requirements for strength and elasticity. The matrix composition of SDFT has been found to differ from that of the common digital extensor tendon (CDET) regarding water and total sulphated glycosaminoglycan content, to allow the SDFT to remain more elastic as a material (Batson *et al.* 2003). Tendons such as the opposing CDET and the deep digital flexor tendon (DDFT), which function to position the limb, have fewer instances of atraumatic injury in the equine athlete than the SDFT (Batson *et al.* 2003).

A frequent clinical finding is partial SDFT rupture with a central core lesion (Wilmink *et al.* 1992). The central fibres tend to rupture at strains lower than that required to rupture the peripheral fibres, owing to differences in crimp characteristics of the collagen fibres of the two areas of the tendon (Wilmink *et al.* 1992). This is particularly so in older horses. This common SDFT injury is a degenerative type of injury, related to cyclical loading, and can be likened to tendinopathy in human athletes. The most common tendinopathies in humans are those of the Achilles, quadriceps and rotator cuff tendons. Tendinopathy is distinct from acute tendinitis, in that the latter is characterised by heat, swelling and pain due to inflammation (Gillis *et al.* 1993; Peers & Lysens 2005). In tendinitis, early tendon inflammation is characterised by decreased echogenicity on sonography, but maintenance of fibre alignment (Reef 2001). Tendinopathy is characterised by local painful thickening and structural changes on imaging (decreased echogenicity or anechoic areas and fibre disruption) and hypertrophy of tendon (Malliaras *et al.* 2006; Reef 2001). Morphological characteristics of tendinopathy include increased glycosaminoglycans, irregular fibre structure and arrangement, and no inflammatory cell infiltrates (Movin *et al.* 1997; Rees *et al.* 2009). The pain in chronic tendinopathy is not inflammatory in nature but its exact origin remains unclear. It is thought that some of the pain may be due to vascularisation into the tendon (Ohberg & Alfredson 2002). In equine literature, it seems tendinopathy is often mistermed tendinitis – it is important to understand the differences in pathology between the two conditions, as they are managed differently, and rehabilitation has a different role in each condition.

Appreciation of the mechanisms involved in the response of normal tendon to training has implications for developing rehabilitation strategies in the management of tendon injuries, particularly the degenerative type injuries caused by repetitive microtrauma (Firth 2006).

Response of equine tendon to exercise

Results of tendon responses to training have been conflicting in the equine literature, highlighting the fact that the level and type of exercise may be critical in rehabilitation.

During the first 4 months of race training, it was found that there was an increase in mean cross-sectional area, and decrease in echogenicity in the SDFT of six young Thoroughbreds, measured ultrasonographically (Gillis *et al.* 1993). Increase in cross-sectional area may lead to an increase in stiffness, thereby reducing the elasticity and energy-storing capacity of the tendon (Marlin & Nankervis 2003). The race training programme involved a gradual increase in speed through trotting to gallop, and at 10 weeks, work at race speed every fifth training day. After the first work at race speed, two horses developed clinical signs involving grade 1 lameness, mild heat and swelling in the mid-metacarpal region of SDFT. Only one of these horses demonstrated histological changes in the tendon, involving increased vascularity and lymphatics.

Another study involved horses being given controlled treadmill exercise for up to 18 months. Changes in cross-sectional area of the extensor tendons were not observed (Birch *et al.* 1999).

Tendon rehabilitation in humans

Much of the rehabilitation of tendinopathy in humans has revolved around eccentric loading of muscle and tendon. Eccentric loading of tendon has had good clinical results over a 12-week training period, but the mechanism behind the results is unknown (Alfredson *et al.* 1998). Eccentric calf muscle training in patients with mid-portion Achilles tendinosis resulted in decreased tendon thickness and normalised structure on imaging (Ohberg *et al.* 2004).

Sustained (3 minutes, three times daily) and intermittent stretching (five sets of 20 seconds, twice daily) increased Achilles tendon flexibility, with a corresponding decrease in pain. There was no significant difference between sustained and intermittent groups over 4 months (Porter *et al.* 2002).

In volleyball players with chronic patellar tendinopathy, eccentric quadriceps training was found to have no effect on knee function after a 12-week programme in which players continued to train (Visnes *et al.* 2005). Tendons of volleyball players undergoing eccentric loading responded variably to the increased load associated with a competitive volleyball season. It was concluded that change in pain and tendon appearance on imaging does not appear to be entirely dependent on load (Malliaras *et al.* 2006).

Implications for rehabilitation of chronic tendon injury in horses

Tendons (especially the SDFT) are already under eccentric load in the normal weight-bearing situation in the horse. As speed of gait increases, there is increased eccentric load on the tendons. Loads will also vary depending on the occupation of the horse, so rehabilitation should be tailored for the load requirements of tendon at return to full performance.

Research suggests that adaptations in equine tendons are already occurring before onset of clinical signs (Gillis *et al.* 1993). In the case of a chronic tendinopathy, a programme of mobilisation is preferable to a programme of immobilisation (Kannus *et al.* 2003). It is beyond the scope of this chapter to prescribe exercise rehabilitation for every situation and occupation in equine athletics, so listed below are some general guidelines for rehabilitation of chronic tendon injury.

From onset of clinical signs, exercise should be restricted to walking. The validity of total box rest may be questioned in these cases – it is up to the discretion of the veterinarian and physiotherapist but prolonged immobilisation may contribute to further detrimental changes in chronic tendon pathology. Evenly distributed, low- to moderate-intensity exercise in young Warmbloods was more effective in developing strong, flexible tendons than single episodes of high-intensity exercise superimposed on box rest (Cherdchutham *et al.* 2001). Keeping the horse in a small paddock or yard, where they can mobilise in a limited way, is paramount. Progression of rehabilitation will depend on astute observation of clinical signs, and diagnostic ultrasonography at regular intervals throughout the rehabilitation (initially and then every 8 weeks (Reef 2001). Eccentric loading can be gradually increased in the following way.

1 Early
  * Standing/walking on varying surfaces, such as springy grass and sand, will increase the loading.
  * Progressing walking into trotting.
  * Walk/trot on a lunge or circle will load different parts of tendon.

2 Mid
  * Progression of in-hand exercise to variable terrain, gentle gradients.
  * Ridden work at trot; straight line then circle – weight of rider will increase tendon load.
  * Graduate into canter; straight line then circle.

3 Late (36 weeks +)
  * Use of slopes and speed work will increase loading and should be brought in towards the end of the programme. Use of either or both will depend on horse's occupation.
  * Jumping horses – slopes, poles and cavalettis should be introduced. Consider that the highest forces are expected in the trailing limb during landing from jumps – fence height affects forces in the SDFT, minimally in the interosseous tendon and did not affect the accessory ligament, therefore reduction in fence height may limit risks for SDFT injury but not affect accessory ligament or interosseous tendon (Meershoek et al. 2001).
  * Consider also the age of the horse – older horses have decreased crimp in the core region (Wilmink et al. 1992), so the rate of change of load that can be applied to the tendon may differ from that of younger horses.

It is recommended that horses with severe tendon injury do not gallop until 6 months post injury, but preferably 9–12 months (Reef 2001).

Implications for rehabilitation of acute tendon injury in horses

As in all acute soft tissue injury, tendinitis involves the acute inflammatory phase, proliferative phase and maturation and remodelling phase (Kannus et al. 2003) (see Chapter 18 for a description of the response to injury at tissue level). In acute injuries, there should be a short period of immobilisation followed by controlled and progressive mobilisation (Kannus et al. 2003). Application of cold may minimise inflammation and limit the action of proteolytic enzymes (Birch et al. 2014). In cases of tendinitis of distal insertion of SDFT, Gibson et al. (1997) found swelling, peritendinous fluid accumulation, disruption of normal fibre alignment and some loss of echogenicity ultrasonographically. As healing progressed, there was return of echogenicity but normal fibre alignment did not return and there was some adhesion formation between branches of the SDFT and adjacent structures. Even though there is a distinct inflammatory phase in tendinitis, the latter may implicate the

importance of mobilisation and exercise from the remodelling phase of the injury.

21.2.3 Bone

Bone has a relatively large elastic zone, and thus is described as a pseudoductile material (Marlin & Nankervis 2003). When rate of bone loading is increased, the behaviour of bone can change from pseudoductile to brittle. A common condition in performance horses, especially young racing Thoroughbred and Quarter Horses, is sore or 'bucked' shins – that is, dorsal metacarpal disease (DMD) involving periostitis of the third metacarpal (MCIII) (Bassage 2014; Marlin & Nankervis 2003).

The presentation of DMD is often bilateral, with swelling, heat and pain over the dorsal surface of the MCIII, and the horse's gait appears 'choppy'. Onset is often after a high-speed workout (Bassage 2014). It has also been found that increasing exercise distances at a canter and high speed in short periods (up to 1 month) are associated with an increased risk of sore shins, as a result of remodelling of bone and associated microdamage (Verheyen et al. 2005). Increasing cumulative exercise distances upon entering training were associated with a decreased risk of disease.

Detection of DMD can be performed by digital palpation of the dorsal surface of the MCIII. Two-year-old Thoroughbreds with a significant pain reaction to such palpation were withdrawn from races, and this was seen to be beneficial to the development of DMD of these horses over a 2-year period, on a Western Australian racetrack (Griffiths et al. 2000).

Treatment of DMD involves rest, reduction of inflammation and modification of the training programme (Bassage 2014). Early signs of sore shins should result in the exercise programme being reduced but not completely stopped (Marlin & Nankervis 2003). This is so that bone can be given time to adapt and remodel.

Implications for rehabilitation for bony injuries
For young Thoroughbred racehorses with shin soreness

In the acute stage of DMD, the horse should be rested and hand-grazed until the soft tissue swelling has subsided (Bassage 2014). Cold hosing/icing the area may help to reduce the soft tissue swelling and tenderness over the dorsal aspect of the MCIII. According to Bassage (2014), the use of NSAIDs and analgesia may impair bony healing, so this is controversial.

In reintroduction and modification of the training programme of young Thoroughbreds, it is suggested that gradual introduction of small amounts of high-speed exercise may be beneficial when designing rehabilitation programmes (Verheyen et al. 2005). This is to gradually emulate the cyclic compressive loads that are experienced during a race (Bassage 2014). Cantering should be kept to a minimum on high-speed work days and large amounts of both canter and high-speed work should be avoided in the early stages of training and rehabilitation (Verheyen et al. 2005). Eventually horses should be worked at or near racing speed no more than twice weekly, for short distances ('breezing') (Bassage 2014). The distance of the speed work is introduced incrementally, and then as speed increases, the distances are shortened slightly. Boston & Nunamaker (2000) showed that 2-year-old Thoroughbred racehorses who had regular short-distance breezing allocated to their training programme had less incidence of DMD that those who had more long gallops.

For shin soreness in other sports and other fracture healing

Exercise should be carried out at gaits that simulate the sport for which the horse is intended (compare racing with dressage). In encouraging bone remodelling, the horse should be exposed to the surfaces and terrain appropriate for the sport. For instance, the surfaces horses compete on in dressage differ greatly from endurance riding and eventing. It is recommended that the more demanding the sport, the smaller the increment in training load increase. Training load should be increased no more than once per 2 weeks. Short periods of high-impact loading are as beneficial as prolonged periods of impact loading, therefore it is unnecessary to spend long periods performing high-impact activity to gain bone remodelling (Marlin & Nankervis 2003).

Studies in rats have found that age does not affect loading and bone strength gains, and the gains were from changes to bone geometry (Bennell et al. 2002). We may extrapolate that bone strength gains can be achieved in all ages of horse. This is particularly applicable for dressage and eventing horses, who tend to be competitive into their teen years.

21.2.4 Cartilage

Articular cartilage is adapted to resist compressive forces, which are taken through the joint surfaces during weight bearing. The weight-bearing joints in the horse that have received the most attention in terms of effect of loading or exercise are the metacarpophalangeal joint and the carpal joint (van Weeren 2014). Some joints, such as the sacroiliac joint and possibly some joints of the vertebral column, are thought to be exposed to shear forces rather than compressive forces (Dalin & Jeffcott 1986).

Degenerative joint disease is a very common cause of wastage in dressage horses (Dyson 2000). Degenerative changes are often seen in the tarsal joints of performance horses, the vertebral column facet joints and sacroiliac joint surfaces. In one study of 36 racehorses, all had degenerative or adaptive changes in the articular facet joints of the vertebral column (Haussler et al. 1999). In a population of horses studied for sacroiliac joint degeneration (SID), dressage and showjumpers were considered to be most at risk of SID (Dyson & Murray 2003). Foals that were subjected to normal pasture and free exercise had better quality articular cartilage in the distal limb than foals subjected to box rest or intermittent exercise (Brama et al. 2002). Similarly there is evidence in humans that cartilage thickness, measured with magnetic resonance imaging, was better in children subjected to vigorous physical activity than sedentary children (Jones et al. 2000).

There is, however, little evidence of the ongoing effect of such early exercise on eventual orthopaedic health (van Weeren 2014). According to van Weeren (2014), too much exercise is more common in the equine industry than too little exercise. Carpal osteoarthritis is frequently seen in 2–3-year-old racehorses and other horses undergoing high-intensity training (Murray et al. 1999). Carpal articular cartilage in strenuously trained horses showed more fibrillation and chondrocyte clusters than cartilage from animals that underwent gentle exercise. Thus, strenuous training may lead to deterioration of cartilage at sites with a high clinical incidence of lesions such as dorsal radial carpal cartilage (Murray et al. 1999).

Implications for rehabilitation of articular cartilage injuries

In support of the case for controlled exercise in rehabilitation of cartilage injury or degeneration, animal studies have shown that unloading of a joint rather than overloading of the joint, combined with poor muscular control and weakness, may be a risk factor in joint degeneration (Herzog et al. 2004; Laurent et al. 2006). In humans with anterior cruciate ligament injury, resulting in instability and often decreased loading at the knee, rapid development of degenerative changes characteristic of osteoarthritis occurs, including damage to type II collagen and an increase in proteoglycan content (Nelson et al. 2006). Strengthening and exercise have a role in increasing joint range of motion and improving joint health – improvement in morphology of articular cartilage – by increasing muscular strength and joint proprioception (Buckwalter 2003). Deficits in neuromuscular reflex pathways as a result of decreased proprioception have been shown to have a detrimental effect on joints. Proprioceptive rehabilitation to facilitate dynamic joint stabilisation is thought to improve the neuromuscular control mechanism (Lephart et al. 1997).

Regarding improvement in morphology of articular cartilage, moderate exercise in human subjects has been shown to improve knee cartilage glycosaminoglycan (GAG) content in individuals at risk of developing osteoarthritis (Roos & Dahlberg 2005). This has also been shown in Beagle dogs, where moderate exercise improved GAG production, and conversely strenuous exercise led to depletion of GAG in high-load areas (Kiviranta et al. 1987). Chondroctyes have been shown to respond to both shear and compressive loading, regarding metabolic regulation and biosynthesis of chondrocytes (Eckstein et al. 1999; Frank et al. 2001).

Thus for weight-bearing joints, such as the carpus, in which the cartilage resists compressive forces, we can extrapolate from equine and human research that moderate exercise has a role in maintaining or improving the status of joints with articular cartilage degeneration. Research suggests this is also the case for joints subjected to shear forces, such as the sacroiliac joint (Eckstein et al. 1999; Frank et al. 2001). It is thought that the

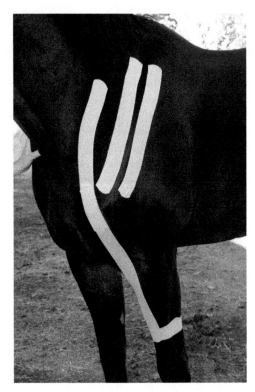

Figure 21.1 Kinesiology taping to the scapular region and biceps of the horse.

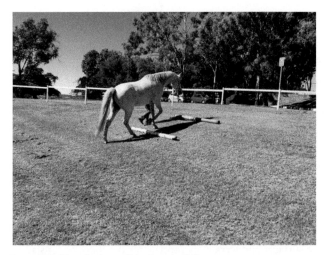

Figure 21.2 Use of poles, walking horse uphill.

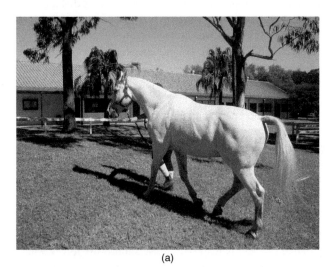

(a)

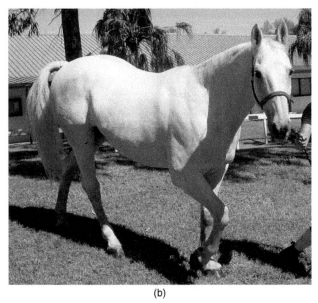

(b)

Figure 21.3 (a) Walking horse up a slope. (b) Walking horse down a slope.

equine musculoligamentous 'sling' and fascial system surrounding the vertebral column and sacroiliac joint (SIJ) may be under proprioceptive control of neural elements within the tissue, as is the case in humans and pigs (Brolinson *et al.* 2003; Indahl *et al.* 1999). Any cause of altered proprioception or altered load transfer through the SIJ or vertebral column may be a reason for development of joint surface changes in horses (Goff *et al.* 2008). Thus exercise designed to improve the neuromotor control around this musculoligamentous sling may be required for articular cartilage health in this area. Use of kinesiology taping and reflex motion to palpatory pressure (both described later in the chapter) may help to improve neuromotor control (Figure 21.1), as well as more global strengthening such as use of cavaletti/poles (Figure 21.2), walking up and down slopes (Figure 21.3) and weight-shift exercises toward pelvic limb with horse standing on various slopes (Figure 21.4).

The cartilage of young horses seems likely to be better able to adapt to mechanical loads than that of older horses (Marlin & Nankervis 2003). Thus the age of the horse should be taken into consideration when designing an exercise rehabilitation programme when articular cartilage is damaged. The older horse may require more gentle exercise over an increased time, before it is prepared to return to sport, as the articular cartilage adapts more slowly.

In summary, specific exercise should be part of the multimodal approach both within physiotherapy modalities and alongside the nutritional (Bruyere *et al.* 2003; Johnson *et al.*

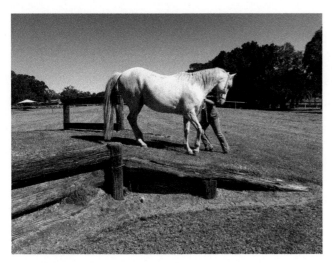

Figure 21.4 Shifting horse's weight to the pelvic limbs, uphill, to engage the musculature of the pelvis and hindlimb.

2001) and veterinary modalities used to enhance articular cartilage, reduce pain and inflammation.

21.2.5 Muscle

Muscle injuries in the athletic horse range from fibre disruption to delayed-onset muscle soreness and problems with neuromuscular control following injury or surgery.

Even though the jury is out on benefits of stretching muscle for injury prevention (Cornwell *et al.* 2002; Herzog *et al.* 2003; Taylor *et al.* 1990), combinations of stretching and strengthening may be of great importance in injury management. In the treatment of grade 2 hamstring injuries, the total time to return to full training was decreased in a group of human athletes exposed to an intensive stretching programme (Malliaropoulos *et al.* 2004). However, progressive general agility and trunk stabilisation exercises were found to be more effective than isolated hamstring stretching and strengthening both in promoting return to sport and reducing injury recurrence in athletes with acute hamstring strain (Sherry & Best 2004). Chronic groin strains in athletes responded more favourably to an 8–12-week strengthening programme, including resistive exercises for agonists and antagonists, proprioceptive training and trunk strengthening, than a programme of stretching and other passive modalities (Holmich *et al.* 1999). Active and passive stretching have been shown to be equally effective for increasing hip flexor range of motion, but the authors were unsure if the results were due to increase in agonist range of motion or improved function of the antagonist muscle group (Winter *et al.* 2004). A systematic review of the literature has found that stretching in humans who do not have a functionally significant contracture of musculature has a convincing effect, but the lasting effect of intensive stretching programmes is yet to be investigated (Harvey *et al.* 2002).

In animal studies, stretching and passive mobilisation to lacerated rat gastrocnemius muscle have been shown to have a strong antifibrotic and muscle regeneration effect, especially when implemented 14 days after laceration (Hwang *et al.* 2006). Another study using rats showed that stretching did not prevent muscle shortening in immobilised soleus but reduced muscle atrophy. Stretching also induced hypertrophic effects in control muscles (Coutinho *et al.* 2004).

It has been shown that increases in strength and an accompanying decrease in pain and disability occurred in women with chronic neck pain who performed intensive training for neck and shoulder musculature. The control group, who performed stretching and aerobic exercise to achieve only minor changes in subjective and functional measures, embarked on a progressive, high-intensity strength training during a second year of rehabilitation. This led to significant improvements in neck strength, and decrease in pain and disability, suggesting that a combination of strength training and stretching may be effective for management of chronic neck pain (Ylinen *et al.* 2006).

In addition to retraining the muscular system for strength and power changes in rehabilitation (Crewther *et al.* 2005), changes in the neuromotor or neuromechanical control are an important contribution to the overall outcome following injury, as well as to enhancing performance.

21.3 Neuromotor control – rehabilitation and performance management

Motor control of equine locomotion and performance may be likened to that in the human, as it also requires an integrated system that has sensory pathways (mechanoreceptors, proprioceptors, stretch receptors, thermoreceptors and nociceptors) to detect the status of the body; a control system to interpret the requirements of stability and motion and plan appropriate responses (central nervous system (CNS)); and the muscles to execute the highly tuned responses required (Hodges 2003). Consideration of all these elements may be the key to successful rehabilitation and performance enhancement. Although not yet reported in the horse, it has been shown in the human spine that even after resolution of acute, first-episode low back pain, multifidus muscle recovery is not automatic (Hides *et al.* 1996). Further, in the human running athlete, altered neuromotor control in the gluteus medius and maximus was evident in males with Achilles tendinopathy, although the causal nature of this is yet to be established (Franettovich Smith *et al.* 2014).

21.3.1 Motor control theories or systems

Two motor control theories or systems exist: the open loop system and the closed loop system.

The *open loop system* implies that movement occurs from a preplanned pathway from the CNS without modification via sensory feedback. These movements are often ballistic and repetitious. Studies of humans and animals with deafferented limbs have shown that movement can occur which is almost indistinguishable from the limb that has normal sensory input, except for fine motor control tasks, which appear clumsy, such as finger motion (Hodges 2003; Taub & Berman 1968). This system occurs when the motion and environmental constraints are predictable: 'an internal system of body dynamics' (Gurfinkel 1994). Owing to a lifetime of experience, the CNS plans in advance the muscle activity required to overcome the predicted movement effects on the body due to the known interaction between the internal and external forces (Cresswell & Thorstensson 1994; Hodges & Richardson 1997a,b; Massion 1992). Thus the CNS tightly couples the feed-forward responses with the predictable demands of control of the system (Hodges & Moseley 2003).

The *closed loop system* implies that when a movement command is generated, the intended motion is compared with feedback regarding the body's status and the relationship with its environment. The motion is continually modulated; if the feedback differs from the command, the performance is corrected, hence sensory feedback is used to mould performance (Schmidt & Lee 1999). This modulator system of the body's segments, posture and overall functional performance encompasses multiple sensory systems: skin, muscle, joint and ligament receptors as well as visual and vestibular systems.

21.3.2 Application of motor control concepts

This closed loop feedback or modulator system can be utilised by the animal physiotherapist very effectively during rehabilitation and performance enhancement in many forms, by tapping into the equine sensory modulation, which includes the mechanoreceptive and proprioceptive systems. Clinically, this can be achieved by using sensory facilitation aids applied directly to the horse's skin or body, for example utilising taping techniques (Figure 21.5a,b), proprioceptive aids such as light chains

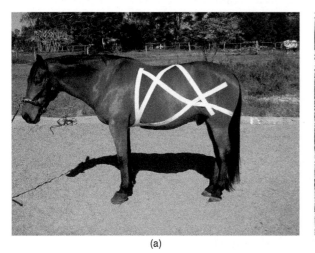

(a)

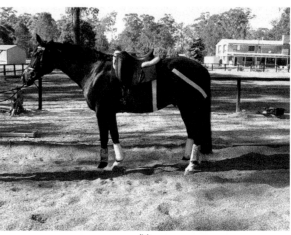

(b)

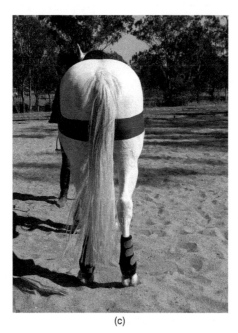

(c)

Figure 21.5 Proprioceptive facilitation techniques. (a) Taping technique for unridden exercise. (b) Taping technique for ridden exercise. (c) Stretch-band technique.

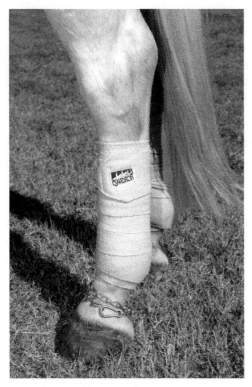

Figure 21.6 Use of proprioceptive chains around the pastern region.

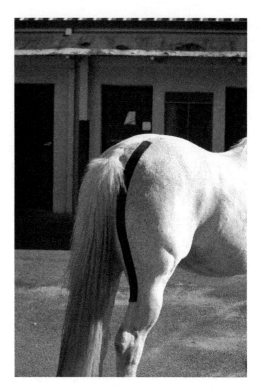

Figure 21.7 Simple application of kinesiology tape designed to facilitate activity in the semitendinosus muscle.

and stretch bandaging (Figure 21.6) and training aids such as stretch-band (Figure 21.5c), the Pessoa lunging system or long-reining techniques. These modalities are highly applicable to the horse as the skin is densely innervated with sensory nerves and the cutaneous trunci muscle system exists. For example, horses are able to feel an insect walking across their back, and twitch their skin in a given area voluntarily! Clinically, and from a neuromotor control perspective, sensory facilitation aids are an extremely valuable clinical tool n equine rehabilitation and performance enhancement.

Kinesiology tape companies offer courses in equine kinesiology taping. As kinesiology tapes are 'stretchy', when applied to the hide of the horse, they can make the horse aware of an area that is taped, and/or give some support to the structure of the musculoskeletal system as well as tapping into the sensory modulation. Application of kinesiology tape is also purported to have an effect on lymphatic and blood flow.

Use of kinesiology tape improves dynamic balance in young male soccer players with functional ankle instability (Lee & Lee 2015). Stimulation of the skin around the human knee, by application of kinesiology tape, was shown to counteract weakness in the quadriceps femoris muscle, due to attenuated afferent activity (Konsihi 2013). Likewise, Han & Lee (2014) suggest that kinesiology taping of the quadriceps and patella reduces fatigue in associated musculature, with respect to body segment repositioning. There has also been support for the beneficial effects of kinesiology taping on scapular reposition in females

(van Herzeele *et al.* 2013) and joint reposition sense around the shoulder (Burfeind & Chimera 2015). Figure 21.1 shows how equine physiotherapists may use kinesiology tape to enhance awareness around the scapular region and biceps mechanism in the horse. There are also purported to be positive effects of kinesiology tape regarding reduction in pain felt during physical activity (Montalvo *et al.* 2014).

There is very little research to date on the effect of kinesiology taping on the equine athlete, so we can only extrapolate from the human. The application of kinesiology tape to the horse can be quite complex, as in Figure 21.5(a), or simple as in Figure 21.7. The horse in the latter picture had a chronic right semitendinosus strain, with a deficit in gait and performance, and visible atrophy of the muscle. The horse had received manual therapy and a rehabilitation programme, including functional strengthening and stretching. The application of this single piece of tape, however, immediately improved the horse's gait. Taping has remained part of this horse's ongoing rehabilitation programme, and tape is worn when the horse is performing.

As there is little evidence to support the use of kinesiology tape in the horse, it is up to the physiotherapist to record and document the sometimes marked and immediate changes seen with the application of kinesiology tape.

As the effects of such taping can be quite dramatic, care should be taken with how the horse is exercised or retested after application. Horses should be lunged with the tape *in situ*, prior to being ridden. Tape should be peeled off, close to the hide, being careful not to let flapping ends startle the horse. Some producers of kinesiology tape suggest that it be applied at least 1 h prior to exercise, for maximum adhesion and effect.

21.4 Stretching for injury prevention and rehabilitation

Stretching is often used for prevention of injury in pre- and postexercise situations, and in the rehabilitation of injuries and conditions that affect soft tissue. There is conflicting evidence, however, regarding effects of stretching and lengthening of the musculotendinous unit in relation to improved performance and injury prevention (Marek *et al.* 2005).

21.4.1 Effects of stretching

The assumption that stretching lengthens muscles and extra-capsular joint structures leading to increased musculoskeletal flexibility has been tested in a number of studies. Fukunaga & Kurokawa (1996) summarise the response of muscle tissue to stretch stimulus as elongation of the muscle fibre by addition of new sarcomeres serially to the ends of existing myofibrils. Woo *et al.* (1982) provide evidence for the lengthening response of tendons and ligaments to stretching. The connective tissue component of a muscle–tendon unit changes in response to exercise stimulus and can thus alter the elasticity of the unit. Stretching may be implicated if the goal of stretching before or after exercise is simply to lengthen the muscle–tendon unit and improve joint range of motion (Hampson *et al.* 2005).

It is agreed that there is increased compliance in the muscle–tendon unit *immediately* following either active or passive stretching (Cornwell *et al.* 2002; Herzog *et al.* 2003; Taylor *et al.* 1990), but it is unclear how long the increased compliance of the tissue is maintained after stretching. It is suggested that four repetitions of a 30-sec passive stretch is the optimal combination for most elongation in the muscle–tendon unit (Taylor *et al.* 1990).

A common belief is that postexercise stretching may reduce or prevent delayed-onset muscle soreness, but a systematic literature review has found no evidence to support this belief, or that of a more rapid return to previous levels of performance (Cheung *et al.* 2003; Herbert & Gabriel 2002). Clinicians should be aware that the combination of heat and/or static stretching has been shown not to reduce soreness, swelling or muscle damage (Jayaraman *et al.* 2004).

Pope *et al.* (2000) provide good evidence that preexercise stretching does not affect injury rate in the type of activities carried out by army recruits. Hennig & Podzielny (1994), Nelson & Kokkonen (2001), Cornwell *et al.* (2002) and Herbert & Gabriel (2002) have all found insufficient evidence to support the use of stretching in relation to injury prevention, delayed-onset muscle soreness and performance. Another study using military recruits has shown that stretching may reduce instances of muscle–tendon injury, but has no effect on prevention of bone and joint injury (Amako *et al.* 2003). However, care must be taken in extrapolating these conclusions to the equine elite athletic population, flat racehorse or eventer, whose performance more closely reaches the limits of physiological capacity, as some of the studies used formerly sedentary people who rose to moderate fitness level over the course of the study.

Implications for stretching in the horse

It has been demonstrated that the type of activity performed by an athlete should be taken into consideration, as stretching before a jumping or lifting type activity, where maximal force and power output is critical, has been shown to be deleterious to performance (Avela *et al.* 2004; Cornwell *et al.* 2002; Hennig & Podzielny 1994). Two mechanisms have been identified as contributing to this diminished performance: depression of muscle activation via neural mechanisms and a decrease in musculotendinous stiffness (Cornwell *et al.* 2002; Kokkonen *et al.* 1998). This has led to better understanding of why conflict exists in the literature (Hampson *et al.* 2005). Cornwell *et al.* (2002) and Wilson *et al.* (1994) offer an equine athlete biomechanical research model, by applying what is known from human exercise physiology and sports science. Using these models, sporting activities can be broadly separated into two types of muscle demand: high-intensity stretch-shortening cycles (HSSC) and low-intensity limited stretch-shortening cycles (LSSC) (Hampson *et al.* 2005).

An example of HSSC activity is the jumping activity of the show jumper or eventer. In this activity, the horse relies on a muscle–tendon unit that is compliant enough to store and release a high amount of elastic energy to enhance performance in the jumping and sprinting phases. This is equally important in landing from height, as an insufficiently compliant muscle–tendon unit may not cope with the energy absorption demands placed on the structures. In the jumping effort, there is an eccentric preloading phase of the prime mover muscles coupled with elastic preloading of passive structures (potential energy) which contributes to an increased power output (kinetic energy) in the concentric lifting phase of the jump. Obviously, a stiff non-compliant musculotendinous unit would be deleterious under these conditions and not only limit performance but contribute to a high injury risk. Consequently, the rationale for performance enhancement and injury prevention in this type of sport is to increase the compliance of the musculotendinous unit through controlled stretching (Hampson *et al.* 2005).

The LSSC activity is well represented by the endurance horse, where locomotion is at a relatively slow, steady pace for an extended period – up to 25+ km. However, in the endurance horse the moderate to slow pace still utilises the extensor apparatus and biceps/lacertus mechanism in a somewhat preloaded manner, as in HSSC exercise. Biomechanically, during LSSC locomotive activity, most of the power generation is by active concentric muscle work, with force generated transferred to the moment arm most efficiently by a non-compliant muscle-tendon unit (Chapter 5). A more compliant muscle–tendon unit in this case would effectively reduce the amount of muscle work converted into external work. Clearly, a stretching programme to lengthen and increase the compliance of the musculotendinous unit would be deleterious to performance in these types of activities (Hampson *et al.* 2005).

Much of the research into the biomechanics of stretching has been carried out on laboratory animals; thus we may extrapolate findings to the equine athlete owing to the similarities in muscle and connective tissue physiology across quadruped species. The value of stretching in HSSC and LSSC situations is likely to be even more relevant than in the human, due to the cursorial locomotor anatomy of the horse which utilises passive structures to aid a more efficient gait (Stashak 2002). For example, in the galloping horse, about 80% of the shoulder extensor moment has been attributed to the biceps/lacertus fibrosis passive elastic storage mechanism (Wilson 2003) (see Chapter 5). Hence, a very compliant and high energy-storing musculotendinous unit would be very beneficial to performance, in reducing energy consumption of gait, and would also assist in injury prevention (prevent overloading the tendon) in any HSSC activity (Hampson *et al.* 2005).

Injury risk of the activity

High-intensity stretch-shortening cycle activities (jumping, sprinting) have a higher soft tissue injury rate than LSSC (steady jogging) activities (Witvrouw *et al.* 2004) due to the less predictable nature, higher impulse loading, and increased soft tissue preloading in the lengthened position, combined with eccentric muscle activity, for the former. However, an accurate assessment for potential injury rate for a particular activity can be determined only by well-designed epidemiology studies; for example, in the Thoroughbred racing industry, specific injury patterns such as the high incidence of suspensory ligament injuries in the racehorses (Brown *et al.* 2003). Such studies will equip the physiotherapist with information that may be used to assess the requirements for a stretching programme.

21.4.2 Types of stretching

Stretching techniques can be divided into four basic categories: ballistic, static, passive and proprioceptive neuromuscular facilitation (PNF). Ballistic stretching is characterised by repeated bouncing movements at the end of range and has been shown to be less beneficial and has been implicated as a causative factor in injury to the muscle–tendon unit (Stanish 1982). Static stretching refers to the subject stretching a muscle to just short of the point of pain and holding this position for 30–60 sec. The technique suggests that the subject is in control of the stretch and it is therefore not realistic in the animal population (Hampson *et al.* 2005). Passive static stretching is performed by a partner, and is stretch applied by an external force. In the horse, a mild

degree of muscle activity is often present because it is standing during treatment. Hence passive stretch may be seen as a variation of the human hold–relax and contract–relax stretching technique. Clinically, this form of stretching enables the physiotherapist to utilise contractile elements or enables eccentric loading of the musculotendinous unit very effectively. If the stretch is performed repeatedly through a full functional range of constant motion, it would be termed a PNF technique, which uses reflex activation and inhibition (Stanish 1982). This may also be termed a neuromechanical mobilisation technique as the therapist is repeatedly stretching the myofascial and neurological systems which can more closely mirror the sport-specific nature of the animal. Hence these stretching methods may prepare the animal's neuromuscular system for performance. Although true PNF is often the technique of choice for human athletes, it requires training and a very compliant horse.

21.4.3 Examples of stretches and sport-specific stretching
Show jumpers

Horses performing at high speeds and/or jumping are classic examples of HSSC activities. There are limited statistics in the literature concerning injury rates in horses performing in jumping events but Pinchbeck *et al.* (2004) report a high injury rate of 8.9% in a large study of hurdle and steeplechase events. Studies on human jumping efforts reveal an interesting pattern (Cornwell *et al.* 2002; Fukunaga & Kurokawa 1996): pre-jump stretching has a deleterious effect on a jump from a standing start but no effect on a lunge jump. The difference is that a lunge jump allows an eccentric preloading of the musculotendinous unit. As discussed earlier, the biomechanics of equine locomotion favour this type of energy production over direct muscle energy transmission. Although no biomechanical studies exist on the effects of prestretching on the equine jumping effort, it can be extrapolated by combining what we know of human jumping and equine locomotion biomechanics that prestretching would certainly not reduce the performance (Hampson *et al.* 2005). Given the extremely high incidence of tendon and ligament overloading injuries below the tarsus and carpus in equine athletes, there is a strong incentive for a very compliant musculotendinous and ligament system. The equine athlete not only has to generate sufficient energy to jump, but requires a compliant musculotendinous system to land safely. Hence, the use of stretching as a training and preevent warm-up technique is highly recommended. The recommendation is strengthened in the presence of previous and existing muscle, tendon and ligament injury.

Dressage

Dressage requires very slow and powerful limb movements with the majority of the joint moments being produced by active muscle contraction (see Chapter 5). In this situation, a low compliant musculotendinous unit is considered desirable. Pre-dressage stretching with the goal of improving performance flexibility would therefore be counterproductive. If, however, the horse were carrying an injury to muscle, tendon or ligamentous tissue which was at risk of further injury, the small potential performance loss would be outweighed by the potential benefit in injury prevention (Hampson *et al.* 2005). In fact, dressage-based 'suppling exercises' are used in many forms of equitation to enhance and optimise performance as well as to prepare the musculoskeletal system for the sport.

Eventing horse

The jumping section of the one- or three-day event can be considered as being applicable to the show jumper above. The cross-country course involves jumping and is not a race, although it is necessary to complete the course within a given time limit. The straights between the jumps could certainly be considered to contain LSSC demands, given the moderate speed and repetitive nature of the gait. However, given the unique locomotor biomechanics of the equine gait and the large role of the passive energy-storing mechanisms, there is a sound argument to exclude the cantering equine from the definition of a LSSC activity. Therefore, the stretching protocol for both sections is covered by that of the show jumper. The first section of the event, the dressage phase, certainly qualifies as an LSCC activity. However, to ensure that the horse was best prepared to complete the three phases intact, most riders would risk a small potential performance loss in the dressage phase, if stretching were to be technically counterproductive. Stretching, then, would probably be part of the everyday training programme, as for the show jumper (Hampson *et al.* 2005).

Racehorses

It is possible that the muscles of these sprinting athletes may suffer repeated strain, which often goes unnoticed, undiagnosed or untreated because the animal cannot verbalise – with the only sign being a poor performance and mild gait changes or subtle stiffness. These muscles work under HSSC conditions and undergo a high eccentric load, particularly the semitendinosus, semimembranosus, middle gluteal and biceps femoris at the end of range. In this case, flexibility is certainly an advantage, particularly when the muscle–tendon unit is probably in a shortened state from previous injury. In terms of injury prevention during training and competition, it is likely that the racehorse would benefit from an activity-based stretching programme during warm-up. It should also be noted that any incidence of muscle injury may also be a result of training error, or more specifically lack of training, and lack of appropriate warm-up.

Examples of stretches

Many riders and practitioners attempt to stretch the 'top line' or epaxial musculature of the horse. This is an active stretch combining both eccentric and concentric activity (a functional

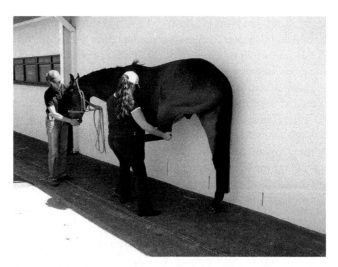

Figure 21.8 Hindlimb stretch.

ballistic stretch). Also called reflex motion to palpatory pressure, it utilises the horse's own biomechanical myofascial and ligamentous 'pulley' system via lengthening the nuchal ligament, thoracolumbar fascia and the complex myofascial attachments of longissimus. To be effective, however, this form of functional stretching requires coordinated neuromotor control, as this would be an ineffective stretch if the hypaxial muscles were inactive. These primarily include the iliopsoas complex, rectus abdominis, subclavius and serratus ventralis to flex actively and dorsally the lumbosacral, thoracolumbar and cervicothoracic regions. It must be noted that in the horse, most of the epaxial, hypaxial and pelvic muscles are myofascially interconnected directly. Hence, stretching often requires a combination of limb and spinal positions to ensure the desired effect occurs, while monitoring for ongoing cheating strategies the animal may adopt to avoid the posture. For example, Figures 21.8, 21.9 and 21.10 demonstrate variations that can be used to stretch

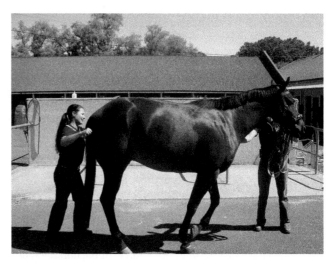

Figure 21.9 Rounding reflex.

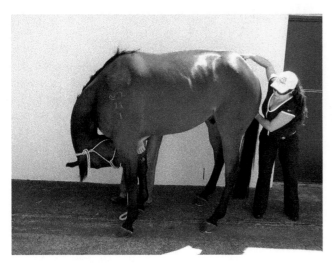

Figure 21.10 Slump stretch.

the pelvic limb and thoracolumbar and lumbosacral complexes. Note that when using the 'slump' to stretch the thoracolumbar and pelvic complex, it is also very important to consider that this position also places the central and peripheral nervous system under tension.

Posterior pelvic limb muscles

To stretch the semimembranosus effectively, the hock must be kept in flexion to wind up the calcaneal tendon or insertion; the limb then needs to be abducted to a greater degree than is shown in Figure 21.8. Biceps femoris would be stretched by adducting the limb from this position. It is important to note the cheating strategies this horse has implemented to prevent a true stretch of the middle gluteal; the muscle is unloaded by pelvic rotation, hitching and thoracolumbar extension and raising of the head and neck. Because of the lumbar attachment of the middle gluteal onto longissimus and the thoracolumbar fascia as far cranially as the first lumbar vertebra, the thoracolumbar and cervical (due to longissimus cervicus) spine must be dorsally flexed as well as the limb (see Figure 21.8).

Thoracolumbar vertebral dorsal flexion stretch

This utilises the rounding response via a noxious stimulus. This stretch, if performed repeatedly on a daily basis, may assist in preventing loss of spinal motion, notably in the facet joints, in all horses but especially those with an increased lordotic posture or conformation (see Figure 21.9).

Equine baited slump stretch (neuromechanical)

This affects many structures, including the nuchal and supraspinous ligament, the entire epaxial myofascial system, thoracolumbar vertebral column and the neurological system (spinal cord, and components of the brachial and lumbosacral plexus and associated fascia) (see Figure 21.10). To place neuromeningeal and myofascial structures on more stretch, unilateral hindlimb protraction may be added.

21.4.4 Summary of implications for rehabilitation of muscle injury in horses

Strengthening has a role in assisting muscle rehabilitation, as has been outlined in cases of both acute and chronic injury (Holmich et al. 1999; Hwang et al. 2006; Sherry & Best 2004). A great deal of literature has investigated the effects of various resistance training programmes on strength and power change in humans, yet the stimuli that effect muscle adaptation are still not fully understood (Crewther et al. 2005). This type of training, where combinations of sets and repetitions of isolated muscle groups are utilised, is not applicable to horses, as we cannot instruct the horse to perform a number of repetitions on an isolated group of muscles as we can in humans. The evidence from Sherry & Best (2004) shows that global trunk strengthening and agility were more useful for return to performance than specific muscle group strengthening and stretching – this may be the most effective path in returning horses to activity following a muscle injury. There is some further evidence in human research that specific stabilisation exercise is effective in reducing pain and disability in chronic back pain, neck pain, cervicogenic headache and pelvic pain as well as reducing recurrence after acute back pain (Ferreira et al. 2006). It may also be the case for muscle-based injury, as regaining neuromuscular control after injury or surgery is necessary for the athlete wishing to return to competition (Lephart et al. 1997).

Should the desired effect of stretching be to improve muscle–tendon compliance in the horse during a bout of activity, then the stretching should be performed immediately before performance, as the lasting effect of stretching is unknown from human studies. The type of activity also needs to be taken into account before implementing a stretching programme, if it is for injury prevention or enhanced performance (Hampson et al. 2005). Factors affecting length of time to hold a passive stretch in a horse are dictated by (a) extrapolation from human studies; (b) the type of stretch that is desired (active versus passive) – there is evidence that both types of stretch are useful in rehabilitation; (c) the length of time a stretch can be physically maintained on a horse by the operator. In the latter case, functional stretches may be of more benefit than isolating a muscle for stretch; for example, standing the horse on an uphill slope with the affected leg in retraction, if the aim is to stretch hip flexors.

In cases where there is moderate contracture of muscle, or potential adhesion formation in a muscle as a result of a laceration, then there is evidence that stretching has a role in enhancing muscle hypertrophy and reducing fibrosis (Coutinho et al. 2004; Hwang et al. 2006).

Despite some conflicting evidence regarding the role of stretching in rehabilitation, particularly in prevention of injury, the physiotherapist should realise that many techniques employed clinically affect the length of muscle, as well as other soft tissue. In our physiotherapy management of the horse, we may use stretching, either alone or in combination with other techniques, to change the range of motion of a segment or limb, with the goal of reducing pain or restriction of motion and/or enhancing performance. Such techniques may include joint mobilisation, neuromeningeal mobilisation, hold-relax technique and even trigger points – this is not an exhaustive list. In the horse, we can also use the closed loop feedback or modulator system, which will cause stretching of some structures whilst facilitating others.

To obtain any benefit when implementing a myofascial stretching programme, the individual horse and its sport-specific functional requirements must always be assessed. This should entail a detailed assessment of the biomechanical requirements of the activity, including the contribution of anatomical and neuromotor control components to the activity. Only then can it be determined if a stretching regime will be beneficial to the performance of the activity, and if so, an accurate regime based on scientific principles can be formulated.

21.5 Assessment of the horse and rider unit

Total rehabilitation of the horse involves assessment and treatment of the horse–rider unit. Horse riding is unique in the world of sports because one of the members of the team is not human and the team must be in absolute harmony to execute even the simplest manoeuvres (Sorli 2000).

Gait in performance horses has been shown to be affected by type of rider (novice versus experienced) (Licka *et al.* 2004). The horse's performance is also affected by the way the rider contacts the horse and the ability of the rider to perform as part of the athletic team. A rider with a lower back problem may have difficulty sitting to a trot due to pain or discomfort. A rider with an ankle injury may have difficulty positioning the foot in the stirrup. More subtle movement dysfunction in the rider can not only cause the rider to look unbalanced but can affect the way a horse moves. An example of the latter is a rider with a mechanical dysfunction of the pelvis causing increased contact through the right ischial tuberosity compared with the left. This will affect delivery of aids, i.e. what the horse is feeling through the epaxial muscles. A rider with poor scapular control, owing to shoulder girdle or cervical spine injury, may have difficulty maintaining position of the upper limb.

21.5.1 Role of equine physiotherapists in rider management
Existing injuries
The physiotherapist should manage existing injuries which result from the equestrian sport as well as concurrent injuries such as lower back pain or other sporting injuries. Common injuries in equestrian sport are as follows (Petridou *et al.* 2004; Sorli 2000; Watt & Finch 1996; Williams & Ashby 1995).
- Head/face
- Upper limb
- Lower limb
- Trunk
- Other

The physiotherapist may need to apply appropriate physiotherapy modalities to maximise function and minimise pain so that the rider can return to their sport and ride to the best of their ability. If the equine physiotherapist does not possess the skills or experience required (such as manual therapy, experience in sports physiotherapy, management of conditions of the vertebral column or neurological problems) then it is their role to refer to a practitioner who can help the rider.

Rider mechanical function
Rider mechanical function needs to be optimised to ensure the best horse–rider integration for optimal equestrian performance. The physiotherapist should assess the following.
- *The mounted rider*. Observe the rider from the back, side and front, when seated on the horse. Look at position of legs, pelvis, trunk, shoulder, neck, arms and head and note asymmetries of posture or muscle bulk (Figure 21.11).

  Question the rider regarding their awareness of contact with the saddle and horse, and symmetry of their own posture. Compare the posture of the horse that you have observed before the rider mounted to after the rider mounted.

  Repeat the same observations when the rider is in motion with the horse moving through various gaits and transitions (Figure 21.12).
- *The rider's 'on-ground' biomechanics*. Assess the rider standing on level ground from behind, front and side and note postural asymmetries and anomalies (including muscle bulk). Compare these findings to what you have seen when the rider is mounted (statically and riding). If the same conditions you see 'on ground' are present when mounted, these may need to be addressed before/concurrently with physiotherapy management of the horse. If the postural anomalies or asymmetries of the rider are more marked when the rider is mounted (particularly in motion) then it may be more pertinent to manage existing biomechanical or musculoskeletal problems in the horse. Then, reassess the horse–rider unit to see if the rider problems remain.

It may not be possible to complete the total assessment and treatment of horse and rider in one session – it is at the discretion of the physiotherapist as to how long is spent in one session. Clinical reasoning may also dictate that only one 'problem' (either horse or rider) is addressed at once.

21.5.2 Contact areas
Contact areas to consider when assessing the rider are as follows.
- Caudal bony landmarks of the pelvis
- Pelvic floor
- Medial surfaces of lower limbs
- Feet
- Hands via the bit

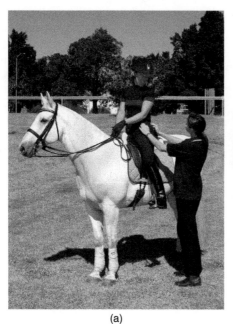
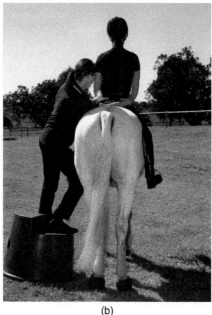

(a)   (b)

Figure 21.11 (a) Assessment of the rider's pelvic position from the side. (b) Assessment of the rider's posterior superior iliac spines.

- Voice
- Mood/temperament
- Other artificial aids

Rider aids are given via subtle change in weight shift or pressure from the rider's seat, positioning and change in pressure via the rider's lower limbs and hands through the bit.

The function and position of the lumbopelvic region of the rider are particularly important to assess when the contact areas with the horse are considered. It is known that the pelvic girdle is important for transfer of forces between legs and trunk (Lee & Vleeming 2000). The lumbopelvic local system stabilises the joints of the spine and pelvis in preparation for or response to external loads (Hodges & Richardson 1996; Hungerford *et al.* 2003). Control of the upper limb and trunk is affected by motor control issues which originate in the lumbopelvic region. It is important that this system functions well in the rider for trunk rotation and stability, head and neck position and motion, and subtle positioning of hands and arms.

Physiotherapists can affect the bony alignment and soft tissue contact of rider contact areas (Huysmans *et al.* 2005), and optimise motor control via coordination of activation of muscles and fascia, neural patterning and awareness (Lee & Vleeming 2000). They also have a role in minimising rider pain and discomfort.

21.6 Conclusion

When providing physiotherapy assessment and treatment of the horse–rider unit, it is important to be able to utilise your physiotherapy skills to restore anatomical position and function of musculoskeletal structures in the rider in addition to treating the horse. If the animal physiotherapist does not have the skills or experience to manage the rider musculoskeletal/neurological conditions, then he/she needs to refer the rider to a practitioner who has the skills/equipment to do so.

Figure 21.12 Assessment of the rider in motion with the horse – note that horse has kinesiology tape applied to the sacroiliac region and abdominal musculature.

References

Alfredson, H., Pietila, T., Jonsson, P. *et al.* 1998, Heavy-load eccentric calf muscle training for the treatment of chronic Achilles tendinosis. *Am. J. Sports Med.* 26: 360–366.

Amako, M., Oda, T., Masuoka, K., et al. 2003, Effect of static stretching on prevention of injuries for military recruits. *Mil. Med.* 168: 442–446.

Avela, J., Finni, T., Liikavainio, T. et al. 2004, Neural and mechanical responses of the triceps surae muscle group after one hour of repeated fast passive stretches. *J. Appl. Physiol.* 96: 2325–2332.

Bassage, L.H. 2014, Metacarpus/metatarsus. In: Hinchcliff, K.W., Kaneps, A.J., Geor, R.J. (eds), *Equine Sports Medicine and Surgery: basic and clinical sciences of the equine athlete*, 2nd edn. Saunders-Elsevier, Philadelphia, pp. 297–322.

Batson, E., Paramour, R., Smith, T. et al. 2003, Are the material properties and matrix composition of equine flexor and extensor tendons determined by their functions? *Equine Vet. J.* 35: 314–318.

Bennell, K., Khan, K., Warmington, S. et al. 2002, Age does not influence bone response to treadmill exercise in female rats. *Med. Sci. Sport Exerc.* 34(12): 1958–1965.

Birch, H.L., McLaughlin, L., Smith, R.K. et al. 1999, Treadmill exercise-induced tendon hypertrophy: assessment of tendons with different mechanical functions. *Equine Vet. J.* 30(suppl): 222–226.

Birch, H.L., Sinclair, C., Goodship, A.E. 2014, Tendon and ligament physiology. In: Hinchcliff, K.W., Kaneps, A.J., Geor, R.J. (eds), *Equine Sports Medicine and Surgery: basic and clinical sciences of the equine athlete*, 2nd edn. Saunders-Elsevier, Philadelphia, pp.107–184.

Boston, R.C., Nunamaker, D.M. 2000, Gait and speed as exercise components of risk factors associated with onset of fatigue injury of the third metacarpal bone in 2-year-old Thoroughbred racehorses. *Am. J. Vet. Res.* 61(6):602–608.

Brama, P.A., Tekoppele, J.M., Bank, R.A. 2002, Development of biochemical heterogeneity of articular cartilage: influences of age and exercise. *Equine Vet J.* 34: 265–269.

Brolinson, P.G., Kozar, A.J., Cibor, G. 2003, Sacroiliac joint dysfunction in athletes. *Curr. Sports Med. Rep.* 2(1): 47–56.

Brown, N.A.T., Pandy, M.G., Kawcak, C.E. et al. 2003, Force- and moment-generating capacities of muscles in the distal forelimb of the horse. *J. Anat.* 203: 101–113.

Bruyere, O., Honore, A., Ethgen, O. 2003, Correlation between radiographic severity of knee osteoarthritis and future disease progression. Results from a 3-year prospective, placebo-controlled study evaluating the effect of glucosamine sulfate. *Osteoarthr. Cartil.* 11: 1–5.

Buckwalter, J. 2003, Sports, joint injury and post-traumatic osteoarthritis. *J. Orthop. Sports Phys. Ther.* 33: 578–588.

Burfeind, S.M., Chimera, N. 2015, Randomized control trial investigating the effects of kinesiology tape on shoulder proprioception. *J. Sport Rehabil.* Jul 13 (epub ahead of print).

Cherdchutham, W., Meershoek, L.S., van Weeren, P.R. et al. 2001, Effects of exercise on biomechanical properties of the superficial digital flexor tendon in foals. *Am. J. Vet Res.* 62(12): 1859–1864.

Cheung, K., Hume, P., Maxwell, L. 2003, Delayed onset muscle soreness: treatment strategies and performance factors. *Sports Med.* 33: 145–164.

Cornwell, A., Nelson, A.G., Sidaway, B. 2002, Acute effects of stretching on the neuromechanical properties of the triceps surae muscle complex. *Eur. J. Appl. Physiol.* 86: 428–434.

Coutinho, E., Gomes, A., Franca, C. et al. 2004, Effect of passive stretching on the immobilized soleus muscle fiber morphology. *Braz. J. Med. Biol. Res.* 37(12): 1853–1861.

Cresswell, A.G., Thorstensson, A. 1994, Changes in intra-abdominal pressure, trunk muscle activation and force during isometric lifting and lowering. *Eur. J. Appl. Physiol.* 68: 315–321.

Crewther, B., Cronin, J., Keogh, J. 2005, Possible stimuli for strength and power adaptation: acute mechanical responses. *Sports Med.* 35(11): 967–989.

Dalin, G., Jeffcott, L.B. 1986, Sacroiliac joint of the horse. 1. Gross morphology. *Anat. Histol. Embryol.* 15(1): 80–94.

Dyson, S. 2000, Lameness and poor performance in the performance horse: dressage, show jumping and horse trials (eventing). *Am. Assoc. Equine Pract.* 46: 308–315.

Dyson, S., Murray, R. 2003, Pain associated with the sacroiliac joint region: a clinical study of 74 horses. *Equine Vet. J.* 35: 240–245.

Eckstein, F., Tieschky, M., Faber, S. et al. 1999, Functional analysis of articular cartilage deformation, recovery and fluid flow following dynamic exercise in vivo. *Anat. Embryol. (Berlin)* 200: 419–424.

Ferreira, P., Ferreira, M., Maher, C. et al. 2006, Specific stabilisation exercise for spinal and pelvic pain: a systematic review. *Aust. J. Physiother.* 52: 79–88.

Firth, E.C. 2006, The response of bone, articular cartilage and tendon to exercise in the horse. *J. Anat.* 208(4): 513–526.

Franettovich Smith, M., Honeywill, C., Wyndow, N. et al. 2014, Neuromotor control of gluteal muscles in runners with achilles tendinopathy. *Med. Sci. Sports Exerc.* 46(3): 594–599.

Frank, J., Quinn, T., Hunizer, E. et al. 2001, Tissue shear formation stimulates proteoglycan and protein biosynthesis in bovine cartilage explants. *Arch. Biochem. Biophys.* 395(1): 41–48.

Fukunaga, T., Kurokawa, S. 1996, Muscle fibre behaviour during drop jump in human. *J. Appl. Physiol.* 80: 158–165.

Gibson, K., Burbidge, H., Anderson, B. 1997, Tendonitis of branches of insertion of superficial digital flexor tendon in horses. *Aust. Vet. J.* 75: 253–256.

Gillis, C., Meagher, D., Pool, R. et al. 1993, Ultrasonographically detected changes in equine superficial digital flexor tendons during the first few months of race training. *Am. J. Vet. Res.* 54: 1797–1802.

Goff, L., Jeffcott, L., Jasiewicz, J. et al. 2008, Structural and biomechanical aspects of equine sacroiliac function and their relationship to clinical disease. *Vet. J.* 176(3): 281–293.

Griffiths, J.B., Steel, C.M, Symons, P.J. et al. 2000, Improving the predictability of performance by prerace detection of dorsal metacarpal disease in thoroughbred racehorses. *Aust Vet J.* 78(7): 466–467.

Gurfinkel, V.S. 1994, The mechanisms of postural regulation in man. *Soviet Scientific Reviews. Section F. Physiology and general biology* 7: 59–89.

Hampson, B., Stubbs, N.C., McGowan, C.M. 2005, Stretching for performance enhancement and injury prevention in animal athletes. *Veterinarian* December: 35–39.

Han, J.T., Lee, J.H. 2014, Effects of kinesiology taping on repositioning error of the knee joint after quadriceps muscle fatigue. *J. Phys. Ther. Sci.* 26(6): 921–923.

Harvey, L., Herbert, R., Crosbie, J. 2002, Does stretching induce lasting increases in joint ROM? A systematic review. *Physiother. Res. Int.* 7: 1–13.

Haussler, K., Stover, S., Willits, N. 1999, Pathological changes in the lumbosacral vertebrae and pelvis in Thoroughbred racehorses. *Am. J. Vet. Res.* 60: 143–153.

Hennig, E.M., Podzielny, S. 1994, Die Auswirkungen von Dehn- und Aufwarmubungen auf die Vertikalsprungleistung (The effect of stretching and warm-up exercises on vertical jump height performance). *Deutsch. Zeitschr. Sportmed.* 45(6): 253–260.

Herbert, R.D., Gabriel, M. 2002, Effects of stretching before and after exercising on muscle soreness and risk of injury: a systematic review. *BMJ* 325: 468.

Herzog, W., Schachar, R., Leonard, T. 2003, Characterization of passive component of force enhancement following active stretching of skeletal muscle. *J. Exp. Biol.* 206: 3635–3643.

Herzog, W., Clark, A., Longino, D. 2004, Joint mechanics in osteoarthritis. *Novartis Foundation Symposium* 260: 79–95.

Hides, J., Richardson, C., Jull, G. 1996, Multifidus muscle recovery is not automatic after resolution of acute, first-episode low back pain. *Spine* 21: 2763–2769.

Hinchcliff, K.W., Kaneps, A.J., Geor, R.J. (eds), *Equine Sports Medicine and Surgery: basic and clinical sciences of the equine athlete*, 2nd edn. Saunders-Elsevier, Philadelphia.

Hodges, P.W. 2003, *Neuromechanical control of the spine. Thesis, Kongl Carlinska Medico Chirurgiska* Institiutet, Stockholm, Sweden.

Hodges, P.W., Moseley, G.L. 2003, Pain and motor control of the lumbopelvic region: effect and possible mechanisms. *J. Electromyogr. Kinesiol.* 13(4): 361–370.

Hodges, P., Richardson, C. 1996, Inefficient muscular stabilisation of the lumbar spine associated with low back pain. *Spine* 21: 26–40.

Hodges, P.W., Richardson, C.A. 1997a, Contraction of the abdominal muscles associated with movement of the lower limb. *Physical Ther.* 77: 132–144.

Hodges, P.W., Richardson, C.A. 1997b, Feed forward contraction of transversus abdominus is not influenced by the direction of arm movement. *Exp. Brain Res.* 114: 362–370.

Holmich, P., Uhrskou, P., Ulnits, L. 1999, Effectiveness of active physical training as treatment for long-standing adductor-related groin pain in athletes: randomized trial. *Lancet* 353: 339–443.

Hungerford, B., Gilleard, W., Hodges, P. 2003, Evidence of altered lumbo-pelvic muscle recruitment in the presence of posterior pelvic pain and failed load transfers through the pelvis. *Spine* 28: 1593–1600.

Huysmans, T., van Audekerke, R., van der Sloten, J. *et al.* 2005, A three-dimensional active shape model for the detection of anatomical landmarks on the back surface. *Proc. Inst. Mech. Eng. J. Eng. Med.* 219: 129–42.

Hwang, J., Ra, Y., Lee, J., Ghil, S. 2006, Therapeutic effect of passive mobilisation exercise on improvement of muscle regeneration and prevention of fibrosis after laceration injury of rat. *Arch. Phys. Med. Rehabil.* 87: 20–26.

Indahl, A., Kaigle, A., Reikeras, O., Holm, S. 1999, Sacroiliac joint involvement in activation of the porcine spinal and gluteal musculature. *J. Spinal Disord.* 12: 325–330.

Jayaraman, R., Reid, R., Foley, J. *et al.* 2004, MRI evaluation of topical heat and static stretching as therapeutic modalitites of the treatment of eccentric exercise-induced muscle damage. *Eur. J. Appl. Physiol.* 93: 30–38.

Jeffcott, L., Dalin, G., Ekman, S. *et al.* 1985, Sacroiliac lesions as a cause of chronic poor performance in competitive horses. *Equine Vet. J.* 17: 111–118.

Johnson, K., Hulse, D., Hart, R. *et al.* 2001, Effects of an orally administered mixture of chondroitin sulfate, glucosamine hydrochloride and manganese ascorbate on synovial fluid chondroitin sulfate 3B3

and 7D4 epitope in a canine cruciate ligament transaction model of osteoarthritis. *Osteoarthr. Cartil.* 9: 14–21.

Jones, G., Glisson, M., Hynes, K. *et al.* 2000, Sex and site differences in cartilage development: a possible explanation for variations in knee osteoarthritis in later life. *Arthritis Rheum.* 43(11): 2543–2549.

Kannus, P., Parkkari, J., Jarvinen, T.L. *et al.* 2003, Basic science and clinical studies coincide: active treatment approach is needed after a sports injury. *Scand. J. Med. Sci. Sports* 13: 150–154.

Kokkonen, J., Nelson, A.G., Cornwell, A. 1998, Acute muscle stretching inhibits maximal strength performance. *Res. Q. Exerc. Sport* 69: 411–415.

Konishi, Y. 2013, Tactile stimulation with kinesiology tape alleviates muscle weakness attributable to attenuation of Ia afferents. *J. Sci. Med. Sport* 16(1): 45–48.

Laurent, D., O'Byrne, E., Wasvary, J. *et al.* 2006, *In vivo* MRI of cartilage pathogenesis in surgical models of osteoarthritis. *Skeletal Radiol.* 35(8): 555–564.

Lee, B.G., Lee, J.H. 2015. Immediate effects of ankle balance taping with kinesiology tape on the dynamic balance of young players with functional ankle instability. *Technol Health Care* March 3: (epub ahead of print).

Lee, D., Vleeming, A. 2000, Current concepts on pelvic impairment. In: Singer, K.P. (ed.), *Proceedings of the 7th Scientific Conference of the IFOMT*, Perth, Australia, November 6–10, pp. 465–491.

Lephart, S.M., Pincivero, D.M., Giraldo, J.L., Fu, F.H. 1997, The role of proprioception in the management and rehabilitation of athletic injuries. *Am. J. Sports Med.* 25(1): 130–137.

Licka, T., Kapaun, M., Peham, C. 2004, Influence of rider on lameness in trotting horses. *Equine Vet. J.* 36: 734–736.

Malliaras, P., Cook, J., Ptasznik, R. *et al.* 2006, Prospective study of change in patellar tendon abnormality on imaging and pain over a volleyball season. *Br. J. Sports Med.* 40: 272–274.

Malliaropoulos, N., Papalexandris, S., Papalada, A. *et al.* 2004, The role of stretching in rehabilitation of hamstring injuries: 80 athletes follow-up. *Med. Sci. Sport Exerc.* 36(5): 756–759.

Marek, S., Cramer, J., Fincher, A. *et al.* 2005, Acute effects of static and proprioceptive neuromuscular facilitation stretching on muscle strength and power output. *J. Athl. Train.* 40: 94–103.

Marlin, D., Nankervis, K. (eds) 2003, Skeletal responses. In: *Equine Exercise Physiology.* Blackwell Science, Malden, MA, pp. 86–93.

Massion, J. 1992, Movement posture and equilibrium: interaction and coordination. *Prog. Neurobiol.* 38: 35–56.

Meershoek, L., Schamhardt, H., Roepstorff, L., Johnston, C. 2001, Forelimb tendon loading during jump landing and the influence of fence height. *Equine Vet. J.* 33(suppl): 6–10.

Montalvo, A.M., Cara E.L., Myer, G.D. 2014, Effect of kinesiology taping on pain in individuals with musculoskeletal injuries: systematic review and meta-analysis. *Phys. Sportsmed.* 42(2): 48–57.

Movin, T., Gad, A., Reinholt, F.P., Rolf, C. 1997, Tendon pathology in long-standing achillodynia. Biopsy findings in 40 patients. *Acta Orthop. Scand.* 68(2): 170–175.

Murray, R.C., Zhu, C.F., Goodship, A.E. *et al.* 1999, Exercise affects the mechanical properties and histological appearance of equine articular cartilage. *J. Orthop. Res.* 17(5): 725–731.

Nelson, A.G., Kokkonen, J. 2001, Chronic stretching and running economy. *Scand. J. Med. Sci. Sports* 115: 260–265.

Nelson, F., Billinghurst, R., Pidoux, I. *et al.* 2006, Early post-traumatic osteoarthritis-like change in human articular cartilage following rupture of the anterior cruciate ligament. *Osteoarthr. Cartil.* 14: 114–119.

Ohberg, L., Alfredson, H. 2002, Ultrasound guided sclerosis of neovessels in painful chronic Achilles tendinosis: pilot study of a new treatment. *Br. J. Sports Med.* 36(3): 173–175.

Ohberg, L., Lorentzon, R., Alfredson, H. 2004, Eccentric training in patients with chronic Achilles tendinosis: normalised tendon structure and decreased thickness at follow up. *Br. J. Sports Med.* 38: 8–11.

Patterson-Kane, J.C., Firth, E.C. 2009, Pathophysiology of exercise-induced superficial digital flexor tendon injury in Thoroughbred racehorses. *Vet. J.* 181(2): 79–89.

Peers, K., Lysens, R. 2005, Patellar tendinopathy in athletes: current diagnostic and therapeutic recommendations. *Sports Med.* 35: 71–87.

Petridou, E., Kediklogou, S., Belechri, M. *et al.* 2004, The mosaic of equestrian-related injuries in Greece. *J. Trauma* 56: 643–647.

Pinchbeck, G.L., Clegg, P.D., Proudman, C.J. *et al.* 2004, A prospective cohort study to investigate risk factors for horse falls in UK hurdle and steeplechase racing. *Equine Vet. J.* 367: 595–601.

Porter, D., Barrill, E., Oneacre, K., May, B.D. 2002, The effects of duration and frequency of Achilles tendon stretching on dorsiflexion and outcome in painful heel syndrome: a randomized, blinded, control study. *Foot Ankle Int.* 23(7): 619–624.

Pope, R.P., Herbert, R.D., Kirwan, J.D. *et al.* 2000, A randomized trial of pre-exercise stretching for prevention of lower-limb injury. *Med. Sci. Sports Exerc.* 322: 271–277.

Reef, V. 2001, Superficial digital flexor tendon healing: ultrasonographic evaluation of therapies. *Vet. Clin. North Am. Equine Pract.* 17: 159–178.

Rees, J., Maffuli, N., Cook, J. 2009, Management of tendinopathy. *Am. J. Sports Med.* 37(9): 1855–1867.

Roos, E., Dahlberg, L. 2005, Positive effects of moderate exercise on glycosaminoglycan content in knee cartilage: a four-month, randomized, controlled trial in patients at risk of osteoarthritis. *Arthritis Rheum.* 52: 3507–3514.

Schmidt, R.A., Lee, T.D. 1999, *Motor Control and Learning: a behavioral emphasis.* Human Kinetics Publishers, Champaign, IL.

Sherry, M., Best, T. 2004, A comparison of 2 rehabilitation programs in the treatment of acute hamstring strains. *J. Orthop. Sports Phys. Ther.* 42: 116–125.

Sorli, J. 2000, Equestrian injuries: a five year review of hospital admission in British Columbia, Canada. *Inj. Prev.* 6: 59–61.

Stanish, W.D. 1982, *Neurophysiology of Stretching: prevention and treatment of running injuries.* Slack, Thorofare, NJ, pp. 135–145.

Stashak, T.S. (ed.) 2002, *Adams' Lameness in Horses*, 5th edn. Lippincott Williams & Wilkins, Baltimore, MD.

Taub, M., Berman, M. 1968, Movement and learning in the absence of sensory feedback. In: Freeman, S.J. (ed.), *Neurophysiology in Spatial Orientated Behavior.* Dorsey Press, Homewood, IL, pp. 173–192.

Taylor, D.C., Dalton, J.D., Seaber, A.V. *et al.* 1990, Viscoelastic properties of muscle-tendon units. The biomechanical effects of stretching. *Am. J. Sports Med.* 183: 300–330.

Treleaven, J., Clamaron-Cheers, C., Jull, G. 2011, Does the region of pain influence the presence of sensorimotor disturbances in neck pain disorders? *Man. Ther.* 16(6): 636–640.

Van Herzeele, M., van Cingel, R., Maenhout, A. *et al.* 2013, Does the application of kinesiotape change scapular kinematics in healthy female handball players? *Int. J. Sports Med.* 34(11): 950–955.

Van Weeren, P.R. 2014, Joint physiology: responses to exercise and training. In: Hinchcliff, K.W., Kaneps, A.J., Geor, R.J. (eds), *Equine Sports Medicine and Surgery: basic and clinical sciences of the equine athlete*, 2nd edn. Saunders-Elsevier, Philadelphia, pp. 213–220.

Verheyen, K., Henley, W., Price, J. *et al.* 2005, Training-related factors associated with dorsometacarpal disease in young Thoroughbred racehorses in the UK. *Equine Vet. J.* 37: 442–448.

Visnes, H., Hoksrud, A., Cook, J. *et al.* 2005, No effect of eccentric training on jumper's knee in volleyball players during the competitive season: a randomized clinical trial. *Clin. J. Sport Med.* 15: 227–234.

Warden, S. 2005, Cyclo-oxygenase-2 inhibitors: beneficial or detrimental for athletes with acute musculoskeletal injuries. *Sports Med.* 35: 271–283.

Watt, G., Finch, C. 1996, Preventing equestrian injuries – locking the stable door. *Sports Med.* 22: 187–197.

Williams, F., Ashby, K. 1995, Horse related injuries. Hazard–Monash University Accident Research Centre, 23, June.

Wilmink, J., Wilson, A., Goodship, A. 1992, Functional significance of the morphology and micromechanics of collagen fibres in relation to partial rupture of the superficial digital flexor tendon in racehorses. *Res. Vet. Sci.* 53: 354–359.

Wilson, A., van den Bogert, A., McGuigan, M. 2000, Optimization of the muscle-tendon unit for economical locomotion in cursorial animals. In: Herzog, W. (ed.), *Skeletal Muscle Mechanics: from mechanism to function.* John Wiley, Chichester, UK, pp. 517–547.

Wilson, A.M. 2003, A catapult action for rapid limb protraction. *Nature* 421: 35–36.

Wilson, G.J., Murphy, A.J., Pryor, J.F. 1994, Musculotendinous stiffness: its relationship to eccentric, isometric and concentric performance. *J. Appl. Physiol.* 76: 2714–2719.

Winter, M., Blake, C., Trost, J. *et al.* 2004, Passive versus active stretching of hip flexor muscles in subjects with limited hip extension. A randomised clinical trial. *Physical Ther.* 84(9): 800–807.

Witvrouw, E., Mahieu, N., Danneels, L. *et al.* 2004, Stretching and injury prevention: an obscure relationship. *Sports Med.* 347: 443–449.

Woo, S.L., Gomez, M.A., Woo, Y.K. 1982, Mechanical properties of tendons and ligaments: the relationship of immobilization and exercise on tissue remodelling. *Biorheology* 19: 397–408.

Wyndow, N., Cowan, S.M., Wrigley, T.V. *et al.* 2013, Triceps surae activation is altered in male runners with Achilles tendinopathy. *J. Electromyogr. Kinesiol.* 23(1): 166–172.

Ylinen, J., Takala, E., Nykanen, M. *et al.* 2006, Effects of twelve-month strength training subsequent to twelve-month stretching exercise in treatment of chronic neck pain. *J. Strength Cond. Res.* 20: 304–308.

CHAPTER 22

Outcome measures in animal physiotherapy

Anna Bergh

Swedish University of Agricultural Sciences, Uppsala, Sweden

Summary

Veterinary surgeons use a variety of methods to diagnose injury and disease, with the aim of describing the pathogenesis, i.e. to find the aetiological or pathoanatomical diagnosis. In animal physiotherapy, a specific assessment of physical function is performed and a functional diagnosis is determined. The functional diagnosis describes the degree of physical dysfunction that the animal demonstrates. A thorough assessment of the animal's function is essential for a correct functional diagnosis. In order to design an optimal rehabilitation protocol, as well as to determine its effect, the protocol must be based on a proper assessment of the animal's physical dysfunction. This chapter briefly describes the indications, validation status, measurement errors and practical implications of a selection of simple, inexpensive outcome measures for everyday physiotherapy practice.

22.1 Introduction

22.1.1 Background

When we speak of animal rehabilitation after injury or disease, we often think of a treatment designed to facilitate the process of recovery to as normal a condition as possible. However, essential for the rehabilitation process is the use of diagnostic tools that provide reliable and reproducible results for understanding the underlying cause of functional deficits and for evaluation of the recovery process.

In everyday clinical examination, veterinary surgeons use a variety of methods to diagnose injury and disease, with the aim of describing the pathogenesis, i.e. to find the aetiological or pathoanatomical diagnosis. In animal physiotherapy, a specific assessment of physical function is added to the conventional examination and a functional diagnosis is set. The functional diagnosis states the type and degree of physical dysfunction of the animal. In an animal with osteoarthritis (OA), the physical dysfunction may manifest as a motion asymmetry due to a decreased joint range of motion in the affected joint. The decreased motion may be caused by osteophytes, but can also have its origin in muscle weakness, soft tissue stiffness or impaired motor control. Finally, physical dysfunction is often accompanied by pain. Thus, the functional diagnosis includes investigation of the manifestation of the injury and disease as well as of the tissues involved.

A thorough assessment of the animal is essential for a correct functional diagnosis (see also Chapter 11). In order to design an optimal rehabilitation protocol, it has to be based on a correct assessment of the animal's physical dysfunction. The assessment will help the clinician to prioritise the clinical findings and set realistic goals. Further, the ability to objectively evaluate and reevaluate the clinical effectiveness of the treatment is fundamental, not only for the sake of the individual animal but also for the building of evidence-based medicine. It increases animal safety, produces a more cost-effective treatment for the animal (and its owner), and demonstrates a higher level of professionalism. Thus, in physiotherapy there is a need for objective, simple and practical outcome measures.

Just as there are many signs of physical dysfunction, there are many possible outcome measures from which to select. It can be difficult to decide which outcome measure to use. Therefore, it is important to understand the types and characteristics of outcome measures to select the one best suited to assessing the specific dysfunction that the animal demonstrates.

The assessment can be direct (the measurement of joint range of motion by goniometer) or indirect (the measurement of pain by pain scales). The measured data may be quantitative (numbers) or qualitative (text). The measurement of physical function includes evaluating specific properties such as passive range of joint motion and muscle condition. These tests can be performed separately or put together into test batteries, in order to obtain a better understanding of the function. However, for the animal to recover optimal performance, it needs to synchronise the function of these separate properties into complex movement. Therefore, there are also functional tests that assess the animal's ability to perform complex movement, with the purpose of ensuring greater practical impact to what is being tested.

22.1.2 Overall validation of outcome measures

Outcome measures have to be tested for reproducibility and accuracy in measuring the function of interest. Regardless of the type of assessment tool, it needs to be valid, reliable and responsive (so-called psychometric properties that relate to the statistical strength of the outcome measure).

Validity is the degree to which the tool measures what it is supposed to measure. It can be determined only in relation to a specific question and a defined population. There are different types of validation.

- *Face validity* is the subjective assessment of how a test appears to measure what it is intended to measure.
- *Content validity* is the degree to which a test includes all the items necessary to represent the concept being measured. If you want to test the weight-bearing function, you might want to do it both during standing and during different gaits.
- *Criterion validity* is assessed when an outcome measure can be compared to a gold standard.
- *Construct validity* is the degree to which a test measures what it claims, or purports, to be measuring. It answers questions like 'Is the scoring system for function testing able to measure what we expect it to?'

Reliability is the extent to which a measurement gives results that are consistent. Several sorts of reliability test exist.

- *Intraexaminer reliability* is the consistency in results measured by one examiner, when the same test is repeated.
- *Interexaminer reliability* is the consistency in results between different examiners.
- *Test-retest reliability* indicates the consistency in test results when the test is performed on more than one occasion (the test-retest reliability is affected by intraexaminer and interexaminer variability).
- *Internal consistency reliability* indicates that in a test composed of several parts, each part produces similar scoring.

Reliability coefficients are used to indicate the level of reliability. According to Landis & Koch (1977), a value of 0 can be considered as 'no agreement (beyond chance)', 0– 0.2 as 'slight agreement', 0.2–0.4 as 'fair agreement', 0.4–0.6 as 'moderate agreement', 0.6–0.8 as 'substantial or high agreement' and 0.8–1.0 as 'almost perfect agreement'.

Finally, responsiveness is the ability of an assessment tool to measure and grade changes. *Internal responsiveness* is the test's ability to detect a change when comparing status before and after a treatment. *External responsiveness* reflects the extent to which changes in a measure relate to changes in other measures of the same function of interest.

A test's *sensitivity* indicates the actual positives which are correctly identified as such and its *specificity* the proportion of negatives which are correctly identified as such.

If a tool or method is to be considered fully validated, it must be tested for all the types of changes that it is supposed to register, in both sound and non-sound animals. Further, its sources of errors and the level of measurement errors must have been defined in order to enable reliable interpretations of results. Today, several outcome measures have fulfilled some parts of the validation process but few are 'fully' validated.

22.1.3 Interpretation of test results

Few assessment tools are perfect and it is of the utmost importance that the examiner performs the test correctly by following a standardised procedure. Studies in humans have shown that a measurement can be biased by the expectations of the clinician performing the test. Thus, the examiner needs to be aware of each method's measuring errors, in order to interpret the results adequately. It is important that the clinician is aware of the test's 'minimal detectable change' (the amount of change needed to exceed measurement error). For example, an increase of 4° in passive joint range of motion is not a significant result if the degree of measurement error for the outcome assessment tool is 5°.

As with any test, a standardised procedure enabling accurate data collection is essential for a reliable result. And with the majority of outcome measures, the animal needs to be acquainted with the testing setting. At a time when there are many new tests introduced to the market, it is also important that the result of a test is closely correlated to its clinical significance. The result should reflect at least a minimal or, rather, a more definitive clinically important difference. It is important to bear in mind that a physical dysfunction, such as motion asymmetry, does not have to be pain induced; the asymmetry can have other origins. And the animal might function really well despite its motion asymmetry.

22.1.4 Practical implications

Outcome measures are important tools for guiding clinical decision making. However, as with all tools, in order to function well they must be used with skill and understanding. There are some questions that the clinician needs to answer before selecting the outcome measure.

- Why are you measuring?
  - What type of question are you trying to answer?
  - Do you want to make a functional diagnosis or evaluate a treatment?
- What are you measuring?
  - Are you interested in some specific physical dysfunction or in performance?
- What kind of animal are you measuring?

Further, you need to know the following.

- If the method is 'partly' or 'fully' validated for the species it is used for.
- Are the results consistent between and within examiners?
- How accurately can it identify and grade the changes you want to measure?
- What are the measurement errors and what magnitude do they have?
- Is there an established correlation with clinical significance?

22.2 Physical dysfunction and its outcome measures

As previously mentioned, signs of physical dysfunction may manifest as:

- pain and tenderness
- motion asymmetry
- swelling
- muscle weakness, tension, stiffness
- neurological dysfunction.

There is a need for objective methods to assess a variety of physical dysfunctions. In the following sections, each outcome measure is listed once under its main purpose area and the focus is on relatively simple, clinically useful outcome measures. However, some methods used only in research settings are also mentioned.

22.3 Pain assessment

In animal physiotherapy, the most common problem for which the animal owner seeks advice is physical dysfunction, often assumed to be either caused by pain or causing pain. Pain may be expressed as changes in both the animal's physiology and its behaviour.

Pain perception, the subjective interpretation of discomfort, involves the transmitted sensory information from the nociceptor through the central nervous system, as well as the modulation of the same information. The sensory information can be both amplified and suppressed on its way to the brain. It is interesting and important to note that through descending neural pathways and competing motivational systems, the pain sensation can be either inhibited or potentiated. Due to this complex pain process, pain assessment and treatment should address both physiological and behavioural components.

Since we cannot ask the animal how much pain it experiences, the methods of assessing pain are indirect. Physiological parameters such as heart and breathing rates are still important measures, often used to assess acute pain. The most common method of pain assessment is response to palpation. Different forms of pain protocols assess the animal's behaviour, using pain scales, ethograms or quality of life/activities of daily living questionnaires. There are also semi-objective methods like the pressure algometer that measures the mechanical nociceptive threshold. Further, analysis of pain mediators may have a role in the future of pain evaluation.

22.3.1 Palpation
Indications

Palpation is a subjective measure and a complex task that requires a combination of knowledge and skills. The major aim with palpation is to detect and quantify the degree of pain, by provoking a pain reaction indicating the location and severity of the pain. However, palpation is also used to detect inflammation by assessing swelling and differences in temperature. It can be used to evaluate different muscle properties (such as muscle tension), soft tissue elasticity and mass, and the quality of joint endfeel. Additionally, palpation plays a fundamental part in specific manual tests (see under 'Manual tests' below; Figure 22.1).

Validation

Palpation, with the aim of assessing pain, has higher intra- than interexaminer reliability. In general, palpation methods used to provoke pain responses are more reliable than palpation methods used to assess joint motion.

A study on horses has shown association between physiotherapy findings and subsequent diagnosis of pelvic or hindlimb fracture in racing Thoroughbreds (Hesse & Verheyen 2010). Studies on horses report a correlation between pain assessments by palpation and by pressure algometry (de Haus *et al.* 2010; Olsén *et al.* 2013; Varcoe-Cocks *et al.* 2006). In the study by de Haus *et al.*, three physiotherapists agreed well in their subjective grading of 'pain', but less for 'temperature' and 'muscle tone' and least for 'mobility', although the results were based on a small number of horses. The aim of a study by Ranner *et al.* (2002) was to investigate the validity of palpation of horses with

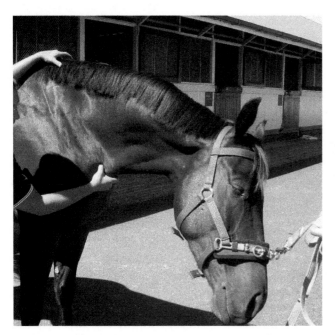

Figure 22.1 Palpation of the brachiocephalicus muscle in a horse and observation of the response (absence of a pain response in this case).

an assumed back problem. Positive palpation agreed with a primary back problem on condition that hindlimb lameness was ruled out and only reproducible painful behaviour was allowed to be interpreted as positive. Hyytiäinen *et al.* (2013) have shown a good correlation between the assessment of muscle atrophy in dogs by palpation and a preset selection of standard outcome measures such as visual gait analysis and force platform measurements. Levine & Goulet (2014) demonstrate that, when palpating the temperature of pads that mimicked skin temperature ranging from healthy to inflamed, clinicians were able to detect temperature differences of 1–5°C. Further, a study on the assessment of swelling (the firmness of an udder in cows) with a four-point palpation scoring system showed high intra- and interexaminer repeatability, although the correlation with dynamometer measurements was moderate (Rees *et al.* 2014).

Measurement errors

It is generally believed that an animal reacts differently to palpation based on its mental awareness, so an animal that is occupied with something like eating will not react as much to palpation as one that is fully concentrating on the examiner. Thus, it is important to examine the animal under the same circumstances. It is also known that the faster the pressure is applied to an animal, the stronger will the pain reaction be.

Practical implications

It is important to give the animal time to get acquainted with the examiner and the examination situation. The force applied to the tissue needs to be gradually increased and adjusted to the type and condition of the tissue examined. The animal's reaction

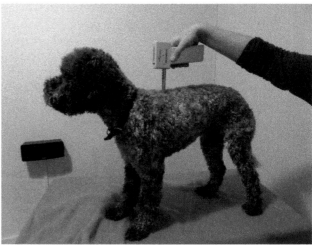

Figure 22.2 Assessment of the mechanical nociceptive threshold in a dog with a pressure algometer.

to the palpation must be carefully monitored. The presence of the owner can be both positive and negative, based on the influence the owner has on the animal's anxiety level. Evaluation and reevaluation should be done by the same examiner and palpation should preferably be used in combination with other methods.

22.3.2 Pressure algometer
Indications

The pressure algometer measures the mechanical nociceptive threshold (MNT) and is a semi-objective tool since it objectively measures pressure, but the threshold point is subjectively assessed by the examiner. In animals, algometry is mainly used to quantify muscle tenderness, but in humans it is also used to measure the overall pain threshold, which is considered to decrease in patients with chronic pain (Figures 22.2 and 22.3).

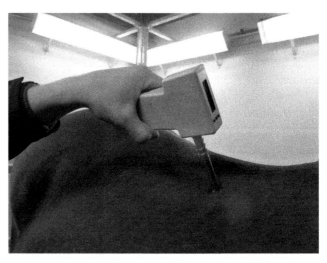

Figure 22.3 Assessment of mechanical nociceptive threshold in a horse with a pressure algometer.

Validation

The method shows moderate to high intraexaminer reliability and low to moderate interexaminer reliability in dogs and horses (Bergh 2010a,b; Coleman *et al.* 2014; Haussler & Erb 2006; Haussler *et al.* 2007). In horses, it correlates with palpation (de Haus *et al.* 2010; Olsén *et al.* 2013; Varcoe-Cocks *et al.* 2006) and EMG measurements (Bergh, unpublished data). A study by Briley *et al.* (2014) reports that the pressure algometer device tested on normal dogs provided repeatable, reliable sensory threshold measurements. However, results from other studies on horses indicate that there are fluctuations in the MNT over time (de Haus *et al.* 2010).

Measurement errors

The results are influenced by variation in speed of pressure applied and the threshold assessment/reading of the avoidance reaction. As with palpation, the level of mental awareness of the animal can influence the results, and there can be adaptation over time (Briley *et al.* 2014; Coleman *et al.* 2014; de Haus *et al.* 2010).

Practical implications

The pressure algometer should have a display demonstrating the speed at which the algometer is applied. The animal should be acquainted with the algometer before the actual testing. The algometer should be applied to soft tissue at a constant speed and with a 90° angle, until the animal reacts with either a clear muscle contraction or an avoidance reaction. To get reliable results, the method should be used on the same animal and by the same examiner. Results over time should be interpreted with caution in case adaptation has occurred.

22.3.3 Pain protocols

Indications

Pain can be assessed with different types of pain protocols, through measurement of behavioural traits by the physiotherapist or the owner. The protocols can be designed for either acute or chronic pain, as well as for specific species and indications. The pain protocols can consist of ethograms, pain faces, specific pain scales such as the visual analogue scale, or 'quality of life' and 'activities of daily living' questionnaires. 'Quality of life' protocols are based on the individual's preferences and with animals that is the owner's interpretations of what their animal prefers, i.e. the situations that make the animal feel comfortable and uncomfortable (Budke *et al.* 2008; Freeman *et al.* 2012; Wiseman-Orr *et al.* 2004).

Validation

There are protocols designed for many species, but the references in this section refer to cats, dogs and horses. Depending on the specific protocol, the validity ranges from low to high (Brown *et al.* 2007, 2013; Burton *et al.* 2009; Hielm-Björkman *et al.* 2011; Hudson *et al.* 2004; Morton *et al.* 2005; Walton *et al.* 2013; Wiseman-Orr *et al.* 2006), the repeatability is moderate

(Bussieres *et al.* 2008; Conzemius *et al.* 1997; Shoening & Bradshaw 2006), the intraexaminer reliability high (Firth & Haldane 1999; Guillot *et al.* 2011; van Loon *et al.* 2010) and the interexaminer reliability moderate (Hielm-Björkman *et al.* 2011; van Loon *et al.* 2010). Some of the protocols have been compared to other methods such as cortisol levels and pain scales (Firth & Haldane 1999).

The simple descriptive scale (SDS), numerical rating scale (NRS) and visual analogue scale (VAS) have been shown to have weak to moderate agreement and an intraexaminer variability that accounted for 35–36% of total variability, indicating that variability among veterinarians accounted for large differences in pain scores (Holten *et al.* 1998; Hudson *et al.* 2004; Quinn *et al.* 2007). The NRS is recommended due to its lower variability.

Examples of specific protocols

The Canine Movement Assessment Questionnaire (CMAQ) consists of 12 questions in VAS format. Studies have shown that the assessment of pain and lameness, among dogs with orthopaedic lameness, is reliable and valid based upon force-plate data (Hudson *et al.* 2004). The study states that no single force could capture all types of lameness. As an example, the question 'play voluntarily' predicted total vertical impulse difference and 'stiff when rising' predicted total peak propulsion difference. The Canine Brief Pain Inventory (CBPI) consists of 11 questions with numerical rating and is used to monitor chronic pain in dogs with, for example, OA and cancer. It has demonstrated high test-retest reliability, internal consistency, responsiveness and construct and convergent validity in several studies (Brown *et al.* 2007, 2008, 2009). The Helsinki Chronic Pain Index has been shown to detect differences in pain in dogs with chronic pain due to OA (Hielm-Björkman *et al.* 2003, 2009, 2011). The Glasgow Composite Pain Scale (Short Form) is one of the more validated scales and has been shown to detect differences in acute pain in dogs measured after pain-relieving treatment (Holton *et al.* 2001; Morton *et al.* 2005; Murrell *et al.* 2008; Reid *et al.* 2007).

The English version of the UNESP-Botucatu-MCPS is regarded as a valid, reliable and responsive instrument for assessing acute pain in cats undergoing ovariohysterectomy, when used by anaesthesiologists or anaesthesia technicians (Brondani *et al.* 2013). Another study on cats describes the use of three questionnaires to differentiate normal cats from those with lameness (Stadig & Bergh 2015). The Feline Musculoskeletal Pain Index (FMPI) has, in some studies, shown appropriate readability, reliability and proven discriminatory ability (Benito *et al.* 2013a; Gruen *et al.* 2014). However, one study has shown neither responsiveness nor criterion validity for cats with degenerative joint disease (Benito *et al.* 2013b).

The PASPAS protocol has been used to assess postoperative pain in horses and the preliminary results state that it has good interexaminer reliability (Graubner *et al.* 2011). A validation of an equine pain scoring system (the Composite Pain Scale,

CPS) showed good agreement with, but better interexaminer reliability than, the postoperative colic pain scoring system devised by Pritchett *et al.* (2003) (van Loon *et al.* 2010).

Measurement errors

One important measurement error is the examiner bias, for instance the physiotherapist's/animal owner's ability to understand and interpret the questions asked. If the protocol has been translated from its original language, it is important to 'translate it back' to make sure the intention of the protocol is the same. Another clinician/owner bias is the interpretation of the animal's behaviour. Further, there is an animal bias, i.e. the animal's level of motivation, how it participates in the test, and the influence that the examination setting has on its behaviour. It is also critical to analyse whether the altered behaviour is related to pain or if it can be explained by other non-pain-related factors.

Practical implications

If the evaluation is performed by the animal owner, make sure that the content of the protocol is understood by the owner. If the evaluation is carried out at the clinic, the animal needs to get acquainted with the examination setting, and the examination setting needs to be the same when reevaluating the animal. It is always valuable, especially when using an ethogram, to film the assessment, which can be easily done at the animal's home by the owner as well.

22.3.4 Pain mediators

Despite the technical possibility of analysing pain mediators such as nociception and substance P, there is not enough data for commercialisation of these tests. Several pain mediators are influenced by things other than pain, such as inflammation and stress.

22.4 Motion assessment

The assessment of motion can be divided into several areas: gait analysis (kinetic and kinematic), weight bearing (static and dynamic), muscle and joint assessment (passive or active).

22.4.1 Gait analysis
Visual lameness examination
Indications

The subjective visual lameness examination is practical and inexpensive and enables assessment of movements other than just ordinary gait, like changing position, jumping and climbing stairs (see also Chapter 7).

Validation

Although visual lameness examination is a common method for assessing motion asymmetry, studies have shown a weak correlation between ratings by experienced clinicians and force-plate measurements. The results apply for both dogs and horses, especially when assessing low- and moderate-grade lameness (Fuller *et al.* 2006; Hewetson *et al.* 2006; Keegan *et al.* 1998, 2010; Quinn *et al.* 2007; Waxman *et al.* 2008). Despite demonstrating a weak correlation between visual evaluations of lameness in dogs compared to force platform measurements, Hyytiäinen *et al.* (2013) reported good intraexaminer reliability.

Visual lameness examination in cats is a challenging task and there are a lack of studies regarding its validation status. In horses, the lameness examination may involve a flexion test. However, the results should not be overinterpreted since studies have shown that the outcome depends on the force applied to the joint and the rather high variability among examiners (Busschers & van Weeren 2001; Keg *et al.* 1997).

Measuring errors

The errors are mainly examiner related, as with the force applied in the flexion test, but the experimental setting can also influence the results.

Practical implications

One way of improving the accuracy of visual lameness examination is to have the animal on a consistent surface at a consistent speed, e.g. on a treadmill or to record the gait using video. The recording enables repeated evaluation and at a slower speed. It is important to be aware of compensatory movement that might mimic lameness.

Two-dimensional and three-dimensional video

The video system is used to measure joint motion during active movement, often by placing reflective markers on preset anatomical landmarks. The 3-D systems are costly and require expertise to handle. The 2-D systems are more affordable and have software that helps with the analysis of data. However, the 2-D system does not register rotations. Although not commercially marketed, it is possible to describe the joint moments and powers by use of an inverse dynamic technique (Headrick *et al.* 2014; Ragetly *et al.* 2010).

Indications

The 2-D technique enables measurement of stride frequency and length, flexion and extension angles, angular acceleration and velocity of joints.

Validation

Studies report that a 2-D video system provided accurate and repeatable data of the sagittal angular motion of canine limbs during walking and that the data had a good correlation to measurements obtained from a 3-D system (Gilette & Angle 2008; Kim *et al.* 2008). This is supported by a study by Feeney *et al.* (2008) showing a high intraexaminer and moderate interexaminer correlation in the evaluation of dogs performing walk and sit to stand. Further, a study comparing two 2-D systems for horses summarised that the systems were consistent at performing repeated measures.

Measurement errors

The results are influenced by the positioning of the reflective markers (Kim *et al.* 2011; Schwenke *et al.* 2012; Torres *et al.* 2011) and the skin displacement of the markers, with a higher degree of displacement of the proximally positioned markers in horses (Bergh *et al.* 2014; van Weeren *et al.* 1988, 1990). Studies have shown poor correlation between skin and pin markers when examining the passive and active motion in the sacroiliac joint in horses (Goff *et al.* 2010). A skin displacement up to 17 cm has been noted in horses (Bergh *et al.* 2014; van Weeren *et al.* 1990).

Practical implications

The positioning of markers needs to be performed by the same investigator and according to a predefined protocol.

Accelerometry, inertial motion capture, activity monitors

The accelerometer measures acceleration in different directions, the most common being the three-axis accelerometer. An inertial motion unit (IMU) consists of accelerometers and a gyroscope, and often a magnetometer, enabling measurement of velocity, orientation and gravitational forces. Further, activity monitors can consist of pedometers, i.e. a pendulum that swings back and forth during movement. It is also possible to track the amount of motion through global position satellite (GPS) techniques.

Indications

The main indication for accelerometers and IMUs is to register motion asymmetry. They can also be used to monitor the level of physical activity, together with pedometers and GPS techniques, such as in rehabilitation or weight loss programmes (see also Chapter 7).

Validation

One study, investigating a pedometer, reported an overestimation of the number of steps of 17% in middle-sized dogs and an underestimation of 7% in small dogs (Chan *et al.* 2005). An accelerometer was considered more reliable than a pedometer in recording the activity of horses (Burla *et al.* 2014). Other studies report good correlation between an accelerometer, used at home for monitoring the level of activity in dogs, and video recordings (Dow *et al.* 2009; Hansen *et al.* 2007; Michel & Brown 2011; Preston *et al.* 2012). Gerencsér *et al.* (2013) used the accelerometer to monitor behaviour and activity in free-running dogs. In a study on cats, Lascelles *et al.* (2008) showed that an accelerometer could be a reliable tool in monitoring activity. Several studies support the conclusion that an inertial sensor system to measure

vertical asymmetry due to lameness in horses has adequate analytic sensitivity for clinical use (Keegan *et al.* 2012; Olsén *et al.* 2013).

Measurement errors

The results are influenced by the positioning of the sensor and the variety in speed of the animal.

Practical implications

The pedometer needs to be calibrated by measuring its accuracy on a set distance. It needs to be secured at a preset position, preferably the elbow in dogs. The ventral portion of the collar was the recommended location for the accelerometer (Hansen *et al.* 2007) or in a harness located between the two scapulae (Preston *et al.* 2012) when used for monitoring the level of activity in dogs. When using accelerometer technique for the measurement of motion asymmetry, make sure that the animal is moving at a constant speed and in a straight line. When reevaluating the same animal, it is important that the measurements are performed at the same velocity.

22.4.2 Weight bearing

Weight-bearing outcome measures investigate how willing the animal is to put weight on its limbs. It can be assessed during static and dynamic conditions. Some outcome measures are subjective, such as observing the animal or letting the animal stand on the examiner's hand. More objective tools are stationary balance systems, bathroom scales, the pressure-sensitive mat technique and the gold standard, the force-plate.

A study by Brown *et al.* (2013) showed no correlation between the scoring of a pain questionnaire (the CBPI) and force-plate measurements in dogs with OA. The authors suggest that animal owners judge the function of their dog in a way that includes more than just stance phase lameness. Another study has shown that 40% of dogs that received placebo were assessed by their owners as better, although the force-plate analysis did not register any difference (Conzemius & Evans 2012). These studies emphasise the importance of using validated outcome measures and having an in-depth knowledge of their specific indications and measurement errors.

Static weight bearing
Bathroom scales
Indications
The use of bathroom scales is the most cost-effective, 'partly validated' outcome measure of static weight bearing.

Validation
In a study by Hyytiäinen *et al.* (2012), measurement of hindlimb weight bearing by force-plate and bathroom scales was compared in dogs with osteoarthritis. The sensitivity was 39% and specificity 85%, indicating that the method can be used in individual dogs but not for comparing different individuals. Further,

the agreement between the bathroom scale measurement and dynamic force platform analysis was slight to moderate.

Measurement errors

The positioning of the animal and the environment greatly influence the results. The magnitude of error due to inadequate positioning can differ between 15% and 30% of bodyweight.

Practical implications

The scales need to be calibrated. It is important that the animal stands with its limbs symmetrically and with its head and tail in a midline position. The method should be used for follow-up of an individual and not for comparing individuals.

There are preliminary studies showing that when lifting one forelimb, the majority of weight transfers to the other forelimb and vice versa for the hindlimb (Bergh, unpublished data).

Computerised stance analysis systems
Indications

The main indication is to investigate the weight distribution between limbs during stance.

Validation

A study has shown high correlation between computerised stance results and force platform results. It suggested that computerised stance analysis was an affordable alternative for objective lameness assessment in dogs (Hicks *et al.* 2005; Millis *et al.* 2012).

Measurement errors

A study on dogs demonstrated the importance of using a standard procedure during measurement since the results are influenced by the handler, the positioning of the animal and the environment (Phelps *et al.* 2007).

Practical implications

To avoid false measurements, it is important that the animal stands with its limbs as symmetrical as possible and with its head and tail in a midline position.

Dynamic weight bearing
Pressure-sensitive mat
Indications

The pressure-sensitive mat registers the vertical ground reaction force and not the horizontal force. It can measure consecutive strides, stride length and time, cadence and average velocity, symmetry indices and centre of gravity. The technique enables immediate feedback (Figure 22.4).

Validation

Oosterlink *et al.* (2010a,b, 2011a, 2012) showed that measurements from a single pressure plate were comparable with those from a force-plate in terms of equine limb symmetry ratios for peak vertical force and vertical impulse (with a 2–7% difference).

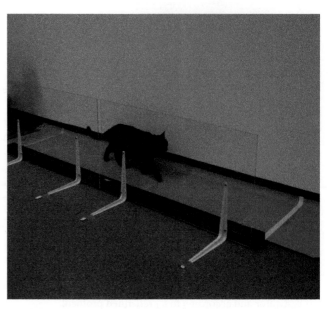

Figure 22.4 Assessment of weight distribution in a cat by use of a pressure-sensitive mat. *Source:* Photo courtesy of Cecilia Ley.

The pressure-sensitive mat technique has been evaluated for use in dogs, demonstrating comparable results with force-plate measurements of symmetry indices, and that vertical forces had a 90% sensitivity and specificity for detecting lameness (Besancon *et al.* 2003; Lascelles *et al.* 2006; Light *et al.* 2010; Oosterlink *et al.* 2011a). The same has been shown for cats, with high agreement of the parameter peak vertical force and vertical impulse (Guillot *et al.* 2013; Lascelles *et al.* 2007; Moreau *et al.* 2013; Stadig & Bergh 2015; Verdugo *et al.* 2013).

Measurement errors

Variations in velocity are a well-known factor that influences the results from both force-plates and pressure mats, since it is correlated to the vertical force (Colborne *et al.* 2006; Voss *et al.* 2010). In a study of cats, the peak vertical force (% bodyweight) increased by a factor of 1.7 when the cat was looking to the side (Stadig & Bergh 2015).

Practical implications

The pressure-sensitive mat produces reliable measures of peak vertical force and vertical impulse, as well as spatiotemporal parameters. The animal should be videoed during measurement, in order to ensure that it is moving at a steady pace and with the body and head in a straight line. When reevaluating the animal, analysis of data should only include trials that have approximately the same velocity as the first measurements.

Force-plate

The force-plate can measure ground reaction forces in three planes; the most used parameters are the peak vertical force, vertical impulse, maximal ground reaction force, total force over time and rate of unloading. To enable the measurement of sequential steps, several force-plates have to be positioned one after another (as in a treadmill). The force-plate is regarded as the gold standard for measuring ground reaction forces but requires a lot of technical input to analyse the data and is rarely used in a clinical setting. The results are influenced by the speed of the animal and the positioning of the animal's head (Nordquist *et al.* 2011; Voss *et al.* 2010).

22.4.3 Muscle assessment

Muscle assessment includes a variety of measurements such as muscle strength and mass, muscle tone, tenderness and stiffness. Muscle tone can be assessed with electromyography (EMG), tenderness can be measured by algometry (see under 'Pain assessment' above) and muscle stiffness indirectly by goniometer (see under 'Joint assessment' below). In cats, there are studies looking at a muscle condition score, which includes palpation and inspection of anatomical landmarks such as scapulae, lumbar vertebrae and pelvic bones (Michel *et al.* 2009).

One study has examined direct muscle strength but the technique used is applicable for research only (Lieber *et al.* 1997). Another method assessed if the animal could lift, for example, a forelimb against gravity. However, this method is not validated. Therefore, in clinical practice, muscle strength may be measured indirectly by use of methods like muscle biopsies, EMG and diagnostic imaging techniques (diagnostic ultrasound, magnetic resonance imaging (MRI), computed tomography (CT)) measuring the muscle cross-sectional area (Orima & Fujita 1997; Weller *et al.* 2007). However, muscle strength is not always correlated to the cross-sectional area of the muscle, since it also depends on the muscle fibre composition and the degree of motor control. Overall muscle strength can also be evaluated by functional tests. It is important to objectively measure muscle strength, as it helps to monitor the progress of the rehabilitation.

Spring-tension tape measure
Indications
Indications include suspicion of inadequate strength, i.e. when the animal shows compensatory movement strategies, imbalance between muscles or overall motion asymmetry (Figures 22.5 and 22.6).

Validation
A study on dogs assessing direct muscle strength also demonstrated a correlation between the cross-sectional area of the muscle and muscle strength (Lieber *et al.* 1997). The cross-sectional area is believed to relate to the overall girth measure of the limb, so muscle strength can be indicated by the limb circumference.

One study compared the results from four types of tape measures; ergonomic, circumference, retractable and spring-tension tape measure (Baker *et al.* 2010). The variability in measurement from the spring-tension tape and the retractable tape was significantly lower than the other two. Interexaminer observations were 3.6 times higher than intraexaminer observations,

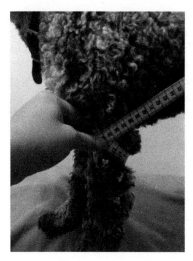

Figure 22.5 Assessment of the circumference of the canine elbow joint with a spring-tension tape measure.

which illustrates the importance of consistency between measurements. Millis *et al.* (1999) reported examiner group mean values that were within 3.5% of each other and that the technique was sensitive enough to determine changes in weight bearing. Single measurements may have less importance but serial measurements over time might give an indication of the progress in muscle strength.

Measurement errors
The results are influenced by the force applied to the measuring tape, the positioning of the tape and the animal while measuring.

Practical implications
The spring-tension tape measure should be used by the same examiner and animal for follow-up. Factors such as precise

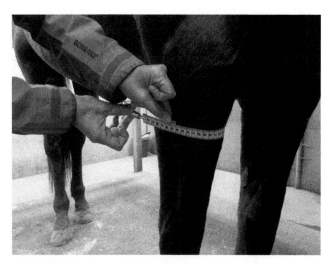

Figure 22.6 Assessment of equine muscle mass with a spring-tension tape measure.

knowledge of measuring procedure, anatomical landmarks and the use of a standardised application force are important. It is essential to have the animal in a standardised position, preferably with the joint in an extended position while measuring, since the level of muscle contraction might influence the results. The recommended location for measurement of hindlimb proximal muscles is 70% of the femur length measured from the greater trochanter to the lateral fabella. The hair coat should be of comparable thickness when repeating measurements (Millis *et al.* 1999).

Electromyography (EMG)

During an EMG, surface electrodes are attached over the muscles to assess changes in electrical voltage that occur during movement and when the muscle is at rest. An EMG can be done in conjunction with a nerve conduction velocity (NCV) test, which measures electrical energy by assessing the nerve's ability to send a signal.

Indications

Recordings of muscle activity, i.e. muscle tone and contractions. It can also be used in neurological cases to detect impairment in nerve function (Wijnberg *et al.* 2003a,b, 2004).

Validation

Surface EMG reflects the force and degree of activity/coordination of a muscle during a gait cycle, revealing bursts of activity when a muscle is active (Butcher *et al.* 2009; Salomons *et al.* 2012).

Measurement errors

Correct positioning and adaption of the electrodes is essential for good measurements. The interelectrode positioning has minor influence on the results if one analyses normalised data; however, the electrode placement in respect of innervation zone had a major influence in humans (Beck *et al.* 2008).

Practical implications

Electromyography produces acceptable measurements for the everyday monitoring of muscle activity, but it is very important that the examiner has in-depth knowledge of muscle anatomy in order to position the electrodes at their proper location.

22.4.4 Joint assessment
Goniometry

Goniometry is a technique that assesses joint range of motion, often as flexion and extension with a universal goniometer (Figure 22.7), but also rotations with a Myrin, gravity-referenced goniometer. Joint motion is a complex motion with additional small motions such as rolling, gliding, compression and distraction, but these cannot be measured. Further, the technique

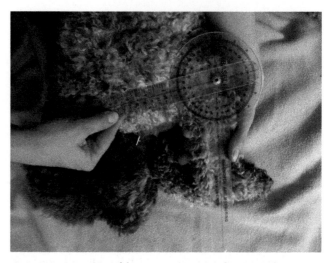

Figure 22.7 Assessment of the passive joint range of motion with a goniometer.

includes assessment of joint quality by evaluating the joint end-feel. This is rather difficult since there is a lack of validated definitions to describe the outcome (like crepitus, pain reaction and snapping). The quality of joint end-feel can be influenced by restrictions in tissues like cartilage, bone spurs, joint capsule and other fibrous tissue.

Indications

Motion asymmetry indicating limited or excessive passive (PROM) and/or active (AROM) joint range of motion. Besides measuring the actual joint range of motion, the results from goniometry technique also give an indication of muscle and joint capsule stiffness.

Validation

Goniometry is partly validated for cats, dogs and horses. It shows better intraexaminer than interexaminer agreement (Corfield *et al.* 2007; Cook *et al.* 2005; Jaegger *et al.* 2002; Liljebrink & Bergh 2010; Thomas *et al.* 2006). There is good correlation between goniometric measures performed on animals compared to those on radiographs (Jaegger *et al.* 2002; Liljebrink & Bergh 2010). And there is no significant difference reported between measurements taken on sedated animals compared to awake. However, a study by Lakey *et al.* (2004) reports significant differences between breeds in eight of 12 joint motions. Studies have not shown a good correlation between goniometry findings, clinical examination and signs on diagnostic imaging techniques of degenerative joint disease in cats (Lascelles *et al.* 2012). However, the authors state that negative goniometry predicts a negative outcome on radiographs.

Measurement errors

The measurement errors are mainly caused by the measurement procedure in regard to the positioning of the goniometer and the adjacent joint, and the force applied to the joint. The measurement error differs between 2° and 10° (equine) and 1° and 6° (dog), depending on the joint (Cook *et al.* 2005; Jaegger *et al.* 2002; Liljebrink & Bergh 2010).

Practical implications

The method should be used by the same examiner and for follow-up of the same animal. When assessing passive range of motion, it is important to have the animal in a relaxed state, the joints and goniometer in a standardised position and to use an equal amount of force while performing measurements.

Specific motion/manual tests

These are tests like the 'springing test', used to assess passive motion in specific joints by use of palpation. The tests assess accessory motion, which can be defined as movement occurring between joint surfaces that are produced by forces applied by the examiner. The examiner assesses the 'joint play', defined as the joint surface movements that are produced by forces applied by the examiner and that are necessary for normal functional movement. The majority of these tests are not validated.

Indications

Motion asymmetries.

Validation

McGowan *et al.* (2010) have studied manual manipulation of the equine pelvis to detect differences in motion or relative sacroiliac movement. The results indicate that the tests were not considered useful as diagnostic tests, and that movement tests were poorly correlated with other clinical factors. However, the article concludes that there are promising batteries of other tests (Goff *et al.* 2006; McGowan *et al.* 2010).

Measurement errors

McGowan *et al.* (2010) showed a tendency by the examiner, during the manual test, to apply more force on one side of the horse than on the other.

Practical implications

Standardise the amount of force applied and interpret the results with caution before further validation has been performed.

22.5 Assessment of swelling and inflammation

There are several ways to directly and indirectly measure inflammation and swelling in soft tissues. The best validated is diagnostic ultrasound, but one can also use water displacement volumetry in the assessment of limb swelling. Assessment of inflammation may be measured with thermography, a technique that uses infrared sensing devices to measure small temperature changes between the two sides of the body. However, in everyday practice

methods like the spring-tension measure tape and slide calliper are more practical.

22.5.1 Thermography

Thermography uses infrared *sensing* devices to detect small temperature changes between the two sides of the body.

Indications

Thermography may be used to detect soft tissue injury.

Validation

A study by Tunley & Henson (2004) suggests that horses may not need time to equilibrate prior to taking thermographic images and that thermographic patterns are reproducible over periods up to 7 days. Time to equilibration was affected by thickness of hair coat and the differences in internal and external environmental temperature. Loughin & Marino (2007) state that thermography can provide consistent images with reproducible thermal patterns in healthy dogs. Clipping decreased the temperature and thermal patterns remained fairly consistent after the coat was clipped.

Measurement errors

The results may be influenced by surrounding objects transmitting heat and by the thickness of the animal's hair coat.

Practical implications

The technique should be used according to a standardised protocol and the external/internal temperatures should be monitored so that the examination setting is the same for repeated measures.

22.5.2 Slide calliper
Indications

The slide calliper measures distances and has a dynamometer that ensures that equal force is applied when testing. It can be used to assess swelling in muscles and joints (Figures 22.8 and 22.9).

Validation

Preliminary results by Bergfors & Bergh (2012) indicate that the method has fair to moderate interexaminer reliability, and moderate to high intraexaminer reliability when assessing the swelling of canine elbow joints. There was a strong correlation between palpation and calliper measurement.

Measurement errors

The measurement error is approximately 0.5 cm when assessing the elbow joint of medium-sized dogs (Bergfors & Bergh 2012).

Practical implications

When using the slide calliper, it is important to follow a standardised protocol with predefined anatomical landmarks and to use a calliper with built-in dynamometer. It is very important

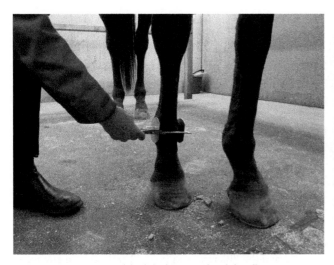

Figure 22.8 Assessment of the fetlock joint with a slide calliper.

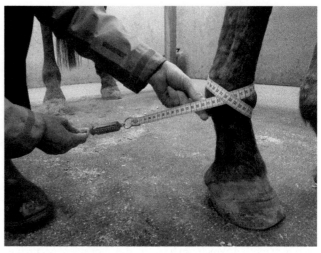

Figure 22.10 Assessment of fetlock joint swelling with a spring-tension tape measure in a figure 8.

that the measurement is performed on soft tissues and not bony prominences.

22.5.3 Spring-tension tape measure (circumference and figure 8)
Indications

Besides assessing muscle strength and mass by measuring girth circumference, the spring-tension tape measure can be used to assess the degree of joint effusion or swelling of soft tissues (Figure 22.10). It is also a practical way of assessing body condition and studies have shown a moderate correlation to body mass (Burkholder 2001).

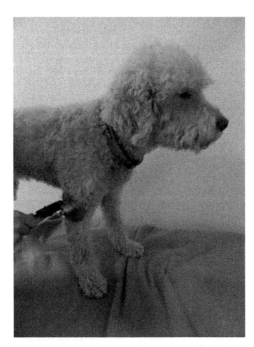

Figure 22.9 Assessment of the canine elbow joint with a slide calliper.

Validation

Preliminary data from Bergfors & Bergh (2012) indicate that the assessment of joint effusion (in the elbow joint of middle-sized dogs) with a spring-tension tape measure has fair to moderate interexaminer reliability and high intraexaminer reliability. The tape was applied either as a measure of circumference or in a figure of 8. There was strong correlation between palpation and tape measurements. Smith *et al.* (2013) report poor to fair intra- and interexaminer reliability.

Measurement errors

The measurement error according to the study by Bergfors & Bergh (2012) was less than 1 cm in medium-sized dogs.

Practical implications

When using the spring-tension tape measure, it is important to follow a standardised protocol with predefined anatomical landmarks.

22.6 Overall functional assessment

22.6.1 Functional tests

Functional tests assess the animal's ability to perform compound movement, instead of just measuring isolated properties such as joint range of motion or muscle tone. The assessment of different tasks like sit to stand can be evaluated according to certain scales (from the lowest level, where the animal requires maximum assistance to maintain balance, to normal where the animal can maintain balance without support and accepts maximum challenge). The better trained the animal is, the more complex tasks will be included. Many of the tests include static and dynamic postures, visual gait examination, evaluation of transitions and transfers, and activities of daily living (ADL) questions. ADL protocols focus on the animal's ability to complete everyday basic life functions like feeding, sleeping and moving. Specific ADL questionnaires can also be used for competing animals, but then the tasks are performance related and have a higher level of motor function. Further, functional tests can also be used to assess neurological deficits.

Indications

To test overall function, after the measurement of separate properties. Suspicion of a neurological disorder, due to clinical signs such as motion dysfunction, lack of coordination, sensory deficits.

Validation

The majority of functional tests are designed for dogs but there are some exercise tests intended for horses.

Measurement errors

The results are influenced by the obedience level of the animal and examiner bias.

Practical implications

It is vital to use standardised procedures and settings. It is highly recommended to video the test situation to enable further analysis after the actual testing.

22.6.2 Examples of specific functional tests

The 6 min walk test determines the distance a dog can walk during 6 minutes. A study comparing healthy dogs with dogs with pulmonary disease showed a difference in walking distance (Swimmer & Rozanski 2011). The interexaminer reliability is considered high. However, the method has several measuring errors such as the motivation of the dog and the handler, and the evaluation on when to stop walking.

The Bioarth functional evaluation scale includes measurement of passive joint range of motion and the evaluation of different tasks like sit to stand. Preliminary data indicate that there is a discrepancy between the assessment of sound dogs (where the inter- and intraexaminer reliability was high) and the assessment of dogs with OA (where the intra- and interexaminer reliability was low to fair) (Bergh, unpublished data).

Canine time up and go test studies have shown high intraexaminer agreement, with gait as a more reliable component than stand (Lamoreaux-Hesbach 2003).

The Texas Spinal Cord Injury Score evaluates gait, proprioception and nociception in dogs with spinal injury (Levine *et al.* 2009). One study describes a functional scoring system for dogs with acute spinal cord injuries (Olby *et al.* 2001).

22.7 Conclusion

To enable the development of evidence-based medicine in animal physiotherapy, it is of the utmost importance to be able to achieve accurate functional diagnoses, design optimal rehabilitation protocols and evaluate the efficacy of treatment. The fundamental basis of this is to increase knowledge in the area and stimulate the use of objective outcome measurements in everyday clinical work. Despite the limited validation of outcome measures assessing physical dysfunction, there are some simple and reliable tools that can be easily used in everyday practice. Generally, the tools are best applied when evaluating and reevaluating the same animal and by the same examiner.

References

Baker, S.G., Roush, J.K., Unis, M.D., Wodiske, T. 2010, Comparison of four commercial devices to measure limb circumference in dogs. *Vet. Compend. Orthopaed. Traumatol.* 23: 406–410.

Beck, T.W., Housh, T.J., Cramer, J.T. *et al.* 2008, Electrode shift and normalization reduce the innervation zone's influence on EMG. *Med. Sci. Sports Exerc.* 40: 1314–1322.

Benito, J., Hansen, B., DePuy, V. *et al.* 2013a, Feline Musculoskeletal Pain Index (FMPI): responsiveness and criterion validity testing. *J. Vet. Intern. Med.* 27: 474–482.

Benito, J., Hardie, E., Zamprogno, H. *et al.* 2013b, Reliability and discriminatory testing of a client-based metrology instrument, Feline Musculoskeletal Pain Index – FMPI, for the evaluation of degenerative joint disease associated pain in cats. *Vet. J.* 196: 368–673.

Bergfors, S., Bergh, A. 2012, Four methods of assessing joint effusion in dogs. Proceedings of the Seventh International Symposium on Rehabilitation and Physical Therapy in Veterinary Medicine.

Bergh, A. 2010a, Mechanical nociceptive threshold in the neck and back of horses after intramuscular injections. Proceedings of the Sixth International Symposium on Rehabilitation and Physical Therapy in Veterinary Medicine.

Bergh, A. 2010b, Mechanical nociceptive threshold in the axial skeleton of dogs. Proceedings of the Sixth International Symposium on Rehabilitation and Physical Therapy in Veterinary Medicine.

Bergh, A., Egenvall, A., Olsson, E., Uhlhorn, M., Rhodin, M. 2014, Evaluation of skin displacement in the equine neck. *Compar. Exerc. Physiol.* doi: http://dx.doi.org/10.3920/CEP143003 (epub ahead of print)

Besancon, M.F., Conzemius, M.G., Derricka, T.R., Ritter, M.J. 2003, Comparison of vertical forces in normal greyhounds between force platform and pressure walkway measurement system. *Vet. Compend. Orthopaed. Traumatol.* 16: 153–157.

Briley, J.D., Williams, M.D., Freire, M., Griffith, E.H., Lascelles, B.D. 2014, Feasibility and repeatability of cold and mechanical quantitative sensory testing in normal dogs. *Vet. J.* 199: 245–250.

Brondani, J.T., Mama, K.R., Luna, S.P. *et al.* 2013, Validation of the English version of the UNESP– Botucatu multidimensional composite pain scale for assessing postoperative pain in cats. *BMC Vet. Res.* 9: 143.

Brown, D.C., Boston, R., Coyne, J., Farrar, J.T. 2007, The Canine BPI: development and psychometric testing of an instrument designed to measure chronic pain in companion dogs with osteoarthritis. *Am. J. Vet. Res.* 68: 631–637.

Brown, D.C., Boston, R.C., Coyne, J. *et al.* 2008, Ability of the Canine Brief Pain Inventory to detect response to treatment in dogs with osteoarthritis. *J. Am. Vet. Med. Assoc.* 233: 1278–1283.

Brown, D.C., Boston, R.C., Coyne, J. *et al.* 2009, A novel approach to the use of animals in studies of pain: validation of the Canine Brief Pain Inventory in canine bone cancer. *Pain Med.* 10: 133–142.

Brown, D.C., Boston, R.C., Farrar, J.T. 2013, Comparison of force plate gait analysis and owner assessment of pain using the Canine Brief Pain Inventory in dogs with osteoarthritis. *J. Vet. Intern. Med.* 27; 22–30.

Budke, C.M., Levine, J.M., Kerwin, S.C., Levine, G.J., Hettlich, B.F., Slater, M.R. 2008, Evaluation of a questionnaire for obtaining owner-perceived, weighted quality-of-life assessments for dogs with spinal cord injuries. *J. Am. Vet. Med. Assoc.* 233: 925–930.

Burkholder, W.J. 2001, Precision and practicality of methods assessing body composition of dogs and cats. *Compend. Contin. Educ. Pract. Vet.* 23: 1–10.

Burla, J.B., Ostertag, A., Westerath, H.S., Hillmann, H. 2014, Gait determination and activity measurement in horses using an accelerometer. *Comput. Electron. Agric. Arch.* 102: 127–133.

Burton, N.J., Owen, M.R., Colborne, G.R., Toscano, M.J. 2009, Can owners and clinicians assess outcome in dogs with fragmented medial coronoid process? *Vet. Compend. Orthopaed. Traumatol.* 22: 183–189.

Busschers, E., van Weeren, P.R. 2001, Use of the flexion test of the distal forelimb in the sound horse: repeatability and effect of age, gender, weight, height and fetlock joint range of motion. *J. Vet. Med. A* 48: 413–427.

Bussières, G., Jacquesa, C., Lainaya, O. *et al.* 2008, Development of a composite orthopaedic pain scale in horses. *Res. Vet. Sci.* 85: 294–306.

Butcher, M.T., Hermanson, J.W., Ducharme, N.G., Mitchell, L.M., Sonderholm, L.V., Bertram, M.J.E.A. 2009, Contractile behavior of the forelimb digital flexors during steady-state locomotion in horses (Equus caballus): an initial test of muscle architectural hypotheses about in vivo function. *Compar. Biochem. Physiol A: Molec. Integr. Physiol.* 152: 100–114.

Chan, C.G., Spierenburg, M., Ihle, S.L. *et al.* 2005, Use of pedometers to measure physical activity in dogs. *J. Am. Vet. Med. Assoc.* 226: 2010–2015.

Colborne, G.R., Walker, A.M., Tattersall, A.J., Fuller, C.J. 2006, Effect of trotting velocity on work patterns on the hind limbs of Greyhounds. *Am. J. Vet. Res.* 67, 1293–1298.

Coleman, K., Schmeidt, C., Kirkby, K. *et al.* 2014, Confounding factors in algometric assessment of mechanical thresholds in normal dogs. *Vet. Surg.* 43: 361–367.

Conzemius, M.G., Evans, R.B. 2012, Caregiver placebo effect for dogs with lameness from osteoarthritis. *J. Am. Vet. Med. Assoc.* 241: 1314–1319.

Conzemius, M.G., Hill, C.M., Sammarco, J.L., Perkowski, S.Z. 1997, Correlation between subjective and objective measures used to determine severity of postoperative pain in dogs. *J. Am. Vet. Med. Assoc.* 210: 1619–1622.

Cook, J.L., Renfro, D.C., Tomlinson, J.L. *et al.* 2005, Measurement of angles of abduction for diagnosis of shoulder instability in dogs using goniometry and digital image analysis. *Vet. Surg.* 34: 463–468.

Corfield, G.S., Read, R.A., Eastley, K.A., Richardson, J.L., Robertson, I.D., Day, R. 2007, Assessment of the hip reduction angle for predicting osteoarthritis of the hip in the Labrador Retriever. *Austr. Vet. J.* 85: 212–216.

De Haus, P.D., van Oossanen, G., van Dierendonck, M.C., Back, W. 2010, A pressure algometer is a useful tool to monitor the effect of palpation by a physiotherapist in warmblood horses. *J. Equine Vet. Sci.* 30: 310–321.

Dow, C., Michel, K.E., Love, M., Brown, D.C. 2009, Evaluation of optimal sampling interval for activity monitoring in companion dogs. *Am. J. Vet. Res.* 70: 444–448.

Feeney, L.C., Lin, C.F, Marcellin-Little, D.J. *et al.* 2008, Validation of two-dimensional analysis of walk and sit-to–stand motions in dogs. *Am. J. Vet. Res.* 68: 277–282.

Firth, A.M., Haldane, S.L. 1999, Development of a scale to evaluate post-operative pain in dogs. *J. Am. Vet. Med. Assoc.* 214: 651–659.

Fuller, C.J., Bladon, B.M., Driver, A.J., Barr, A.R.S. 2006, The intra- and inter-assessor reliability of measurement of functional outcome by lameness scoring in horses. *Vet. J.* 171: 281–286.

Gerencsér, L., Vásárhelyi, G., Nagy, M., Vicsek, T., Miklósi, A. 2013, Identification of behaviour in freely moving dogs (Canis familiaris) using inertial sensors. *PLoS One* 8: e77814.

Gilette, R.L., Angle, T.C. 2008, Recent developments in canine locomotion – a review. *Vet. J.* 178: 167–176.

Goff, L.M., Jasiewicz, J., Jeffcott, L.B., Condie, P., McGowan, T.W., McGowan, C.M. 2006, Movement between the equine ilium and sacrum – in vivo and in vitro studies. *Equine Vet. J.* 36(suppl): 457–461.

Goff, L.M., van Weeren, P.R., Jeffcott, L., Condie, P., McGowen, C. 2010, Quantification of equine sacral and iliac motion during gait: a comparison between motion capture with skin-mounted and bone-fixated sensors. *Equine Vet. J.* 42: 468–474.

Graubner, C., Gerber, V., Doherr, M., Spadavecchia, C. 2011, Clinical application and reliability of a post abdominal surgery pain assessment scale (PASPAS) in horses. *Vet. J.* 188: 178–183.

Gruen, M., Griffith, E., Thomson, A., Simpson, W., Lascelles, B.D.X. 2014, A novel approach to the detection of clinically relevant pain relief in cats with degenerative joint disease associated pain. *J. Vet. Intern. Med.* 28: 346–350.

Guillot, M., Rialland, P., Nadeau, M.E. *et al.* 2011, Pain induced by a minor medical procedure (bone marrow aspiration) in dogs: comparison of pain scales in a pilot study. *J. Vet. Intern. Med.* 25: 1050–1056.

Guillot, M., Moreaua, M., Heitb, M., Martel-Pelletier, J., Pelletier, J.P., Troncya, E. 2013, Characterization of osteoarthritis in cats and meloxicam efficacy using objective chronic pain evaluation tools. *Vet. J.* 196: 360–367.

Hansen, B.D., Lascelles, B.D.X, Keene, B.W., Adams, A.K., Thomson, A.E. 2007, Evaluation of an accelerometer for at-home monitoring of spontaneous activity in dogs. *Am. J. Vet. Res.* 68: 468–475.

Haussler, K.K., Erb, H.N. 2006, Mechanical nociceptive thresholds in the axial skeleton of horses. *Equine Vet. J.* 38: 70–75.

Haussler, K.K., Hill, A.E., Frisbie, D.D., McIlwraith, C.W. 2007, Determination and use of mechanical nociceptive thresholds of the thoracic limb to assess pain associated with induced osteoarthritis of the middle carpal joint in horses. *Am. J. Vet. Res.* 68: 1167–1176.

Headrick, J.F., Zhang, S., Millard, R.P., Rohrbach, B.W., Weigel, J.P., Millis, D.L. 2014, Use of an inverse dynamics method to describe the motion of the canine pelvic limb in three dimensions. *Am. J. Vet. Res.* 75: 544–553.

Hesse, K.L., Verheyen, K.L. 2010, Associations between physiotherapy findings and subsequent diagnosis of pelvic or hindlimb fracture in racing Thoroughbreds. *Equine Vet. J.* 42: 234–239.

Hewetson, M., Christley, R.M., Hunt, I.D., Voute, L.C. 2006, Investigations of the reliability of observational gait analysis for the assessment of lameness in horses. *Vet. Rec.* 158: 852–857.

Hicks, D.A., Millis, D.L., Arnold, G.A. *et al.* 2005, Comparison of weight bearing at a stance vs. trotting in dogs with rear limb lameness. Proceedings of the 32nd Veterinary Orthopedic Society, Snowmass, CO, March, p. 12.

Hielm-Bjorkman, A.K., Kuusela, E., Liman, A. *et al.* 2003, Evaluation of methods for assessment of pain associated with chronic osteoarthritis in dogs. *J. Am. Vet. Med. Assoc.* 222: 1552–1558.

Hielm-Björkman, A.K., Rita, H., Tulamo, R. 2009, Psychometric testing of the Helsinki chronic pain index by completion of a questionnaire in Finnish by owners of dogs with chronic signs of pain caused by osteoarthritis. *Am. J. Vet. Res.* 70: 727–734.

Hielm-Björkman, A.K., Kapatkin, A.S., Rita, H.J. 2011, Reliability and validity of a visual analogue scale used by owners to measure chronic pain attributable to osteoarthritis in their dogs. *Am. J. Vet. Res.* 72, 601–607.

Holten, L.L., Scott, E.M., Nolan, A. *et al.* 1998, Comparison of three methods used for assessment of pain in dogs. *J. Am. Vet. Med. Assoc.* 212: 61–66.

Holton, L., Reid, J., Scott, E.M., Pawson, P., Nolan, A. 2001, Development of a behaviour-based scale to measure acute pain in dogs. *Vet. Rec.* 148: 525–531.

Hudson, J.T., Slater, M.R., Taylor, L., Scott, H.M., Kerwin, S.C. 2004, Assessing repeatability and validity of a visual analogue scale questionnaire for use in assessing pain and lameness in dogs. *Am. J. Vet. Res.* 65: 1634–1643.

Hyytiäinen, H.K., Molsa, S.H., Junnila, J.T. *et al.* 2012, Use of bathroom scales in measuring asymmetry of hindlimb static weight bearing in dogs with osteoarthritis. *Vet. Compend. Orthopaed. Traumatol.* 25: 390–396.

Hyytiäinen, H.K., Mölsä, S.H., Junnila, J.T., Laitinen-Vapaavuori, O.M., Hielm-Björkman, A.K. 2013, Ranking of physiotherapeutic evaluation methods as outcome measures of stifle functionality in dogs. *Acta Vet. Scand.* 55: 29.

Jaegger, G.H., Marcellin-Little, D.J., Levine, D. 2002, Reliability of goniometry in Labrador retrievers. *Am. J. Vet. Res.* 63; 979–986.

Keegan, K.G., Wilson, D.A., Wilson, D.J. *et al.* 1998, Evaluation of mild lameness in horses trotting on a treadmill by clinicians and interns or residents and correlation of their assessments with kinematic gait analysis. *Am. J. Vet. Res.* 59: 1370–1377.

Keegan, K.G., Dent, E.V., Wilson, D.A. *et al.* 2010, Repeatability of subjective evaluation of lameness in horses. *Equine Vet. J.* 42: 92–97.

Keegan, K.G., MacAllister, C.G., Wilson, D.A. *et al.* 2012, Comparison of an inertial sensor system with a stationary force plate for evaluation of horses with bilateral forelimb lameness. *Am. J. Vet. Res.* 73: 368–374.

Keg, P.R., van Weeren, P.R., Back, W. *et al.* 1997, Influence of the force applied and its period of application on the outcome of flexion test of the distal forelimb of the horse. *Vet. Rec.* 141: 463–466.

Kim, J., Rietdyk, S., Breur, G.J. 2008, Comparison of two-dimensional and three-dimensional systems for kinematic analysis of the sagittal motion of canine hindlimbs during walking. *Am. J. Vet. Res.* 69: 1116–1122.

Kim, S.Y., Kim, J.Y., Hayashi, K., Kapatkin, A.S. 2011, Skin movement during the kinematic analysis of the canine pelvic limb. *Vet. Comp. Orthop. Traumatol.* 5: 226–232.

Lakey, S., Smith, M., Benson, C. *et al.* 2004, A comparison of canine range of motion measurements between two breeds of disparate body type. APTA CSM.

Lamoreaux-Hesbach, A. 2003, A proposed canine movement performance test: the canine timed up and go test (CTUG). *Orthoped. Phys. Ther. Pract.* 15: 26.

Landis, J.R., Koch, G.G. 1977, The measurement of observer agreement for categorical data. *Biometrics* 33: 159–174.

Lascelles, B.D., Roe, S.C., Smith, E. *et al.* 2006, Evaluation of a pressure walkway system for measurement of vertical limb forces in clinically normal dogs. *Am. J. Vet. Res.* 67: 277–282.

Lascelles, B.D., Findley, K., Correa, M., Marcellin-Little, D., Roe, S. 2007, Kinetic evaluation of normal walking and jumping in cats, using a pressure-sensitive walkway. *Vet. Rec.* 160: 512–516.

Lascelles, B.D., Hansen, B.D., Thomson, A., Pierce, C.C., Boland, E., Smith E.S. 2008, Evaluation of a digitally integrated accelerometer-based activity monitor for the measurement of activity in cats. *Vet. Anaesth. Analg.* 35: 173–183.

Lascelles, B.D., Dong, Y.H., Marcellin-Little, D.J., Thomson, A., Wheeler, S., Correa, M. 2012, Relationship of orthopedic examination, goniometric measurements, and radiographic signs of degenerative joint disease in cats. *BMC Vet. Res.* 27: 10.

Levine, D., Goulet, R. 2014, The ability to assess temperature differences by palpation. Proceedings of the Eighth International Symposium on Rehabilitation and Physical Therapy in Veterinary Medicine, p.149.

Levine, G.J., Levine, J.M., Budke C.M. *et al.* 2009, Description and repeatability of a newly developed spinal cord injury scale for dogs. *Prevent. Vet. Med.* 89: 121–127.

Lieber, R.L., Jacks, T.M., Mohler, R.L. *et al.* 1997, Growth hormone secretagogue increases muscle strength during remobilization after canine hindlimb immobilization. *J. Orthopaed. Res.* 15: 519–527.

Light, V.A., Steiss, J.E., Montgomery, R.D. *et al.* 2010, Temporal-spatial gait analysis by use of a portable walkway system in healthy Labrador Retrievers at a walk. *Am. J. Vet. Res.* 71: 997–1002.

Liljebrink, Y., Bergh, A. 2010, Goniometry: is it a reliable tool to monitor passive joint range of motion in horses? *Equine Vet. J.* 38(suppl): 676–682.

Loughin, C.A., Marino, D.J. 2007, Evaluation of thermographic imaging of the limbs of healthy dogs. *Am. J. Vet. Res.* 68: 1064–1069.

McGowan, C., Goff, L., McGowan, T., Jaseiwicz, J., Condie, P., Jeffcott, L. 2010, *Studies of the Movement of the Equine Pelvis: Sacroiliac Kinematics.* RIRDC Publication No 10/157. Rural Industries Research and Development Corporation, Barton, ACT, Australia.

Michel, K.E., Brown, D.C. 2011, Determination and application of cut points for accelerometer–based activity counts of activities with differing intensity in pet dogs. *Am. J. Vet. Res.* 72, 866–870.

Michel, K.E., Anderson, W., Cupp, C. *et al.* 2009, Validation of a subjective muscle mass scoring system for cats. *J. Anim. Physiol. Anim. Nutr.* 93: 806.

Millis, D., Westling, M., Westling Kapler, W. 2012, Comparison of weightbearing at a stance vs. trotting in dogs with lameness. Poster presentation, ISVRPT, Vienna, 17 August.

Millis, D.L., Scroggs, L., Levine D. *et al.* 1999, Variables affecting thigh circumference measurements in dogs. Proceedings of the First International Symposium on Rehabilitation and Physical Therapy in Veterinary Medicine, p.157.

Moreau, M., Guillot, M., Pelletier, J.P., Martel-Pelletier, J., Troncy, E. 2013, Kinetic peak vertical force measurement in cats afflicted by coxarthritis: data management and acquisition protocols. *Res. Vet. Sci.* 95: 219–224.

Morton, C.M., Reid, J., Scott, E.M., Holton, L.L., Nolan, A.M. 2005, Application of a scaling model to establish and validate an interval level pain scale for assessment of acute pain in dogs. *Am. J. Vet. Res.* 66: 2154–2166.

Murrell, J., Psatha, E., Scott, E., Reid, J., Hellebrekers, L.J. 2008, Application of a modified form of the Glasgow pain scale in a veterinary teaching centre in the Netherlands. *Vet. Rec.* 162: 403–408.

Nordquist, B., Fischer, J., Kim, S.Y. *et al.* 2011, Effects of trial repetition, limb side, intraday and inter-week variation on vertical and craniocaudal ground reaction forces in clinically normal labrador retrievers. *Vet. Compend. Orthopaed. Traumatol.* 24: 435–444.

Olby, N.J., de Risio, L., Munana, K.R. *et al.* 2001, Development of a functional scoring system in dogs with acute spinal cord injuries. *Am. J. Vet. Res.* 62: 1624–1628.

Olsen, E., Andersen, P.H., Pfau, T. 2012, Accuracy and precision of equine gait event detection during walking with limb and trunk mounted inertial sensors. *Sensors (Basel, Switzerland)* 126: 8145–8156.

Olsén, L., Bremer, H., Olofsson, K. *et al.* 2013, Intramuscular administration of sodium benzylpenicillin in horses as an alternative to procain benzylpenicillin. *Res. Vet. Sci.* 95: 212–218.

Oosterlinck, M., Pille, F., Back, W., Dewulf, J., Gasthuys, F. 2010a, Use of a stand-alone pressure plate for the objective evaluation of forelimb symmetry in sound ponies at walk and trot. *Vet. J.* 183: 305–309.

Oosterlinck, M., Pille, F., Huppes, T., Gasthuys, F., Back, W. 2010b, Comparison of pressure plate and force plate gait kinetics in sound Warmbloods at walk and trot. *Vet. J.* 186: 347–351.

Oosterlinck, M., Pille, F., Back, W., Dewulf, J., Gasthuys, F. 2011a, A pressure plate study on fore and hindlimb loading and the association with hoof contact area in sound ponies at the walk and trot. *Vet. J.* 190: 71–76.

Oosterlinck, M., Bosmans, T., Gasthuys, F. *et al.* 2011b, Accuracy of pressure plate kinetic asymmetry indices and their correlation with visual gait assessment scores in lame and nonlame dogs. *Am. J. Vet. Res.* 72: 820–825.

Oosterlinck, M., Pille, F., Sonneveld, D.C., Oomen, A.M., Gasthuys, F., Back, W. 2012, Contribution of dynamic calibration to the measurement accuracy of a pressure plate system throughout the stance phase in sound horses. *Vet. J.* 193: 471–474.

Orima, H., Fujita, M. 1997, Computed tomographic findings of experimentally induced neurogenic muscular atrophy in dogs. *J. Vet. Med. Sci.* 59: 729–731.

Phelps, H.A., Ramos, V., Shires, P.K. *et al.* 2007, The effect of measurement method on static weight distribution to all legs in dogs using the Quadraped Biofeedback System. *Vet. Compend. Orthopaed. Traumatol.* 20: 108–112.

Preston, T., Baltzera, W., Trost, S. 2012, Accelerometer validity and placement for detection of changes in physical activity in dogs under controlled conditions on a treadmill. *Res. Vet. Sci.* 93: 412–416.

Pritchett, L.C., Ulibarri, C., Roberts, M.C., Schneider, R.K., Sellon, D.C. 2003, Identification of potential physiological and behavioral indicators of postoperative pain in horses after exploratory celiotomy for colic. *Appl. Animal Behav. Sci.* 80: 31–43.

Quinn, M.M., Keuler, N.S., Lu, Y. *et al.* 2007, Evaluation of agreement between numerical rating scales, visual analogue scoring scales, and force plate gait analysis in dogs. *Vet. Surg.* 36: 360–367.

Ragetly, C.A., Griffon, D.J., Mostafa, A.A., Thomas, J.E., Hsiao-Wecksler, E.T. 2010, Inverse dynamics analysis of the pelvic limbs in Labrador retrievers with and without cranial cruciate ligament disease. *Vet. Surg.* 39: 513–522.

Ranner, W., Gerhards, H., Klee, W. 2002, Diagnostic validity of palpation in horses with back problems. *Berl. Munch. Tierarztl. Wochenschr.* 115: 420–424.

Rees, A., Fischer-Tenhagen, C., Heuwieser, W. 2014, Evaluation of udder firmness by palpation and a dynamometer. *J. Dairy Sci.* 97: 3488–3497.

Reid, J., Nolan, A.M., Hughes, J.M.L. *et al.* 2007, Development of the short-form Glasgow Composite Measure Pain Scale (CMPS-SF) and derivation of an analgesic intervention score. *Anim. Welfare* 16(suppl 1).

Salomons, K.K., Tnibar, A., Harrison, A.P. 2012, Surface electromyography during both standing and walking in m. Ulnaris lateralis of diversely trained horses. In: Schwartz, M. (ed.), *EMG Methods for Evaluating Muscle and Nerve Function.* InTech, Croatia, pp. 209–224.

Schoening, B., Bradshaw, J.W.S. 2006, Applying ethological measures to quantify a dog's temperament: are ethograms a valid instrument? *J. Vet. Behav.* 2: 84.

Schwencke, M., Smolders, L.A., Bergknut, N. *et al.* 2012, Soft tissue artifact in canine kinematic gait analysis. *Vet. Surg.* 41: 829–837.

Smith, T.J., Baltzer, W.I., Jelinski, S.E., Salinardi, B.J. 2013, Inter- and intratester reliability of anthropometric assessment of limb circumference in labrador retrievers. *Vet. Surg.* 42: 316–321.

Stadig, S., Bergh, A. 2015, Gait and jump analysis in healthy cats using a pressure mat system. *J. Feline Med. Surg.* 17: 523–529.

Swimmer, R.A., Rozanski, E.A. 2011, Evaluation of the 6-minute walk test in pet dogs. *J. Vet. Intern. Med.* 25: 405–406.

Thomas, T.M., Marcellin-Little, D.J., Roe, S.C., Lascelles, B.D., Brosey, B.P. 2006, Comparison of measurements obtained by use of an electrogoniometer and a universal plastic goniometer for the assessment of joint motion in dogs. *Am. J. Vet. Res.* 67: 1974–1979.

Torres, B.T., Whitlock, D., Reynolds, L.R *et al.* 2011, The effect of marker location variability on noninvasive canine stifle kinematics. *Vet. Surg.* 40: 715–719.

Tunley, B.V., Henson, F.M. 2004, Reliability and repeatability of thermographic examination and the normal thermographic image of the thoracolumbar region in the horse. *Equine Vet. J.* 36: 306–312.

Van Loon, J.P.A.M., Back, W., Hellebrekers, L.J., van Weeren, P.R. 2010, Application of a composite pain scale to objectively monitor horses with somatic and visceral pain under hospital conditions. *J. Equine Vet. Sci.* 30: 641–649.

Van Weeren, P.R., van der Bogert, A.J., Barneveld, A. 1988, Quantification of skin displacement near the carpal, tarsal and fetlock joints of the horse. *Equine Vet. J.* 10: 203–208.

Van Weeren, P.R., van der Bogert, A. J., Barneveld, A. 1990, Quantification of skin displacement in the proximal parts of the limbs of the walking horse. *Equine Vet. J.* 9: 110–118.

Varcoe-Cocks, K., Sagar, K.N., Jeffcott, L.B., McGowan, C.M. 2006, Pressure algometry to quantify muscle pain in racehorses with suspected sacroiliac dysfunction. *Equine Vet. J.* 38: 558–562.

Verdugo, M.R., Rahal, S.C., Agostinho, F.S, Govoni, V.M., Mamprim, M.J., Monteiro, F.O. 2013, Kinetic and temporospatial parameters in male and female cats walking over a pressure sensing walkway. *BMC Vet. Res.* 27: 129.

Voss, K., Galeandro, L., Wiestner, T., Haessig, M., Montavon, P.M. 2010, Relationships of body weight, body size, subject velocity, and vertical ground reaction forces, in trotting dogs. *Vet. Surg.* 39: 863–869.

Walton, M.B., Cowderoy, E., Lascelles, D., Innes, J.F. 2013, Evaluation of construct and criterion validity for the 'Liverpool Osteoarthritis in Dogs' (LOAD) clinical metrology instrument and comparison to two other instruments. *PLoS One* 83: e58125.

Waxman, A.S., Robinson, D.A., Evans, R.B., Hulse, D.A., Innes, J.F., Conzemius, M.G. 2008, Relationship between objective and subjective assessment of limb function in normal dogs with an experimentally induced lameness. *Vet. Surg.* 37: 241–246.

Weller, R., Pfau, T., Ferrari, M., Griffith, R., Bradford, T., Wilson, A. 2007, The determination of muscle volume with a freehand 3D ultrasonography system. *Ultrasound Med. Biol.* 33: 402–407.

Wijnberg, I.D., Franssen, H., van der Kolk, J.H. 2003a, Influence of age of horse on results of quantitative electromyograhic needle examination of skeletal muscles in Dutch Warmblood horses. *Am. J. Vet. Res.* 64: 70– 75.

Wijnberg, I.D., van der Kolk, J.H., Franssen, H., Breukink, H.J. 2003b, Needle electromyography in the horse compared with its principles in man: a review. *Equine Vet. J.* 35: 9–17.

Wijnberg, I.D., Back, W., de Jong, M., Zuidhof, M.C., van den Belt, A.J.M., van der Kolk, J. 2004, The role of electromyography in clinical diagnosis of neuromuscular locomotor problems in the horse. *Equine Vet. J.* 36: 718–722.

Wiseman-Orr, M.L., Nolan, A.M., Reid, J., Scott, E.M. 2004, Development of a questionnaire to measure the effects of chronic pain on health-related quality of life in dogs. *Am. J. Vet. Res.* 65: 1077–1084.

Wiseman-Orr, M.L., Scott, E.M., Reid, J., Nolan, A.M. 2006, Validation of a structured questionnaire as an instrument to measure chronic pain in dogs on the basis of effects on health-related quality of life. *Am. J. Vet. Res.* 67: 1826–1836.

Index